PULMONARY REHABILITATION

LUNG BIOLOGY IN HEALTH AND DISEASE

Executive Editor

Claude Lenfant
Director, National Heart, Lung and Blood Institute
National Institutes of Health
Bethesda, Maryland

1. Immunologic and Infectious Reactions in the Lung, *edited by Charles H. Kirkpatrick and Herbert Y. Reynolds*
2. The Biochemical Basis of Pulmonary Function, *edited by Ronald G. Crystal*
3. Bioengineering Aspects of the Lung, *edited by John B. West*
4. Metabolic Functions of the Lung, *edited by Y. S. Bakhle and John R. Vane*
5. Respiratory Defense Mechanisms (in two parts), *edited by Joseph D. Brain, Donald F. Proctor, and Lynne M. Reid*
6. Development of the Lung, *edited by W. Alan Hodson*
7. Lung Water and Solute Exchange, *edited by Norman C. Staub*
8. Extrapulmonary Manifestations of Respiratory Disease, *edited by Eugene Debs Robin*
9. Chronic Obstructive Pulmonary Disease, *edited by Thomas L. Petty*
10. Pathogenesis and Therapy of Lung Cancer, *edited by Curtis C. Harris*
11. Genetic Determinants of Pulmonary Disease, *edited by Stephen D. Litwin*
12. The Lung in the Transition Between Health and Disease, *edited by Peter T. Macklem and Solbert Permutt*
13. Evolution of Respiratory Processes: A Comparative Approach, *edited by Stephen C. Wood and Claude Lenfant*
14. Pulmonary Vascular Diseases, *edited by Kenneth M. Moser*
15. Physiology and Pharmacology of the Airways, *edited by Jay A. Nadel*
16. Diagnostic Techniques in Pulmonary Disease (in two parts), *edited by Marvin A. Sackner*
17. Regulation of Breathing (in two parts), *edited by Thomas F. Hornbein*
18. Occupational Lung Diseases: Research Approaches and Methods, *edited by Hans Weill and Margaret Turner-Warwick*
19. Immunopharmacology of the Lung, *edited by Harold H. Newball*
20. Sarcoidosis and Other Granulomatous Diseases of the Lung, *edited by Barry L. Fanburg*
21. Sleep and Breathing, *edited by Nicholas A. Saunders and Colin E. Sullivan*
22. *Pneumocystis carinii* Pneumonia: Pathogenesis, Diagnosis, and Treatment, *edited by Lowell S. Young*

23. Pulmonary Nuclear Medicine: Techniques in Diagnosis of Lung Disease, *edited by Harold L. Atkins*
24. Acute Respiratory Failure, *edited by Warren M. Zapol and Konrad J. Falke*
25. Gas Mixing and Distribution in the Lung, *edited by Ludwig A. Engel and Manuel Paiva*
26. High-Frequency Ventilation in Intensive Care and During Surgery, *edited by Graziano Carlon and William S. Howland*
27. Pulmonary Development: Transition from Intrauterine to Extrauterine Life, *edited by George H. Nelson*
28. Chronic Obstructive Pulmonary Disease: Second Edition, Revised and Expanded, *edited by Thomas L. Petty*
29. The Thorax (in two parts), *edited by Charis Roussos and Peter T. Macklem*
30. The Pleura in Health and Disease, *edited by Jacques Chrétien, Jean Bignon, and Albert Hirsch*
31. Drug Therapy for Asthma: Research and Clinical Practice, *edited by John W. Jenne and Shirley Murphy*
32. Pulmonary Endothelium in Health and Disease, *edited by Una S. Ryan*
33. The Airways: Neural Control in Health and Disease, *edited by Michael A. Kaliner and Peter J. Barnes*
34. Pathophysiology and Treatment of Inhalation Injuries, *edited by Jacob Loke*
35. Respiratory Function of the Upper Airway, *edited by Oommen P. Mathew and Giuseppe Sant'Ambrogio*
36. Chronic Obstructive Pulmonary Disease: A Behavioral Perspective, *edited by A. John McSweeny and Igor Grant*
37. Biology of Lung Cancer: Diagnosis and Treatment, *edited by Steven T. Rosen, James L. Mulshine, Frank Cuttitta, and Paul G. Abrams*
38. Pulmonary Vascular Physiology and Pathophysiology, *edited by E. Kenneth Weir and John T. Reeves*
39. Comparative Pulmonary Physiology: Current Concepts, *edited by Stephen C. Wood*
40. Respiratory Physiology: An Analytical Approach, *edited by H. K. Chang and Manuel Paiva*
41. Lung Cell Biology, *edited by Donald Massaro*
42. Heart–Lung Interactions in Health and Disease, *edited by Steven M. Scharf and Sharon S. Cassidy*
43. Clinical Epidemiology of Chronic Obstructive Pulmonary Disease, *edited by Michael J. Hensley and Nicholas A. Saunders*
44. Surgical Pathology of Lung Neoplasms, *edited by Alberto M. Marchevsky*
45. The Lung in Rheumatic Diseases, *edited by Grant W. Cannon and Guy A. Zimmerman*
46. Diagnostic Imaging of the Lung, *edited by Charles E. Putman*
47. Models of Lung Disease: Microscopy and Structural Methods, *edited by Joan Gil*
48. Electron Microscopy of the Lung, *edited by Dean E. Schraufnagel*

49. Asthma: Its Pathology and Treatment, *edited by Michael A. Kaliner, Peter J. Barnes, and Carl G. A. Persson*
50. Acute Respiratory Failure: Second Edition, *edited by Warren M. Zapol and Francois Lemaire*
51. Lung Disease in the Tropics, *edited by Om P. Sharma*
52. Exercise: Pulmonary Physiology and Pathophysiology, *edited by Brian J. Whipp and Karlman Wasserman*
53. Developmental Neurobiology of Breathing, *edited by Gabriel G. Haddad and Jay P. Farber*
54. Mediators of Pulmonary Inflammation, *edited by Michael A. Bray and Wayne H. Anderson*
55. The Airway Epithelium, *edited by Stephen G. Farmer and Douglas Hay*
56. Physiological Adaptations in Vertebrates: Respiration, Circulation, and Metabolism, *edited by Stephen C. Wood, Roy E. Weber, Alan R. Hargens, and Ronald W. Millard*
57. The Bronchial Circulation, *edited by John Butler*
58. Lung Cancer Differentiation: Implications for Diagnosis and Treatment, *edited by Samuel D. Bernal and Paul J. Hesketh*
59. Pulmonary Complications of Systemic Disease, *edited by John F. Murray*
60. Lung Vascular Injury: Molecular and Cellular Response, *edited by Arnold Johnson and Thomas J. Ferro*
61. Cytokines of the Lung, *edited by Jason Kelley*
62. The Mast Cell in Health and Disease, *edited by Michael A. Kaliner and Dean D. Metcalfe*
63. Pulmonary Disease in the Elderly Patient, *edited by Donald A. Mahler*
64. Cystic Fibrosis, *edited by Pamela B. Davis*
65. Signal Transduction in Lung Cells, *edited by Jerome S. Brody, David M. Center, and Vsevolod A. Tkachuk*
66. Tuberculosis: A Comprehensive International Approach, *edited by Lee B. Reichman and Earl S. Hershfield*
67. Pharmacology of the Respiratory Tract: Experimental and Clinical Research, *edited by K. Fan Chung and Peter J. Barnes*
68. Prevention of Respiratory Diseases, *edited by Albert Hirsch, Marcel Goldberg, Jean-Pierre Martin, and Roland Masse*
69. *Pneumocystis carinii* Pneumonia: Second Edition, Revised and Expanded, *edited by Peter D. Walzer*
70. Fluid and Solute Transport in the Airspaces of the Lungs, *edited by Richard M. Effros and H. K. Chang*
71. Sleep and Breathing: Second Edition, Revised and Expanded, *edited by Nicholas A. Saunders and Colin E. Sullivan*
72. Airway Secretion: Physiological Bases for the Control of Mucous Hypersecretion, *edited by Tamotsu Takishima and Sanae Shimura*
73. Sarcoidosis and Other Granulomatous Disorders, *edited by D. Geraint James*
74. Epidemiology of Lung Cancer, *edited by Jonathan M. Samet*
75. Pulmonary Embolism, *edited by Mario Morpurgo*

76. Sports and Exercise Medicine, *edited by Stephen C. Wood and Robert C. Roach*
77. Endotoxin and the Lungs, *edited by Kenneth L. Brigham*
78. The Mesothelial Cell and Mesothelioma, *edited by Marie-Claude Jaurand and Jean Bignon*
79. Regulation of Breathing: Second Edition, Revised and Expanded, *edited by Jerome A. Dempsey and Allan I. Pack*
80. Pulmonary Fibrosis, *edited by Sem Hin Phan and Roger S. Thrall*
81. Long-Term Oxygen Therapy: Scientific Basis and Clinical Application, *edited by Walter J. O'Donohue, Jr.*
82. Ventral Brainstem Mechanisms and Control of Respiration and Blood Pressure, *edited by C. Ovid Trouth, Richard M. Millis, Heidrun F. Kiwull-Schöne, and Marianne E. Schläfke*
83. A History of Breathing Physiology, *edited by Donald F. Proctor*
84. Surfactant Therapy for Lung Disease, *edited by Bengt Robertson and H. William Taeusch*
85. The Thorax: Second Edition, Revised and Expanded (in three parts), *edited by Charis Roussos*
86. Severe Asthma: Pathogenesis and Clinical Management, *edited by Stanley J. Szefler and Donald Y. M. Leung*
87. *Mycobacterium avium*–Complex Infection: Progress in Research and Treatment, *edited by Joyce A. Korvick and Constance A. Benson*
88. Alpha 1–Antitrypsin Deficiency: Biology • Pathogenesis • Clinical Manifestations • Therapy, *edited by Ronald G. Crystal*
89. Adhesion Molecules and the Lung, *edited by Peter A. Ward and Joseph C. Fantone*
90. Respiratory Sensation, *edited by Lewis Adams and Abraham Guz*
91. Pulmonary Rehabilitation, *edited by Alfred P. Fishman*
92. Acute Respiratory Failure in Chronic Obstructive Pulmonary Disease, *edited by Jean-Philippe Derenne, W. A. Whitelaw, and Thomas Similowski*

ADDITIONAL VOLUMES IN PREPARATION

Environmental Impact on the Airways: From Injury to Repair, *edited by Jacques Chrétien and Daniel Dusser*

Tissue Oxygen Deprivation: From Molecular to Integrated Function, *edited by Gabriel G. Haddad and George Lister*

Primary Pulmonary Hypertension, *edited by Lewis J. Rubin and Stuart Rich*

Inhalation Aerosols: Physical and Biological Basis for Therapy, *edited by Anthony J. Hickey*

Parasitic Lung Diseases, *edited by Adel A. F. Mahmoud*

Nitric Oxide and the Lung, *edited by Warren Zapol and Kenneth D. Bloch*

The Genetics of Asthma, *edited by Stephen B. Liggett and Deborah A. Meyers*

Topical Glucocorticoids in Asthma: Mechanisms and Clinical Actions, *edited by Robert P. Schleimer, William W. Busse, and Paul M. O'Byrne*

Pulmonary and Cardiac Imaging, *edited by Caroline Chiles and Charles E. Putman*

PULMONARY REHABILITATION

Edited by

Alfred P. Fishman

University of Pennsylvania Medical Center
Philadelphia, Pennsylvania

Marcel Dekker, Inc. **New York • Basel • Hong Kong**

Library of Congress Cataloging-in-Publication Data

Pulmonary rehabilitation / edited by Alfred P. Fishman.
p. cm. — (Lung biology in health and disease ; 91)
Includes bibliographical references and index.
ISBN 0-8247-9673-X (hardcover : alk. paper)
1. Respiratory organs — Diseases — Patients — Rehabilitation.
I. Fishman, Alfred P. II. Series.
[DNLM: 1. Lung Diseases — rehabilitation. W1 LU62 v.91 1996 / WF 600 P9862 1996]
RC732.P87 1996
616.2'403—dc20
DNLM/DLC
for Library of Congress 95-52986
CIP

The publisher offers discounts on this book when ordered in bulk quantities. For more information, write to Special Sales/Professional Marketing at the address below.

This book is printed on acid-free paper.

Marcel Dekker, Inc., 270 Madison Avenue, New York, New York 10016

Current printing (last digit):
10 9 8 7 6 5 4 3 2 1

PRINTED IN THE UNITED STATES OF AMERICA

INTRODUCTION

Use strengthens, disuse debilitates.
—Hippocrates, 460–377 B.C.

It would appear from this statement that the underlying concept of medical rehabilitation has been known for a very long time. The word "rehabilitation" is itself an interesting one; it is derived from the Latin *habilitatus,* which means "made fit," by way of the French *habileté,* which translates into "skillfulness or capability."

Yet, utilization of rehabilitation by the medical community has been slow in coming. It appears to have begun in the late 1700s in France and in England with the use of electrotherapy, which later was used in the United States to relieve indigestion and nervousness. The electrotherapists (as they were called) were very aggressive and mounted attacks on their competitors, especially surgeons and neurologists. As reported by Gritzer and Arluke (1), "The electrotherapists called for a halt in this lust for operative surgery and the replacement of surgical procedures with safer and more effective physical therapies such as electricity, hot air and water." It is not hard to imagine that such an approach was not well received by the conventional medical community. Eventually, very early in the twentieth century, the electrotherapists were rebuffed by the American Medical Association, which went on to create a section on physical therapeutics to establish the legitimacy of the methods used by physical therapists.

As one looks back at the history of rehabilitation and at its acceptance by the medical community, especially the academic one, it seems that other factors impeded its recognition as well. Beginning with the twentieth century, medicine shifted from being an art to being a science, and rehabilitation medicine was perceived to be lacking in the scientific basis on which medicine rested. This newly developed scientific basis was grounded in the emergence of fundamental disciplines such as biochemistry, physiology, and pathophysiology. Rehabilitation medicine was and still is the forerunner of a multidisciplinary approach based on fundamental and clinical knowledge, but also on behavioral and social sciences.

Against this background, pulmonary rehabilitation developed and emerged as the clinical science that we know today. The extraordinary acquisition of understanding of respiratory psysiology—particularly respiratory mechanics and gas exchange—that came during the pre– and post–World War II era was used by astute and compassionate clinicians to help their patients. One of them, Alvin L. Barach, knew very well that "a man would do nothing if he waited until he could do it so well that no one would find fault with what he has done" (2).

And then, during the ensuing years, more and more clinicians and public service entities recognized and adopted the precept and the teaching of these pioneers. Yet, the scientific basis of pulmonary rehabilitation, as well as the interest of the scientific community in pulmonary rehabilitation, remains rudimentary. As a consequence, as Alfred Fishman says in his Preface, "Debates continue about the effectiveness of pulmonary rehabilitation."

This book is bound to start a renewal. It presents a comprehensive state of the art, but also poses questions and, in so doing, paves the way for new investigations. Today's research is almost by definition multidisciplinary and so is the science of rehabilitation. The selection, the interest, and past accomplishments of the contributors illustrate very well the breadth with which rehabilitation must be investigated.

Alfred Fishman brings to rehabilitative cardiopulmonary medicine an encyclopedic knowledge of cardiopulmonary medicine and vast experience in its study. His acceptance of my invitation to edit this monograph for the series Lung Biology in Health and Disease represented not only a testimony to our friendship, but also one of the best moments in the development of the series of monographs. As it goes to print, the book itself is ample proof of this.

I am greatly appreciative of the efforts that Dr. Fishman and his colleagues put into this volume. Undoubtedly, it constitutes a new landmark in the series.

Claude Lenfant, M.D.
Bethesda, Maryland

References

1. Gritzer G, Arluke A. The Making of Rehabilitation. Berkeley: University of California Press, 1985.
2. Attributed to Cardinal Newman by William Miller, in Barach AL. A Treatment Manual for Patients with Pulmonary Emphysema. New York: Grune & Stratton, 1969.

PREFACE

As a therapeutic modality, pulmonary rehabilitation extends far beyond the boundaries of chronic pulmonary care. Because of its emphasis on functional outcome and quality of life, not only chest physicians, but a variety of other health professionals, engage in the rehabilitative process.

The purpose of this book is to sort out pulmonary care from pulmonary rehabilitation and to help the various professionals to define their respective roles. Consequently, it is anticipated that this book will have a wide audience that includes chest physicians, respiratory therapists, physical therapists, nurses, psychologists, social workers, and vocational rehabilitationists.

This list is not exhaustive. In institutions where lung transplantation is being performed, exercise physiologists often join the team. Those concerned with health care costs, effectiveness, and delivery will find useful information relevant to their interests in the chapters that follow. As another example, the comprehensive sweep of pulmonary rehabilitation is amply illustrated by chapters concerning pulmonary rehabilitation in the intensive care setting.

Debates continue about the effectiveness of pulmonary rehabilitation. In large measure, these debates stem from the use of inappropriate criteria to measure outcome. For example, conventional pulmonary function tests often fail to display much improvement after the patient has undergone pulmonary rehabilitation. The debates along this line would end if the pulmonary abnormalities were accepted as a relatively fixed set of physical impairments, accurately reflected in the pulmonary function tests, and if the outcome of pulmonary rehabilitation was more meaningfully measured in terms of quality of life and functional capacity.

In addition to addressing the respective roles of the various health specialists who engage in pulmonary rehabilitation, this book provides useful information to general physicians who take care of patients with chronic pulmonary disease. By recognizing the comprehensive nature of pulmonary rehabilitation and taking cognizance of its concepts, protocols, and practices, practitioners can greatly enlarge the scope and quality of care administered to their patients with pulmonary disease.

Alfred P. Fishman

CONTRIBUTORS

John R. Bach, M.D. Vice Chairman and Professor, Department of Physical Medicine and Rehabilitation, University of Medicine and Dentistry–New Jersey Medical School, Newark, New Jersey

Michael J. Belman, M.D. Associate Director, Division of Pulmonary Medicine, Cedars Sinai Medical Center, and Associate Professor of Medicine, UCLA School of Medicine, Los Angeles, California

Kathy Lee Bishop, M.S., P.T., C.C.S. Cardiopulmonary Clinical Team Leader, Department of Physical Therapy, University of Pennsylvania Medical Center, Philadelphia, Pennsylvania

Richard Casaburi, Ph.D., M.D. Professor of Medicine, Division of Respiratory and Critical Care Physiology and Medicine, Harbor–UCLA Medical Center, Torrance, California

Bartolome R. Celli, M.D. Professor of Medicine, Tufts University School of Medicine, and Chief, Pulmonary and Critical Care Medicine, St. Elizabeth's Medical Center, Boston, Massachusetts

Sandra S. Cole, Ph.D. Professor and Director, Sexuality Training Center, Department of Physical Medicine and Rehabilitation, University of Michigan Medical Center, Ann Arbor, Michigan

Theodore M. Cole, M.D. Professor and Chairman, Department of Physical Medicine and Rehabilitation, University of Michigan Medical School, Ann Arbor, Michigan

David B. Coultas, M.D. Associate Professor and Director, Epidemiology and Cancer Control, Department of Internal Medicine, University of New Mexico Health Sciences Center, Albuquerque, New Mexico

Gerard J. Criner, M.D. Associate Professor of Medicine and Director of Pulmonary and Critical Care Medicine, Temple University School of Medicine, Philadelphia, Pennsylvania

J. Randall Curtis, M.D., M.P.H. Acting Assistant Professor, Division of Pulmonary and Critical Care, Department of Medicine, University of Washington, Seattle, Washington

Susan M. Czajkowski, M.D. Social Service Analyst, Behavioral Medicine Branch, National Heart, Lung, and Blood Institute, National Institutes of Health, Bethesda, Maryland

André De Troyer, M.D., Ph.D. Professor of Medicine, Chest Service, Erasme University Hospital, and Director, Laboratory of Cardiorespiratory Physiology, Brussels School of Medicine, Brussels, Belgium

Michael Donahoe, M.D. Assistant Professor of Medicine, Department of Medicine, University of Pittsburgh School of Medicine, Pittsburgh, Pennsylvania

Marc Estenne, M.D. Assistant Professor of Medicine, Chest Service, Erasme University Hospital, and Brussels School of Medicine, Brussels, Belgium

Alfred P. Fishman, M.D. William Maul Measey Professor of Medicine, Department of Rehabilitation Medicine, University of Pennsylvania Medical Center, Philadelphia, Pennsylvania

Harmeet S. Gill, M.D. Instructor in Medicine, Pulmonary Department, St. Elizabeth's Medical Center, and Tufts University School of Medicine, Boston, Massachusetts

Roger S. Goldstein, M.D. Associate Professor, and Director, Divisional Programme in Respiratory Rehabilitation, Division of Respiratory Medicine, Department of Medicine, University of Toronto, Toronto, Ontario, Canada

Michael J. Hall, M.D. Consultant Physician, Department of Medicine, Monash University, Alfred Hospital, Melbourne, Australia

Andrew Harver, Ph.D. Associate Professor of Psychology, University of North Carolina at Charlotte, Charlotte, North Carolina

Nicholas S. Hill, M.D. Professor of Medicine, Brown University, and Director, Respiratory Care Unit, Division of Pulmonary and Critical Care Medicine, Rhode Island Hospital, Providence, Rhode Island

John E. Hodgkin, M.D. Director, Respiratory Care and Pulmonary Rehabilitation, St. Helena Hospital, Deer Park, and Clinical Professor of Medicine, University of California, Davis, Davis, California

Ira E. Holland, M.A. President, Concepts of Independence, Inc., New York, New York

Carol J. Hossler, B.S., P.T. Physical Therapist, Department of Physical Medicine and Rehabilitation, University of Michigan Medical Center, Ann Arbor, Michigan

Lisa Isaac, Ph.D. Director, Behavioral Medicine Division, Department of Medicine, Mercy Catholic Medical Center, Darby, Pennsylvania

Robert M. Kaplan, Ph.D. Professor and Chief, Division of Health Care Sciences, Department of Family and Preventive Medicine, University of California, San Diego, San Diego, California

Lewis E. Kazis, Sc.D. Senior Scientist, Bedford VA Health Services Research and Development Field Program, Edith Nourse Rogers Memorial Veterans Hospital, Bedford, and Associate Professor of Public Health, Health Services, Boston University School of Public Health, Boston, Massachusetts

Steven G. Kelsen, M.D. Professor of Medicine, Division of Pulmonary Disease and Critical Care Medicine, Department of Medicine, Temple University School of Medicine, Philadelphia, Pennsylvania

Karen T. Labuhn, M.S.N., M.P.H., Ph.D. Associate Professor, College of Nursing, Wayne State University, Detroit, Michigan

Paul N. Lanken, M.D. Associate Professor of Medicine, Division of Pulmonary and Critical Care Medicine, and Medical Director, Medical Intensive Care Unit, University of Pennsylvania Medical Center, Philadelphia, Pennsylvania

Donald A. Mahler, M.D. Associate Professor of Medicine, Section of Pulmonary and Critical Care Medicine, Department of Medicine, Dartmouth Medical School, Lebanon, New Hampshire

A. John McSweeny, Ph.D. Professor, Department of Psychiatry, Medical College of Ohio, Toledo, Ohio

Richard P. Millman, M.D. Associate Professor of Medicine, Brown University, and Director, Sleep Disorders Center, Division of Pulmonary and Critical Care Medicine, Rhode Island Hospital, Providence, Rhode Island

Richard K. Murray, M.D. Pulmonary and Critical Care Division, Department of Medicine, University of Pennsylvania Medical Center, Philadelphia, Pennsylvania

Virginia Simson Nelson, M.D., M.P.H. Chief, Pediatric and Adolescent Service, Department of Physical Medicine and Rehabilitation, C. S. Mott Children's Hospital, University of Michigan Medical Center, Ann Arbor, Michigan

Richard S. Novitch, M.D. Assistant Professor of Medicine, Cornell University Medical College, New York, and Assistant Director of Pulmonary Medicine, Burke Rehabilitation Hospital, White Plains, New York

Reynold A. Panettieri, Jr., M.D. Assistant Professor of Medicine, Pulmonary and Critical Care Division, Department of Medicine, University of Pennsylvania Medical Center, Philadelphia, Pennsyvlania

Andrew L. Ries, M.D., M.P.H. Professor of Medicine, Division of Pulmonary and Critical Care Medicine, University of California, San Diego, San Diego, California

Dudley F. Rochester, M.D. Professor Emeritus, Division of Pulmonary and Critical Care Medicine, University of Virginia School of Medicine, Charlottesville, Virginia

Robert M. Rogers, M.D. Professor of Medicine, Division of Pulmonary, Allergy, and Critical Care Medicine, University of Pittsburgh School of Medicine, Pittsburgh, Pennsylvania

Jonathan M. Samet, M.D. Professor and Chairman, Department of Epidemiology, School of Public Health and Hygiene, The Johns Hopkins University, Baltimore, Maryland

Alfredo J. Selim, M.D. Research Associate, Health Services Research and Development Field Program, Veterans Administration, Edith Nourse Rogers Memorial Veterans Hospital, Bedford, Massachusetts

Arthur A. Siebens, M.D. Professor Emeritus, The Johns Hopkins University, and Director, Pharyngology Rehabilitation and Research, Milton J. Dance, Jr., Center, Greater Baltimore Medical Center, Baltimore, Maryland

Peggy M. Simon, M.D. Assistant Professor of Medicine, Division of Pulmonary and Critical Care Medicine, Mayo Clinic, Rochester, Minnesota

Heidi C. Squier, M.S. Doctoral Candidate, Medical Clinical Psychology, UCSD/SDSU Joint Doctoral Program in Clinical Psychology, University of California, San Diego, and San Diego State University, San Diego, California

Bruce A. Staats, M.D. Associate Professor of Medicine, Division of Pulmonary and Critical Care Medicine, Mayo Clinic, Rochester, Minnesota

Henry M. Thomas III, M.D. Professor of Clinical Medicine, Cornell University Medical College, New York, and Chief, Pulmonary Division, Will Rogers Pulmonary Research Laboratory, Burke Rehabilitation Hospital, White Plains, New York

Cynthia Coffin Zadai, M.S., P.T. Director, Rehabilitation Services, Beth Israel Hospital, and Assistant Professor, Department of Physical Therapy, Massachusetts General Institute, Boston, Massachusetts

CONTENTS

Part Three THERAPEUTIC INTERVENTIONS

FOREWORD

Dr. Alvin Barach dropped in shortly after I moved uptown. I was fresh from the Cardiopulmonary Laboratory and Chest Service at Bellevue Hospital. In contrast, the Medical Center had long been home to Dr. Barach and he was held in high esteem as a chest physician and as a charming, creative, and inventive individual. Everyone there knew of his contributions to the treatment of chronic lung disease using oxygen therapy and positive-pressure breathing. Often in his company were Drs. Beck and Bickerman, also notable chest specialists, whose activities centered more around the Goldwater Memorial Hospital, which provided a large population of patients with chronic lung disease for treatment and study. To round out the entourage was Mr. Eckman, a kind of mechanical genius who could picture, and then turn into practical reality, the mechanical devices envisaged by Barach, Beck, and Bickerman.

All of this went through my mind as I lifted my eyes to gaze at Dr. Barach in the doorway. What I did not appreciate was the extent to which our paths would diverge in the years to come: his was to lead to pulmonary rehabilitation, mine to scientific pulmonary medicine. Nor could I imagine that after a long stretch of going their own ways, the two paths would converge.

Once in the room, Dr. Barach paced back and forth and around. He paid no heed to the small space, the unopened boxes, the clutter on the desktop. As he walked, he gesticulated with his right hand, cigarette between two fingers. Occasionally, without breaking stride, he would take a puff—almost invariably breaking his train of thought to reassure me that he was not inhaling.

His topic was diaphragmatic breathing and how it could be improved by diaphragmatic exercises. Indeed, he could show how effective it could be if we were to walk over to the Harkness Pavilion where he would show me a patient to illustrate his point. The patient proved to be a young woman, an opera singer, hospitalized for some nonpulmonary condition. For some months, to improve her singing, she had been practicing diaphragmatic breathing under Dr. Barach's tutelage. Willingly, she exposed her abdomen and lower thorax so that we could witness their excursions. Dr. Barach and I watched from the side of the bed. There was no doubt that she and Dr. Barach were convinced that her diaphragm was functioning better as a result of the breathing exercises. Since I had not seen the patient before, I could only marvel at the large abdominal excursions. But I left unconvinced.

This experience was to exemplify my relationship with Dr. Barach and his colleagues in the years to come: they would show, patient by patient, living proof that some ingenious interventions had greatly improved the patient's functioning and quality of life. Their enthusiasm was contagious. But, invariably, as in the *Rubáiyát* of Omar Khayyám, I went out by the same door as the one by which I entered—wishing for more objective evidence and more controls.

For years thereafter, Dr. Barach and I pursued neighboring but parallel paths at the Columbia-Presbyterian Medical Center. He and his colleagues continued to develop new mechanical devices and empirical strategies that were forerunners of pulmonary rehabilitation; my clinic and laboratory provided clinical care, often using Barach's devices, that were rooted in physiology, pathophysiology, and pathology.

Then, long after I had left the Columbia-Presbyterian Medical Center, the two paths became one: I was invited to build an academic department of rehabilitation medicine at the University of Pennsylvania. Because of my training and experience, I explored the possibilities of focusing on pulmonary and cardiac rehabilitation. In the process, I rediscovered the contributions of Dr. Barach. At about the same time that I began to explore the possibilities of cardiopulmonary rehabilitation, the National Institutes of Health was about to take the same tack: the National Heart, Lung, and Blood Institute joined forces with the newly formed Center for Medical Rehabilitation Research to sponsor a conference on the current state of research in pulmonary rehabilitation. I was invited to chair the meeting; it was an eye-opener. One message was clear: for pulmonary rehabilitation to prosper, it needed scientific underpinnings. True, these underpinnings could not be compared to physiology, biochemistry, and pathology; they had to include other sciences, such as the psychosocial sciences, biostatistics, and epidemiology, to do justice to the comprehensive nature of the field. Moreover, each science had to be assessed not in the manner of the traditional basic sciences, but by its own professional standards for research.

Looking back, I can now appreciate that Barach's creativity was coupled with a remarkable foresight that enabled him to see beyond the clinic, the hospital bedside, and physiological measurements. His vision took in the whole patient, not only in the hospital and clinic, but also in the home, family, community, and workplace. It is true that this time was not ripe for functional assessment, outcomes research, and dissociation of the underlying pathology and pathophysiology from such overtones as psychosocial influences and physical deconditioning. But, it is equally true that the time has now come to apply scientific principles to all aspects of pulmonary rehabilitation.

The pages that follow indicate the present state of diverse aspects of pulmonary rehabilitation. I am grateful for the time, effort, and talent of the contributors. I also realize that this book would not have started without the seminal conference arranged under the auspices of the National Institutes of Health, and it would not have materialzied without the guiding lights of Drs. Suzanne Hurd and Sri Ram, of the National Heart, Lung, and Blood Institute, and Drs. Duane Alexander, Marcus Fuhrer, and Louis Quatrano, of the Center for Medical Rehabilitation Research.

Others played different roles in the genesis of this book. Ms. Alice K. Glover orchestrated the flow of material and helped to package it properly. Ms. Betsy Ann Bozzarello freed my time from other duties to make editing possible. Last but not least, my wife, Linda, and daughter, Hannah, provided the environment and set a frame of mind that made possible the translation of the idea of a book on pulmonary rehabilitation into the reality that follows.

Alfred P. Fishman

Part One

OVERVIEW

1

Rehabilitation Medicine

A Framework for Pulmonary Rehabilitation

THEODORE M. COLE

University of Michigan Medical School
Ann Arbor, Michigan

I. The Need

Between 35 million and 43 million Americans have a disability, a total roughly equivalent to the combined populations of the nation's two most populous states, California and Florida. Almost one in 20 Americans has a disability so severe that it prohibits carrying out a major life activity. An additional one in 20 is restricted in a major activity, and approximately another one in 20 is limited in other types of activities. The penalty on human functioning imposed by disability has enormous economic consequences. It is estimated that losses to the country's economy exceed \$170 billion dollars a year, approximately 6.5% of the gross national product (1). Disability is arguably the nation's largest health problem. On April 14, 1969, in his first speech as a U.S. Senator, Robert Dole harkened back to another April 14, 24 years earlier during World War II, when he involuntarily became a member of a minority group, the exceptional group of people who have physical disabilities (2). He suggested the creation of a presidential task force or commission to review what the public and private sectors were doing and to recommend how we could do it better. He particularly lamented the economic, employment, and health care problems of people with disabilities. Twenty-five years later, we are only beginning to realize the potential for people with physical disabilities to experience improvement through medical rehabilitation.

What is medical rehabilitation? Rehabilitation medicine is the diagnosis and treatment of impairments, disabilities, and handicaps resulting from illness, injury, and developmental processes that begin before birth and continue until the last stages of life. It focuses on health-related improvement in human functioning—physical, cognitive, behavioral, and social (1). Cole likened rehabilitation to a tree (3). The earth from which the tree grows is likened to the sciences from which rehabilitation grows; the roots correspond to research; the ever-widening trunk is likened to medical practice, which is shaped by opportunity; the branches correspond to all the disciplines in rehabilitation; the leaves, which appear and depart in cycles, are compared to the practitioners; and, the flowers and fruits of the tree correspond to the students. They are the brightest ornament of the tree.

II. A Framework for Pulmonary Rehabilitation

Rehabilitation medicine is the medical practice of the specialist in physical medicine and rehabilitation, or the physiatrist. Rehabilitation medicine might be considered a framework for pulmonary rehabilitation. The discipline was formed in 1923 when the American College of Radiology and Physiotherapy was founded. However, it was not until 1937 that the American Medical Association gave recognition to the first rehabilitation organization in the United States, the American Congress of Physical Therapy. Since that time and over many name changes, the field of medical rehabilitation has grown. The first medical journal in the field was established in 1954 and a second journal, also devoted exclusively to medical rehabilitation, in 1988. Now over 4000 physicians are trained in the specialty of rehabilitation medicine, but the demand still grows. The specialty is just now coming of age as a scientific discipline. This development comes none too soon, as the medical sciences attempt to address the consequences of chronic illness, impairment, and disability. The reader who is interested in the 50 years of developments in rehabilitation medicine is referred to the special issue of the *Archives of Physical Medicine and Rehabilitation* of October 1988 (4).

Rounds made on the wards and in the clinics of any major medical rehabilitation center will reveal patients with major pulmonary problems. These children and adults are most frequently being treated for pulmonary insufficiency due to neuromuscular diseases or central nervous system injuries to the brainstem or the spinal cord. Consequently, it is not uncommon to see mechanical ventilation machines and pulmonary therapies in use on a rehabilitation inpatient unit, and to see staff trained and experienced in proper management, interventions, and technologies. In many hospitals the rehabilitation unit is the only place, other than intensive care and step-down units, where one sees sophisticated approaches to pulmonary problems that threaten life or limit function.

Although there are over 600,000 physicians in the United States, less than 1% specialize in medical rehabilitation. It is necessary that they be joined by physicians from other specialties who are also interested in physical disability and its management. In the case of pulmonary rehabilitation, it is likely that the medical services will be delivered by physicians specializing in chest medicine, aided by an interdisciplinary team of health practitioners. Table 1 shows the diversity of the physicians currently practicing one or another aspect of medical rehabilitation.

In recent years, there has been a broadening of both the effects on medical rehabilitation and the effects from it. These changes include the following (1): (1) there has been a recent expansion of public and private agencies serving people with physical disabilities; (2) legislation has now established not only the civil rights of people with disabilities, but also the criteria by which disabled people can receive reimbursable services; (3) evaluations of the economics of health care have affected the availability and accessibility of intensive and often expensive rehabilitation services; (4) emphasis has moved away from the process and toward the outcomes of medical rehabilitation; (5) medical care has moved outside of institutions and into the communities; (6) independent living is now emphasized as a goal for the disabled and aging populations.

As has been the case for medical rehabilitation, pulmonary rehabilitation will have to deal with the social conflicts that are associated with growth and change. Centralized control is being displaced by individual empowerment of the patient. Single, small health delivery units are being replaced by large corporate organizations. Not-for-profit medical centers are being replaced by entrepreneurial, for-profit organizations. Process is being replaced by product lines.

Table 1 Diversity of Physicians in Rehabilitation

Burn surgeons	Orthopedists
Cardiologists	Pediatricians
General internists	Physiatrists
Geriatrists	Plastic surgeons
Neurologists	Pulmonologists
Neurosurgeons	Urologists

It is interesting to note that emphasis is being placed on pulmonary rehabilitation at a time when health care and its component services are witnessing the emergence of new health industries. One such industry is managed care, which is an effort to contain cost and control directions taken by providers, their services, and the people they serve. The Washington Business Group on Health proposes the development of organized systems of care (5) that will impel four paradigm shifts: (1) health care will change from fragmented to integrated and changes in practice standards will be combined with outcomes; (2) the patient role will change from passive to active in order to take responsibility for health-promoting behaviors; professionals will respect the patients' preferences; (3) the paradigm will shift from an emphasis on health services to the concept of value, here defined as necessary care provided at reasonable costs; (4) another change will be from shifting responsibility to taking responsibility. Consumers have wanted physicians to make them well and they want employers and government to pay. Providers want to exercise their skills while remaining free from external intrusion. Payers have wanted providers to reduce costs as they continue to shift their own costs. It is believed that consumers, providers, and payers will all shoulder a share of these responsibilities in the future.

Practitioners of medical rehabilitation will find some comfort in the proposed organized systems of care. There are many parallels between medical rehabilitation and managed care. A new spinal cord injury book (6) documents 20 years of accomplishments by a national system of care for people with spinal cord injury, illustrating that medical rehabilitation has utilized managed care paradigms for over two decades.

III. Elements of Medical Rehabilitation

A. Measurement of Function and Outcome

The care systems of the future are likely to be those that will document patient outcome measured in terms of human function, as well as in other terms. At its core, medical rehabilitation is focused on functional outcomes. While the measurement of functional status in some of the body's systems is quite advanced, as in the case of vision and hearing, the measurement of impairment caused by multisystem disease is still controversial (7–13). It has been taken on faith that improvement in organ function would decrease the levels of disability and handicap. We now know that this is not the entire picture. Today consumers and payers demand that medical providers document the effectiveness of their interventions. To do this requires measurement of impairment, functional limitation, disability, and quality of life before and after rehabilitation. With enactment of Public Law 101-129, the U.S. Congress and the President have endorsed the funding of health care services that document the effectiveness of interventions as the basis for decisions on whether specific services are warranted. Public Law 101-129 has established a major program of research on the effectiveness and outcomes of health care services.

Functional assessment of impairments produced by pulmonary diseases is clearly necessary to measure the effects of rehabilitation interventions. A variety of clinical assessment tools have been developed in an attempt to measure function. Among these, the most frequently used tool in medical rehabilitation is the Functional Independence Measure (FIM) of the Uniform National Data System for Medical Rehabilitation (UNDSMR) (14–16). A Functional Independence score can be a measure of what an individual is capable of doing in a particular activity, or it can express what the person customarily does in the usual course of each day, given circumstances, resources, and competing demands upon his/her energy reserves. The summary FIM score is comprised of six subsections or activities of daily living: self-care, sphincter control, mobility transfer, locomotion, communication, and social cognition. These activities apply to all people and are important to measure no matter what the medical diagnosis or disease. The same disability can be caused by different disease entities.

B. Quality of Life

Ability is linked to quality of life. Disability, or limitation in one's ability to function effectively in a chosen setting, is therefore an aspect of health-related quality of life (HRQL). Health care practitioners are striving to provide necessary and helpful services to improve or maintain HRQL. A workshop sponsored by the National Institutes of Health studied quality-of-life assessments (17). It reported that HRQL can be conceptualized as a three-part model that includes: (1) clinical status or biological functioning; (2) disease-specific and treatment-specific symptoms and problems; and (3) general health measures that focus on various aspects of functioning and general health perceptions. The definition of general health measures includes physical, functional, and emotional status; cognitive functions; performance and social roles; and general well-being. These parameters are reflected in the FIM assessment tool.

Three aspects of HRQL are especially important to patients. First is the increasing predominance of chronic disease and the need to limit disabling consequences rather than cure the disease. Second, there is greater emphasis on preventive care. The third factor is the growing number of comparably effective therapeutic options for the same problem. Clearly, one of the trends in modern medicine will be improving human function in an effort to improve the overall quality of life for the individual.

C. Interdisciplinary Team

Working alongside the physician are nonphysicians who contribute to the broad field of medical rehabilitation. What started as a tight family of rehabilitationists has now become an extended family of professionals from many disciplines and all academic levels (Table 2).

The interdisciplinary health team is the holy grail of traditional medical rehabilitation. Even the word "interdisciplinary," rather than "multidisciplinary," is important to medical rehabilitation professions. The word explicitly identifies the interactive and collegial nature of the team members. Although a physician is often assigned a leadership role in hospital settings, each member strives to understand and respect the uniqueness and contribution of the other team members. A traditional hierarchical model is replaced with one that values the contribution of each team member. This atmosphere is essential in order to create an ambiance in which the patient and the patient's family can play active roles in the healing and rehabilitation process. They become members of the team. The atmosphere also facilitates the educational role of the professional team, which constantly works to educate the patient and keep family and other significant parties fully informed so they can carry out their supportive roles in rehabilitation. Rehabilitationists believe that adjustment to the changed physical status of disability is best done in a more horizontal and less pyramidal structure. Even the word "patient," appropriate in the acute hospital setting, is often replaced with the word "client," "consumer," or "customer," depending on where the individual is situated in the continuum of health care. These terms help to empower the person seeking rehabilitation services and allow a more active commitment to the rehabilitation process. These are not trivial distinctions. They are so important that the National Institute on Disability and Reha-

Table 2 Diversity of Nonphysicians in Rehabilitation

Case managers	Orthotists/prosthetists
Educators	Physical therapists
Engineers	Physician assistants
Independent living specialists	Psychologists
Job coaches	Sexologists
Nurses	Social workers
Nutritionists	Speech and language pathologists
Occupational therapists	Vocational counselors
Personal care attendants	

bilitation Research (NIDRR) funded a project undertaken by the interdisciplinary American Congress of Rehabilitation Medicine to study team processes and develop training methods for interdisciplinary staff (18). It follows that physicians, too, must work collegially and effectively with fellow team members.

D. Systems Approach to Medical Rehabilitation

Specialists in medical rehabilitation subscribe to a systems approach in the rehabilitation process (19). Terminology varies as the process for creating uniform terms develops. However, all conceptual models are based on earlier work by the World Health Organization (20), Nagi (21), and Melvin and Nagi (22). The National Advisory Board to the National Center for Medical Rehabilitation Research (NCMRR) modified their earlier work and further extended the previous constructs (23). In this model of disability, there are five separate definitions which, together, embody the entire spectrum of disability and its effects on people: (1) The model begins with pathophysiology, which is the underlying cause of the disease or injury. Pathophysiology focuses on the cells and tissues. It is the interruption of or interference with normal physiological and developmental processes or structures. Pathophysiology may produce impairment, which focuses on the level of the organ. (2) Impairment is the loss or abnormality of cognitive, emotional, physiological, or anatomical structure or function, not just those attributable to the initial pathophysiology. Impairment may produce functional limitation(s). The focus of functional limitation is on the whole person who is affected by loss or abnormality. (3) Functional limitation is a restriction or lack of ability to perform an action in the manner or within the range consistent with the purpose of an organ or organ system. The functional limitation may yield a disability, which is the interface between the individual and his/her environment. (4) A disability is the inability or limitation in performing tasks, activities, and roles to levels expected within physical and social context. The NCMRR's unique contribution was in defining a fifth level of disability, namely societal limitation. (5) Societal limitation is restriction attributable to social policy or barriers (structural or attitudinal) which limits fulfillment of roles or denies access to services and opportunities that are associated with full participation in society.

E. Primary Health Care

As discussion of health care reform progresses, many medical disciplines are reconsidering their role in primary health care. Some ask if primary health care for individuals with severe physical disabilities belongs in the province of primary care physician. Or, should primary health care in some circumstances be delivered by specialists who have in-depth understandings of unusual or complicated medical conditions, but lack training or experience in primary health care?

DeJong and others reviewed the primary health care complaints of persons with physical disabilities in a conference conducted in 1989 by the National Rehabilitation Hospital Research Center and the National Institute on Disability and Rehabilitation Research (NIDRR) (24). McGinnis et al. (25) further substantiated these complaints in their report of 240 patients discharged from three Boston-area medical rehabilitation programs. Patients complained that they often had to use numerous providers in attempting to resolve a single health problem. They concluded that there is little effective case management to resolve the basic health problems of persons with major physical disabilities. Litvak and co-workers (26) reported that many persons with disabilities require the services of a personal attendant to assist them with their basic physical needs. They found that self-care, whether performed by the disabled person or a personal attendant, is a major part of preventive health care for many people with disabilities. Attendants can often assist the disabled person in creating good health habits, including exercise and nutrition, and they are frequently the early observers of health problems. The lack of access to personal care assistants may increase the disabled person's vulnerability toward secondary disabilities. Furthermore, when a person with a physical disability incurs a new health problem, often the consequences are worse than for an able-bodied counterpart. New health problems often increase the functional dependence and further compromise the person's ability to work and to live independently. Whereas able-bodied people can employ many strategies to offset acute illness and can utilize community resources, the disabled person frequently cannot independently pursue optimum health habits such as independent exercise and healthy social interactions. If avoidable stress is coupled with avoidable nutritional problems and avoidable social isolation, further secondary disabilities may ensue. Thus, there is a need to provide primary care services to people with disabilities, including the disability caused by severe, chronic pulmonary disease.

Early workers in primary health care have been trying to provide managed health care services to working-age disabled people for the past decade (27). Recently, the Rehabilitation Institute of Michigan has been participating in a statewide project to evaluate the effectiveness of a primary health care clinic, wherein physiatrists and internists combine to meet patients' medical and rehabilitative needs for primary care. The effectiveness of these programs is yet to be fully understood. Their success will be measured by their ability to satisfy patients' and families' needs for primary health care while avoiding unnecessary hospitalizations and medical procedures, as well as social and vocational deterioration that could otherwise be prevented.

IV. Implications for Pulmonary Rehabilitation

Pulmonary rehabilitation is not a new field, but its potential for new growth is significant in this decade. To realize its potential, advocates will pursue many of the directions and recommendations that have emerged in the field of medical rehabilitation. Pulmonary rehabilitation will increasingly focus its activities on enhancing the quality of life for people with chronic lung diseases. This will be done through pursuing research on improvement of physiological functions, and on replacement, enhancement, or prevention of functional deterioration. We must gain involvement and cooperation of scientists who are interested in and have the technical expertise to improve the knowledge base in the field of pulmonary rehabilitation. They will improve clinical practice and develop technical advances on behalf of people with severe pulmonary diseases.

Bringing the health-related problems of people with pulmonary diseases to the attention of our best scientists is necessary to reduce the costs of pulmonary disease to the individual and to society. It will be necessary to apply rigorous scientific methods to open the promising field of pulmonary rehabilitation, with all its new opportunities and uncertainties, to the people with or at risk for chronic pulmonary disability. Definitions in this expanding field will need to be settled, priorities set, measurement tools developed, interventions scrutinized, and outcomes assessed.

HRQL will be benefited as we learn how to elicit patient preferences for health status and quality-of-life outcomes. Survey instruments and data collection strategies for subpopulations must be adopted. Societal norms will have to be identified to deal with variations of individual preferences in response to changes in disease state and changes in affect during the course of illness. Measures that incorporate duration of survival, functional status, and patient preferences in a single index number will have to be developed. We must also examine the relationship between patients' responses and the responses of family, friends, and caregivers. All this must be done in an atmosphere where we can feel secure that our conclusions and actions are determined with scientific validity.

References

1. Cole TM, Edgerton VR. Report on the Task Force on Medical Rehabilitation Research. Huntvalley, MD: National Institutes of Health, 1990.
2. Congressional Record, Vol 115, Monday, April 14, 1969.
3. Cole TM. The greening of physiatry in a golden era of rehabilitation. Arch Phys Med Rehabil 1993; 74:231–237.
4. Arch Phys Med Rehabil 1988; 69(Special Issue):1–68.

5. Strategy 2000. Chicago: Paralyzed Veterans of America 1992:20–25.
6. Stover SL, DeLisa JA, Whiteneck GG, eds. Spinal Cord Injury: Clinical Outcomes from the Model Systems. Gaithersburg, MD: Aspen (in press).
7. Feinstein AR, Josephy BR, Wells CK. Scientific and clinical problems in indexes of functional disability. Ann Intern Med 1986; 105:413–420.
8. Ben-Yishay Y, Gerstman L, Diller L, Haas A. Prediction of rehabilitation outcomes from psychometric parameters in left hemiplegics. J Clin Psychol 1970; 34:436–441.
9. Carey RG, Seibert JH, Posavac EJ. Who makes the most progress in inpatient rehabilitation? An analysis of functional gain. Arch Phys Med Rehabil 1988; 69:37–43.
10. Granger CV, Hamilton BB, Gresham GE, Kramer AA. The stroke rehabilitation outcome study. II. Relative merits of the total Barthel Index Score and a four-item subscore in predicting patient outcomes. Arch Phys Med Rehabil 1989; 70:100–103.
11. Johnson MV, Keith RA, Hinderer SR. Measurement standards for interdisciplinary medical rehabilitation. Arch Phys Med Rehabil 1992; 73:S3–23.
12. Champion HR, Copes WS, Sacco WJ, et al. The Major Trauma Outcome Study: establishing national norms for trauma care. J Trauma 1990; 30:1356.
13. Baker S, O'Neill B, Haddon W, et al. Injury Severity Score: a method for describing patients with multiple injuries and evaluating emergency care. J Trauma 1974; 215:2771.
14. Linacre JM, Heinemann AW, Wright BD, Granger CV, Hamilton BB. The structure and stability of the Functional Independence Measure. Arch Phys Med Rehabil 1994; 75:127–132.
15. Heinemann AW, Linacre JM, Wright BD, Hamilton BB, Granger CV. Prediction of rehabilitation outcomes with disability measures. Arch Phys Med Rehabil 1994; 75:133–143.
16. Wrigley JM, Yoels WC, Webb CR, Fine PR. Social and physical factors in the referral of people with traumatic brain injuries to rehabilitation. Arch Phys Med Rehabil 75:149–155.
17. Quality of Life Assessment: Practice, Problems, Promise. Proceedings of a Workshop, National Institutes of Health, Bethesda, MD, October 15–17, 1990.
18. Campbell L, Eisenberg M, Elliott T, et al. Guide to Interdisciplinary Practice in Rehabilitation Settings. Chicago, IL: American Congress of Rehabilitation Medicine, 1992.
19. Cole TM. Prevention of secondary disabilities after brain injury and spinal cord injury: implications for future research. J Prev Med 1994; 23:670–675.
20. World Health Organization. International Classification of Impairments, Disabilities, and Handicaps: A Manual of Classification Relating to the Consequences of Disease. Geneva: World Health Organization, 1980.
21. Nagi SZ. An epidemiology of disability among adults in the United States. Milbank Mem Fund 1976; 54:439–467.
22. Melvin JL, Nagi SZ. Factors in behavioral responses to impairments. Arch Phys Med Rehabil 1970; 51:552–557.

23. Wood PHN, Bradly EM. People with Disabilities: Toward Acquiring Information Which Reflects More Sensitively Their Problems and Needs. New York: World Rehabilitation Fund, 1980.
24. Meeting the Primary Health Care Needs of Persons with Physical Disabilities; Setting the Agenda Proceedings of the NRH National Invitational Conference on Primary Care Disability, Washington DC, December 28, 1989.
25. McGinnis G, Osberg JS, DeJong G, Seward M, Branch L. Predicting charges for inpatient medical rehabilitation services using severity, DRG, age and function. Am J Public Health 1987; 77:827–829.
26. Litvak S, Zukas H, Heumann J. Attending to America; Personal Assistance for Independent Living. Berkeley, CA: Wold Institute on Disability, 1987.
27. Meyers AR, Couple A, Lederman RI, et al. A prospective evaluation of the effect of managed care on medical care utilization among severely disabled independently living adults. Med Care 1987; 25:1057–1068.

2

Pulmonary Rehabilitation: From Empiricism to Science

ALFRED P. FISHMAN

University of Pennsylvania Medical Center
Philadelphia, Pennsylvania

Pulmonary rehabilitation is governed by the same guiding principles as rehabilitation medicine in general. However, it has not been easy to prove that pulmonary rehabilitation is as effective and efficient as other subsets of rehabilitation medicine, e.g., musculoskeletal, simply because the degree of clinical benefit is usually not very dramatic and objective measures are more difficult to quantify. As a result, not all chest physicians are true believers in the value of pulmonary rehabilitation as part of the therapeutic armamentarium.

I. The Misgivings of the Chest Physician

The traditional model on which the chest physician is born and bred relies almost exclusively on the patient-doctor relationship. In contrast, the rehabilitation model depends on an interplay among a team of health professionals, on the one hand, and the patient and family, on the other. No preset number of health professionals, e.g., physical therapists, respiratory therapists, nurses, comprise the team. Indeed, the number and nature of these professionals may vary considerably in the course of the disease. Not entirely clear to the chest physician may be the role that each other professional can play and how to sort out the contributions of the team from those of an individual subset, e.g., physical therapy.

A second area of discomfort for the chest physician is with the goals of rehabilitation medicine. By its very nature, rehabilitation medicine is more ambitious and comprehensive than acute or chronic care medicine: it aspires not only to restore the individual to the optimal state of health, but also to optimize the individual's functioning at home, in the community, and in the workplace, thereby improving the individual's quality of life. To accomplish these sweeping goals, rehabilitation may come on stage at different times in the course of the patient's illness. As a rule, the time of entry is after the patient's illness has stabilized and the focus is on minimizing the disability that the pathological process has produced (Table 1). However, rehabilitation can also be helpful in the acute setting, e.g., in the intensive care unit, where it can prevent physical deconditioning. Or, it may play a role in preventing disease, e.g., in promoting the cessation of smoking. Moreover, as noted above, different health professionals may be involved at different times.

A third type of misgiving is inherent in the usual training of the chest physician. The chest physician has been raised on a heavy diet of scientific medicine, i.e., with heavy reliance on the physiology and pathophysiology of the lung. As a result, the chest physician has developed great faith in pulmonary function tests as a measure of the success of an intervention. By this criterion, pulmonary rehabilitation is generally a failure since pulmonary function tests are often unchanged after a course of pulmonary rehabilitation even though the patient feels better, enjoys life more, and is functioning better.

Finally, the therapeutic goals and expectations of chest physicians usually fall far short of those of rehabilitation physicians. As a rule, the therapeutic interventions of the chest physician are directed at arresting, reversing, or lim-

Table 1 Domains Relevant to Pulmonary Rehabilitation in Patients with Dyspnea[a]

Domain	Example
Pathophysiology	Obstructive airways disease
Impairment	Breathless, cough, sputum; malnutrition; depression
Functional limitation	Limited exercise tolerance; requires O_2 for the activities of daily life and sleep; weakness
Disability	Cannot do constructive work; deterioration of sex life and intimate relationships; loss of recreation
Societal limitation	Cannot find employment; difficulty with health, life, and/or disability insurance; architectural barriers

[a]For patient with COPD.
Source: Modified from Table 3, p. 35 in Ref. 24.

iting the initiating pathology and pathogenetic mechanisms, whereas the rehabilitation physician generally is obliged to assume that the impairment has stabilized and to direct attention to improving the functional capacity of the individual and the health-related quality of life.

One partial remedy by which many of these misgivings could be dispelled would be to include the concepts and practice of rehabilitation medicine in the training of the chest physician. This approach affords another bright prospect. At present, almost all lessons about pulmonary rehabilitation derive from experience with chronic obstructive disease of the airways, especially COPD (chronic bronchitis and emphysema). This preoccupation with COPD has been justified on the grounds of its prevalence. However, extrapolation from the experience with rehabilitation medicine in COPD to other respiratory disorders, e.g., musculoskeletal disorders, sleep apnea syndromes, difficulty in weaning, and pre- and post-lung transplantation, need not be direct. If we include the principles and practice of rehabilitation medicine in the training of the chest physician, a larger and more diverse population will become available for assessing the value of pulmonary rehabilitation in different types of lung disease.

II. What Is Pulmonary Rehabilitation?

At a recent workshop on pulmonary rehabilitation, sponsored as a collaborative effort by two components of the National Institutes of Health—the Lung Division of the National Heart, Lung, and Blood Institute, and the Center for Medical Rehabilitation Research—the crowded room of participants and audience was asked to examine the textbook definition of pulmonary rehabilitation as originally defined by a committee of the American College of Chest Physicians and subsequently endorsed by the American Thoracic Society:

> Pulmonary rehabilitation may be defined as an *art* of medical practice wherein an individually tailored, multidisciplinary program is formulated which through accurate diagnosis, therapy, emotional support, and education, stabilizes or reverses both the physio- and psychopathology of pulmonary diseases and attempts to return the patient to the highest possible functional capacity allowed by his pulmonary handicap and overall life situation (1,2).

The designation of pulmonary rehabilitation as an "art" provoked animated discussion. To many, the rubric "art" was a refuge that exempted pulmonary rehabilitation from critical scientific evaluation. Instead of resorting to this type of nonquantifiable term, the consensus was that each specialty involved in pulmonary rehabilitation should define its own criteria by which its particular contribution to pulmonary rehabilitation could be assessed.

One suggested alternative to "art" was the word "process," used as follows:

> Pulmonary rehabilitation may be defined as a *process* by which health professionals and specialists, working in conjunction with the chest physician, the patient with pulmonary disease, and the patient's family, interact as a team to improve the functional capabilities and the health-related quality of the patient's life. The size and composition of the team as well as the specific therapeutic measures are tailored to the physical, emotional, and societal needs of the patient.

III. Assessment of Outcomes

Outcomes of interventions designed to improve the lot of individuals have been assessed in different ways: in terms of disability, function, cost-effectiveness, and quality of life (health status) (Table 2). In clinical trials, mortality and decrease in the number of hospitalizations or visits to the clinic are commonly used to measure outcome, often with little regard to morbidity, disability, functional status, and quality of life (3–5). These usual end-points do little to address the major goals of rehabilitation medicine, i.e., improvement in functional capacity and in the health-related quality of life. Nor do they take into

Table 2 Components of Functional Status

Impairment. Loss or abnormality of psychological, physiological, or anatomical structure or function (6).

Disability. Effects of one or more impairments on an individual's normal level of skill or ability. Disabilities can be of different kinds, e.g., difficulty in feeding oneself, turning over in bed, dressing, walking independently, tending to personal hygiene, and communicating appropriately. The Functional Independency Measure (FIM) is one commonly used measure of disability.

Functional status. Assessment involves beginning with inventory of ability to satisfy the basic body needs (defined above under "Disability"). It can then extend to include psychosocial functioning, e.g., cognition and behavior, daily living, work, and leisure (7). It can be expanded further to include the instrumental activities of daily living, e.g., cooking, shopping, working around the house, taking medications, and using transportation. Determined by a constellation of factors: the abilities of the individual, limits on function, demands, support from environment, financial, and social systems; relationships with family and significant others; social roles; motivation; attitude. The greater the disability, the more the functional status is likely to be influenced by factors other than abilities (8). Functional assessment can serve multiple purposes in addition to providing an instrument for assessing patient's capabilities, a measure of outcome, planning health care, reimbursement, and prevention.

Quality of life or health status. Includes perception of individual about his/her health and how the perceived health affects his/her activities and attitudes in general. Functional assessment plays a key role in evaluating the quality of life.

account the cost-effectiveness of therapeutic interventions or regimens (6). In essence, a major problem for pulmonary rehabilitation is a lack of consensus about optimal measures of functional, as well as physiological, outcomes. Moreover, since multiple and diverse therapeutic modalities are generally applied concomitantly, it would be helpful to sort out the respective contributions of each component of the rehabilitation program to the outcome.

A. Functional Assessment

The assessment of function extends far beyond the testing of pulmonary function (7–15). In essence, it evaluates the individual's ability to carry out the activities of daily life. These may extend from basic elements, such as getting in and out of bed, dressing, and walking, on the one hand, to activities associated with a greater degree of independence, such as shopping, using the telephone, doing work around the house, and driving or taking public transportation. The need for supplemental oxygen to carry out these activities has to be included in the evaluation. In addition to these physical functions, psychosocial functioning, such as cognition and behavior, has to be included. A major problem in functional assessment is in ensuring proper content of items to be measured and the accuracy and reproducibility of the measurements.

Two general approaches have been taken to functional assessment: generic and specific. *Generic instruments* for evaluation of general health status have the advantage of being reducible to a single or a small number of scores and applicable to a variety of conditions. Their disadvantage is that they may not deal adequately with specific aspects of health status, such as dyspnea.

Disease-specific or *symptom-specific instruments* have the advantage of being closely related to the clinical manifestations of a particular disorder, so they are more responsive than general instruments to changes effected by intervention (2,13). Moreover, physiological measurements can be related to specific functions, e.g., the O_2 cost of dressing in patients with COPD.

B. Health-Related Quality of Life

Because the goal of pulmonary rehabilitation is to ameliorate not only the physical disabilities, but also their emotional and social consequences, functional assessment has to identify unmet medical, psychosocial, and environmental needs for the sake of improving the health-related quality of life (16,17). One battery for assessing health-related quality of life in chronic obstructive lung disease includes four dimensions: emotional functioning, social role functioning, activities of daily life, and recreation (7).

C. Dyspnea

Because it is usually the major cause of disability in patients with chronic pulmonary disease, dyspnea is used not only for functional assessment, but also as an essential target of programs directed at improving functional capacities and quality of life. Not infrequently, the disability originating with dyspnea is aggravated by physical deconditioning and malnutrition; easy fatigability is usually more of a prospect than a reality because shortness of breath and physical deconditioning generally preclude taxing levels of activity. As dyspnea intensifies in the course of progressive pulmonary disease, it increasingly limits the activities of daily life, conversation, and self-care. Not infrequently it calls for oxygen to provide relief not only while awake and during activity, but also during sleep (18–22).

Quantification of dyspnea holds considerable appeal for those engaged in pulmonary rehabilitation because of several bright prospects: insights into the pathogenesis and pathophysiology of dyspnea, a basis for addressing functional limitations, definition of realistic (achievable) goals in the process of pulmonary rehabilitation, specification of appropriate therapeutic interventions, and the evaluation of outcomes.

One problem in dealing with dyspnea is its subjective nature. Coupled with uncertainties about its mechanism(s) of production, it typifies "an enigma wrapped in a mystery." Attempts at quantification are seriously handicapped by psychological overtones to the physiological derangements (23).

Various disease-specific indices are currently in use for quantifying dyspnea, e.g., the Borg Dyspnea Rating Scale, the Chronic Respiratory Questionnaire, and the Baseline and Transition Dyspnea Indices (2). A recent approach to assessing outcomes in terms of dyspnea is illustrated by the algorithm developed by the National Center for Medical Research and Rehabilitation (24). This algorithm is based on the following five domains: pathophysiology, impairment, functional limitation, disability, and societal limitation (Fig. 1).

The severity of the dyspnea when the patient/client is first seen generally plays a critical role in shaping the program. For example, in the person who is severely breathless at rest and depends on others for the activities of daily life, the continuous administration of oxygen, the use of energy-conserving measures, and education directed at promoting psychological well-being are often all that can be afforded (21–28). In those less compromised, exercise training programs, the administration of oxygen during exercise, and education about energy-conserving measures may not only prevent physical and mental deterioration, but greatly improve functional capacity and enhance the health-related quality of life (29).

PATHOPHYSIOLOGY →	IMPAIRMENT →	FUNCTIONAL LIMITATION →	DISABILITY →	SOCIETAL LIMITATION
Interruption of, or interference with, normal physiological and developmental processes or structures.	Loss and/or abnormality of cognitive, emotional, physiological, or anatomical structure or function. Impairment includes all losses or abnormalities, not just those attributable to the initial pathology and pathophysiology.	Restriction or lack of ability to perform an action in the manner, or within a range, consistent with the purpose of an organ or organ system.	Inability or limitation in performing tasks, activities, and roles to levels expected within physical and social contexts.	Restriction, attributable to social policy or barriers (structural or attitudinal), which limits fulfillment of roles, or denies access to services and opportunities, that are associated with full participation in society.

Example: Chronic Obstructive Pulmonary Disease

Adult with chronic bronchitis and emphysema.	Shortness of breath upon limited activity; easy fatigability; malnutrition; depression.	Difficulties with activities of daily living, such as eating, dressing, personal hygiene; requires supplemental oxygen during sleep and activity.	Activities of daily life require extra time and assistance; cannot do work mechanic; cannot do hobbies and recreational activities; not independent with family and peers.	Difficulties in finding employment; lack of involvement in social activities; health insurer limits home care; limited access to recreational facilities.

Figure 1 Terminology of rehabilitation medicine as applied to chronic obstructive pulmonary disease. (Modified from Table 3, Research Plan for the National Center for Medical Rehabilitation Research, National Institutes of Health, National Institute of Child Health and Development, NIH Publication No. 93-3509, March 1993, p. 35.)

IV. Physiological Bases for Therapeutic Interventions

The impairment that led to the disability is generally either irreparable or held in a steady state by medical management. However, a firm grasp of the derangement underlying disability can provide the basis for physiological interventions that can minimize the disability. For example, exercise training holds the prospect of improving the health-related quality of life. Also, prolonged assisted ventilation can be tailored to provide optimal comfort and mobility. A third example is weaning from mechanical ventilation. Finally, the use of oxygen therapy is deeply vested in physiological principles.

A. Exercise Training

Physical exercise training has been shown to improve exercise capacity, ability to walk, and sense of well-being, even in hypercapnic patients. Moreover, different types of exercise have proved to be effective, e.g., high intensity at low frequency, on the one hand, and low intensity at high frequency on the other; also useful is exercise involving legs, arms, cycling, walking, and stair climbing (30–38).

However, many questions remain: Does training have any effect when pulmonary impairment is severe? What are optimal regimens for initial conditioning and for its maintenance? What types of exercise, e.g., arm, leg, or combinations of exercise, are optimal for different categories of patients/clients? What are the effects of exercise training on dyspnea, capacity for activities of daily living, and overall psychological, functional, and societal status?

Respiratory muscle strength and endurance improve in response to inspiratory muscle resistive training or threshold load training. However, dyspnea is only marginally relieved and the capacity for the activities of daily living is only slightly improved. The value of other breathing exercises has not been assessed in controlled studies. Unique types of breathing training (glossopharyngeal breathing, cough training) are applicable in special situations. Certain questions can be identified (39,40): Are combinations of respiratory muscle training regimens, e.g., strength, endurance, and increase in tidal volume, more effective than conventional regimens? Does combining respiratory muscle training with physical exercise training confer more benefit? Is it possible to increase diaphragmatic excursion by training? Does respiratory muscle training delay the onset of ventilatory failure? Is it possible by training to increase the effectiveness of the cough mechanism? How effective are breathing exercises?

B. Prolonged Mechanical Ventilation

Patients with pulmonary disorders in whom the ventilatory reserve is low require mechanical ventilatory support for prolonged periods. This is particularly true in patients with neuromuscular and chest wall diseases (41). Interest is particularly high in avoiding intubation of the trachea and in devising schedules of ventilatory support that alternate with spontaneous breathing. Techniques available for this purpose include negative-pressure body devices, positive-pressure masks and lip seals, rocking beds, and pneumatic belts. Other mechanical aids under investigation include continuous positive airway pressure (CPAP) and the Barach exsufflator (cough machine). Some key questions about the choice of the method used for mechanical ventilation are: How should patients be selected for exposure to newly discovered and rediscovered techniques? What pattern of mechanical ventilation is most comfortable, and why? What are the optimal ways of delivering mechanical ventilation to different types of patients? What psychological factors determine a person's acceptance of any given mode of mechanical ventilation?

Long-term mechanical ventilation poses a new set of questions: What are the clinical, physiological, and psychological criteria for initiating long-term ventilatory support? What is the optimum schedule for which type of patient? What are the most important outcomes? What factors most interfere with long-term ventilatory support, and how can they be ameliorated? Similar questions can be posed with regard to other forms of mechanical support, e.g., CPAP and the cough machine.

C. Weaning from Mechanical Ventilation

Numerous articles have been written about the troublesome issues of weaning from mechanical ventilation, and various strategies have been advocated to accomplish this goal. All agree that a steady state of the respiration, circulation, and metabolism are prerequisite for success. For pulmonary rehabilitation, this continues to be a major concern as well as an opportunity (6).

D. Oxygen Therapy

The most successful therapeutic intervention of pulmonary rehabilitation based on sound physiological principles is the use of supplemental oxygen. Of all the physiologically based interventions in current use, only the administration of oxygen has been shown to prolong life. Most of the data on the therapeutic use of oxygen comes from patients with COPD. Its use in other types of patients, e.g., those with neuromuscular or chest wall disease, is not as well documented (18–20,28).

V. Education

The education of patients and their families is a necessary part of any rehabilitation program (42). Understanding of the illness for which the patient is being treated can help to relieve anxiety and improve the quality of life. However, no studies have systematically tested the effects of providing different types of information, e.g., different materials, modes of delivery, and so forth, to patients with chronic pulmonary disease.

VI. Psychosocial Factors in Pulmonary Rehabilitation

Psychosocial factors that are important in the recovery and rehabilitation process ("psychosocial assets") include emotional and personality characteristics, as well as environmental factors, that enhance a patient's ability to cope with chronic illness. The patient/client with enhanced psychosocial assets adapts better to stressful life events, has more positive responses to psychological interventions such as group therapy, and is more likely to adhere to medical and behavioral regimens than is the less endowed patient. In terms of pulmonary rehabilitation, these patients have less dyspnea, require less medication, adapt more readily to emotionally based physiological changes in ventilation, and survive longer than do patients with few psychosocial assets (16,23,42,43).

The attitudes of those engaged in pulmonary rehabilitation may influence the outcome. The training of physicians rarely provides for exposure to the concepts and practice of pulmonary rehabilitation. Little is known about the beliefs, attitudes, and behaviors of physicians (pulmonary and primary care) and other health professionals with respect to patients with chronic pulmonary disease, particularly COPD. It is also unclear how these attributes of health care providers affect the quality of health care.

A. Psychosocial Interventions

"Psychosocial interventions" are designed to enhance patients' psychosocial assets. They afford the prospect of enhancing the patient's health-related quality of life and psychosocial functioning, increasing adherence to behavioral and medical treatment regimens, and/or enhancing physical recovery and survival. Among the psychosocial interventions are education of patients and family members as to the nature of the disease and the use of preventive and self-management strategies, counseling and therapy, stress management and relaxation techniques, specific cognitive and behavioral modification techniques, and the provision of support to patients and their families (17,44–46).

B. Cognitive and Behavioral Interventions

An important factor in achieving positive outcomes in patients with COPD is the use of coping skills, whether cognitive, e.g., enhancing self-confidence and positive attitudes, or behavioral, e.g., appropriate use of disease management strategies (44). Interventions focused on enhancing coping skills are directed at increasing the patient's ability to meet the cognitive and behavioral demands imposed by the disease, thereby enhancing feelings of mastery and control, with concomitant improvement in physiological and psychological functioning.

Patients with pulmonary disease in the critical care setting, and those with severe disease or dependent on life support technology, e.g., ventilator-dependent patients, have special psychological needs and problems related to the stresses associated with their disease and treatment environment. These patients tend to be severely depressed and show psychological and cognitive deficits that can pose challenges within the rehabilitation setting. For these patients, special psychological interventions are needed. Ventilator-dependent patients can benefit from an in-depth psychosocial evaluation that includes assessment of behavioral problems, cognitive function, and environmental influences. Interventions aimed at increasing mobility of the patient, minimizing sleep disturbances, facilitating communication, and increasing interactions with others in their environment, can be helpful in decreasing psychological disturbances and enhancing psychosocial functioning.

C. The Affective Component of Dyspnea

As indicated above, dyspnea is the most frequent and distressing symptom for patients with pulmonary disease. Although dyspnea often cannot be fully relieved, interventions directed at changing the affective component, i.e., the patient's response to the symptom, may change the patient's perception of the intensity of the symptom without changes in the physiological cause. A decrease in the intensity of dyspnea and the distress associated with the symptom may be one of the most significant goals for patients in pulmonary rehabilitation (47).

Certain emotional states (fear, anxiety, anger) can increase dyspnea. The increase in breathlessness is accompanied by an increase in energy expenditure, ventilation, oxygen consumption, and skeletal muscle tension. In turn, the increase in dyspnea promotes greater anxiety, which contributes to its pathophysiological underpinnings. Clearly, psychosocial interventions at the emotional level would have as their goal the interruption of this destructive cycle.

Patients with COPD seem to be able to differentiate the sensory component of dyspnea, i.e., the intensity of the symptom, from its affective component (the distress and anxiety associated with the symptom). The patients' self-efficacy (defined as the belief in one's capability to perform a specific task) is related to dyspnea. Increasing patients' self-efficacy and confidence through systematic desensitization, or "guided mastery" techniques, holds promise for decreasing both the intensity of dyspnea and the distress associated with it.

Several aspects of the affective component warrant investigation: Should health care providers continue to focus on the affective component of dyspnea (which includes the patient's/client's response to the sensation)? What kinds of interventions decrease the affective component of dyspnea? Does decreasing the affective component improve outcome? And finally, what is the optimal "dose" (intensity and time) of various components of pulmonary rehabilitation, e.g., exercise, education, needed to decrease dyspnea and make significant differences in psychological outcomes?

D. Depression

Although depression is a prevalent complication in patients/clients with chronic pulmonary disease, little is known about the natural history of depression in such patients and its effects on rehabilitation outcomes (48). Among the uncertainties are the following: What factors are predictors of depression in patients/clients with COPD? Does it help to treat their depression, and what are the optimal strategies for treatment, i.e., pharmacological, nonpharmacological, combination of the two? Should depression be treated prior to, or within, the rehabilitation program? Are current measures capable of distinguishing between somatic symptoms and depression, or will new measures be needed?

E. Smoking Cessation

Quitting smoking is critical for the patient with pulmonary disease (4,49,50). This topic is considered elsewhere in this book. However, a recent study, the Lung Health Study (LHS), merits special note. This was a multicenter intervention trial sponsored by the National Heart, Lung, and Blood Institute to determine whether smoking cessation and bronchodilator therapy can influence the course of subjects without clinical illness who are at high risk for the development of COPD (51). A total of 4887 smokers, aged 35–60, who had signs of early impairment of pulmonary function were recruited into this study. This study underscores the importance of early intervention in arresting the downhill course of individuals en route to the development of COPD.

F. Other Aspects of Psychosocial Interventions

Lack of social support and the stresses of life predict the number of hospitalizations better than any other factor, including demographic characteristics, severity of illness, and previous hospitalizations.

Although social support improves outcomes for individuals with pulmonary disease, the optimal way to use social support in pulmonary rehabilitation is unclear (45). Can the patient/client be trained to take better advantage of available supports? What methods are most suited to provide support for spouses and other caregivers? What is the impact of COPD on family functioning? Are interventions involving group support for family members beneficial to both the family and patient?

A relationship exists between marital status and exercise tolerance in COPD: married COPD patients have a better exercise tolerance than do unmarried patients—even when controlled for age and disease severity. The existence of a supportive spouse has been credited with an important role in successful coping by individuals with COPD.

The spouses of patients with pulmonary disease also require social support. They often show levels of depression and loneliness that are similar to those of COPD clients/patients. Indeed, spouses are generally less satisfied with their social networks than are the clients/patients (32).

Because of their interactions, psychosocial interventions need to be integrated with physiological interventions in pulmonary rehabilitation programs. However, it is unclear which psychosocial interventions produce the best outcomes. It would be helpful to learn if there is a minimal psychosocial intervention or set of interventions that can be incorporated into pulmonary rehabilitation programs for all patients, i.e., a "core" set of interventions. Other questions also need answering: Which psychosocial interventions are most effective and most cost-effective, either alone or along with physiological interventions? Are interventions that improve the health-related quality of life for patients/clients or caregivers also cost-effective, e.g., due to decreases in emergency services and hospitalizations?

Adherence to behavioral and medical regimens is necessary for patients/clients to benefit fully from rehabilitation programs (44). What interventions are most effective in increasing the individual's adherence to behavioral or medical regimens? What are the major barriers to the adherence of the patient/client to specific components of rehabilitation, e.g., exercise, medications?

Although motivation is generally held to be an important predictor of outcomes, an understanding of the construct of motivation and its effects is lacking. Who is a "motivated" patient/client? Are patients/clients who are traditionally labeled as "unmotivated" simply motivated toward different values/outcomes? Can standard criteria be developed to determine who is motivated and who is not, or who is differently motivated?

Little also is known about the proper timing of psychosocial interventions. How early in the course of pulmonary rehabilitation should psychosocial interventions be started? For example, when should psychosocial support be provided in the intensive care unit? What is the optimal length of psychosocial intervention and follow-up?

Nutritional repletion rebuilds muscles, improves function of vital organ systems, and restores immune competence. Many questions remain about proper nutritional support as part of pulmonary rehabilitation. For example, what is the optimal prescription for repletion? How to maintain the gains of repletion? What are the optimal routes of administration? What are the relative contributions in repletion of restoring nitrogen versus potassium? What factors prevent patients from complying with nutritional repletion and/or maintenance?

Other supportive measures include treatment with anabolic agents (steroids, growth hormone, or growth factor). Modest improvements in strength and body weight have been reported from these interventions, but the functional and long-term benefits have not been defined. The risks of excessive nutritional repletion and overdosage of anabolic steroids are known, but neither the optimal initial and maintenance prescriptions nor the long-term risks of the usual doses of anabolic substances have as yet been defined.

VII. Concluding Comments

This introductory chapter will have served its purpose if it has succeeded in illustrating the differences between the medical and rehabilitation models, the implications of these differences for pulmonary rehabilitation, their goals in treatment, the comprehensive nature of rehabilitation medicine, the importance of nonphysiological factors in determining the outcomes of pulmonary rehabilitation, and finally, the many unanswered questions in rehabilitation medicine in general and in pulmonary rehabilitation in particular. The chapters that follow enlarge upon these themes, provide details, and indicate in their reference lists the likely sources of additional information.

References

1. American Thoracic Society. Position statement on pulmonary rehabilitation. Am Rev Respir Dis 1981; 124:663–666.
2. Hodgkin JE, Connors GL, Bell CW. Pulmonary Rehabilitation. Guidelines to Success. Philadelphia: JB Lippincott, 1993 (pg 6 is statement of AACP), 619 pp.
3. Ikegami N. Functional assessment and its place in health care. N Engl J Med 1994; 331–332.
4. McSweeny AJ, Labuhn KT. Chronic obstructive pulmonary disease. In: Spilker B, ed. Quality of Life Assessments in Clinical Trials. New York: Raven Press, 1990:391–417.
5. Make BJ, ed. Pulmonary rehabilitation. Clin Chest Med 1986; 7:519–540.
6. Nicol J, Hodgkin JE, Connors G, et al. Strategies for developing a cost-effective pulmonary rehabilitation program. Respir Care 1983; 28:1451–1455.

7. Guyatt GH, Berman LB, Townsend M. Long-term outcome after respiratory rehabilitation. Can Med Assoc J 1987; 137:1089–1095.
8. Kaplan RM, Atkins CJ, Timms R. Validity of a quality of well-being scale as an outcome measure in chronic obstructive pulmonary disease. J Chronic Dis 1984; 37:85–95.
9. Hodgkin JE, Zorn EG, Connors GL, eds. Pulmonary Rehabilitation—Guidelines to Success, 2d ed. Boston: Butterworth, 1993.
10. McSweeny AJ, Grant I, Heaton RK, Adams KM, Timms RM. Life quality of patients with chronic obstructive pulmonary disease. Arch Intern Med 1982; 142:473–478.
11. Petty TL, MacIlroy ER, Swigert MA, Brink GA. Chronic airway obstruction, respiratory insufficiency, and gainful employment. Arch Environ Health 1970; 21:71–78.
12. Prigatano GP, Wright EC, Levin D. Quality of life and its predictors in patients with mild hypoxemia and chronic obstructive pulmonary disease. Arch Intern Med 1984; 144:1613–1619.
13. Ries AL. Pulmonary rehabilitation. In: Fishman AP, ed. Pulmonary Diseases and Disorders, 2d ed. New York: McGraw-Hill, 1988:1325–1331.
14. Ries AL, Farrow JT, Clausen JL. Pulmonary function tests cannot predict exercise-induced hypoxemia in chronic obstructive pulmonary disease. Chest 1988; 93:454–459.
15. Sahn SA, Nett LM, Petty TL. Ten-year follow-up of a comprehensive rehabilitation program for severe COPD. Chest 1980; 77:311–314.
16. Dudley DL, Glaser EM, Jorgenson BN, Logan DL. Psychosocial concomitants to rehabilitation in chronic obstructive pulmonary disease. Part 1. Psychosocial and psychological considerations. Part 2. Psychosocial treatment. Part 3. Dealing with psychiatric disease (as distinguished from psychosocial or psychophysiologic problems). Chest 1980; 77:413–420, 544–551, 677–684.
17. Glaser EM, Dudley DL. Psychosocial rehabilitation and psychopharmacology. In: Hodgkin JE, Petty TL, eds. Chronic Obstructive Pulmonary Disease: Current Concepts. Philadelphia: WB Saunders, 1987:128–153.
18. Anthonisen NR. Long-term oxygen therapy. Ann Intern Med 1983; 99:519–527.
19. Longo AM, Moser KM, Luchsinger PC. The role of oxygen therapy in rehabilitation of patients with chronic obstructive pulmonary disease. Am Rev Respir Dis 1971; 103:690–697.
20. Nocturnal Oxygen Therapy Trial Group. Continuous or nocturnal oxygen therapy in hypoxemic chronic obstructive lung disease: a clinical trial. Ann Intern Med 1980; 93:391–398.
21. Petty TL, Finigan MM. Clinical evaluation of prolonged ambulatory oxygen therapy in chronic airway obstruction. Am J Med 1968; 45:242–252.
22. Tiep BL. Oxygen therapy for the mobile patient. J Cardiopulm Rehabil 1988; 11:412–418.
23. Light RW, Merrill EJ, Despars JA, Gordon GH, Mutalipassi LR. Prevalence of depression and anxiety in patients with COPD: relationship to functional capacity. Chest 1985; 87:35–38.

24. National Institute of Child Health and Human Development. Research Plan for the National Center for Medical Rehabilitation Research. Bethesda, MD: National Institute of Child Health and Human Development, National Institutes of Health, 1993, publication no. 93-3509.
25. Davidson AC, Leach R, George RJD, Geddes DM. Supplemental oxygen and exercise ability in chronic obstructive airways disease. Thorax 1988; 43:965–971.
26. Foster S, Lopez D, Thomas HM. Pulmonary rehabilitation in COPD patients with elevated Pco_2. Am Rev Respir Dis 1988; 138:1519–1523.
27. Tiep BL, Lewis MI. Oxygen conservation and oxygen-conserving devices in chronic lung disease: a review. Chest 1987; 92:263–272.
28. Zack MB, Palange AV. Oxygen supplemental exercise of ventilatory and non-ventilatory muscles in pulmonary rehabilitation. Chest 1985; 88:669–675.
29. Belman MJ. Exercise in chronic obstructive pulmonary disease. Clin Chest Med 1986; 7:585–597.
30. Casaburi R. Exercise training in chronic obstructive lung disease. In: Casaburi R, Petty TL, eds. Principles and Practice of Pulmonary Rehabilitation. Philadelphia: WB Saunders, 1993:204–224.
31. Rochester DF, Goldberg SK. Techniques of respiratory physical therapy. Am Rev Respir Dis 1980; 122(Suppl):133–146.
32. Ries AL. Scientific basis of pulmonary rehabilitation. J Cardiopulm Rehabil 1990; 10:418–439.
33. Pardy RL, Reid WD, Belman MJ. Respiratory muscle training. Clin Chest Med 1988; 9:287–296.
34. Harver A, Mahler DA, Daubenspeck JA. Targeted inspiratory muscle training improves respiratory muscle function and reduces dyspnea in patients with chronic obstructive pulmonary disease. Ann Intern Med 1989; 111:117–124.
35. Hughes RL, Davison R. Limitations of exercise reconditioning in COPD. Chest 1983; 83:241–249.
36. Bach JR, Barnett V. Ethical considerations in the management of individuals with severe neuromuscular disorders. Am J Phys Med Rehabil 1994; 73:134–140.
37. Casaburi R, Wasserman K. Exercise training in pulmonary rehabilitation. N Engl J Med 1986; 314:1509–1511.
38. Celli BR. Importance of the respiratory muscles in rehabilitation. Problems Respir Care 1990; 3:459–482.
39. Similowski T, Yan S, Gauthier AP, Macklem PT, Bellemare F. Contractile properties of the human diaphragm during chronic hyperinflation. N Engl J Med 1991; 325:917–923.
40. Kirilloff LH, Owens GR, Rogers RM, Mazzocco MC. Does chest physical therapy work? Chest 1985; 88:436–444.
41. Foster S, Thomas HM. Pulmonary rehabilitation in lung disease other than chronic obstructive pulmonary disease. Am Rev Respir Dis 1990; 141:601–604.
42. Howland J, Nelson EC, Barlow PB, et al. Chronic obstructive airway disease: impact of health education. Chest 1986; 90:233–238.
43. Sandhu HS. Psychosocial issues in chronic obstructive pulmonary disease. Clin Chest Med 1986; 7:629–642.

44. Dales RE, Spitzer WO, Schechter MT, Suissa S. The influence of psychological status on respiratory symptom reporting. Am Rev Respir Dis 1989; 139:1459–1463.
45. Gilmartin ME. Patient and family education. Clin Chest Med 1986; 7:619–627.
46. Williams SJ. Chronic respiratory illness and disability: a critical review of the psychosocial literature. Soc Sci Med 1989; 28:791–803.
47. Tandon MK. Adjunct treatment with yoga in chronic severe airways obstruction. Thorax 1978; 33:514–517.
48. Light RW, Merrill EJ, Despars JA, Gordon GH, Mutalipassi LR. Prevalence of depression and anxiety in patients with COPD: relationship to functional capacity. Chest 1985; 87:35–38.
49. Crofton J, Bjartveit K. Smoking as a risk factor for chronic airways disease. Chest 1989; 96(Suppl):307s–312s.
50. The Lung Health Study. Design of the trial and recruitment of participants. Controlled Clin Trials 1993; 14:2S.
51. The Health Consequences of Smoking: Chronic Obstructive Lung Disease: A Report of the Surgeon General. Rockville, MD: Department of Health and Human Services, PHS Office on Smoking and Health, 1984.

3

Benefits of Pulmonary Rehabilitation

JOHN E. HODGKIN

St. Helena Hospital
Deer Park, California
and University of California, Davis
Davis, California

Pulmonary rehabilitation programs utilize a variety of treatment modalities, which are tailored to meet the individual's needs. Table 1 lists the components of a pulmonary rehabilitation program. The overall benefits reported for pulmonary rehabilitation programs and the demonstrated benefits for each individual component of care are discussed in this chapter.

I. Overall Benefits of Pulmonary Rehabilitation

While many benefits have been reported by pulmonary rehabilitation teams (1–5), information is still accumulating concerning the specific benefits of the various individual components. A summary of the overall benefits that have been reported is included in Table 2. Most individuals report an improvement in respiratory manifestations such as dyspnea and cough, and many have a reduction in anxiety and depression and an improvement in self-confidence (ego strength) (6–8). Also routinely reported for patients completing a pulmonary rehabilitation program are an improved ability to perform activities of daily living (ADL) (9–20), enhanced exercise capacity (21–45), and a better quality of life (9–20,46,47). Although many of the individuals who enter a pulmonary

Table 1 Components of Pulmonary Rehabilitation

General factors
Patient and family education
Proper nutrition including weight control
Avoidance of smoking and other inhaled irritants
Immunization and avoidance of infection
Proper environment
Adequate hydration
Medications
Bronchodilators
Expectorants
Antimicrobials
Corticosteroids
Cromolyn sodium/nedocromil sodium
Digitalis
Diuretics
Psychopharmacological agents
Respiratory therapy techniques
Aerosol therapy
Oxygen therapy
Home use of ventilators
Physical therapy modalities
Relaxation training
Breathing retraining
Chest percussion and postural drainage
Deliberate coughing and expectoration
Exercise conditioning
Occupational therapy
Evaluate activities of daily living
Outline energy-conserving maneuvers
Psychosocial rehabilitation
Vocational rehabilitation

rehabilitation program are either retired or very close to retirement, some younger individuals have been able to continue or return to gainful employment (9,12,48–51).

Many groups have reported a significant decrease in the number of hospital days required by individuals with chronic obstructive pulmonary disease (COPD) following their participation in a pulmonary rehabilitation program (4,7,14,19,52–58). Patients at Loma Linda University Medical Center (Loma Linda, CA) had a reduction from approximately 19 days of hospitalization in

Table 2 Demonstrated Benefits of Pulmonary Rehabilitation

Reduction in respiratory symptoms
Reversal of anxiety and depression and improved ego strength
Enhanced ability to carry out activities of daily living
Increased exercise ability
Better quality of life
Reduction in hospital days required
Prolongation of life for some patients

the year before the pulmonary rehabilitation program to slightly over 6 days of hospitalization per year in the first year after completion of the program (52). This trend continued for the 8 years for which follow-up data are available (4). It would be natural to think that this reduction in days of hospitalization simply reflects the deaths of the sickest patients during the initial years of follow-up. However, the hospital days required over the 8-year period for only those patients surviving for the entire 8 years was very similar to the hospital days required when all of the patients' data were included (Fig. 1). This reduction in the need for hospitalization provides a substantial economic savings.

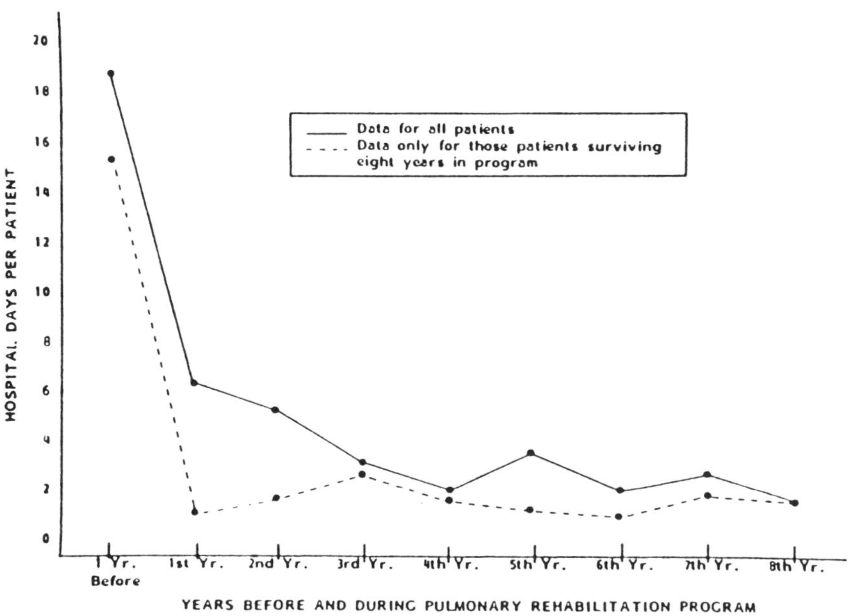

Figure 1 Analysis of hospital days before and during pulmonary rehabilitation program at Loma Linda University Medical Center.

The forced expiratory volume in 1 sec (FEV_1) has been reported to decrease by approximately 20–30 ml/year in individuals with no lung disease (59,60). In patients with COPD, the yearly decrease in FEV_1 has been reported to be 40–80 ml/year (61–68). No pulmonary rehabilitation program has claimed to significantly alter the yearly decrease in spirometric values in COPD patients as a result of rehabilitation per se.

For many years, it has been presumed that although pulmonary rehabilitation, i.e., good comprehensive care, helps patients feel and function better, they do not live longer. It is clear that oxygen therapy significantly improves survival in COPD patients who are seriously hypoxemic (69,70), and there have been an increasing number of reports suggesting that the process of pulmonary rehabilitation itself can lead to improved survival. Haas and Cardon (12) reported on 252 COPD patients undergoing pulmonary rehabilitation compared with 50 control subjects selected from an outpatient clinic. They reported 5-year death rates from respiratory failure of 22% in the rehabilitated patients compared with 42% in the control subjects.

Petty and associates (61) reported on 182 patients with COPD (mean FEV_1 0.94 L) who participated in a pulmonary rehabilitation program between 1966 and 1968. The individuals who participated in this program in Denver had a significantly improved survival at 2.5 years when compared with the only other study of COPD patients residing at a similar high altitude, i.e., the Veterans Administration (VA) cooperative study by Renzetti and co-workers (67). Survival at 2½ years in the Petty study was 67% compared with 50% in the VA cooperative study. Petty has also reported slightly better survival in patients undergoing pulmonary rehabilitation compared with matched control patients who received "ordinary care" in the same community (71).

Hodgkin and associates (72,73) reported significantly better long-term survival than in most previous reports in patients participating in a university hospital–based pulmonary rehabilitation program. These patients had a mean FEV_1 of 1.53 L. Participants had chronic bronchitis and/or emphysema; patients thought to have asthma were excluded from the study. Patients from the study by Hodgkin and associates with an FEV_1 above 1.24 L were compared with patients with a similar level of pulmonary impairment from the Burrows Chicago study (62,74). Patients in the Burrows study (62,74) did not participate in a formal pulmonary rehabilitation program, and their treatment was not standardized; they did, of course, receive appropriate care and hospitalization when needed. These patients from the study of Hodgkin and associates with more mild pulmonary impairment had a significantly better survival rate at 2–5 years of follow-up than patients with similar impairment in the Burrows study, suggesting that the comprehensive care, including careful follow-up, provided by the pulmonary rehabilitation program might be responsible for some of the improved survival compared with that in earlier studies.

Burns and colleagues reported on patients (mean FEV_1 0.97 L) completing a pulmonary rehabilitation program between 1977 and 1987 (75). Subjects in this study had chronic bronchitis and/or emphysema.

The survival curves for COPD patients reported from five large series (61,72–76) are shown in Figure 2. Characteristics of patients from these studies are shown in Table 3. Patients in the Burns study (75) were somewhat older than the patients in the other studies. In the Postma study (76), 90% of the patients showed a greater than 10% increase in the FEV_1 following bronchodilator inhalation, and oral corticosteroid therapy seemed to significantly reduce the rate of deterioration, suggesting that a considerable number of these individuals had a component of reactive airway disease. Patients in the Postma study were also younger than those in the other studies. Patients in the Hodgkin study (72,73) had milder obstructive airway disease at the time they entered the pulmonary rehabilitation program. Individuals in the Petty study (61) resided at higher altitude, i.e., in Denver, Colorado.

Sneider and colleagues (58) reported on the experience of patients participating in their pulmonary rehabilitation program between 1976 and 1987. Al-

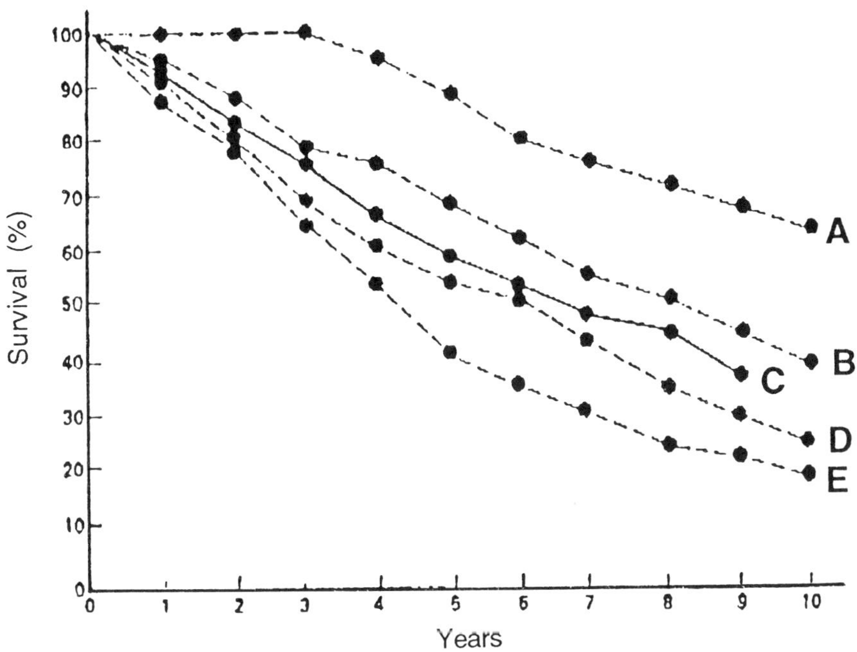

Figure 2 Comparison of survival curves in patients with COPD from (A) Hodgkin and colleagues (72, 73), (B) Postma and Sluiter (76), (C) Burns and colleagues (75), (D) Burrows and colleagues (62, 74), (E) Petty and colleagues (61).

Table 3 Studies Comparing Survival

Investigator	No. patients	Age[a]	$FEV_1(L)$[a]	Survival (%) 5 year	10 year
Burns (75)	240	64.9	0.89	58	38
Burrows (62,74)	200	59.1	1.04	52	23
Hodgkin (72,73)	75	59.9	1.53	86	64
Petty (61)	182	61	0.94	41	17
Postma (76)	129	54	0.61	69	40

[a]Mean.

though 1592 patients were evaluated during this period, only 212 patients (mean FEV_1 1.19 L) completed the entire pulmonary rehabilitation program. Patients with a reactive airway disease component were not specifically excluded from this study. Survival at 5 and 10 years was 86% and 66%, respectively. Sneider and associates compared the 212 patients completing the pulmonary rehabilitation program with the 921 individuals with similar impairment who did not complete the program and with a group of 100 randomly selected patients with similar pulmonary impairment who died of COPD at the hospital over a 10-year period (58). Five- and 10-year survival was significantly better in those completing the full pulmonary rehabilitation program than in the other two groups from the same community, cared for at the same hospital.

The largest study to suggest that good comprehensive care may improve survival in patients with COPD is the National Institutes of Health Intermittent Positive Pressure Breathing Trial (NIH/IPPB) (77,78). A total of 985 patients with COPD (mean FEV_1 1.03 L) participated in this study. Asthmatics were excluded. The age and level of pulmonary impairment were similar to those of subjects in the Burrows Chicago study (74). Patients in the NIH/IPPB study were compared with those from the Burrows Chicago group. Survival was similar in patients with the least obstruction (postbronchodilator FEV_1 above 42.5% of predicted), but as shown in Figure 3, in patients with more severe obstruction survival was greater in the NIH/IPPB patients than in the Burrows Chicago group. One potential explanation for this would seem to be that the Burrows group did not exclude severely hypoxemic patients as was done in the NIH/IPPB study. The first 3 years of the Burrows study preceded the widespread use of home oxygen therapy, which was given to patients in the NIH/IPPB study who became significantly hypoxemic during the study. This would be a reasonable explanation for survival differences among patients with the most severe obstruction (FEV_1 below 30.5% of predicted); 22% of the NIH/IPPB patients in this category eventually received home oxygen therapy. However,

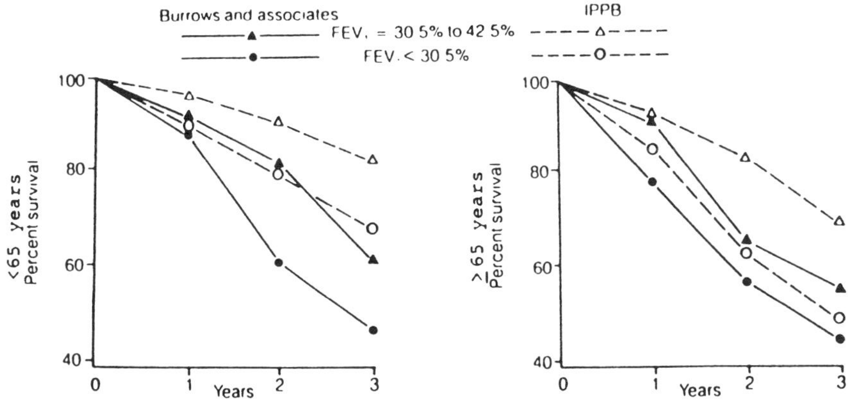

Figure 3 Comparison of survival in the NIH/IPPB trial (open symbols) with that of patients in the Burrows Chicago study (closed symbols). (Left) Patients <65 years of age at the start of the studies; (right) patients ≥65 years of age. (Circles) Patients with baseline postbronchodilator FEV_1 < 30.5% predicted; (triangles) patients with baseline postbronchodilator FEV_1 30.5–42.5% predicted. (From Ref. 78, with permission. Courtesy of the American Lung Association.)

only 12% of the less obstructed patients (FEV_1 of 30.5–42.5% of predicted) in the NIH/IPPB study received home oxygen, so this is not likely to account for mortality differences between these two groups. It seems reasonable that survival was better in the NIH/IPPB patients because of the careful assessment, education, treatment, and follow-up they received in this clinical trial.

In COPD patients, the postbronchodilator FEV_1 and age have been reported to be the best predictors of survival (71,78,79). COPD patients with comparable FEV_1s have similar survival between hypoxemic and nonhypoxemic patients when the hypoxemia is corrected by long-term oxygen therapy (78,79). It seems reasonable that if one is going to slow the rate of deterioration in respiratory function and achieve significant prolongation of life, the principles of pulmonary rehabilitation must be applied to individuals earlier in the course of their disease, rather than waiting until severe, irreversible impairment of function is present.

II. Benefits of Individual Components of Care

A. Education

Teaching patients about their disease process and its treatment is an integral part of pulmonary rehabilitation (3,80,81). Hopp and colleagues (82) have developed and validated a pulmonary rehabilitation knowledge test. Education of COPD patients has been reported to improve their knowledge of their disease process and its treatment (81,83).

B. Nutrition

A careful assessment of patients' diet patterns and nutritional needs is an important part of pulmonary rehabilitation. A weight reduction program in obese individuals can lessen the work of breathing, resulting in reduced dyspnea. In those patients with ongoing weight loss, a high-protein diet with multiple small feedings can help prevent or reverse the problem. Poorly nourished individuals have been shown to have reduced respiratory muscle strength (84). Good nutrition can aid in resisting respiratory infections (85) and has been reported to help restore the ventilatory response to hypoxemia (86) and hypercapnia (87) in severely malnourished patients.

Body weight has been shown to help predict survival, independent of the FEV_1 (88). COPD patients who are underweight have a worse survival than their colleagues with an equal level of impairment but with normal weight. (See Fig. 4.) Whether adequate nutrition support in undernourished patients with COPD can improve survival or not is yet to be determined. Further studies to help answer the question are justified (89,90).

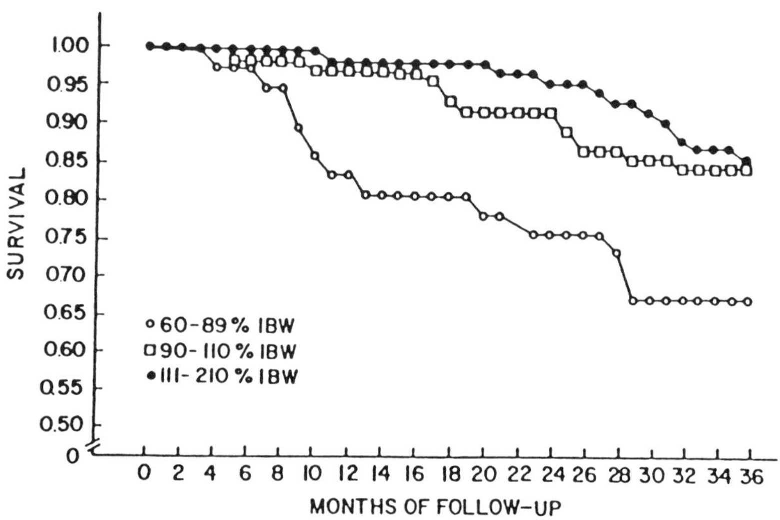

Figure 4 Survival of patients with FEV_1 > 47% predicted by % ideal body weight (IBW) category. (From Ref. 88, EC, et al. Body weight in chronic obstructive pulmonary disease, with permission. Courtesy of the American Lung Association.)

C. Smoking Cessation

Cessation of smoking is one of the most important interventions for patients with COPD. Improved appetite, reduced dyspnea, reduction in cough and sputum, and improved pulmonary function are all demonstrated benefits of smoking cessation (91,92). Individuals who smoke are more prone to influenza infection (93). Postma and Sluiter (76) clearly showed that smoking cessation can improve survival in patients with significant COPD. (See Fig. 5.)

D. Medications

The appropriate use of medications is crucial for patients with COPD. All of these agents have significant side effects and if not used properly can lead to a

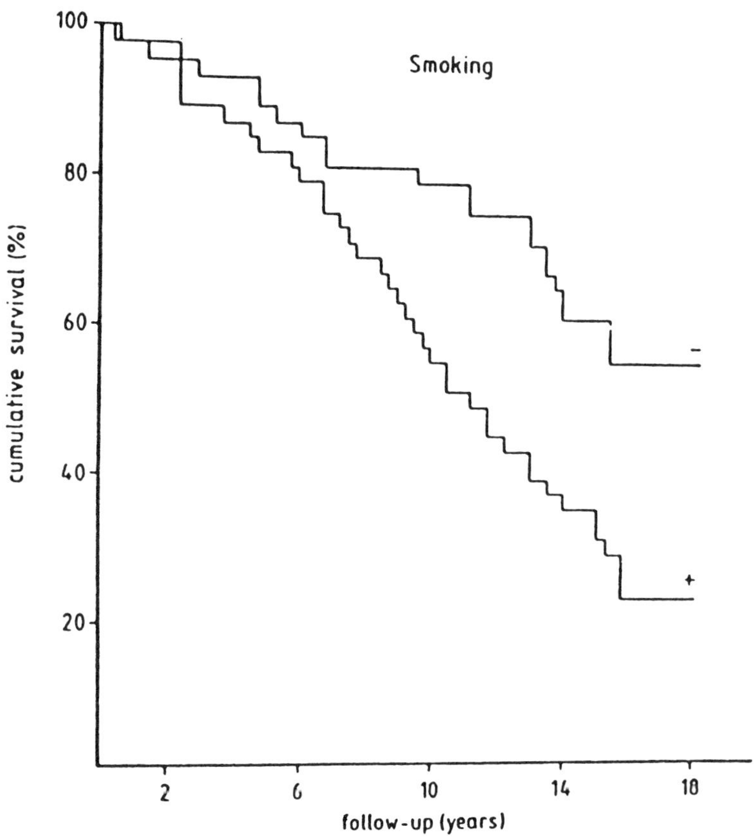

Figure 5 Cumulative survival curves of continuing smokers (+) and ex-smokers (−). (From Ref. 76, with permission. Courtesy of the American Lung Association.)

worsening of the patient's status. The proper use of pharmacological agents in patients with respiratory disease is reviewed in this book, as well as in other publications (94).

E. Aerosol Therapy

A variety of devices have been used to aerosolize bronchodilators, corticosteroids, mucolytic agents, bland mist, and antimicrobials. While there is little support for the aerosolization of the latter three agents in asthma or COPD patients, clearly inhalation of bronchodilators and corticosteroids is of benefit. Inhalation of β-sympathomimetic agents results in much faster bronchodilation than the use of oral agents, with fewer systemic side effects. Inhalation of steroids accomplishes much of the corticosteroid benefit, while avoiding systemic side effects. Recently, the aerosolization of dornase alfa (Pulmozyme) has been shown to be of major benefit in patients with cystic fibrosis (95).

F. Oxygen Therapy

Supplemental oxygen has been shown to lessen the adverse effects of significant hypoxemia, such as pulmonary hypertension, polycythemia, and neuropsychological dysfunction in COPD patients. In addition, patients with COPD and severe hypoxemia live significantly longer with continuous oxygen as compared to nocturnal oxygen only or room air (69,70). Patients who develop significant hypoxemia during exercise testing can improve their exercise performance by using supplemental oxygen during exercise training (21,95–99). Patients with hypoxemia associated with sleep apnea and those with arrhythmias resulting from nocturnal hypoxemia benefit from nocturnal oxygen (100–102). The use of supplemental oxygen in COPD patients with severe hypoxemia results in a survival rate similar to that of patients with similar levels of airway obstruction but without severe hypoxemia (78). (See Fig. 6.)

G. Intermittent Positive-Pressure Breathing (IPPB)

There is no evidence that in COPD patients the outpatient use of IPPB therapy has any advantage over less expensive and simpler methods of aerosol therapy, such as cartridge inhalers or compressor nebulizers. The NIH-sponsored study comparing IPPB therapy with compressor nebulizers in outpatients with COPD showed no difference in morbidity or mortality between subjects in the two groups (77). This evaluation in 985 patients did not demonstrate any role for periodic IPPB treatments in outpatients with COPD. The continuous use of positive-pressure breathing, i.e., mechanical ventilation in patients with chronic respiratory failure, has been reported to be of benefit as part of the rehabilita-

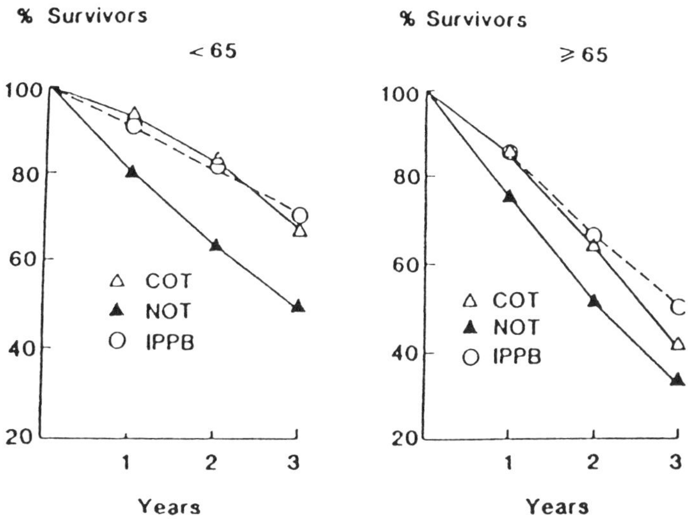

Figure 6 Comparison of survival in the NIH/IPPB and NOTT trials. All patients had baseline $FEV_1 < 30\%$ predicted. (Left) Data from patients <65 years of age at the beginning of the studies; (right) patients ≥65 years of age. (Circles) Patients in the IPPB trial; (open triangles) hypoxemic patients receiving continuous oxygen therapy; (closed triangles) hypoxemic patients receiving 12 hr of nocturnal oxygen therapy. (From Ref. 78, with permission. Courtesy of the American Lung Association.)

tion process for those individuals requiring outpatient ventilator assistance (102).

H. Relaxation Training

Relaxation techniques such as biofeedback and listening to soothing music can help individuals reduce fear and tension and are particularly recommended for individuals with high fear and high anxiety (103). Relaxation exercises, such as contracting and then relaxing skeletal muscle groups, has been reported to reduce dyspnea and anxiety in patients with COPD (104). Other demonstrated benefits of relaxation include a slowing of the respiratory rate and heart rate and a lowering of oxygen consumption (105,106).

I. Breathing Retraining

Training COPD patients to slow their respiratory rate with a prolonged exhalation (with or without the use of pursed lips) helps control dyspnea and results in improved ventilation, increased tidal volume, decreased respiratory rate, and a reduced alveolar-arterial oxygen difference (107–112). This type of breathing pattern helps relieve dyspnea and enhances the patient's ability to exercise and perform activities of daily living more comfortably.

Improved respiratory muscle strength and endurance have been demonstrated through voluntary normocapnic hyperpnea (113–117) and inspiratory resistive loading (118). Although ventilatory muscle training has been reported to improve exercise capacity in some COPD patients (116–119), the role of such training remains to be defined. It is yet to be shown that respiratory muscle training adds to the improved activity level and quality of life that has been demonstrated through exercise training of the upper and lower extremities.

J. Deliberate Cough, Chest Percussion, and Postural Drainage

Program team members routinely teach patients how to cough properly so they can achieve more effective expectoration. The forced expiratory technique for coughing has been recommended for expectorating sputum more successfully (120,121). Postural drainage, accompanied by chest percussion or vibration, has also been recommended for many years to help clear secretions from patients with obstructed airways. The role of chest physical therapy is reviewed in this book, as well as in other publications (122). Postural drainage in outpatients should be reserved for those individuals with large amounts of sputum, i.e., greater than 30 ml/day (123). There is no evidence that postural drainage is useful in COPD patients with smaller amounts of sputum during acute exacerbations of COPD (124) or in those with uncomplicated pneumonia (125).

K. Exercise Conditioning

Exercise training is an integral component of all pulmonary rehabilitation programs. There have been many reports of improved exercise capacity following general conditioning exercises such as walking, bicycle riding, and swimming (21–45,126). Exercise conditioning allows patients to do more work for any given oxygen consumption. For many years, COPD patients have been encouraged to exercise; however, it is only recently that such patients have been shown to have the capacity to exercise at a considerably higher percentage of their maximal exercise capacity than has been used in the past (127–129). Exercise training accomplished above the anaerobic threshold in those COPD patients who are able to achieve this level of intensity has been reported to achieve more benefit than training at a lower intensity level (130–132). Adding upper-extremity exercise training to lower-extremity training has been shown to provide additional benefit for COPD patients (133–135).

L. Activities of Daily Living

Each individual participating in a pulmonary rehabilitation program should have a careful assessment to determine his/her ability to perform routine activities of daily living. Patients can then be taught how to perform such activities while conserving energy.

M. Psychosocial Rehabilitation

COPD patients commonly exhibit such reactions as depression, fear, anxiety, hostility, and denial, all of which impair functional capacity (6). Neuropsychological benefits of pulmonary rehabilitation include significant reduction in depression and anxiety and improvement in general well-being (6–8,136). Psychotherapy, sometimes requiring a psychologist or psychiatrist, and the appropriate use of psychopharmacological agents can help such patients better cope with their disease process. Improved sexual function can also be achieved with proper counseling and advice (137).

N. Vocational Rehabilitation

Many individuals coming to pulmonary rehabilitation programs have already quit their jobs or retired; however, some patients can be helped to continue working in their current occupations or to change to an occupation that requires less energy and oxygen. Possible goals to be considered include (138):

- Returning the patient to the job he or she is holding
- Returning the patient to the same occupational field or plant, but in a different job or location
- Changing the occupational field to a totally different one in which the patient can use previous training or existing skills
- Job retraining and reemployment
- Entering the patient in a sheltered workshop program
- Retraining the individual in daily self-care with an eye to conservation of effort and efficiency of motion

III. Summary

A careful assessment to help determine a patient's needs and limitations is essential to outlining an appropriate treatment program. It is through this comprehensive assessment that proper goals can be established. The potential benefits reviewed in this chapter clearly make the process of pulmonary rehabilitation worthwhile and, in fact, essential for patients with chronic respiratory impairment.

References

1. Hodgkin JE, ed. Chronic obstructive pulmonary disease: current concepts in diagnosis and comprehensive care. Park Ridge, IL: American College of Chest Physicians, 1979.
2. Make BJ. Pulmonary rehabilitation: myth or reality? Clin Chest Med 1986; 7(4):519.
3. Hodgkin JE, Farrell MJ, Gibson SR, et al. Pulmonary rehabilitation: official ATS statement. Am Rev Respir Dis 1981; 124:663.
4. Hodgkin JE. Pulmonary rehabilitation: structure, components, and benefits. In: Hodgkin JE, ed. Pulmonary rehabilitation symposium. J Cardiopulm Rehabil 1988; 8:423.
5. Ries AL. Position paper of the American Association of Cardiovascular and Pulmonary Rehabilitation. Scientific basis of pulmonary rehabilitation. J Cardiopulm Rehabil 1990; 10:418.
6. Dudley DL, Glaser EM, Jorgenson BN, Logan DL. Psychosocial concomitants to rehabilitation in chronic obstructive pulmonary disease. Chest 1980; 77:413, 544, 677.
7. Agle DP, Baum GL, Chester EH, Wendt M. Multidiscipline treatment of chronic pulmonary insufficiency. 1. Psychologic aspects of rehabilitation. Psychosom Med 1973; 35:41.
8. Fishman DB, Petty TL. Physical, symptomatic, and psychological improvement in patients receiving comprehensive care for chronic airway obstruction. J Chronic Dis 1971; 14:775.
9. Kass I, Dyksterhuis JE. The Nebraska COPD Rehabilitation Project: A Program to Identify the Factors Involved in the Rehabilitation of Patients with Chronic Obstructive Pulmonary Disease: A Multidisciplinary Study of 140 Patients. Final Report, Social and Rehabilitation Service, DHEW Project RD-2517-m. Omaha: University of Nebraska, December 1971.
10. Daughton DM, Fix AJ, Kass I, Patil KD, Bell CW. Physiological-intellectual components of rehabilitation success in patients with chronic obstructive pulmonary disease (COPD). J Chronic Dis 1979; 32:405.
11. Miller WF, Taylor HF, Pierce AK. Rehabilitation of the disabled patient with chronic bronchitis and pulmonary emphysema. Am J Public Health 1963; 53(Suppl):18.
12. Haas A, Cardon H. Rehabilitation in chronic obstructive pulmonary disease: a five-year study of 252 male patients. Med Clin North Am 1969; 53:593.
13. Cherniack RM, Handford RG, Svanhill E. Home care of chronic respiratory disease. JAMA 1969; 208:821.
14. Petty TL, Nett LM, Finigan MM, Brink GA, Corsello PR. A comprehensive care program for chronic airway obstruction: methods and preliminary evaluation of symptomatic and functional improvement. Ann Intern Med 1969; 70:1109.
15. Kimbel P, Kaplan AS, Alkalay I, Lester D. An in-hospital program for rehabilitation of patients with chronic obstructive pulmonary disease. Chest 1971; 60(Suppl):6S.

16. Shapiro BA, Vostinak-Foley E, Hamilton BB, Buehler JH. Rehabilitation in chronic obstructive pulmonary disease: a two-year prospective study. Respir Care 1977; 22:1045.
17. White B, Andrews JL Jr, Mogan JJ, Downes-Vogel P. Pulmonary rehabilitation in an ambulatory group practice setting. Med Clin North Am 1979; 63:379.
18. Krumholz RA. Pulmonary outpatient rehabilitation: a four-year follow-up. Ohio State Med J 1973; 69:680.
19. Moser RM. Rehabilitation of the COPD Patient. Lesson 40 in Weekly Update: Pulmonary Medicine. Princeton, NJ: Biomedia, 1979.
20. Balchum OJ. Rehabilitation in chronic obstructive pulmonary disease. Arch Environ Health 1968; 16:614.
21. Pierce AK, Paez PN, Miller WF. Exercise therapy with the aid of a portable oxygen supply in patients with emphysema. Am Rev Respir Dis 1965; 91:653.
22. Miller WF. Rehabilitation of patients with chronic obstructive lung disease. Med Clin North Am 1967; 51:349.
23. Woolf CR, Suero JT. Alterations in lung mechanics and gas exchange following training in chronic obstructive lung disease. Dis Chest 1969; 55:37.
24. Bass H, Whitcomb JF, Forman R. Exercise training: therapy for patients with chronic obstructive pulmonary disease. Chest 1970; 57:116.
25. Woolf CR. A rehabilitation program for improving exercise tolerance of patients with chronic lung disease. Can Med Assoc J 1972; 106:1289.
26. Rusk HA. Pulmonary problems. In: Rehabilitation Medicine, 3rd ed. St. Louis: CV Mosby, 1971.
27. Schrijen F, Jezek V. Haemodynamic variables during repeated exercise in chronic lung disease. Clin Sci Mol Med 1978; 55:485.
28. Nicholas JJ, Gilbert R, Gabe R, Auchincloss JH Jr. Evaluation of an exercise therapy program for patients with chronic obstructive pulmonary disease. Am Rev Respir Dis 1970; 102:1.
29. Unger KM, Moser KM, Hansen P. Selection of an exercise program for patients with chronic obstructive pulmonary disease. Heart Lung 1980; 9:68.
30. Brundin A. Physical training in severe chronic obstructive pulmonary disease. Scand J Respir Dis 1974; 55:25.
31. Wasserman K, Whipp BJ. Exercise physiology in health and disease. Am Rev Respir Dis 1973; 112:219.
32. Degre S, Sergysels R, Messin R, et al. Hemodynamic responses to physical training in patients with chronic lung disease. Am Rev Respir Dis 1974; 110: 395.
33. Alpert JS, Bass H, Szucs MM, Banas JS, Dalen JE, Dexter L. Effects of physical training on hemodynamics and pulmonary function at rest and during exercise in patients with chronic obstructive pulmonary disease. Chest 1974; 66:647.
34. Shephard RJ. Exercise and chronic obstructive lung disease. Exerc Sport Sci Rev 1976; 4:263.
35. Hughes RL, Davison R. Limitations of exercise reconditioning in COLD. Chest 1983; 83:241.
36. Mall RW, Medeiros M. Objective evaluation of results of a pulmonary rehabilitation program in a community hospital. Chest 1988; 94:1156.

37. Cockcroft AE, Saunders MT, Berry G. Randomized controlled trial of rehabilitation in chronic respiratory disability. Thorax 1981; 36:200.
38. McGavin CR, Gupta SP, Lloyd EL, McHardy JR. Physical rehabilitation of chronic bronchitis: results of a controlled trial of exercises in the home. Thorax 1977; 32:307.
39. Sinclair DJM, Ingram CG. Controlled trial of supervised exercise training in chronic bronchitis. Br Med J 1980; 280:519.
40. Busch AJ, McClements JD. Effects of a supervised home exercise program on patients with severe chronic obstructive pulmonary disease. Phys Ther 1988; 68:469.
41. Strijbos JH, Koeter GH, Meinesz AF. Home care rehabilitation and perception of dyspnea in chronic obstructive pulmonary disease (COPD) patients. Chest 1990; 97:109S.
42. Chester EF, Belman MJ, Bahler RC, et al. Multidisciplinary treatment of chronic pulmonary insufficiency. 3. The effect of physical training on cardiopulmonary performance in patients with chronic obstructive pulmonary disease. Chest 1977; 72:695.
43. Carter R, Nicotra B, Clark L, et al. Exercise conditioning in the rehabilitation of patients with chronic obstructive pulmonary disease. Arch Phys Med Rehabil 1988; 69:118.
44. Holle RHO, Williams DV, Vandree JC, Starks GL, Schoene RB. Increased muscle efficiency and sustained benefits in an outpatient hospital-based pulmonary rehabilitation program. Chest 1988; 94:1161.
45. Tydeman DE, Chandler AR, Graveling BM, Culot A, Harrison BDW. An investigation into the effects of exercise tolerance training on patients with chronic airways obstruction. Physiotherapy 1984; 70:261.
46. Atkins CJ, Kaplan RM, Timms RM, Reinsch S, Lofback K. Behavioral exercise programs in the management of chronic obstructive pulmonary disease. J Consult Clin Psychol 1984; 52:591.
47. Guyatt GH, German LB, Townsend M. Longterm outcome after respiratory rehabilitation. Can Med Assoc J 1987; 137:1089.
48. Petty TL, MacIlroy ER, Swigert MA, Brink GA. Chronic airway obstruction, respiratory insufficiency, and gainful employment. Arch Environ Health 1970; 21:71.
49. Lustig FM, Haas A, Castillo R. Clinical and rehabilitation regime in patients with chronic obstructive pulmonary disease. Arch Phys Med Rehabil 1971; 53:315.
50. Kass I, Dyksterhuis JE, Rubin H, Patil KD. Correlation of psychophysiological variables with vocational rehabilitation outcome in patients with chronic obstructive pulmonary disease. Chest 1975; 67:433.
51. Fix AJ, Daughton D, Kass I, et al. Personality traits affecting vocational rehabilitation success in patients with chronic obstructive pulmonary disease. Psychol Rep 1978; 43:939.
52. Burton GG, Gee G, Hodgkin JE, Dunham JL. Respiratory care warrants studies for cost-effectiveness. Hospitals 1975; 49:61.
53. Hudson LD, Tyler ML, Petty TL. Hospitalization needs during an outpatient rehabilitation program for severe chronic airway obstruction. Chest 1976; 70:606.

54. Lertzman MM, Cherniack RM. Rehabilitation of patients with chronic obstructive pulmonary disease. Am Rev Respir Dis 1976; 114:1145.
55. Jensen PS. Risk, protective factors, and supportive interventions in chronic airway obstruction. Arch Gen Psychiatry 1983; 40:1203.
56. Johnson HR, Tanzi F, Balcham OJ, et al. Inpatient comprehensive pulmonary rehabilitation in severe COPD. Respir Ther 1980; May/June:15.
57. Nichol J, Hodgkin JE, Connors G, et al. Strategies for developing a cost-effective pulmonary rehabilitation program. Respir Care 1983; 28:1451.
58. Sneider R, O'Malley JA, Kahn M. Trends in pulmonary rehabilitation at Eisenhower Medical Center: an 11-years' experience (1976–1987). In: Hodgkin JE, ed. Pulmonary rehabilitation symposium. J Cardiopulm Rehabil 1988; 11:453.
59. Ferris BG Jr, Anderson DO, Zickmantel R. Prediction values for screening tests of pulmonary function. Am Rev Respir Dis 1965; 91:252.
60. Kory RC, Callahan R, Boren HG, Syner JC. Veterans Administration–Army cooperative study of pulmonary function. I. Clinical spirometry in normal men. Am J Med 1961; 30:243.
61. Sahn SA, Nett LM, Petty TL. Ten-year follow-up of a comprehensive rehabilitation program for severe COPD. Chest 1980; 77(Suppl):311.
62. Burrows B, Earle RH. Course and prognosis of chronic obstructive pulmonary disease. N Engl J Med 1969; 280:397.
63. Boushy SF, Thompson HK, North LB, Beale AR, Snow TR. Prognosis in chronic obstructive pulmonary disease. Am Rev Respir Dis 1973; 108:1373.
64. Diener CF, Burrows B. Further observations on the course and prognosis of chronic obstructive lung disease. Am Rev Respir Dis 1975; 111:719.
65. Emergil C, Sobol BJ. Longterm course of chronic obstructive pulmonary disease: a new view of the mode of functional deterioration. Am J Med 1971; 51:504.
66. Postma DS, Burema J, Gimeno F, et al. Prognosis in severe chronic obstructive pulmonary disease. Am Rev Respir Dis 1979; 119:357.
67. Renzetti AD Jr, McClement JH, Litt BD. The Veterans Administration cooperative study of pulmonary function. III. Mortality in relation to respiratory function in chronic obstructive pulmonary disease. Am J Med 1966; 41:115.
68. Davis AL, McClement JH. The course and prognosis of chronic obstructive pulmonary disease. In: Current Research in Chronic Respiratory Disease. Proceedings of the 11th Aspen Emphysema Conference. Arlington, VA: DHEW, 1968:219.
69. Medical Research Council Working Party. Longterm domiciliary oxygen therapy in chronic hypoxic cor pulmonale complicating chronic bronchitis and emphysema. Lancet 1981; 1:681.
70. Nocturnal Oxygen Therapy Trial Group. Continuous or nocturnal oxygen therapy in hypoxemic chronic obstructive pulmonary disease: a clinical trial. Ann Intern Med 1980; 93:391.
71. Petty TL. Pulmonary rehabilitation. Am Rev Respir Dis 1979; 122(Suppl):159.
72. Bebout DE, Hodgkin JE, Zorn EG, Yee AR, Sammer EA. Clinical and physiological outcomes of a university-hospital pulmonary rehabilitation program. Respir Care 1983; 28:1468.
73. Hodgkin JE, Branscomb BV, Anholm JD, Gray LS. Benefits, limitations and the future of pulmonary rehabilitation. In: Hodgkin JE, Zorn EG, Connors GL,

eds. Pulmonary Rehabilitation: Guidelines to Success. Boston: Butterworths, 1984.
74. Traver GA, Cline MG, Burrows B. Predictors of mortality in chronic obstructive pulmonary disease. Am Rev Respir Dis 1979; 119:895.
75. Burns MR, Sherman B, Madison R, et al. Pulmonary rehabilitation outcome. Respir Ther 1989;2:25.
76. Postma DS, Sluiter HJ. Prognosis of chronic obstructive pulmonary disease: the Dutch experience. Am Rev Respir Dis 1989:140(Suppl):S100.
77. Intermittent Positive Pressure Breathing Trial Group. Intermittent positive pressure breathing therapy of chronic obstructive pulmonary disease. Ann Intern Med 1983; 99:612.
78. Anthonisen NR, Wright EC, Hodgkin JE, et al. Prognosis in chronic obstructive pulmonary disease. Am Rev Respir Dis 1986; 133:14.
79. Hodgkin JE. Prognosis in chronic obstructive pulmonary disease. In: Hodgkin JE, ed. Chronic obstructive pulmonary disease. Clin Chest Med 1990; 11(3):555.
80. Gilmartin ME. Patient and family education. Clin Chest Med 1986; 7:619.
81. Neish CM, Hopp JW. The role of education in pulmonary rehabilitation. In: Hodgkin JE, ed. Pulmonary rehabilitation symposium. J Cardiopulm Rehabil 1988; 11:439.
82. Hopp JW, Lee JW, Hills R. Development and validation of a pulmonary rehabilitation knowledge test. J Cardiopulm Rehabil 1989; 7:273.
83. Ashikaga T, Vacek PM, Lewis SO. Evaluation of a community-based education program for individuals with chronic obstructive pulmonary disease. J Rehabil Res Dev 1980; 46:23.
84. Arora NS, Rochester DF. Respiratory muscle strength and maximal voluntary ventilation in undernourished patients. Am Rev Respir Dis 1981; 126:5.
85. Wilson DO, Rogers RM, Hoffman RM. Nutrition and chronic lung disease: state of the art. Am Rev Respir Dis 1985; 132:1347.
86. Doekel RC Jr, Zwillich CW, Scoggin CH, Kryger M, Weil JV. Clinical semistarvation: depression of hypoxic ventilatory response. N Engl J Med 1976; 295:358.
87. Askanazi J. Weissman C, La Sala PA, Milic-Emili J, Kinney JM. Effect of protein intake on ventilatory drive. Anesthesiology 1984; 60:106.
88. Wilson DO, Rogers RM, Wright EC, Anthonisen NR. Body weight in chronic obstructive pulmonary disease. The National Institutes of Health Intermittent Positive Pressure Breathing Trial. Am Rev Respir Dis 1989; 139:1435.
89. Wilson DO, Rogers RM, Pennock BE, Keilly J. Nutritional intervention in malnourished emphysema patients. Am Rev Respir Dis 1985; 131(part 2):61.
90. Efthimiou J, Fleming J, Gomes C, Spiro SG. The effect of supplementary oral nutrition in poorly nourished patients with chronic obstructive pulmonary disease. Am Rev Respir Dis 1988; 137:1075.
91. Buist AS, Nagy JM, Sexton GJ. Effect of smoking cessation on pulmonary function: a 30-month follow-up to two smoking cessation clinics. Am Rev Respir Dis 1979; 120:953.
92. Camilli AE, Burrows B, Knudson RJ, et al. Longitudinal changes in forced expiratory volume in one second in adults. Am Rev Respir Dis 1987; 135:794.

93. Kark JD, Legiush M, Rannon L. Cigarette smoking as a risk factor for epidemic A (HI,NI) in influenza in young men. N Engl J Med 1982; 307:1042.
94. Glaser EM, Dudley DL. Psychosocial rehabilitation and psychopharmacology. In: Hodgkin JE, Petty TL, eds. Chronic Obstructive Pulmonary Disease: Current Concepts. Philadelphia: WB Saunders, 1987.
95. Ramsey BW, Astley SJ, Aitken ML, et al. Efficacy and safety of short term administration of aerosolized recombinant human deoxy-ribonuclease in patients with cystic fibrosis. Am Rev Respir Dis 1993; 148:145.
96. Cotes JE, Gilson JC. Effect of oxygen on exercise ability in chronic respiratory insufficiency. Lancet 1956; 1:872.
97. Barach AL. Ambulatory oxygen therapy: oxygen inhalation at home and out-of-doors. Dis Chest 1959; 35:229.
98. Leggett RJE, Flenley DC. Portable oxygen and exercise tolerance in patients with chronic hypoxic cor pulmonale. Br Med J 1977; 2:84.
99. Stein DA, Bradley BL, Miller WC. Mechanisms of oxygen effects on exercise in patients with chronic obstructive pulmonary disease. Chest 1982; 81:6.
100. Kearley R, Wynne JW, Block AJ, et al. The effect of low flow oxygen on sleep disordered breathing and oxygen saturation. Chest 1980; 78:682.
101. Tirlapur VG, Mir MA. Nocturnal hypoxemia and associated electrocardiographic changes in patients with chronic obstructive airways disease. N Engl J Med 1982; 306:125.
102. Tiep BL. Longterm home oxygen therapy. In: Hodgkin JE, ed. Chronic obstructive pulmonary disease. Clin Chest Med 1990; 11:505.
103. Sexton DL. Relaxation techniques and biofeedback. In: Hodgkin JE, Petty TL, eds. Chronic Obstructive Pulmonary Disease: Current Concepts. Philadelphia: WB Saunders, 1987:99.
104. Renfroe KL. Effect of progressive relaxation on dyspnea and anxiety in patients with chronic obstructive pulmonary disease. Heart Lung 1988; 17: 408.
105. Benson H. The Relaxation Response. New York: Morrow, 1975.
106. Benson H, Kotch JB, Crassweller KD. The relaxation response: a bridge between psychiatry and medicine. Med Clin North Am 1977; 61:929.
107. Mueller RE, Petty TL, Filley GF. Ventilation and arterial blood gas changes induced by pursed lip breathing. J Appl Physiol 1970; 28:784.
108. Motley HL. The effects of slow deep breathing on the blood gas exchange in emphysema. Am Rev Respir Dis 1963; 88:484.
109. Paul G, Eldridge F, Mitchell J, Fiene T. Some effects of slowing respiration rate in chronic emphysema and bronchitis. J Appl Physiol 1966; 21:877.
110. Sergysels R, Willeput R, Lenders D, et al. Low frequency breathing at rest and during exercise in severe chronic obstructive bronchitis. Thorax 1979; 34:536.
111. Thoman RL, Stoker GL, Ross JC. The efficacy of pursed-lip breathing in patients with chronic obstructive pulmonary disease. Am Rev Respir Dis 1966; 93:100.
112. Tiep BL, Burns M, Kao D, Madison R, Herrera J. Pursed lips breathing training using ear oximetry. Chest 1986; 90:218.

113. Leith DE, Bradley ME. Ventilatory muscle strength and endurance training. J Appl Physiol 1976; 41:508.
114. Peress L, McClean P, Woolf C, Zamel N. Respiratory muscle training in severe chronic obstructive pulmonary disease. Am Rev Respir Dis 1979; 119(4,part 2):157.
115. Celli BR. Respiratory muscle function. Clin Chest Med 1986; 7:567.
116. Pardy RL, Reid WD, Belman MJ. Respiratory muscle training. Clin Chest Med 1988; 9(2):287.
117. Belman MJ, Mittman D, Weir R. Ventilatory muscle training improves exercise capacity in chronic obstructive pulmonary disease patients. Am Rev Respir Dis 1980; 121:273.
118. Pardy RL, Rivington RN, Despas PJ, Macklem PT. The effects of inspiratory muscle training on exercise performance in chronic airflow limitation. Am Rev Respir Dis 1981; 123:426.
119. Larson JL, Kim MJ, Sharp JT, Larson DA. Inspiratory muscle training with a pressure threshold breathing device in patients with chronic obstructive pulmonary disease. Am Rev Respir Dis 1988; 138:689.
120. Pryor JA, Webber BA, Hodson ME, Batten JC. Evaluation of the forced expiration technique as an adjunct to postural drainage in treatment of cystic fibrosis. Br Med J 1979; 2:417.
121. Sutton PP, Parker RA, Webber BA, et al. Assessment of the forced expiration technique, postural drainage and directed coughing in chest physiotherapy. Eur J Respir Dis 1983; 64:62.
122. Faling LJ. Chest physical therapy. In: Burton GG, Hodgkin JE, Ward JJ, eds. Respiratory Care: A Guide to Clinical Practice, 3rd ed. Philadelphia: JB Lippincott, 1991:625.
123. Murray JF. The ketch-up bottle method. N Engl J Med 1979; 300:1155.
124. Anthonisen P, Riis P, Sogaard-Andersen T. The value of lung physiotherapy in the treatment of acute exacerbations in chronic bronchitis. Acta Med Scand 1964; 175:715.
125. Graham WGB, Bradley GA. Efficacy of chest physiotherapy and intermittent positive-pressure breathing in the resolution of pneumonia. N Engl J Med 1978; 299:624.
126. Barach AL, Gickerman HA, Beck GJ. Advances in treatment of nontuberculous pulmonary disease. Bull NY Acad Med 1952; 28:353.
127. Hodgkin JE, Litzau KL. Exercise training target heart rates in chronic obstructive pulmonary disease. Chest 1988; 94:30S.
128. Punzal PA, Ries AL, Kaplan RM, Prewitt LM. Maximum intensity exercise training in patients with chronic obstructive pulmonary disease. Chest 1991; 100:618.
129. Carter R, Nicotra B, Clark L, et al. Exercise conditioning in the rehabilitation of patients with chronic obstructive pulmonary disease. Arch Phys Med Rehabil 1988; 69:118.
130. Casaburi R, Wasserman K, Patessio A, et al. A new perspective in pulmonary rehabilitation: anaerobic threshold as a discriminant in training. Eur Respir J 1989; 2(Suppl 7):618S.

131. Casaburi R, Patessio A, Ioli F, et al. Reductions in lactic acidosis and ventilation as a result of exercise training in patients with obstructive lung disease. Am Rev Respir Dis 1991; 143:9.
132. Casaburi R. Principles of exercise training. Chest 1992; 101:263S.
133. Couser Jr JI, Martinez FJ, Celli BR. Pulmonary rehabilitation that includes arm exercise reduces metabolic and ventilatory requirements for simple arm elevation. Chest 1993; 103:37.
134. Ries AL, Ellis B, Hawkins RW. Upper extremity exercise in chronic obstructive pulmonary disease. Chest 1988; 93:688.
135. Ellis B, Ries AL. Upper extremity exercise training in pulmonary rehabilitation. Cardiopulm Rehabil 1991; 11:227.
136. Emery CF, Leatherman NE, Burker EJ, MacIntyre NR. Psychological outcomes of a pulmonary rehabilitation program. Chest 1991; 100:613.
137. Selecky PA. Sexuality and the COPD patient. In: Hodgkin JE, Petty TL, eds. Chronic Obstructive Pulmonary Disease: Current Concepts. Philadelphia: WB Saunders, 1987.
138. Matzen RV. Vocational rehabilitation: the culmination of physical reconditioning. Chest 1971; 60(Suppl):21S.

4

The Team Concept in Pulmonary Rehabilitation

ANDREW L. RIES

University of California, San Diego
San Diego, California

HEIDI C. SQUIER

University of California, San Diego
and San Diego State University
San Diego, California

Pulmonary rehabilitation is directed at decreasing the disability caused by lung disease and restoring the individual to the highest possible level of independent function. For the individual patient, the objectives of pulmonary rehabilitation focus not only on the physical aspects of health, but also on psychological and social functioning. In patients disabled by chronic lung disease, pulmonary rehabilitation looks beyond the traditional medical model of treatment and cure by a physician and brings together a number of other skilled allied health professionals who contribute their expertise and work toward common goals.

The primary purpose of the team is to utilize the talents of a variety of health care professionals collectively to increase the effectiveness of overall treatment efforts for optimal patient care (1,2). The overall goal of the rehabilitation team is to aid the patient in the attainment of increased quality of life, functional ability, and independence.

Team responsibilities for successful rehabilitation include the ability and competence to fulfill the following tasks: adequately evaluate patients for relevant treatment; set goals that are realistic, albeit challenging, for the patient and significant others; arrange and administer appropriate treatments; assess progress; document plans for assessment and treatment; individualize a maintenance program; and provide liaison services for the patient's referring physician and other relevant health care providers.

Rehabilitation is a well-established therapeutic option not only for chronic lung disease, but also for a wide variety of other diseases, including cardiovascular disease, stroke, spinal cord injury, arthritis, and chronic pain (3–16). Such conditions lend themselves to the approach of rehabilitation medicine because of the complex interactions of physical, psychological, social, and environmental factors in the pathogenesis of the patient's disability. With this broader understanding of the whole individual and of the contributing factors that are multifactorial and interrelated, it is difficult for any one specialty alone to provide the required comprehensive care (2). Such conditions are best treated with input from multiple specialties acting collaboratively with the shared goal of satisfying the needs of the individual patient (1,2,10,16–19).

Successful pulmonary rehabilitation programs have been established in a variety of settings using different team structures and various combinations of health professionals. No one correct model or structure has been proven to be the most effective. One type of successful pulmonary rehabilitation program may center around one key health professional who, with the support of a medical director, serves as the program coordinator, bringing together other professionals on site who have complementary skills. This key individual may come from a variety of health professions such as nursing, respiratory therapy, physical therapy, or exercise science.

The purpose of this chapter is to review the basic concepts of team organization and structure that pertain to a comprehensive pulmonary rehabilitation program. Regardless of the size or makeup of a particular team, some common principles of team function serve to define such program. The focus of this discussion is on the interdisciplinary team, which is a common organizational approach used in medical rehabilitation. Using a variety of outcome measures, this model of care has proven to be effective for pulmonary as well as other types of patients (1–3,10–19). However, other approaches may work as well. In developing a rehabilitation team, the behavioral features of the health professionals to be engaged in pulmonary rehabilitation are of critical importance: working with individuals disabled by pulmonary disease—who often have complex medical, psychological, and social problems—poses a special challenge that requires special attributes.

I. Pulmonary Rehabilitation

The rehabilitation of patients with lung disease entails extensive knowledge of both pulmonary and rehabilitation medicine (20). Until recently in pulmonary medicine, the typical combination of a close physician-patient relationship and of long-term care has often precluded the inclusion of other specialists in the delivery of health care (20). However, the complexity of medical problems for such patients, the changing forces in medical practice, and the increasing emphasis on health outcomes other than physiological parameters, such as functional status, psychosocial variables, and quality of life, have led to an increasing interest in pulmonary rehabilitation as a standard of care for symptomatic patients with chronic lung diseases (20–24).

The comprehensive therapy entailed in pulmonary rehabilitation has been shown to produce substantial benefits for patients with chronic lung diseases (3): increase in physical activity, exercise tolerance, and endurance, as well as decrease in breathlessness and psychosocial dysfunction (e.g., fear, depression)—important elements of quality of life for these patients. By gaining knowledge and understanding of their disease, the patients are better able to cope with their own problems (3,25–28). Moreover, the national economic burden imposed by the growing number of such patients is lessened.

The current practice of comprehensive pulmonary rehabilitation consists of several basic components: patient evaluation, including physical and psychosocial evaluation and diagnostic testing, and the programmatic components, which include instruction in chest physiotherapy, supervised exercise training, and psychosocial support (4–8). Increasingly, rehabilitation teams are being used to deliver these services (17–19).

II. Types of Rehabilitation Teams

Several models for team structure in rehabilitation have been used; they can be classified as multidisciplinary, interdisciplinary, and transdisciplinary (1,2). The terms are often used interchangeably, and pulmonary rehabilitation teams may well incorporate elements of more than one model. Nevertheless, it is useful to understand the conceptual differences of these three approaches.

A. Multidisciplinary Team

The most common form used today is a multidisciplinary team. It includes a group of professionals from varying specialties who work in parallel with the same patients, often in the same health care setting (1,2). Using this approach, each member of the team conducts his/her own assessment and treatment but communicates results, recommendations, and plans to the other team members at regular conferences.

For each patient, this model generally includes both a team leader, who coordinates and directs the team, and a "case manager." Thus, decisions are typically made primarily by one or two team members with significant input from the other disciplines.

One advantage of a multidisciplinary team in rehabilitation is input from several different specialties, which can be integrated at team meetings into a plan for the care and management of the particular patient (1,2). A disadvantage of this approach is that team members work independently with each patient. The end result of the multidisciplinary team is that the treatment plan and outcome can become the aggregate of individual contributions from different specialties, rather than the product of an integrated team effort, thereby fragmenting the care of the patient and diminishing the cost-effectiveness of the rehabilitation team (1).

B. Interdisciplinary Team

The second model for team organization in rehabilitation medicine is the interdisciplinary team. The terms "multidisciplinary" and "interdisciplinary" are sometimes used interchangeably; some regard interdisciplinary teams as a subgroup of multidisciplinary teams. The main differences relate to the extent of team collaboration and coordination in planning and carrying out treatment goals. The interdisciplinary team emphasizes a total team approach to decision making and goal setting at a patient's case conference (1,2). In this model, although professionals in each specialty conduct separate assessments of the patient, they all converge to set goals, plan treatment, and evaluate the patient's progress (1). In addition, the patient and his/her family or significant others are often included in this process. Although this type of structure may be more time-consuming, it can actually be more cost-effective due to greater efficiency in the utilization of staff, greater patient and staff satisfaction, fewer errors in conceptualizing the therapeutic program, and overall decrease in personnel and other health care costs (1).

The use of the interdisciplinary team in medical rehabilitation is mandated by legislation for programs that seek federal reimbursement for services (1). Also, both the Joint Commission on Accreditation of Health Care Organizations (29) and the Commission on Accreditation of Rehabilitation Facilities (30) require the use of the interdisciplinary team approach to patient care. Therefore, this model of treatment has been widely adopted at a variety of sites, including rehabilitation units, agencies, and skilled nursing facilities (31).

C. Transdisciplinary Team

The transdisciplinary model is the most integrated and novel, but least frequently used, form of team organization in rehabilitation (1). In this model, team members work across boundaries of their professional disciplines: each team member shares responsibility for all areas of patient care, based on practical issues and individual expertise rather than on specialty training or formal disciplines (1). This model enables the involved health care professionals, along with the patient and significant others, to fulfill their responsibilities interchangeably in assessment, treatment, and evaluation. Each team member comes to view his/her profession as a "pulmonary rehabilitation specialist" rather than as a nurse, therapist, or other specialist based on formal training, degree, license, or official certification.

III. Structure of a Medical Rehabilitation Team

One useful way to characterize the components of an interdisciplinary team is to distinguish between core members, extended members, and consultants (2).

Core team members work together and interact daily in the same program unit. In smaller programs, the core may include only a medical director and program coordinator, but often other health professionals are involved (2,18).

Extended members are those who participate regularly in team activities and conferences, but are not necessarily involved on a daily basis. They typically have other clinical duties and responsibilities and may interact with several teams simultaneously. Typically included are professionals brought in to complement the expertise of core team members. Traditional pulmonary rehabilitation professionals include nurses, respiratory and physical therapists, and exercise specialists. Psychologists, dietitians, pharmacists, social workers, occupational therapists, vocational rehabilitation counselors, and others may also be included (2).

Consultants are primarily involved at the invitation of the core and extended team members. Such individuals may provide input at team conferences, either in person, by written report, or by discussions with other team members.

IV. Members of the Interdisciplinary Pulmonary Rehabilitation Team

Because of the complexity of many lung diseases and their treatment (17), pulmonary rehabilitation teams often operate on the interdisciplinary team model. In both inpatient and outpatient settings, an autonomous, well-functioning team can have a considerable impact on the health outcome of the patient (32). Roles for the members of the team often overlap, a desirable and important element in the interdisciplinary setting. Some of the responsibilities and common functions of core, extended, and consultant members of a pulmonary rehabilitation team are described below.

A. Medical Director

The medical director is usually a pulmonary specialist who also has an interest in pulmonary rehabilitation. He/she prescribes the rehabilitation program and oversees its implementation. He also serves as a consultant concerning issues in medical management and provides insight into the physiological derangements of the patient (1,17). In these roles, the medical director does not serve as the patient's primary care physician (17). Instead, he/she interacts, when appropriate, with the patient's primary care provider.

B. Program Coordinator

A key component of a pulmonary rehabilitation team is a designated program coordinator who is responsible for organizing and facilitating the group/team process. As a rule, this individual is also responsible for administration of the rehabilitation program as well as for patient recruitment and marketing. He/she may come from any of the related health professions that make up the pulmonary rehabilitation team and it is helpful for this individual to be a full-time employee of the program.

The coordinator is responsible for scheduling and coordinating team conferences and, particularly in smaller programs, may serve as the case manager who oversees development and implementation of individual patient goals and treatment plans.

C. Other Team Members

In addition to the program coordinator, any number of other health care professionals may participate in an interdisciplinary pulmonary rehabilitation team. As a rule, other members serve to complement the coordinator's professional qualifications. Accordingly, one or more of the following may be included in the team: pulmonary nurse, respiratory therapist, physical therapist, exercise specialist, clinical psychologist, psychiatrist, dietitian, pharmacist, occupational and vocational therapist, and/or social worker.

D. Pulmonary Nurse

A nurse with specialty training in pulmonary care often functions as a core or extended member of the pulmonary rehabilitation team. This individual brings to the team special knowledge in clinical evaluation, physical examination and diagnosis, use of medications, comorbid conditions, and self-assessment skills.

He/she generally shares with other team members responsibilities for managing the patient's rehabilitation treatment plan, including exercise training.

E. Respiratory Therapist

A respiratory therapist experienced in dealing with patients with chronic lung diseases may also function as a core or extended member of the pulmonary rehabilitation team. This individual brings to the team expert knowledge in the clinical evaluation and treatment of the pulmonary patient, use of respiratory therapy modalities such as techniques of breathing retraining (e.g., pursed-lip and diaphragmatic breathing), methods for control of secretions (e.g., postural drainage, coughing, chest percussion, and vibration), and equipment (e.g., oxygen, metered-dose inhalers, nebulizers, etc.). The respiratory therapist is also involved in implementing the rehabilitation treatment plan and in supervising the exercise training program including the use of supplemental oxygen.

F. Physical Therapist

A physical therapist with specialized interest and training in cardiopulmonary care is often included in a pulmonary rehabilitation team and may function as a core, extended, or consultant team member. This individual brings to the team expert knowledge in the application of exercise or physical activity programs, as well as stretching routines. He/she is also responsible for the care of patients who are limited in their ability to exercise due to conditions such as musculoskeletal abnormalities.

G. Exercise Specialist

A professional with training and experience in exercise physiology or exercise science is frequently included as part of an interdisciplinary pulmonary rehabilitation team. This individual may function as a core or extended team member. He/she brings expert knowledge in the principles of exercise testing, training, and prescription and the application of physical activity programs of normals as well as for various disease populations. This person will share with other team members in supervising the exercise training program and may participate actively in other team functions.

H. Clinical Psychologist or Psychiatrist

A mental health professional in a comprehensive pulmonary rehabilitation program usually functions in an extended member or consultant role, involved in patient contact, but not in day-to-day clinical activities. He/she may conduct patient support group meetings, which are included in some programs. These sessions are helpful in encouraging patients to discuss the often difficult associated emotional symptoms that accompany their medical illnesses. He/she may also be responsible for evaluating individual patients to identify psychological and emotional problems in need of professional follow-up.

I. Dietitian

A dietitian may serve as a consultant to provide nutrition instruction, paying special attention to the unique needs of pulmonary patients and providing information on foods that may exacerbate or relieve the patients' symptoms of dyspnea and/or fatigue. He/she may also be used to evaluate and counsel individual patients regarding diet and nutrition. This is particularly important for pulmonary patients who are markedly over or under ideal body weight.

J. Pharmacist

A pharmacist may serve as a consultant to provide instruction regarding medications commonly used by pulmonary patients. This information is typically taught in group sessions that describe indications, side effects, interactions, and techniques of administration for medications.

K. Occupational and Vocational Therapist

These specialized therapists are used as consultants in some programs for group teaching and individual counseling regarding energy-saving techniques, hobby and job retraining, and travel. They may be particularly helpful in evaluating and counseling patients who are becoming more disabled for their usual work responsibilities and having difficulty adjusting to reduced levels of function.

L. Social Worker

Some teams provide the services of a clinical social worker for patient and family issues that require a more comprehensive and systems-based approach to intervention. This professional can be particularly helpful in assisting patients in coping with the social handicaps imposed by their illness and in making referrals to community agencies or organizations that provide access to support groups and/or other services.

It should be emphasized again that there is no one formula for success in developing and building a pulmonary rehabilitation team. The exact makeup of each team will depend on the individuals and disciplines available in a given setting. A key common denominator is an interested and committed medical director and program coordinator.

V. The Future of the Pulmonary Rehabilitation Team

The use of the team approach in pulmonary rehabilitation follows in the footsteps of other successful medical rehabilitation programs that have been shown to provide important benefits for patients (1,2,4–12,15–17). As anyone who has worked with pulmonary patients can attest, these patients present challenges that exceed the ability and expertise of any one type of health professional. Chronic lung diseases encompass a variety of conditions with different pathophysiological derangements. The preponderance of experience in pulmonary rehabilitation has been with patients with chronic obstructive pulmonary diseases. These patients are often in the older age ranges with other concomitant diseases that challenge and stretch even the best-trained health professional. However, many patients with other conditions such as the various restrictive lung diseases and pulmonary vascular disorders, in addition to lung transplant candidates and recipients, can benefit from such preventive health programs.

References

1. Lyth JR. Models of the team approach. In: Fletcher GF, Banja JD, Jann BB, Wolf SL, eds. Rehabilitation Medicine: Contemporary Clinical Perspectives. Philadelphia: Lea & Febinger, 1992:225–242.
2. Cole KD, Ramsdell JW. Issues in interdisciplinary team care. In: Kemp B, Brummel-Smith K, Ramsdell JW, eds. Geriatric Rehabilitation. Boston: Little, Brown, 1990:371–385.
3. Ries AL. Position paper of the American Association of Cardiovascular and Pulmonary Rehabilitation: scientific basis of pulmonary rehabilitation. J Cardiopulm Rehabil 1990; 10:418–441.
4. Connors G, Hilling L, eds. Guidelines for Pulmonary Rehabilitation Programs. Champaign, IL: Human Kinetics, 1993.
5. Hodgkin JE, Connors GL, Bell CW, eds. Pulmonary Rehabilitation Guidelines to Success, 2d ed. Philadelphia: JB Lippincott, 1993.
6. Casaburi R, Petty TL, eds. Principles and Practice of Pulmonary Rehabilitation. Philadelphia: WB Saunders, 1993.
7. Ries AL. Pulmonary rehabilitation. In: Tierney DF, ed. Current Pulmonology. Vol 15. St. Louis: CV Mosby, 1994:441–467.
8. Ries AL. Pulmonary Rehabilitation. In: Fishman AP, ed. Pulmonary Diseases and Disorders, 2d ed. New York: McGraw-Hill, 1988:1325–1331.
9. American Association of Cardiovascular and Pulmonary Rehabilitation. Guidelines for Cardiac Rehabilitation Programs, 2d ed. Champaign, IL: Human Kinetics, 1995.
10. Pashkow FJ, Dafoe WA, eds. Clinical Cardiac Rehabilitation: A Cardiologist's Guide. Baltimore: Williams & Wilkins, 1990.

11. Pollock ML, Schmidt DH, eds. Heart Disease and Rehabilitation, 2d ed. New York: Wiley, 1986.
12. Wilson PK, Fardy PS, Froelicher VF. Cardiac Rehabilitation, Adult Fitness and Exercise Testing. Philadelphia: Lea & Febiger, 1981.
13. Greenland P, Chu JS. Efficacy of cardiac rehabilitation services. Ann Intern Med 1988; 109:650–663.
14. Oldridge N. Guyatt G, Jones J, et al. Effects on quality of life with comprehensive rehabilitation after acute myocardial infarction. Am J Cardiol 1991; 67:1084–1089.
15. Kemp B, Brummel-Smith K, Ramsdell JW, eds. Geriatric Rehabilitation. Boston: Little, Brown, 1990.
16. Fordyce WE. Behavioral Methods for Chronic Pain and Illness. St. Louis: CV Mosby, 1976:103–119.
17. Tiep BL. Pulmonary rehabilitation program organization. In: Casaburi R, Petty TL, eds. Principles and Practice of Pulmonary Rehabilitation. Philadelphia: WB Saunders, 1993:302–316.
18. Connors G, Hilling L. Program management. In: Connors G, Hilling L, eds. Guidelines for Pulmonary Rehabilitation Programs. Champaign, IL: Human Kinetics, 1993:63–71.
19. Beytas LJR, Connors GL. Organization and management of a pulmonary rehabilitation program. In: Hodgkin JE, Connors GL, Bell CW, eds. Pulmonary Rehabilitation Guidelines to Success, 2d ed. Philadelphia: Lippincott, 1993:32–49.
20. Fishman AP. Pulmonary rehabilitation research. Am J Respir Crit Care Med 1994; 149:825–833.
21. Kaplan RM, Bush JW. Health-related quality of life measurement for evaluation of research and policy analysis. Health Psychol 1982; 1:61–80.
22. Kaplan RM, Anderson JP. The general health policy model: update and applications. Health Serv Res 1989; 23:203–235.
23. Toshima MT, Kaplan RM, Ries AL. Experimental evaluation of rehabilitation in chronic obstructive pulmonary disease: short-term effects on exercise endurance and health status. Health Psychol 1990; 9:237–252.
24. Kaplan RM, Ries AL, Atkins CJ. Behavioral management of chronic obstructive pulmonary disease. Ann Behav Med 1985; 7:5–10.
25. Ries AL, Kaplan RM, Limberg TM, Prewitt LM. Clinical trial of pulmonary rehabilitation vs education in COPD. Am J Respir Crit Care Med 1994; 149:A595.
26. Toshima MT, Blumberg E, Ries AL, Kaplan RM. Does rehabilitation reduce depression in patients with chronic obstructive pulmonary disease? J Cardiopulm Rehabil 1992; 12:261–269.
27. Kaplan RM, Eakin EA, Ries AL. Psychosocial issues in the rehabilitation of patients with chronic obstructive pulmonary disease. In: Casaburi R, Petty TL, eds. Principles and Practice in Pulmonary Rehabilitation. Philadelphia: WB Saunders, 1993:351–365.
28. Ojanen M. Lahdensuo A, Laitinen J, Karvonen J. Psychosocial changes in patients participating in a chronic obstructive pulmonary disease rehabilitation program. Respiration 1993; 60:96–102.

29. Accreditation Manual for Hospitals, Joint Commission on Accreditation of Healthcare Organizations. Oakbrook Terrace, IL: JCAH, 1991:194–195.
30. Commission on Accreditation of Rehabilitation Facilities, Standards Manual for Organizations Serving People with Disabilities. Tucson, AZ: Commission on Accreditation of Rehabilitation Facilities, 1991:45–60.
31. Melvin JL. Status report on interdisciplinary medical rehabilitation. Arch Phys Med Rehabil 1989; 70:273–276.
32. Knaus WA, Draper EA, Wagner DP, Zimmerman JE. An evaluation of outcome from intensive care in major medical centers. Ann Intern Med 1986; 104:410–418.

5

Physiological Basis for Pulmonary Rehabilitation

DUDLEY F. ROCHESTER

University of Virginia School of Medicine
Charlottesville, Virginia

I. Goals of Pulmonary Rehabilitation

The overall objective of pulmonary rehabilitation is to facilitate transition from a lower to a higher functional class. This includes reducing or abolishing dependence on mechanical ventilation, as well as improving capacities for physical exercise and activities of daily living. Ventilatory limitation and dyspnea limit exercise, lead to ventilatory failure, and worsen quality of life. Thus, specific aims for pulmonary rehabilitation are to enhance ventilatory endurance, increase tidal volume, minimize dyspnea, and improve quality of life.

II. Historical Background

Pulmonary rehabilitation has been practiced for over four decades (1). Almost all of the rehabilitation efforts have been directed toward patients with chronic obstructive pulmonary disease (COPD), with less attention given to patients with cystic fibrosis and asthma. In neuromuscular and chest wall diseases, most efforts have focused on developing techniques for prolonged, intermittent mechanical ventilation. Other forms of pulmonary rehabilitation have been used sparsely in obesity, chest wall, and neuromuscular diseases. Oxygen therapy and physical exercise training have been identified as valuable components of rehabilitation programs from the beginning. Breathing exercises, with emphasis on pursed-lips breathing, relaxation, and "diaphragmatic breathing," were also found to be helpful. In addition, some early work addressed improvement of the position of the diaphragm, using the head-down posture or therapeutic pneumoperitoneum.

Since 1976, other rehabilitation modes have emerged, notably training specific to the respiratory muscles and respiratory muscle rest. The usual training techniques involve voluntary isocapnic hyperpnea and an inspiratory flow-resistive or threshold load. A few programs utilize mechanical aids such as continuous positive airway pressure (CPAP), as well as various types of relaxation techniques. Prolonged, intermittent respiratory muscle rest can be provided by negative-pressure body devices, positive pressure via endotracheal tube or face mask, as well as by the abdominal pneumobelt and the rocking bed.

Pulmonary rehabilitation has two components, ventilatory rehabilitation and general rehabilitation. The purposes of this chapter are to review the physiological basis for interventions in these two areas, to consider their outcomes, and to suggest future directions for physiological interventions in pulmonary rehabilitation. The focus is on the impacts of interventions on the respiratory muscles and the significance of these effects to the patient.

III. Respiratory System Responses to Disease

A. The Normal Respiratory Pump

The components of the respiratory system are the lungs and airways, the chest wall, the respiratory (ventilatory) muscles that comprise the air pump, and their neural control apparatus. Among the inspiratory muscles, the diaphragm has the greatest capacity to shorten. For example, over the vital capacity (VC), it descends 10 cm and displaces 60% of the inspired VC volume (2–4). The parasternal, lateral intercostal, and scalene muscles shorten much less (5), but owing to their effect on rib angles and thoracic diameters (6), they account for 40% of the VC. The most important expiratory muscles are the transversus abdominis and the internal and external obliques (7).

The strength of the respiratory muscles can be assessed by measuring maximal inspiratory and expiratory pressures at the mouth (PImax, PEmax), during maximal voluntary efforts against a closed airway (8). Typically, PImax is approximately -100 cmH_2O, and PE max is $+150$ cmH_2O. Physically fit subjects have stronger respiratory muscles, and respiratory muscle strength in women is approximately 75% of that in men. Special techniques may be used to measure the strength of the diaphragm; these involve placing balloon catheters in the esophagus and stomach to sample pleural and abdominal pressures, respectively. The difference between positive abdominal and negative pleural pressure is the transdiaphragmatic pressure (Pdi). To circumvent the problem of voluntary effort, diaphragmatic strength may be assessed from Pdi responses to phrenic nerve stimulation (9–11).

The normal respiratory system performs with great ease and minimal energy expenditure to provide the minute ventilation ($\dot{V}E$) needed to support a wide range of tasks. There is a high degree of coordination among its component parts. Interactions among the respiratory muscles (Table 1) are so well synchronized that there is little distortion of the chest wall at all but the most strenuous efforts (12). The diaphragm contributes to inspiration either by moving downward or by elevating and flaring the lower rib cage (13). Which effect predominates depends on whether it is easier to move the lower rib cage or the abdomen (14). The diaphragm accounts for approximately 70% of the tidal volume at the normal breathing position, but at higher lung volumes the diaphragm contributes less and other inspiratory muscles contribute more (3).

Normal patterns of respiratory muscle recruitment enable the respiratory system to continue its smooth operation despite constraints posed by changes in posture, lung volume, and ventilatory load. In thc supinc position the diaphragm and parasternal, intercostal, and the scalene muscles are the only active muscles (Table 1) (14). Shifting from supine to upright posture is associated

Table 1 Respiratory Muscle Interactions and Recruitment

Inspiratory muscles
Diaphragmatic contraction lowers dome and lifts and flares lower rib cage; dome action predominates in supine posture.
Diaphragm, parasternal, and scalene muscles are active at rest, in supine position.
Diaphragm shortens, and parasternal and scalene muscles are further activated on assuming erect posture.
Inspiratory muscles are activated more with increasing $\dot{V}E$.
Recruitment of other rib cage and neck inspiratory muscles at high lung volume or with inspiratory resistance.
Expiratory muscles
Quiet at supine rest, activated on standing.
Expiratory recruitment at high level of $\dot{V}E$, high lung volume or with resistive loads; diaphragm length normalizcd.
Early inspiratory relaxation of abdominal muscles initiates inspiration before diaphragm contracts.

with greater activation of the scalenes and recruitment of parasternal intercostal muscles, as well as recruitment of abdominal muscles (15). The intercostal and neck inspiratory muscles and abdominal muscles are recruited even more when $\dot{V}E$ is increased, when breathing at high lung volume, or when inspiring through resistive or elastic loads (16,17).

Examples of the extraordinary flexibility of respiratory recruitment patterns are afforded by experiments in which normal subjects inspired through flow-resistive loads to the point where they developed inspiratory muscle fatigue. With the load in place, subjects developed an oscillating pattern of breathing that shifted the load between the diaphragm and the other inspiratory muscles (18). After the load was removed and subjects were challenged by rebreathing carbon dioxide, they were again able to shift the work of breathing away from the diaphragm and onto the upper rib cage and neck inspiratory muscles and to the abdominal muscles (19). Indeed, end-expiratory contraction of abdominal muscles followed by their abrupt relaxation at the onset of inspiration accounted for nearly half the tidal volume (19). This pattern of respiratory muscle contraction is virtually the same as seen in patients with severe COPD.

The significance of the way that respiratory muscles are coordinated and recruited lies in two areas. First, breathing proceeds with minimal actual and perceived effort, despite constraints posed by movements of the torso and limbs during a variety of activities ranging from walking and running to swimming and rowing, and at heavy labor such as digging and chopping. Second, the patterns of breathing seen in disease are "hard-wired" into the system, to help the respiratory center cope with an increased ventilatory load, and to minimize the load on any one respiratory muscle group. Thus, the obvious use of neck inspiratory and abdominal muscles and asynchronous movements of the chest and abdomen seen in asthma attack or severe COPD (20) are not intrinsically abnormal. Rather, they reflect a normal response to the increases in airway resistance and lung volume.

B. The Respiratory Pump in Disease

The hallmarks of diseases such as asthma and COPD are reductions in forced expiratory volume in 1 sec (FEV_1), forced vital capacity (FVC), and FEV_1/FVC, coupled with increases in residual volume (RV), functional residual capacity (FRC), and total lung capacity (TLC). Yet the degree of airflow limitation during inspiration appears to be more important than expiratory airflow limitation in the development of CO_2 retention (21). That is, the correlations between partial pressure of carbon dioxide in arterial blood (Pa_{CO_2}) and either peak inspiratory airflow or inspired vital capacity are much higher than between Pa_{CO_2} and the FEV_1. The total respiratory system impedance, as estimated from the ratio of mouth occlusion pressure to mean inspiratory flow rate, is twice as high in COPD as in normals (22).

COPD increases the work and energy cost of breathing. The oxygen cost per liter of $\dot{V}E$ is approximately five times normal (23,24). Respiratory muscle oxygen consumption ($RMvo_2$) during quiet breathing is normally less than 3% of the total oxygen consumption ($\dot{V}o_2$), whereas it is nearly 20% of the total in COPD (23, 24). The ventilatory load is very high owing to increases in airway resistance and lung volume. Recruitment of the rib cage and abdominal muscles contributes to the increase in energy expenditure (20,25). The severe impairment of gas exchange makes it necessary for patients with COPD to breathe nearly twice as much as the normal individual to maintain $Paco_2$ normal (26).

In COPD, the ability of the respiratory muscles to handle the increased load is compromised. Normal subjects breathe at approximately 50% of their TLC, but patients with severe asthma, cystic fibrosis, and COPD breathe at 70–100% of their predicted TLC. Almost all of the hyperinflation is at the expense of the diaphragm (6), which is displaced downward, passively shortened, and at a significant mechanical disadvantage. Inspiratory muscle strength is inversely related to lung volume (27,28) but is directly proportional to diaphragm length (27). Mechanical disadvantage impairs neuromuscular coupling, as judged from the ratio of mouth occlusion pressure to the rate of rise of inspiratory muscle electrical activity; the ratio was one-third of normal in eucapnic COPD patients and only one-tenth of normal in hypercapnic patients (22). In addition, patients with COPD often have significant generalized muscle weakness consequent to malnutrition or other conditions, which is shared by the respiratory muscles (27,28).

The work and energy cost of breathing are also high in kyphoscoliosis and morbid obesity; again the oxygen cost per liter of $\dot{V}E$ is approximately five times normal (23,29,30). The increased work is related to the degree of spinal distortion in kyphoscoliosis and to the mass loading in obesity (29,31). Respiratory muscle weakness occurs in kyphoscoliosis, but is related to age more than to the degree of spinal deformity (32). Respiratory muscle strength is near normal in uncomplicated obesity (33), but there is moderate inspiratory weakness in the obesity-hypoventilation syndrome (34). When patients with the obesity-hypoventilation syndrome are supine, the diaphragm may be at a mechanical disadvantage from being overstretched (35).

Neuromuscular diseases commonly involve the respiratory muscles, and respiratory muscle weakness is often severe enough to cause ventilatory failure. For example, patients with proximal myopathies and normal lungs retain CO_2 when respiratory muscle strength is less than 30% of normal, whereas patients with myopathy and concomitant lung disease and patients with COPD retain CO_2 when inspiratory muscle strength falls below 50% of normal (27,36). The $Paco_2$ is also negatively correlated with expiratory muscle strength (37). Severe generalized and respiratory muscle weakness also results from complications of critical or chronic illness, such as metabolic disarray, sepsis, neuropathy, myopathy from alcohol or steroids, disuse, malnutrition, and cachexia (26).

C. Respiratory Muscle Fatigue, Dyspnea, and Ventilatory Failure

The balance between the effort required to breathe and the capacity of the respiratory muscles to sustain breathing can be quantified by relating the pressure needed to inspire a breath (Pbreath) to the maximal static inspiratory pressure (PImax). Pbreath/PImax is elevated by mechanical impediments to breathing, as in chest wall and obstructive lung diseases, by respiratory muscle weakness, as in neuromuscular disease and critical or chronic illness, and by combinations of mechanical impediments and weakness, especially in chest wall disease and COPD. Another relevant variable in breathing is the duration of inspiration (Ti) in relation to the duration of the breath (Ttot). The fraction Ti/Ttot is referred to as the inspiratory duty cycle. The product [(Pbreath/PImax) × (Ti/Ttot)] is referred to as the inspiratory pressure-time index (PTI). Experiments with normal volunteers and patients with COPD indicate that inspiratory muscle fatigue would occur when the PTI surpasses a critical level of 0.15 (38,39). Patients with COPD may enter into a fatiguing pattern of breathing merely by engaging in slow, deep breathing (39), and a fatiguing pattern of breathing often develops with exercise (40), in ventilatory failure, and during weaning from mechanical ventilation (41,42). Although PTI often exceeds the fatigue threshold, overt fatigue is uncommon (43). Part of the reason is that it takes several hours to develop overt fatigue when the PTI is just over the fatigue threshold (38).

The dominant term in the PTI is Pbreath/PImax. The inspiratory muscles may become fatigued when Pbreath is more than 30–40% of PImax (18). In fatigue experiments, the subjects are asked to maintain the targetted Pbreath and Ti until they fatigue. In the absence of such coaching, the natural response to an increase in Pbreath/PImax is to adopt a rapid, shallow pattern of breathing (26,44). The minimizes dyspnea and reduces the probability of fatigue in the clinical setting. However, the small breath leads to CO_2 retention (26,42,44,45).

Typical values for respiratory rate, tidal volume, and $P_{0.1}$ in eucapnic patients are summarized in Table 2. The normal tidal volume is 7–8 ml/kg of body weight during quiet breathing, somewhat larger in eucapnic patients with COPD, and substantially smaller in neuromuscular and chest wall diseases (26). Rapid, shallow breathing is characteristic of hypercapnic patients with COPD (45,46), acute ventilatory failure (42), kyphoscoliosis (47), and neuromuscular disease (48,49). This phenomenon is associated with an increase in neural drive to breathe, as manifest by the mouth occlusion pressure ($P_{0.1}$)

Table 2 Ventilatory Drive and Pattern of Breathing[a]

Condition	$P_{0.1}$ (cmH_2O)	RR (br/min)	VT (L)
Normal	0.9	11	0.7
COPD	4.4	18	0.7
Kyphoscoliosis	2.8	24	0.5
Neuromuscular disease	1.5	23	0.4

[a]Mouth occlusion pressure and respiratory rate are higher in normocapnic patients with COPD and chest wall and neuromuscular diseases, and tidal volume is lower in chest wall and neuromuscular diseases.
$P_{0.1}$ = mouth occlusion pressure; RR = respiratory rate; VT = tidal volume; br = breaths.
Source: Data from Refs. 22, 48, 50.

(22,48–50). Indeed, there is an inverse correlation between $P_{0.1}$ and tidal volume such that increasing $P_{0.1}$ is associated with decreasing tidal volume (50). Patients with neuromuscular disease and chest wall diseases who have relatively normal lungs can tolerate a tidal volume as low as 3 ml/kg, but patients with COPD and other conditions that disrupt gas exchange retain CO_2 when tidal volume falls below 5 ml/kg (26).

Dyspnea in normal subjects and in chronic lung disease is closely linked to the pattern of respiratory muscle contraction (51–53) as well as to the degree of lung hyperinflation (54). Dyspnea is severe when a hemidiaphragm is displaced downward by pleural effusion, and thoracentesis relieves the dyspnea (55). Dyspnea can be abolished by mechanical ventilation when inspiratory muscle activity is suppressed (56–58). Dyspnea during exercise is related to Pbreath/PImax (52,53), to $\dot{V}E$, tidal volume, and peak tidal inspiratory flow (59), and to asynchronous movements of the chest and abdomen (60,61). Dyspnea is worse in arm exercise because inspiratory muscles are involved in stabilization of the torso (62–65). Dyspnea is related more to recruitment of the rib cage and neck inspiratory muscles than to activity of the diaphragm (66,67). As a corollary, dyspnea is also related to the intensity of the neural drive to breathe (68). It has been shown by factor analysis that dyspnea ratings from questionnaires, PImax, and spirometric assessment of lung function each give independent information about the condition of patients with COPD (69).

D. Respiratory Muscles and Exercise Capacity

Oxygen consumption at maximal exercise ($\dot{V}o_2max$) in COPD and other conditions is shown in Table 3. The values in disease are expressed as ml/kg and as percent of normal values for the same age and sex distribution (70). Several

Table 3 Exercise $\dot{V}O_2max$ in Patients with Chest Wall Diseases, Morbid Obesity, and Neuromuscular Diseases

Condition	$\dot{V}O_2max$ (ml/kg)	$\dot{V}O_2max$ (% normal)
COPD, moderate	16	48
COPD, severe	13	39
Interstitial lung disease	22	56
Kyphoscoliosis	32	73
Ankylosing spondylitis	23	56
Morbid obesity	28	60
Neuromuscular disease	27	54

$\dot{V}O_2max$ = maximal oxygen consumption during progressive exercise.
Source: Data in various diseases are from references 74, 77, 85–91. Values in disease are compared to normal values for age and sex distribution from Ref. 70.

aspects of respiratory muscle dysfunction are responsible for limiting exercise in COPD (Table 4). The mechanical disadvantage to the diaphragm impairs its ability to increase inspired tidal volume. Ventilation at maximal exercise ($\dot{V}Emax$) is correlated with FEV_1 and peak inspiratory flow rate, which in turn is correlated with PImax (71). Respiratory muscle weaknesss contributes to the reduction in maximal voluntary ventilation (MVV) independently of the influence of airway conductance (72), and MVV is a major determinant of maximal exercise capacity (73,74). PImax and the diffusing capacity are key determinants of bicycle ergometric work capacity and 6-min walk distance (6MWD) (75). PImax, severity of airway obstruction (FEV_1/FVC), and respiratory im-

Table 4 Causes of Reduced Exercise Capacity in COPD

Respiratory muscle limitation
Mechanical disadvantage to the diaphragm
Respiratory muscle weakness contributes to reduction in MVV
$RM\dot{V}O_2$ limits oxygen available to the exercising muscles
High Pbreath/PImax predisposes to dyspnea and fatigue
Respiratory muscles stabilize torso during arm exercise
Pulmonary limitation
Low DLco with loss of capillary surface area
Dynamic compression of airways aggravates hyperinflation and dyspnea
Disproportionately high VT/VC in severely obstructed patients
Circulatory limitation
Fatigue of exercising extremities (arms, legs)
Low cardiac index with low mixed venous blood oxygen tension

pedance (ratio of mouth occlusion pressure to mean inspiratory flow rate) are major determinants of maximal power output during bicycle ergometry (76). In COPD, RM$\dot{V}O_2$ is 40% of total $\dot{V}O_2$ at exercise (24). Yet the relation between total $\dot{V}O_2$ and mechanical work done in exercise is the same in patients with COPD as in normals (77). In other words, a high of RM$\dot{V}_{O_2}$ makes less oxygen available for nonrespiratory muscles (24,78). The effects of RM$\dot{V}O_2$ and hypercapnia on oxygen available for activity in COPD are presented in Table 5.

E. Other Determinants of Exercise Capacity

Other factors that limit exercise in COPD are related to the abnormal airway and lung mechanics, and to loss of capillary surface area (Table 4). Thus, $\dot{V}O_2$max can be predicted from the diffusing capacity and the ratio of dead space to tidal volume (VD/VT) as well as the MVV (73). Patients with COPD and matched normal subjects experienced the same intensity of dyspnea and leg effort during bicycle ergometry, although the maximal power output was only 60% of predicted in the COPD patients versus 98% in the normals (79). The tidal volume at maximal exercise is higher in COPD patients with the most abnormal resting mechanics (80,81). Dynamic compression of the airways curtails expiratory flow, aggravates dyspnea, increases intrinsic PEEP, and leads to dynamic hyperinflation of the lungs during exercise (54,82). Dynamic hyperinflation and intrinsic PEEP are added burdens on the inspiratory muscles, but the progressive increase in lung volume worsens the mechanical disadvantage to the diaphragm.

Table 5 Total and Respiratory Muscle Oxygen Consumption, and Oxygen Available for Activity, in Normal Subjects and Patients with COPD[a]

Variable	Normal	COPD-A	COPD-B
$PaCO_2$ (torr)	40	40	60
$\dot{V}A/\dot{V}E$	0.7	0.4	0.4
Oxygen cost (ml/L)	1.0	10.5	10.5
Total $\dot{V}O_2$ (ml/min)	1230	690	1050
RM$\dot{V}O_2$ (ml/min)	30	300	300
$\dot{V}O_2$ available (ml/min)	1200	390	750

[a]Hypercapnic COPD-B has lower RM$\dot{V}_{O_2}$ and more O_2 available for activity, even though $\dot{V}A/\dot{V}E$ and oxygen cost are the same as in COPD-A.

$PaCO_2$ − partial pressure of carbon dioxide in arterial blood, $\dot{V}A$ − effective alveolar ventilation; $\dot{V}E$ = minute ventilation; $\dot{V}O_2$ = oxygen consumption; RM$\dot{V}_{O_2}$ respiratory muscle oxygen consumption; $\dot{V}O_2$ = oxygen available for physical activity. Values of RM$\dot{V}_{O_2}$, total $\dot{V}O_2$, and O_2 available for activity are calculated for VE of 30 L/min.

Source: Adapted from Ref. 78.

The presence of circulatory limitation to exercise in COPD (Table 4) can be inferred from the observation that COPD patients often have no evidence of respiratory muscle fatigue during exercise (83). Among 55 patients with severe COPD, half had a low mixed venous Po_2, i.e. less than 35 mmHg, at rest (84). The cardiac index in the patients with the low mixed venous Po_2 averaged 2.7 L/min/m^2 versus 3.1 L/min/m^2 in patients whose mixed venous Pv_{O_2} was normal. The low mixed venous Po_2 was accurately predicted by a Pao_2 less than 65 mmHg in eucapnic patients and less than 50 mmHg in hypercapnic patients (84). These patients were not studied at exercise, but it is likely that as many as a third of patients with severe COPD have a significant circulatory limitation to exercise.

Exercise impairment in restrictive diseases of the chest wall (Table 3) is for the most part consistent with muscle weakness and physical deconditioning. The low $\dot{V}o_2$max for obesity in Table 3 results from using the observed weight. In absolute terms, the $\dot{V}o_2$ for a given of exercise in obese subjects is much higher than normal (85,86). In kyphoscoliosis the $\dot{V}o_2$max and work capacity are moderately reduced (87,88). The ventilatory responses to exercise are appropriate for the exercise, and anaerobic threshold is attained (87,88). Work capacity does not correlate with the severity of scoliosis (88), but is related to muscularity, ventilatory impairment, and physical deconditioning (87,88). Similar results are found in ankylosing spondylitis (89). Patients with neuromuscular diseases have limited exercise capacity, but their ventilatory and oxygen consumption responses are appropriate for the of exercise (90,91).

IV. Physiological Interventions to Reduce Ventilatory Load

A. Oxygen

Physiological interventions in pulmonary rehabilitation are summarized in Table 6. Hypoxia curtails respiratory muscle endurance (92), and giving oxygen to exercising COPD patients improves respiratory muscle and exercise endurance (40). Oxygen also ameliorates dyspnea (93), but maximal exercise capacity increases in less than half the patients (94,95). Administration of oxygen relieves dyspnea at rest in hypoxemic patients with COPD or pulmonary fibrosis (96). In interstitial lung disease, breathing 60% oxygen increases maximal work, $\dot{V}o_2$max, and exercise endurance time by 15–20% (97). The mechanisms of increased exercise performance with supplemental oxygen are mainly a reduction in ventilatory equivalents for oxygen or carbon dioxide ($\dot{V}E/\dot{V}o_2$, $\dot{V}E/\dot{V}co_2$), an increase in $Paco_2$, and improvement in arterial oxyhemoglobin saturation (94,95,97).

Table 6 Physiological Interventions in Pulmonary Rehabilitation

Reduce ventilatory load	
	Oxygen therapy
	Mechanical support using PEEP or CPAP
Respiratory muscle training	
	Slow respiratory rate using pursed-lips breathing
	Enlarge tidal volume by repetitive deep inspirations
	Increase respiratory muscle strength (PImax, PEmax)
Physical exercise training	
	Walking and stair-climbing exercises to enhance mobility
	High-intensity exercise of arms and legs (to increase MSVC, $\dot{V}E$ during exercise should exceed 70% MVV)
	Support training with oxygen and CPAP as needed
Occupational therapy training	
	Stratgegies for using limb, trunk, and respiratory muscles during ADL
	Enhance endurance for activities of daily living
Combinations of regimens	
	Concurrent use of regimens to maximize benefit in multiple areas

B. Intermittent Mechanical Ventilation

Patients whose ventilatory endurance is limited to a few days or less need intermittent mechanical ventilatory support. In patients with neuromuscular or chest wall disease, prolonged intermittent mechanical ventilation improves blood gas composition and prolongs life (98–100). Negative-pressure ventilation does not work well for the majority of patients with COPD (101,102). Nonetheless, some patients with COPD and cystic fibrosis receive benefits such as increases in PImax by approximately 10 cmH_2O and significantly better arterial blood gas composition (103–106). There may also be a reduction in dyspnea (58,107,108) and an increase in 12MWD (58,103,109). The mechanism underlying these changes remains unclear. It is unlikely to be relief of respiratory muscle fatigue, but relief of dyspnea and improved sleep architecture may be contributing factors (108,110).

C. PEEP and CPAP

Even when mechanical support is limited to positive end-expiratory pressure (PEEP) or continuous positive airway pressure (CPAP) without ventilation, the load on the inspiratory muscles is substantially reduced (111,112). CPAP and PEEP maintain the patency of lower airways during expiration. Thus, PEEP and CPAP have also been used in COPD to minimize dyspnea during exercise (113,114). Proportional assist ventilation, a technique that is intermediate between CPAP and positive-pressure ventilation, also enhances physical exercise capacity in COPD (115). Supplemental oxygen and/or CPAP should be used as needed during physical exercise training (113). Both oxygen therapy and physical exercise training reduce the $\dot{V}E$ needed for a given activity (116).

V. Physical Exercise Training

A. Lower-Extremity Exercise

Walking training may be carried out using a treadmill or a free-style course (117,118). Alternatively, exercise training may be accomplished using a bicycle ergometer (116). Training can be set at low intensity with long duration or high intensity with short duration per session (116,118). Training is usually carried out for 30–60 min, once or twice per day, for 3–4 days per week, for at least 4 weeks. Performance can be tested by measuring the distance walked in 6 or 12 min (6MWD, 12MWD), by climbing stairs (119), or by determining maximal ventilatory, circulatory, and gas exchange responses in a progressive exercise test. The $\dot{V}Emax$ and $\dot{V}o_2max$ of patients with COPD are similar in bicycle and treadmill tests, but $\dot{V}Emax$ and $\dot{V}o_2max$ are higher and more variable in a step-climbing test (120). Many patients with severe COPD are able to reach an anaerobic threshold during progressive exercise (116,118). Factors that predict inability to attain the anaerobic threshold include higher resting airway resistance (Raw), Raw/PImax, Pbreath/PImax, and PTI (121). In other words, the patients who cannot reach the anaerobic threshold are those whose inspiratory muscles are more stressed during quiet breathing.

B. Upper-Extremity Exercise

Arm elevation and arm exercise require a higher of $\dot{V}E$ and produce more dyspnea than leg exercise, for a given of energy expenditure (62–65). Several forms of upper-extremity training have been devised, including repetitive arm motion, weight lifting, arm cycling, and exercises with dowels (122,123). Many activities of daily living require proficiency at arm exercise, and arm exercise is good training for patients who are unable to tolerate much walking (122). Other examples of upper-extremity exercise training include swimming and canoeing (124) and weight lifting (125,126).

C. Results of Physical Exercise Training

All COPD patients who underwent 8 weeks of training five times weekly on a bicycle ergometer exhibited some training benefit, although half used a short-duration, high-intensity regimen and half used a long-duration, low-intensity regimen (116). The benefits were much greater in the high-intensity trainers, who improved their exercise endurance by 73% and decreased their $\dot{V}E$ and lactate levels for a given exercise intensity. The low-intensity trainers had a much smaller increase in endurance and no reductions in $\dot{V}E$ or lactate (116). Other COPD patients who underwent 8 weeks of high-intensity treadmill training had 10% increases in $\dot{V}Emax$ and $\dot{V}O_2max$, a 32% increase in maximal treadmill load, and an 83% increase in exercise endurance time (118). Patients with cystic fibrosis had increases in exercise tolerance and maximal $\dot{V}O_2$ and lower heart rates at submaximal loads, after 3 months of training by running (127).

Physical exercise training programs that last 4–8 weeks improve walk capacity by 25–100%, even in chronically hypercapnic COPD patients (117,128–130), but occasionally a month of exercise training has no benefit in terms of 12MWD or exercise endurance time (131). The magnitude of improvement in 12MWD is negatively correlated with initial 12MWD and positively correlated with initial FEV_1 (130). A program of unsupervised home exercise for 6 weeks substantially reduced dyspnea, both as measured during a maximal treadmill workload and in the transitional dyspnea index scores (132). Training the arms and legs by weight lifting for 8 weeks increased limb muscle strength and exercise endurance time on the bicycle ergometer, but had a borderline effect on 6MWD (126). Upper extremity exercise training, especially unsupported arm exercise, increases arm exercise endurance time (122,123). Arm exercise training reduces the energy and ventilatory costs of arm elevation (133), as well as perceptions of dyspnea and fatigue (122).

D. Effect of Exercise Training on Respiratory Muscles

Exercise training often affects respiratory muscle function to a modest degree. In normal subjects, running for 20 weeks increased PImax and maximal sustainable ventilatory capacity (MSVC) by 15% (134). Endurance exercise training in older normals lowered the ventilatory equivalent for oxygen ($\dot{V}E/\dot{V}O_2$) (135), which translates to less respiratory muscle work for a given of exercise. Twelve weeks of swim training increased PImax by 20% and inspiratory muscle endurance by 113% in young women (136). Swimming and canoeing for 4 weeks increased MSVC of patients with cystic fibrosis by 57% (124), and a 3-month running program increased ventilatory endurance by 50% (127). Exercise training increased the MVV of COPD patients by about 10% (137), and arm or leg exercise increased the MSVC by 10% in patients with COPD (138). A 4-week program for COPD patients yielded small, but significant, improvements in PImax and $Paco_2$ (117). Unsupported arm exercise improved inspiratory muscle strength and endurance (123), but other forms of upper-extremity exercise had no effect on the respiratory muscles (122,126,128,133).

VI. Breathing Exercises and Respiratory Muscle Training

A. Measures to Increase Tidal Volume

Early efforts to improve diaphragmatic excursion and tidal volume in patients with COPD utilized the head-down position (139) and therapeutic pneumoperitoneum (140,141). Diaphragm excursion and vital capacity increased, and respiratory rate decreased, but tidal volume did not change. These techniques fell out of favor because they were cumbersome and often not well tolerated. Nonetheless, it is of interest that diaphragmatic excursion could increase by 3–4 cm in patients with chronic hyperinflation of the lungs.

When untrained patients with COPD adopt a slower, deeper pattern of breathing, the diaphragmatic PTI increases beyond the fatigue threshold (39). In contrast, pursed-lip breathing increases inspiratory recruitment of rib cage and neck muscles and expiratory recruitment of abdominal muscles (142). Pursed-lip breathing also decreased the respiratory rate and the inspiratory duty cycle (142). The net result of these effects is to improve ventilation while sparing the diaphragm. Inspiratory incentive spirometers use targets based on inspiratory flow rate or tidal volume; training COPD patients with such a device increased their tidal volume, as compared to no change in the untrained COPD controls (143). Training with breathing exercises such as pursed-lip and "diaphragmatic" breathing increased tidal volume of COPD patients by 30–40%, as well as increasing their diaphragmatic excursion by 3 cm (137,144–146). Diaphragmatic breathing exercises increased Pdi by 30% (147). However, abdominal situp or weight exercises had no significant effect on respiratory muscle function (148).

Biofeedback and relaxation techniques may reduce the perception of ventilatory effort and dyspnea, even when the ventilatory load is unchanged. Tidal volume training combined with relaxation feedback helped patients to wean from mechanical ventilation and increased tidal volume by 40% (149). Biofeedback training using signals from abdominal and neck inspiratory muscles was associated with improvements in FEV_1 and $FEF_{25\text{-}75}$ in patients with cystic fibrosis (150). Proprioceptive musculoskeletal education for normal subjects relieves habitual muscle tension and postural abnormalities, with concomitant increases of approximately 10% in peak expiratory flow, MVV, PImax, and PEmax, as compared to no changes in the controls (151).

B. Ventilatory Endurance Training

Ventilatory endurance (MSVC) can be increased by breathing at approximately 70% of MVV. Exercise is the most physiological and practical way to hyperventilate, but patients with COPD or other lung, chest wall, or neuromuscular disease may have trouble exercising to a level high enough to bring their training $\dot{V}E$ into the effective range (138). Voluntary hyperventilation may be used instead of exercise. Hypocapnia is prevented by providing a CO_2 supplement, or by breathing through added dead space with an O_2 supplement. Voluntary hyperventilation for 15–30 min, several times per day, for 4–6 weeks increases the MSVC by 20–30% in normal subjects (124,152,153). Voluntary hyperventilation training also increases MSVC by approximately 30–45% in patients with cystic fibrosis or COPD (124,154–156). Physical exercise training increases MSVC about half as much as hyperventilation training (157). In physical exercise training the ventilatory training stimulus is usually inadequate, since the level of $\dot{V}E$ generally does not exceed 50–60% of MVV (157). Training normal subjects by repetetive inhalations to TLC increases VC, possibly by increasing inspiratory muscle shortening capacity (158).

C. Respiratory Muscle Strength Training

It has been shown in normal subjects that inspiratory muscle training is highly specific to the training conditions of pressure, flow, and lung volume. Training for strength by repeating inspiratory and expiratory pressures leads to 50% increases in PImax and PEmax with no change in MSVC (152). Conversely, hyperventilation training to increase MSVC is without effect on respiratory muscle strength. Training with repetetive PImax maneuvers at low lung volumes improves inspiratory strength over a wider range of lung volumes than similar training at high lung volume (159). Training by maximal unobstructed inspirations increased maximal inspiratory flow rate by 17% with no effect on PImax, whereas training with repetetive PImax maneuvers increased PImax 37% but had no effect on peak inspiratory flow rate (160). Subjects who trained with an inspiratory resistive device that imposed intermediate pressure and flow loads had lesser improvements in both PImax and maximal inspiratory flow rate. In normal subjects, strength training for 6–18 weeks increased PImax by 50% and reduced dyspnea at maximal exercise (161). In contrast, inspiratory load training at 30% of PImax for 4 weeks increased PImax by 30%, but had no effect on dyspnea (162). Strength training is as effective in patients with severe, chronic lung disease as it is in normal subjects (163).

D. Respiratory Muscle Strength and Endurance Training

The strength and endurance of inspiratory muscles can be enhanced by inspiring through external flow-resistive or threshold loads. In order to increase PImax, the training load must cause Pbreath to exceed 30% of pretraining PImax (157), and the pattern of breathing must be controlled so that there is a constant training effect with each breath (164–166). Typically, inspiratory load training is carried out 30 min twice a day, 5–7 days a week, for at least 4 weeks, but results are better if training continues for 8–12 weeks (167–169). Results are virtually identical with inspiratory flow-resistive and threshold loading.

Inspiratory load training improves inspiratory muscle strength and endurance for the training load, but has no effect on MSVC (157). Inspiratory load training has variable effects on exercise performance, some studies showing improvement (131,169,170) and others not (171–173). There is some indication that inspiratory load training works best for patients who demonstrate evidence of inspiratory muscle fatigue during exercise (83). Inspiratory load training can reduce dyspnea (168,174,175), but it is of little or no benefit in terms of capacity for activities of daily living (157,176). Patients with asthma who trained at a threshold load equal to 60% of PImax had a 27% increase in PImax, a 38% increase in inspiratory muscle endurance, and a substantial reduction in asthma-related symptoms of cough, chest tightness, and wheeze, as compared to asthmatic controls (177). Uncontrolled studies suggest that inspiratory load training may facilitate weaning from mechanical ventilation (178,179).

Inspiratory muscle training is of benefit in neuromuscular disease, but the outcome varies with diagnosis. Inspiratory load training increased PImax by 37% and inspiratory muscle endurance by 110% in quadriplegic patients (167). In muscular dystrophy and other diffuse neuromuscular diseases, inspiratory load training did not increase PImax, although inspiratory muscle endurance improved (180–182). A combination of inspiratory load and strength training increased PImax by 70% in 10 of 15 muscular dystrophy patients in the training group, as compared to no change in the five training dropouts and the 15 non-trained controls (183). Of interest, the improvement in the 10 patients who completed the 6-month training program lasted for 6 months after training was stopped.

E. Combined Physical Exercise and Inspiratory Muscle Training

The combination of exercise training with inspiratory muscle load training has been tested in one uncontrolled and two controlled studies involving 129 patients with COPD whose FEV_1 averaged 43% predicted (174,184,185). The combination of inspiratory muscle and exercise training yielded substantially better results than exercise training alone, with regard to exercise endurance and walk capacity. With the combined regimen, the average increase in PImax was 18 cmH_2O (+39%), 12MWD increased by 267 m (+38%), and cycle exercise endurance time increased by 17–150%. COPD patients who performed breathing exercises plus physical exercise training improved their maximal exercise capacity by 9–32% (145,146). Indeed, exercise capacity improved more with combined breathing exercise and general exercise training than in controls who trained with physical exercise alone (146).

VII. Summary and Recommendations

A. Ventilatory Rehabilitation

Ventilatory rehabilitation comprises breathing training to reduce dyspnea and restore ventilatory capacity. This should involve specific measures such as pursed-lips breathing and deep breathing to increase tidal volume and improve gas exchange, the hyperventilation of high-intensity exercise training for ventilatory endurance, and strength training for inspiratory and expiratory muscles to enhance respiratory muscle endurance and ameliorate dyspnea. Supplemental measures to support training may include oxygen and CPAP.

Rapid, shallow breathing is the final common pathway for ventilatory failure in obstructive lung, chest wall, and neuromuscular diseases. Training to increase tidal volume would complement pursed-lips breathing to slow the respiratory rate. Older reports indicate it is possible to achieve a meaningful increase in tidal volume, but optimal training techniques have not been identified. Simply repeating deep inspirations with the aid of an inspiratory incentive spirometer may be as easy and effective as other methods, but the effect of physical exercise training on tidal volume should also be determined. Biofeedback and relaxation techniques may also have a useful role in training to increase tidal volume. Since dyspnea sometimes results from downward displacement of the diaphragm, it would also be of interest to determine whether improvement of diaphragmatic excursion has any bearing on breathlessness.

The simplest way to train for ventilatory endurance would be to use the physiological stimulus of exercise hyperventilation. A good argument for high-intensity exercise training is that $\dot{V}E$ during training is likely to be close to the level needed to successfully increase ventilatory endurance. It would be helpful to know if the pleural, abdominal, and transdiaphragmatic inspiratory and expiratory pressure swings during high-intensity physical exercise training are high enough to increase respiratory muscle strength. The relative effects on ventilatory endurance of upper-extremity versus lower-extremity exercise should also be assessed.

Respiratory system responses to increased ventilatory loads involve expiratory as well as inspiratory muscles. Global respiratory muscle weakness is common in COPD as well as in chest wall and neuromuscular diseases. Increasing respiratory muscle strength may enhance exercise capacity and alleviate dyspnea. Thus, the strength of both inspiratory and expiratory muscles should be tested, and both groups should be trained. Respiratory muscle strength training can be done easily at home, merely by repeating maximal inspiratory and expiratory efforts against a closed airway.

B. General Rehabilitation

General rehabilitation focuses on increasing the capacity for physical exercise and activities of daily living. It utilizes exercise and occupational therapy training techniques. Exercise training should include high-intensity exercises designed to train the respiratory and circulatory systems as well as the arms and legs, plus walking and stair climbing to improve motility. Occupational therapy should be used to help develop strategies to cope with activities of daily living in ways that minimize energy expenditure and dyspnea.

Exercise is often limited in patients with COPD, obesity, chest wall, and neuromuscular diseases by muscular deconditioning. Such patients should benefit substantially from physical exercise programs. It is important to identify which COPD patients suffer from circulatory versus ventilatory limitation to exercise. To this end, easier ways to predict mixed venous oxygen tension and the potential for respiratory muscle fatigue during exercise will have to be developed. More patients with morbid obesity, chest wall disease, and neuromuscular diseases should be enrolled in rehabilitation programs, and the outcomes of rehabilitation should be examined. Once respiratory muscle and exercise training have been completed, patients should participate in maintenance regimens, but there is little information on the optimal characteristics of maintenance regimens.

Research in the area of occupational therapy should be directed toward determining how various respiratory and other muscle groups are used during activities of daily living and exploring how some patients with severe airflow limitation are able to perform surprisingly high levels of activity. Patients should be evaluated during specific activities, such as dressing, housework, shopping, light work, and recreational pursuits. Training regimens should be developed to help with the physical maneuvers that are utilized in activities of daily living.

C. Analysis of Outcomes

The physiological outcomes of most forms of respiratory muscle training are well understood, whereas the physiological benefits of training to improve tidal volume and diaphragmatic excursion are currently hypothesized but not proven. Comprehensive respiratory muscle training may delay the onset of ventilatory failure or help reverse it. It is far easier to investigate the latter proposition. The physiological outcomes of exercise training are also well understood, but there are areas for future research, especially in regard to the effects of high-intensity exercise on respiratory muscle strength and ventilatory endurance. Research into physiological strategies to improve performance of activities of daily living might be especially rewarding.

Other important outcomes such as cost-benefit analysis, positive and negative psychological effects of training, and impacts of training on quality of life, sense of mastery, and societal role function are beyond the scope of this chapter. They are addressed elsewhere in this book, and they must be kept in mind when new programs in pulmonary rehabilitation are devised or old programs modified.

References

1. Barach AL, Bickerman HA, Beck G. Advances in the treatment of non-tuberculous pulmonary disease. Bull NY Acad Med 1952; 28:353–384.
2. Wade OL. Movements of the thoracic cage and diaphragm in respiration. J Physiol 1954; 124:193–212.
3. Rochester DF, Farkas GA, Lu J-Y. Contractility of the in situ human diaphragm: assessment based on dimensional analysis. In: Sieck GC, Gandevia SC, Cameron WE, eds. Respiratory Muscles and Their Neuromotor Control. New York: Alan R Liss, 1987:327–336.
4. Verschakelen JA, Deschepper K, Demedts M. Relationship between axial motion and volume displacement of the diaphragm during VC maneuvers. J Appl Physiol 1992; 72:1536–1540.
5. Sharp JT, Beard GAT, Sunga M, et al. The rib cage in normal and emphysematous subjects: a roentgenographic approach. J Appl Physiol 1986; 61:2050–2059.
6. Walsh JM, Webber CL Jr, Fahey PJ, Sharp JT. Structural change of the thorax in chronic obstructive pulmonary disease. J Appl Physiol 1992; 72:1270–1278.
7. De Troyer A, Estenne M, Ninane V, Van Gansbeke D, Gorini M. Transversus abdominis muscle function in humans. J Appl Physiol 1990; 68:1010–1016.
8. Rochester DF. Tests of respiratory muscle function. Clin Chest Med 1988; 9:249–261.
9. Aubier M, Murciano D, Lecocguic Y, Vlires N, Pariente R. Bilateral phrenic stimulation: a simple technique to assess diaphragmatic fatigue in humans. J Appl Physiol 1985; 58:58–64.
10. Yan S, Gauthier AP, Similowski T, Macklem PT, Bellemare F. Evaluation of human diaphragm contractility using mouth pressure twitches. Am Rev Respir Dis 1992; 145:1064–1069.
11. Yan S, Gauthier AP, Similowski T, Faltus R, Macklem PT, Bellemare F. Force-frequency relationships of in vivo human and in vitro rat diaphragm using paired stimuli. Eur Respir J 1993; 6:211–218.
12. Grassino AE, Goldman MD. Respiratory muscle coordination. In: Mecklam PT, Mead J, eds. Handbook of Physiology. Section 3. The Respiratory System. Vol III. Mechanics of Breathing, Part 2. Bethesda: American Physiological Society, 1986:463–480.

13. Mead J, Loring SH. Analysis of volume displacement and length changes of the diaphragm during breathing. J Appl Physiol 1982; 53:750–755.
14. De Troyer A, Estenne M. Coordination between rib cage muscles and diaphragm during quiet breathing in humans. J Appl Physiol 1984; 57:899–906.
15. Druz WS, Sharp JT. Activity of the respiratory muscles in upright and recumbent humans. J Appl Physiol 1981; 51:1552–1561.
16. Loring SH, Mead J. Abdominal muscle use during quiet breathing and hyperpnea in uninformed subjects. J Appl Physiol 1982; 52:700–704.
17. DiMarco AF, Supinski GS, Budzinska K. Inspiratory muscle interaction in the generation of changes in airway pressure. J Appl Physiol 1989; 66:2573–2578.
18. Roussos C, Fixley M, Gross D, Macklem PT. Fatigue of inspiratory muscles and their synergic behavior. J Appl Physiol 1979; 46:897–904.
19. Yan S, Sliwinski P, Gauthier AP, Lichros I, Zakynthinos S, Macklem PT. Effect of global inspiratory muscle fatigue on ventilatory and respiratory muscle responses to CO_2. J Appl Physiol 1993; 75:1371–1377.
20. Martinez FJ, Couser JI, Celli BR. Factors influencing ventilatory muscle recruitment in patients with chronic airflow obstruction. Am Rev Respir Dis 1990; 142:276–282.
21. Molho M, Shulimzon T, Benzaray S, Katz I. Importance of inspiratory load in the assessment of severity of airways obstruction and its correlation with CO_2 retention in chronic obstructive pulmonary disease. Am Rev Respir Dis 1993; 147:45–49.
22. Gorini M, Spinelli A, Ginanni R, Duranti R, Gigliotti F, Scano G. Neural respiratory drive and neuromuscular coupling in patients with chronic obstructive pulmonary disease (COPD). Chest 1990; 98:1179–1186.
23. Fritts HW Jr, Filler J, Fishman AP, Cournand A. The efficiency of ventilation during voluntary hyperpnea: studies in normal subjects and in dyspneic patients with either chronic pulmonary emphysema or obesity. J Clin Invest 1959; 38:1339–1348.
24. Levison H, Cherniack RM. Ventilatory cost of exercise in chronic obstructive pulmonary disease. J Appl Physiol 1968; 25:21–27.
25. Ninane V, Rypens F, Yernault J-C, De Troyer A. Abdominal muscle use during breathing in patients with chronic airflow obstruction. Am Rev Respir Dis 1992; 146:16–21.
26. Rochester DF. Respiratory muscles and ventilatory failure: 1993 perspective. Am J Med Sci 1993; 305:394–402.
27. Rochester DF, Braun NMT. Determinants of maximal inspiratory pressure in chronic obstructive pulmonary disease. Am Rev Respir Dis 1985; 132:42–47.
28. Lands L, Desmond KJ, Demizio D, Pavilanis A, Coates AL. The effects of nutritional status and hyperinflation on respiratory muscle strength in children and young adults. Am Rev Respir Dis 1990; 141:1506–1509.
29. Bergofsky EH, Turino GM, Fishman AP. Cardiorespiratory failure in kyphoscoliosis. Medicine (Baltimore) 1959; 38:263–317.
30. Cherniack RM, Guenter CA. The efficiency of the respiratory muscles in obesity. Can J Biochem Physiol 1961; 39:1215–1222.

31. Rochester DF, Enson Y. Current concepts in the pathogenesis of the obesity-hypoventilation syndrome. Am J Med 1974; 57:402–420.
32. Lisboa C, Moreno R, Fava M, Ferretti R, Cruz E. Inspiratory muscle function in patients with severe kyphoscoliosis. Am Rev Respir Dis 1985; 132:48–52.
33. Kelly TM, Jensen RL, Elliott CG, Crapo RO. Maximum respiratory pressures in morbidly obese subjects. Respiration 1988; 54:73–77.
34. Rochester DF, Arora NS. Respiratory failure from obesity. In: Mancini M, Lewis B, Contaldo F, eds. Medical Complications of Obesity. New York: Academic Press, 1979:183–190.
35. Sharp JT, Druz WS, Kondragunta VR. Diaphragmatic responses to body position changes in obese patients with obstructive sleep apnea. Am Rev Respir Dis 1986; 133:32–37.
36. Braun NMT, Arora NS, Rochester DF. Respiratory muscle and pulmonary function in polymyositis and other proximal myopathies. Thorax 1983; 38:616–623.
37. Corrado A, Bruscoli G, De Paola E, Ciardi-Dupre GF, Baccini A, Taddei M. Respiratory muscle insufficiency in acute respiratory failure of subjects with severe COPD: treatment with intermittent negative pressure ventilation. Eur Respir J 1990; 3:644–648.
38. Bellemare F, Grassino A. Effect of pressure and timing of contraction on human diaphragm fatigue. J Appl Physiol 1982; 53:1190–1195.
39. Bellemare F, Grassino A. Force reserve of the diaphragm in patients with chronic obstructive pulmonary disease. J Appl Physiol 1983; 55:8–15.
40. Bye PTP, Esau SA, Levy RD, et al. Ventilatory muscle function during exercise in air and oxygen in patients with chronic air-flow limitation. Am Rev Respir Dis 1985; 132:236–240.
41. Cohen CA, Zagelbaum G, Gross D, Roussos C, Macklem PT. Clinical manifestations of inspiratory muscle fatigue. Am J Med 1982; 73:308–316.
42. Jabour ER, Rabil DM, Truwit JD, Rochester DF. Evaluation of a new weaning index, based on ventilatory endurance and the efficiency of gas exchange. Am Rev Respir Dis 1991; 144:531–537.
43. Efthimiou J, Fleming J, Spiro SG. Sternomastoid muscle function and fatigue in breathlessness patients with severe respiratory disease. Am Rev Respir Dis 1987; 136:1099–1105.
44. Oliven A, Cherniack NS, Deal EC, Kelsen SG. The effects of acute bronchoconstriction on respiratory activity in patients with chronic obstructive pulmonary disease. Am Rev Respir Dis 1985; 131:236–241.
45. Begin P, Grassino A. Inspiratory muscle dysfunction and chronic hypercapnia in chronic obstructive pulmonary disease. Am Rev Respir Dis 1991; 143:905–912.
46. Loveridge B, West A, Kryger MH, Anthonisen NR. Alteration in breathing pattern with progression of chronic obstructive pulmonary disease. Am Rev Respir Dis 1986; 134:930–934.
47. Kafer ER. Idiopathic scoliosis-gas exchange and the age dependence of arterial blood gases. J Clin Invest 1976; 58:825–833.
48. Baydur A. Respiratory muscle strength and control of ventilation in patients with neuromuscular disease. Chest 1991; 99:330–338.

49. Spinelli A, Marconi G, Gorini M, Pizzi A, Scano G. Control of breathing in patients with myasthenia gravis. Am Rev Respir Dis 1992; 145:1359–1366.
50. Ramonatxo M, Milic-Emili J, Prefaut C. Breathing pattern and load compensatory responses in young scoliotic patients. Eur Respir J 1988; 1:421–427.
51. Killian KJ, Jones NL. Respiratory muscles and dyspnea. Clin Chest Med 1988; 9:237–248.
52. LeBlanc P, Summers E, Inman MD, Jones NL, Campbell EJM, Killian KJ. Inspiratory muscles during exercise: a problem of supply and demand. J Appl Physiol 1988; 64:2482–2489.
53. LeBlanc P, Bowie DM, Summers E, Jones NL, Killian KJ. Breathlessness and exercise in patients with cardiorespiratory disease. Am Rev Respir Dis 1986; 133:21–25.
54. O'Donnell DE, Webb KA. Exertional breathlessness in patients with chronic airflow limitation. The role of lung hyperinflation. Am Rev Respir Dis 1993; 148:1351–1357.
55. Estenne M, Yernault JC, De Troyer A. Mechanism of relief of dyspnea after thoracocentesis in patients with large pleural effusions. Am J Med 1983; 74.813–819.
56. Rochester DF, Braun NT, Laine S. Diaphragmatic energy expenditure in chronic respiratory failure. Am J Med 1977; 223–232.
57. Bott J, Carroll MP, Conway JH, et al. Randomised controlled trial of nasal ventilation in acute ventilatory failure due to chronic obstructive airways disease. Lancet 1993; 341:1555–1557.
58. Renston JP, DiMarco AF, Supinski GS. Respiratory muscle rest using nasal BiPAP ventilation in patients with stable severe COPD. Chest 1994; 105:1053–1060.
59. Noseda A, Carpiaux J-P, Schmerber J, Valente F, Yernault J-C. Dyspnoea and flow-volume curve during exercise in COPD patients. Eur Respir J 1994; 7:279–285.
60. Sharp JT, Druz WS, Moisan T, Foster J, Machnach W. Postural relief of dyspnea in severe chronic obstructive pulmonary disease. Am Rev Respir Dis 1980; 122:201–211.
61. Delgado HR, Braun SR, Skatrud JB, Reddan WG, Pegelow DF. Chest wall and abdominal motion during exercise in patients with chronic obstructive pulmonary disease. Am Rev Respir Dis 1982; 126:200–205.
62. Celli B, Criner G, Rassulo J. Ventilatory muscle recruitment during unsupported arm exercise in normal subjects. J Appl Physiol 1988; 64:1936–1941.
63. Couser JI, Martinez FJ, Celli BR. Respiratory response and ventilatory muscle recruitment during arm elevation in normal subjects. Chest 1992; 101:336–340.
64. Celli BR, Rassulo J, Make BJ. Dyssynchronous breathing during arm but not leg exercise in patients with chronic airflow obstruction. N Engl J Med 1986; 314:1485–1490.
65. Martinez FJ, Couser JI, Celli BR. Respiratory response to arm elevation in patients with chronic airflow obstruction. Am Rev Respir Dis 1991; 143:476–480.
66. Ward ME, Eidelman D, Stubbing DG, Bellemare F, Macklem PT. Respiratory

sensation and pattern of respiratory muscle activation during diaphragm fatigue. J Appl Physiol 1988; 65:2181–2189.
67. Breslin EH, Garoutte BC, Kohlman-Carrieri V, Celli BR. Correlations between dyspnea, diaphragm and sternomastoid recruitment during inspiratory resistance breathing in normal subjects. Chest 1990; 98:298–302.
68. Altose MD. Assessment and management of breathlessness. Chest 1985; 88:77S–82S.
69. Mahler DA, Harver A. A factor analysis of dyspnea ratings, respiratory muscle strength, and lung function in patients with chronic obstructive pulmonary disease. Am Rev Respir Dis 1992; 145:467–470.
70. Fairbarn MS, Blackie SP, McElvaney NG, Wiggs BR, Pare PD, Pardy RL. Prediction of heart rate and oxygen uptake during incremental and maximal exercise in healthy adults. Chest 1994; 105:1365–1369.
71. Dillard TA, Piantadosi S, Rajagopal KR. Prediction of ventilation at maximal exercise in chronic air-flow obstruction. Am Rev Respir Dis 1985; 132:230–235.
72. Aldrich TK, Arora NS, Rochester DF. The influence of airway obstruction and respiratory muscle strength on maximal voluntary ventilation in lung disease. Am Rev Respir Dis 1982; 126:195–199.
73. Carlson DJ, Ries AL, Kaplan RM. Prediction of maximum exercise tolerance in patients with COPD. Chest 1991; 100:307–311.
74. LoRusso TJ, Belman MJ, Elashoff JD, Koerner SK. Prediction of maximal exercise capacity in obstructive and restrictive pulmonary disease. Chest 1993; 104:1748–1754.
75. Wijkstra PJ, Ten Vergert EM, van der Mark Th, et al. Relation of lung function, maximal inspiratory pressure, dyspnoea, and quality of life with exercise capacity in patients with chronic obstructive pulmonary disease. Thorax 1994; 49:468–472.
76. Loiseau A, Dubreuil C, Loiseau P, Pujet JC, Georges R, Saumon G. Exercise tolerance in chronic obstructive pulmonary disease: importance of active and passive components of the ventilatory system. Eur Respir J 1989; 2:522–527.
77. Lewis MI, Belman MJ, Monn SA, Elashoff JD, Koerner SK. The relationship between oxygen consumption and work rate in patients with chronic airflow obstruction. Chest 1994; 106:366–372.
78. Rochester DF, Arora NS, Braun NMT, Goldberg SK. The respiratory muscles in chronic obstructive pulmonary disease (COPD). Bull Eur Physiopathol Respir 1979; 15:951–975.
79. Killian KJ, LeBlanc P, Martin DH, Summers E, Jones NL, Campbell EJM. Exercise capacity and ventilatory, circulatory, and symptom limitation in patients with chronic airflow limitation. Am Rev Respir Dis 1992; 146:935–940.
80. Vaz Fregoso CA, Clark T, Kotch A. The tidal volume response to incremental exercise in COPD. Chest 1993; 103:1438–1441.
81. Marin J, Hussain SNA, Gibbons WJ, Polverino M, Levy RD, Cosio MG. Relationship of resting lung mechanics and exercise pattern of breathing in patients with chronic obstructive lung disease. Chest 1993; 104:705–711.
82. O'Donnell DE, Sanii R, Anthonisen NR, Younes M. Effect of dynamic airway

compression on breathing pattern and respiratory sensation in severe chronic obstructive pulmonary disease. Am Rev Respir Dis 1987; 135:912–918.
83. Pardy RL, Rivington RN, Despas PJ, Macklem PT. The effects of inspiratory muscle training on exercise performance in chronic airflow limitation. Am Rev Respir Dis 1981; 123:426–433.
84. Mithoefer JC, Ramirez C, Cook W. The effect of mixed venous oxygenation on arterial blood in chronic obstructive pulmonary disease. Am Rev Respir Dis 1978; 117:259–264.
85. Dempsey JA, Reddan W, Balke B, Rankin J. Work capacity determinants and physiologic cost of weight-supported work in obesity. J Appl Physiol 1966; 21:1815–1820.
86. Kollias J, Boileau RA, Bartlett HL, Buskirk ER. Pulmonary function and physical conditioning in lean and obese subjects. Arch Environ Health 1972; 25:146–150.
87. Kesten S, Garfinkel SK, Wright T, Rebuck AS. Impaired exercise capacity in adults with moderate scoliosis. Chest 1991; 99:663–666.
88. Kearon C, Viviani GR, Killian KJ. Factors influencing work capacity in adolescent idiopathic thoracic scoliosis. Am Rev Respir Dis 1993; 148:295–303.
89. Fisher LR, Cawley MI, Holgate ST. Relation between chest expansion, pulmonary function, and exercise tolerance in patients with ankylosing spondylitis. Ann Rheum Dis 1990; 49:921–925.
90. Poppius H, Varpela E, Korhonen O. Respiratory function and exercise tolerance in relaxation of the diaphragm. Scand J Respir Dis 1969; 50:68–75.
91. Lyager S, Noeraa N, Pedersen OF. Cardiopulmonary response to exercise in patients with neuromuscular diseases. Respiration 1984; 45:89–99.
92. Jardim J, Farkas G, Prefaut C, Thomas D, Macklem PT, Roussos CH. The failing inspiratory muscles under normoxic and hypoxic conditions. Am Rev Respir Dis 1981; 124:274–279.
93. Dean NC, Brown JK, Himelman RB, Doherty JJ, Gold WM, Stulbarg MS. Oxygen may improve dyspnea and endurance in patients with chonic obstructive pulmonary disease and only mild hypoxemia. Am Rev Respir Dis 1992; 146:941–945.
94. Light RW, Mahutte CK, Stansbury DW, Fischer CE, Brown SE. Relationship between improvement in exercise performance with supplemental oxygen and hypoxic ventilatory drive in patients with chronic airflow obstruction. Chest 1989; 95:751–756.
95. Corriveau ML, Rosen BJ, Dolan GF. Oxygen transport and oxygen consumption during supplemental oxygen administration in patients with chronic obstructive pulmonary disease. Am J Med 1989; 87:633–637.
96. Swinburn CR, Mould H, Stone TN, Corris PA, Gibson GJ. Symptomatic benefit of supplemental oxygen in hypoxemic patients with chronic obstructive lung disease. Am Rev Respir Dis 1991; 143:913–915.
97. Harris-Eze AO, Sridhar G, Clemens RE, Gallagher CG, Marciniuk DD. Oxygen improves maximal exercise performance in interstitial lung disease. Am J Respir Crit Care Med 1994; 150:1616–1622.
98. Goldstein RS, Molotiu N, Skrastins R, et al. Reversal of sleep induced hypoventi-

lation and chronic respiratory failure by nocturnal negative pressure ventilation in patients with restrictive ventilatory impairment. Am Rev Respir Dis 1987; 135:1049–1055.
99. Sawicka EH, Loh L, Branthwaite MA. Domiciliary ventilatory support: an analysis of outcome. Thorax 1988; 43:31–35.
100. Jackson M, Kinnear W, King M, Hockley S, Shneerson J. The effects of five years of nocturnal cuirass-assisted ventilation in chest wall disease. Eur Respir J 1993; 6:630–635.
101. Celli B, Lee H, Criner G, et al. Controlled trial of external negative pressure ventilation in patients with severe chronic airflow obstruction. Am Rev Respir Dis 1989; 140:1251–1256.
102. Shapiro SH, Ernst P, Gray-Donald K, et al. Effect of negative pressure ventilation in severe chronic obstructive pulmonary disease. Lancet 1993; 340:1425–1429.
103. Gutierrez M, Beroiza T, Contreras G, et al. Weekly cuirass ventilation improves blood gases and inspiratory muscle strength in patients with chronic air-flow limitation and hypercarbia 1–4. Am Rev Respir Dis 1988; 138:617–623.
104. Scano G, Gigliotti F, Duranti R, Spinelli A, Gorini M, Schiavina M. Changes in ventilatory muscle function with negative pressure ventilation in patients with severe COPD. Chest 1990; 97:322–327.
105. Piper AJ, Parker S, Torzillo PJ, Sullivan CE, Bye PTP. Nocturnal nasal IPPV stabilizes patients with cystic fibrosis and hypercapnic respiratory failure. Chest 1992; 102:846–850.
106. Gigliotti F, Spinelli A, Duranti R, Gorini M, Goti P, Scano G. Four-week negative pressure ventilation improves respiratory function in severe hypercapnic COPD patients. Chest 1994; 105:87–94.
107. Waldhorn RE. Nocturnal nasal intermittent positive pressure ventilation with bilevel positive airway pressure (BiPAP) in respiratory failure. Chest 1992; 101:516–521.
108. Hill NS, Eveloff SE, Carlisle CC, Goff SG. Efficacy of nocturnal nasal ventilation in patients with restrictive thoracic disease. Am Rev Respir Dis 1992; 145:365–371.
109. Goldstein RS, De Rosie JA, Avendano MA, Dolmage TE. Influence of noninvasive positive pressure ventilation on inspiratory muscles. Chest 1991; 99:408–415.
110. Hill NS. Noninvasive ventilation. Does it work, for whom, how? Am Rev Respir Dis 1993; 147:1050–1055.
111. Appendini L, Patessio A, Zanaboni S, et al. Physiologic effects of positive end-expiratory pressure and mask pressure support during exacerbations of chronic obstructive pulmonary disease. Am J Respir Crit Care Med 1994; 149:1069–1076.
112. Mezzanotte WS, Tangel DJ, Fox AM, Ballard RD, White DP. Nocturnal nasal continuous positive airway pressure in patients with chronic obstructive pulmonary disease. Influence on waking respiratory muscle function. Chest 1994; 106:1100–1108.

113. O'Donnell DE, Sanii R, Younes M. Improvement in exercise endurance in patients with chronic airflow limitation using continuous positive airway pressure. Am Rev Respir Dis 1988; 138:1510–1514.
114. O'Donnell DE, Sanii R, Giesbrecht G, Younes M. Effect of continuous positive airway pressure on respiratory sensation in patients with chronic obstructive pulmonary disease during submaximal exercise. Am Rev Respir Dis 1992; 138:1185–1191.
115. Younes M, Puddy A, Roberts D, et al. Proportional assist ventilation. Results of an initial clinical trial. Am Rev Respir Dis 1992; 145:121–129.
116. Casaburi R, Patessio A, Ioli F, Zanaboni S, Donner CF, Wasserman K. Reductions in exercise lactic acidosis and ventilation as a result of exercise training in patients with obstructive lung disease. Am Rev Respir Dis 1991; 143:9–18.
117. Foster S, Lopez D, Thomas HM III. Pulmonary rehabilitation in COPD patients with elevated Pco_2. Am Rev Respir Dis 1988; 138:1519–1523.
118. Punzal PA, Ries AL, Kaplan RM, Prewitt LM. Maximum intensity exercise training in patients with chronic obstructive pulmonary disease. Chest 1991; 100:618–623.
119. Johnson AN, Cooper DF, Edwards RHT. Exertion of stair climbing in normal subjects and in patients with chronic obstructive bronchitis. Thorax 1977; 32:711–716.
120. Swinburn CR, Wakefield JM, Jones PW. Performance, ventilation, and oxygen consumption in three different types of exercise test in patients with chronic obstructive lung disease. Thorax 1985; 40:581–586.
121. Wanke T, Formanek D, Lahrmann H, Merkle M, Rauscher H, Zwick H. Inspiratory muscle performance relative to the anaerobic threshold in patients with COPD. Eur Respir J 1993; 6:1186–1191.
122. Ries AL, Ellis B, Hawkins RW. Upper extremity exercise training in chronic obstructive pulmonary disease. Chest 1988; 93:688–692.
123. Martinez FJ, Vogel PD, Dupont DN, Stanopoulos I, Gray A, Beamis JF. Supported arm exercise vs unsupported arm exercise in the rehabilitation of patients with severe chronic airflow obstruction. Chest 1993; 103:1397–1402.
124. Keens TG, Krastins IRB, Wannamaker EM, Levison H, Crozier DN, Bryan AC. Ventilatory muscle endurance training in normal subjects and patients with cystic fibrosis. Am Rev Respir Dis 1977; 116:853–860.
125. Estenne M, Knoop C, Vanvaerenbergh J, Heilporn A, De Troyer A. The effect of pectoralis muscle training in tetraplegic subjects. Am Rev Respir Dis 1989; 139:1218–1222.
126. Simpson K, Killian K, McCartney N, Stubbing DG, Jones NL. Randomised controlled trial of weightlifting exercise in patients with chronic airflow limitation. Thorax 1992; 47:70–75.
127. Orenstein DM, Franklin BA, Doershuk CF, et al. Exercise conditioning and cardiopulmonary fitness in cystic fibrosis. The effects of a three-month supervised running program. Chest 1981; 80:392–398.
128. Lake FR, Henderson K, Briffa T, Openshaw J, Musk AW. Upper-limb and lower-limb exercise training in patients with chronic airflow obstruction. Chest 1990; 97:1077–1082.

129. Niederman MS, Clemente PH, Fein AM, et al. Benefits of a multidisciplinary pulmonary rehabilitation program. Improvements are independent of lung function. Chest 1991; 99:798–804.
130. ZuWallack RL, Patel K, Reardon JZ, Clark BA III, Normandin EA. Predictors of improvement in the 12-minute walking distance following a six-week outpatient pulmnary rehabilitation program. Chest 1991; 99:805–808.
131. Pardy RL, Rivington RN, Despas PJ, Macklem PT. Inspiratory muscle training compared with physiotherapy in patients with chronic airflow limitation. Am Rev Respir Dis 1981; 123:421–425.
132. Reardon J, Awad E, Normandin E, Vale F, Clark B, ZuWallack RL. The effect of comprehensive outpatient pulmonary rehabilitation on dyspnea. Chest 1994; 105:1046–1052.
133. Couser JI, Martinez FJ, Celli BR. Pulmonary rehabilitation that includes arm exercise reduces metabolic and ventilatory requirements for simple arm elevation. Chest 1993; 103:37–41.
134. Robinson EP, Kjeldgaard JM. Improvement in ventilatory muscle function with running. J Appl Physiol 1982; 52:1400–1406.
135. Yerg YE II, Seals DR, Hagberg JM, Holloszy JO. Effect of endurance training on ventilatory function in older individuals. J Appl Physiol 1985; 58:791–794.
136. Clanton TL, Dixon GF, Drake J, Gadek JE. Effects of swim training on lung volumes and inspiratory muscle conditioning. J Appl Physiol 1987; 62:39–46.
137. Miller WF. A physiologic evaluation of the effects of diaphragmatic breathing training in patients with chronic pulmonary emphysema. Am J Med 1954; 17:471–484.
138. Belman MJ, Kendregan BA. Physical training fails to improve ventilatory muscle endurance in patients with chronic obstructive pulmonary disease. Chest 1982; 81:440–443.
139. Barach AL, Beck GJ. The ventilatory effects of the head-down position in pulmonary emphysema. Am J Med 1954; 16:55–60.
140. Gaensler EA, Carter MG. Ventilation measurements in pulmonary emphysema treated with pneumoperitoneum. J Lab Clin Med 1950; 35:945–959.
141. Kory RC, Roehm DC, Meneeley GR, Goodwin RA Jr. Pulmonary function and circulatory dynamics in artificial pneumoperitoneum. II. Studies on patients with pneumoperitoneum as a therapeutic measure in emphysema. Dis Chest 1953; 23:608–620.
142. Breslin EH. The pattern of respiratory muscle recruitment during pursed-lip breathing. Chest 1992; 101:75–78.
143. Gregg BL. Inspiratory muscle training with a weighted incentive spirometer in subjects with chronic airways obstruction. Respir Care 1989; 34:860–867.
144. Sinclair JD. The effect of breathing exercises in pulmonary emphysema. Thorax 1955; 10:246–249.
145. Gimenez M, Uffholtz H, Ferrara G, Plouffe P, Lacoste J. Exercise training with oxygen supply and directed breathing in patients with chronic airway obstruction. Respiration 1979; 37:157–166.
146. Casciari RJ, Fairshter RD, Harrison A, Morrison JT, Blackburn C, Wilson AF.

Effects of breathing retraining in patients with chronic obstructive pulmonary disease. Chest 1981; 79:393–398.
147. Ioli F, Donner CF, Fracchia C. Transdiaphragmatic pressure in the assessment of diaphragmatic and abdominal breathing exercise. Bull Eur Physiopathol Respir 1982; 18 (Suppl 4):177–180.
148. Merrick J, Axen K. Inspiratory muscle function following abdominal weight exercises in healthy subjects. Phys Ther 1981; 61:651–656.
149. Holliday JE, Hyers TM. The reduction of weaning time from mechanical ventilation using tidal volume and relaxation biofeedback. Am Rev Respir Dis 1990; 141:1214–1220.
150. Delk KK, Gevirtz R, Hicks DA, Carden F, Rucker R. The effects of biofeedback assisted breathing retraining on lung functions in patients with cystic fibrosis. Chest 1993; 105:23–28.
151. Austin JHM, Ausubel P. Enhanced respiratory muscular function in normal adults after lessons in proprioceptive musculoskeletal education without exercises. Chest 1992; 102:486–490.
152. Leith DE, Bradley M. Ventilatory muscle strength and endurance training. J Appl Physiol 1976; 41:508–516.
153. Belman MJ, Gaesser GA. Ventilatory muscle training in the elderly. J Appl Physiol 1988; 64:899–905.
154. Belman MJ, Mittman C. Ventilatory muscle training improves exercise capacity in chronic obstructive pulmonary disease patients. Am Rev Respir Dis 1980; 121:273–280.
155. Levine S, Weiser P, Gillen J. Evaluation of a ventilatory muscle endurance training program in the rehabilitation of patients with chronic obstructive pulmonary disease. Am Rev Respir Dis 1986; 133:400–406.
156. Ries AL, Moser KM. Comparison of isocapnic hyperventilation and walking exercise training at home in pulmonary rehabilitation. Chest 1986; 90:285–289.
157. Pardy RL, Rochester DF. Respiratory muscle training. Semin Respir Med 1992; 13:53–62.
158. Fanta CH, Leith DE, Brown R. Maximal shortening of inspiratory muscles: effect of training. J Appl Physiol 1983; 54:1618–1623.
159. Tzelepis GE, Vega DL, Cohen ME, McCool FD. Lung volume specificity of inspiratory muscle training. J Appl Physiol 1994; 77:789–794.
160. Tzelepis GE, Vega DL, Cohen ME, Fulambarker AM, Patel KK, McCool FD. Pressure-flow specificity of inspiratory muscle training. J Appl Physiol 1994; 77:795–801.
161. Redline S, Gottfried SB, Altose MD. Effects of changes in inspiratory muscle strength on the sensation of respiratory force. J Appl Physiol 1991; 70:240–245.
162. Suzuki S, Yoshiike Y, Suzuki M, Akahori T, Hasegawa A, Okubo T. Inspiratory muscle training and respiratory sensation during treadmill exercise. Chest 1993; 104:197–202.
163. Lecoq A, Delhez L, Janssens F, Petit JM. Reentrainement de la fonction motrice ventilatoire chez des insuffisants respiratoires chroniques. Acta Tub Pneum Belg 1970; 61:63–69.

164. Chen H-I, Dukes R, Martin BJ. Inspiratory muscle training in patients with chronic obstructive pulmonary disease. Am Rev Respir Dis 1985; 131:251–255.
165. Belman MJ, Shadmehr R. Targeted resistive ventilatory muscle training in chronic obstructive pulmonary disease. J Appl Physiol 1988; 65:2726–2735.
166. Larson JL, Kim MJ, Sharp JT, Larson DA. Inspiratory muscle training with a pressure threshold breathing device in patients with chronic obstructive pulmonary disease. Am Rev Respir Dis 1988; 138:689–696.
167. Gross D, Ladd HW, Riley EJ, Macklem PT, Grassino A. The effect of training on strength and endurance of the diaphragm in quadriplegia. Am J Med 1980; 68:27–35.
168. Harver A, Mahler DA, Daubenspeck JA. Targeted inspiratory muscle training improves respiratory muscle function and reduces dyspnea in patients with chronic obstructive pulmonary disease. Ann Intern Med 1989; 111:117–124.
169. Preusser BA, Winningham ML, Clanton TL. High- vs low-intensity inspiratory muscle training in patients with COPD. Chest 1994; 106:110–117.
170. Sawyer EH, Clanton TL. Improved pulmonary function and exercise tolerance with inspiratory muscle conditioning in children with cystic fibrosis. Chest 1993; 104:1490–1497.
171. Asher MI, Pardy RL, Coates AL, Thomas E, Macklem PT. The effects of inspiratory muscle training in patients with cystic fibrosis. Am Rev Respir Dis 1982; 126:855–859.
172. Noseda A, Carpiaux JP, Vandeput W, Prigogine T, Schmerber J. Resistive inspratory muscle training and exercise performance in COPD patients. A comparative study with conventional breathing retraining. Bull Eur Physiopathol Respir 1987; 23:457–463.
173. Flynn MG, Barter CE, Nosworthy JC, Pretto JJ, Rochford PD, Pierce RJ. Threshold pressure training, breathing pattern, and exercise performance in chronic airflow obstruction. Chest 1989; 95:535–540.
174. Weiner P, Azgad Y, Ganam R. Inspiratory muscle training combined with general exercise reconditioning in patients with COPD. Chest 1992; 102:1351–1356.
175. Lisboa C, Munoz V, Beroiza T, Leiva A, Cruz E. Inspiratory muscle training in chronic airflow limitation: comparison of two different training loads with a threshold device. Eur Respir J 1994; 7:1266–1274.
176. Smith K, Cook D, Guyatt GH, Madhavan J, Oxman AD. Respiratory muscle training in chronic airflow limitation: a meta-analysis. Am Rev Respir Dis 1992; 145:533–539.
177. Weiner P, Azgad Y, Ganam R, Weiner M. Inspiratory muscle training in patients with bronchial asthma. Chest 1992; 102:1357–1361.
178. Lerman RM, Weiss MS. Progressive resistive exercises in weaning high quadriplegics from the ventilator. Paraplegia 1987; 25:130–135.
179. Aldrich TK, Karpel JP, Uhrlass RM, Sparapani MA, Eramo D, Ferranti R. Weaning from mechanical ventilation: adjunctive use of inspiratory muscle resistive training. Crit Care Med 1989; 17:143–147.
180. DiMarco AF, Kelling JS, DiMarco MS, Jacobs I, Shields R, Altose MD. The

effects of inspiratory resistive training on respiratory muscle function in patients with muscular dystrophy. Muscle Nerve 1985; 8:284–290.
181. Martin AJ, Stern L, Yeates J, Lepp D, Little J. Respiratory muscle training in Duchenne muscular dystrophy. Dev Med Child Neurol 1986; 28:314–318.
182. Estrup C, Lyager S, Noeraa N, Olsen C. Effect of respiratory muscle training in patients with neuromuscular diseases. Respiration 1986; 50:36–43.
183. Wanke T, Toifl K, Merkle M, Formanek D, Lahrmann H, Zwick H. Inspiratory muscle training in patients with Duchenne muscular dystrophy. Chest 1994; 105:475–482.
184. Zack MB, Palange AV. Oxygen supplemented exercise of ventilatory and non-ventilatory muscles in pulmonary rehabilitation. Chest 1985; 88:669–675.
185. Dekhuijzen PNR, Folgering HTM, van Herwaarden CLA. Target-flow inspiratory muscle training during pulmonary rehabilitation in patients with COPD. Chest 1991; 99:128–133.

6

Dyspnea

DONALD A. MAHLER

Dartmouth Medical School
Lebanon, New Hampshire

ANDREW HARVER

University of North Carolina at Charlotte
Charlotte, North Carolina

Over the past two decades there has been a gradual shift in the recognition of the importance of dyspnea in pulmonary rehabilitation medicine. In a comprehensive review entitled "Rehabilitation of Patients with Chronic Obstructive Pulmonary Disease" published in 1976 the term "dyspnea" appeared exactly twice, once in conjunction with recommendations about low-flow oxygen therapy, and in the other instance Lertzman and Cherniack (1) cautioned that "the . . . reduction of dyspnea described in many reports should not be dismissed too lightly." In the summary of the recent National Institutes of Health Workshop on Pulmonary Rehabilitation Research, "dyspnea," the most frequent symptom reported by patients with chronic respiratory disease, is used 48 times (2). In this context dyspnea was acknowledged both as a primary interest in pulmonary rehabilitation research and as a critical component of outcomes assessment. With language much stronger than that used 20 years ago, Fishman (2) proposed that a "decrease in the intensity of dyspnea . . . may be one of the most significant goals for patients in pulmonary rehabilitation."

In this chapter we review briefly the symptom and the language of dyspnea. Clinical instruments and exercise ratings used to measure or quantify the intensity of dyspnea are described. We summarize published studies that have evaluated dyspnea as an outcome in trials of pulmonary rehabilitation. Finally, we present the approach of using dyspnea ratings obtained during exercise testing as a target for patients to monitor their exercise intensity during training. As evident in this review, most published studies of pulmonary rehabilitation involve patients with chronic obstructive pulmonary disease (COPD).

I. The Symptom of Dyspnea

Most discussions on the topic of dyspnea use terms including breathlessness and shortness of breath to characterize the subjective complaint of difficult, labored breathing. For simplicity and the purposes of this chapter, we will use the words "dyspnea" and "breathlessness" as synonyms. However, dyspnea may be conceived of as a broad class of experiences, and separate feelings of tightness, suffocation, heaviness, and other similar physical sensations likely represent unique experiences.

Normal breathing is an unconscious act. But when respiration becomes disturbed, an individual may become acutely aware of inappropriate discomfort or distress associated with breathing. As a sensory experience, dyspnea is frequently compared to the sensation of pain. The experience of difficult, labored breathing is not painful in the usual sense of the word (3), but dyspnea, like pain, is a multidimensional experience, varying along dimensions that are not intuitively obvious (4). Like any other symptom, dyspnea is subjective and apparent only to the affected individual. Like pain, dyspnea is a symptom that frequently signals the need for medical attention. However, dyspnea is localized to the cardiopulmonary system (5). The person who experiences increasingly acute episodes of breathlessness, especially on exertion, usually seeks medical evaluation as the severity of the symptom results in reductions in, or limits altogether, performance of daily activities.

The ability of an individual to discriminate the symptom of breathlessness depends on the awareness, the appropriate interpretation, as well as the response to changes in breathing. Individual sensitivity to changes in internal state varies widely, and a considerable literature exists concerned with the perception of physiological sensations (6). Errors in the discrimination process can occur and may result from various cognitive, behavioral, physiological, environmental, and physical events (7). For most individuals the acute onset of intense breathlessness appears life-threatening. But some patients, especially those with asthma, have difficulty recognizing the development of acute bronchoconstriction (i.e., they are "poor perceivers"), and may thereby be "at risk" for serious morbidity and even death (8,9). A particularly critical point is that acute fluctuations in airflow are not always readily perceived. The initial observations of Rubinfeld and Pain (10) demonstrated that some patients report no symptoms despite marked levels of airway obstruction. Additional investigations have confirmed that various patients have difficulty in estimating the severity of airflow obstruction (11,12).

Patients with COPD may readily recognize the presence of exertional dyspnea but they may incorrectly attribute the symptom to "getting old" or "being out of shape." Elderly individuals are likely to assume that mild chronic symptoms are due to aging (13). Once the physiological signal is referenced accurately, however, reactions to the occurrence of symptoms may subsequently serve to modify the presence or level of the sensation and, accordingly, health care decisions. The patient who recognizes increasing shortness of breath on exertion can easily avoid the sensory experience and minimize its impact by a change in behavior (e.g., by using the elevator rather than climbing stairs). Years ago Comroe (14) noted that dyspnea "involves both perception of the sensation by the patient and the reaction to the sensation."

How an individual reacts to the experience of dyspnea may be affected by both motivational and emotional factors (15). Breathing and the perception of breathing sensations are substantially affected by emotions (15). Both anger and anxiety are associated with hyperventilation and the feeling that breathing is hard and fast; depression is associated with hypoventilation and the feeling that breathing is heavy and difficult (16). Emotional quantities are also important in the self-rating of symptoms. Levels of mood, well-being, and distress affect both a person's view of his or her health status and the interpretation of physical sensations. Bodily sensations such as pain or dyspnea may be reactivated under times of emotional stress or may intensify when combined with an emotional interpretation to create more diffuse sensory experiences (5).

The affective component of breathlessness can substantially contribute to the disability experienced by many patients with chronic respiratory disease. Perhaps the most severe consequence of increasing breathlessness is profound reductions in activity. Activity may initiate an unpleasant chain reaction comprised of the interactions among fear, anxiety, and dyspnea that may quickly accelerate and contribute to exercise limitations (5,16–18). The subsequent sedentary life-style may contribute to progressive muscular deconditioning, which leads to greater breathlessness. Because of the fear of eliciting a dyspneic episode, patients may avoid the expression or experience not only of negative emotions such as anger and anxiety, but also of positive emotions such as euphoria and general excitement (5).

II. The Language of Breathlessness

Many patients find it difficult to describe their physical sensations, and they vary in terms of the accuracy or precision of their reports, particularly in the description of the causes of their symptoms (19). Because symptoms are private and subjective events, we depend on the verbal reports of persons to characterize the nature of their experience. Various descriptions of the sensation of dyspnea by patients convey an extremely heterogeneous set of experiences, which can be differentially influenced by the underlying pathophysiology. For example, patients with dyspnea may complain of uncomfortable sensations arising from the chest or lungs, an inability to get enough air in, chest tightness, or chest congestion. In addition, the experience of dyspnea may occur in parallel with multiple, collateral sensations. The simultaneous presence of fatigue, numbness, headache, tingling, pain, exhaustion, muscular aching, apprehension, or dizziness further increases the range of symptom reports (19).

A variety of descriptors have been used by clinicians and researchers to refer to a complex sensation that involves a range of qualities and attributes. Such attempts illustrate the complexity of experiences assumed by the word "dyspnea." For example, Comroe (20), described five types of breathlessness, including awareness of increased ventilation, hindered breathing, suffocation, shortness of breath ("harder to get one's breath"), and the sensation at the breaking point of breath holding. Guz (21) described four different types of respiratory sensations, including breath-holding sensations, irritation of the tracheobronchial tree, obstructed breathing, and the inability to get in enough air. Campbell and Guz (22) emphasized four elemental sensations of chest tightness or irritation, awareness of excessive ventilation, excessive frequency of breathing, and difficulty in the act of breathing that "singly or in combination underlie breathlessness." Although many of the several meanings of dyspnea include the role of increased ventilation, breathlessness is clearly associated with an "unpleasant" (3,14) or "uncomfortable" (14) experience for most affected individuals.

Recently, Simon and colleagues (23) demonstrated that normal volunteers in whom dyspnea was induced by various stimuli (e.g., breath holding, CO_2 inhalation, breathing with a resistive load) could distinguish different sensations of breathlessness. In a subsequent report Simon et al. (24) studied 53 patients with seven different conditions who selected descriptions that applied to their "uncomfortable awareness of breathing" from among a list of 19 descriptors. These investigators showed that the different descriptors grouped into 14 discrete clusters and that various descriptors were preferred by patients with different types of cardiorespiratory abnormalities. For example, the 16 patients with COPD chose the phrases "my breathing requires effort" and "my breathing requires more work"—which characterize the cluster *work*—and, "I feel a hunger for more air," "I feel out of breath," and "I cannot get enough air"—which characterize the cluster *hunger*—to describe their sense of breathlessness. Each disease was associated with a unique set of clusters, suggesting that the composite of sensations that comprise the experience of dyspnea varies reliably with specific pathophysiological conditions (Table 1). The observations of Elliott and colleagues (25) are consistent with these expectations. They reported

Table 1 Descriptors of Dyspnea in Patients with Various Cardiorespiratory Diseases

Cluster	PVD	NM	CHF	ILD	A	COPD
1. Rapid	—		—			
2. Exhalation					—	
3. Shallow		—				
4. Work		—		—	—	—
5. Suffocating			—			
6. Hunger			—			—
7. Tight					—	

PVD = pulmonary vascular disease ($n=6$); NM = neuromuscular disease ($n=5$); CHF = congestive heart failure ($n=5$); ILD = interstitial lung disease ($n=9$); A = asthma ($n=7$); COPD = chronic obstructive pulmonary disease ($n=16$).
Source: From Ref. 24, with permission.

on the selection of descriptors by 169 patients of breathing discomfort related to exertion. A cluster analysis revealed that: patients with COPD identified distress; those with asthma selected wheeziness; patients with restrictive disease reported rapid breathing; and the group with cardiac disease described a need to sigh (25). Prospective application of the shortened list of 15 descriptors developed by Simon et al. (24) has been reported in two preliminary investigations involving 82 patients (26,27). These observations, summarized in Table 2, virtually replicate the work of Simon and colleagues (24) and provide additional support that predictable differences may exist for sensations of dyspnea experienced by patients with diverse respiratory diseases. Possibly, extensions of this line of research may be useful to examine the mechanisms of breathlessness and to assist the health care provider in establishing a specific diagnosis.

III. Measurement of Dyspnea

A. Clinical Instruments

Clinical ratings of dyspnea provide information that characterizes or relates the condition of patients with respiratory disease independent of physiological function (28,29). Over the past 40 years a variety of clinical instruments have been developed for measuring or quantifying dyspnea (30,31). Based on measurement criteria and current clinical practice, different instruments are appropriate for either acute or chronic evaluation of breathlessness. For an acute evaluation (e.g., to assess an intervention over a brief time period) the visual analog scale (VAS) or the category-ratio 0–10 scale (CR-10) is most commonly used. The VAS is a horizontal or vertical line, usually 100 mm in length, that

Table 2 Preliminary Data that Characterize Descriptors of "Uncomfortable Awareness of Breathing" with Activities

Disease	*n*	Cluster	Descriptor (% of patients[a])
Asthma[b]	18	Work	"Feel out of breath" (39%)
			"Cannot get enough air" (39%)
		Tight	"Chest feels tight" (39%)
COPD[b]	45	Work	"Feel out of breath" (60%)
			"Requires effort" (47%)
			"Requires more work" (33%)
ILD[c]	19	Work	"Feel out of breath" (58%)
			"Requires effort" (32%)
			"Breathing is rapid" (32%)
		Hunger	"Cannot get enough air" (32%)

Each patient selected items from a list of 15 descriptors of breathlessness developed by Simon et al. (24) and then chose the "best three" that applied to his/her experience. A k means cluster analysis was performed to identify groupings of these descriptors.
[a]percentage of patients who identified these descriptors as one of the "best three" that applied to their breathing difficulty
Source: (b) From Ref. 26. (c) From Ref. 27.

is frequently anchored at each end by the descriptors "no breathlessness" and "greatest breathlessness" (Fig. 1) (32). By requesting patients to place a mark on the line that reflects their subjective experience, the physician can use the VAS to grade the intensity of dyspnea associated with a specific task or activity. The CR-10 scale developed by Borg (33) consists of verbal descriptors adjacent to specific numbers; the spacing of the numbers and corresponding descriptors essentially provides a category scale with ratio properties. Figure 2 depicts a modified CR-10 scale for the measurement of dyspnea. A rating above 10 can be used to represent more severe dyspnea than the individual has ever previously experienced. Written instructions are important for the patient to read prior to using either of the two scales.

Another approach to assess an acute change (increase or decrease) in the intensity of respiratory sensation is a category scale with descriptors corresponding to a range of values (+5 to −5) that reflect "markedly harder" to "markedly easier" breathing (Fig. 3) (34). For example, a patient could indicate whether breathing was easier, harder, or the same following a specific intervention by selecting a number on the scale. An advantage of this instrument is that it incorporates a spectrum of possible responses to assess transient changes in dyspnea.

For chronic evaluation of dyspnea (i.e., to observe changes or to assess an intervention over a sustained time period such as weeks or months), multidi-

Figure 1 Visual analog scale for measuring dyspnea. (From Ref. 32, with permission.)

0	Nothing at all
0.5	Very, very slight (just noticeable)
1	Very slight
2	Slight (light)
3	Moderate
4	Somewhat severe
5	Severe (heavy)
6	
7	Very severe
8	
9	
10	Very, very severe (almost max)
•	Maximal

Figure 2 Modified 0–10 category-ratio scale for measuring dyspnea.

mensional instruments such as the Baseline (BDI) and Transition (TDI) Dyspnea Indexes or the dyspnea component of the Chronic Respiratory Questionnaire (CRQ) are recommended. In 1984 Mahler et al. (35) developed the BDI/TDI, which includes three dimensions that affect breathlessness: functional impairment, magnitude of task, and magnitude of effort. Each dimension is com-

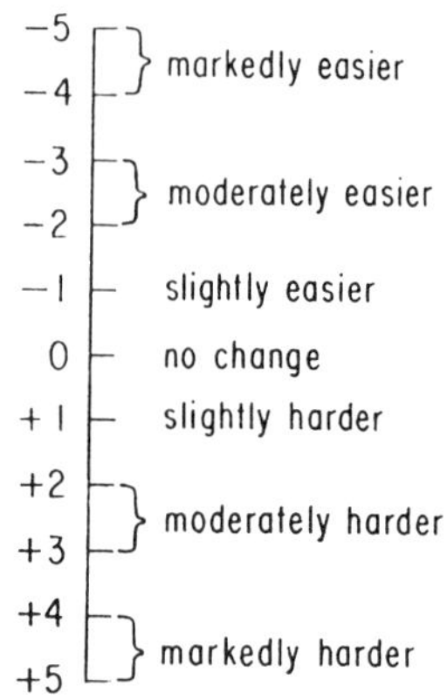

Figure 3 +5 to −5 category scale for measuring dyspnea. A positive score indicates breathing was easier and a negative score indicates breathing was harder. (From Ref. 34, with permission.)

prised of five grades or levels (Table 3). An interviewer selects a grade for each dimension based on the patient's responses to questions as part of the medical history. The TDI includes specific criteria for changes in dyspnea for each dimension compared to an initial or baseline state. In 1987 Guyatt and colleagues (36) devised the CRQ, a quality of life instrument designed specifically for use in patients with lung disease. The CRQ evaluates four components of functional status including dyspnea, fatigue, emotional function, and mastery (the extent to which a patients feels control over the disease and its effects). For the dyspnea evaluation, patients indicate the severity of dyspnea using a 1–7 scale for the five most important activities that affect their daily lives (Table 4).

The validity, reliability, and responsiveness of the VAS, the CR-10, the Baseline and Transition Dyspnea Indices, and the CRQ component to measure dyspnea in patients with respiratory disease have been demonstrated (30,31,37). However, the exact relationship between dyspnea and everyday activities, and between dyspnea and more general assessment of health status, requires additional investigation (38,39). Because the measurement of dyspnea provides independent information that complements physiological data, we encourage clinicians and investigators to apply routinely one or more of these instruments to quantify dyspnea in patients.

B. Exercise Ratings

Exercise testing simulates the physical challenges of daily activities that may provoke breathlessness in a patient. More importantly, it provides an opportu-

Table 3 Dyspnea Indexes

Component	Grade
Baseline Dyspnea Index (BDI)	
Functional impairment	0 to 4
Magnitude of task	0 to 4
Magnitude of effort	0 to 4
BDI Focal Score	0 to 12
Transition Dyspnea Index (TDI)	
Change in functional impairment[a]	−3 to +3
Change in magnitude of task[a]	−3 to +3
Change in magnitude of effort[a]	−3 to +3
TDI Focal Score	−9 to +9

An interviewer selects a grade for each component of dyspnea based on the patient's responses to questions as part of the medical history.
[a]Change from baseline state.

nity to measure physiological responses as well as the perception of sensations in a controlled environment. Dyspnea ratings during exercise, in both healthy individuals and patients with respiratory disease, vary over a wide range (40). Many investigators have focused on ratings of dyspnea at peak exercise. In practice, most patients select submaximal values (e.g., 5–8 on the CR-10 scale) for the intensity of dyspnea at peak exercise performance (40–45), and peak ratings of dyspnea are similar regardless of the type of chronic respiratory disease (e.g., asthma, COPD, or interstitial lung disease). For most patients with severe COPD, dyspnea is reported to be the major "limiting" symptom in performing daily activities. In contrast, Killian et al. (40) have demonstrated that during actual exercise testing patients with mild to moderate COPD frequently report that leg discomfort/effort is more severe than breathlessness.

However, measurement of ratings at peak exertion provides limited information. For example, Figure 4 shows dyspnea ratings during two different progressive incremental exercise tests in a patient with COPD before and after completion of a rehabilitation program that included exercise training. Although there is no difference in peak ratings of dyspnea, ratings at comparable submaximal work intensities are lower after reconditioning. This illustration demonstrates the value of considering a continuum of dyspnea responses. In this way, the principles of psychophysics can be applied to examine a stimulus-response relationship. Although the exact stimulus for dyspnea during exercise is unknown, it is reasonable to consider that either the work performed, or power produced, during exercise is a general stimulus for breathlessness

Table 4 Dyspnea Component of Chronic Respiratory Questionnaire (CRQ)

A. Patient determines 5 most important activities that cause dyspnea and affect daily life by:
   1. self-selection
   2. review of a list of 26 activities (e.g., bending, eating, cleaning, shopping)

B. For each activity severity of dyspnea is measured using a 1 ("extremely short of breath") to 7 ("not at all short of breath") scale

Activity	*Score*
A	1–7
B	1–7
C	1–7
D	1–7
E	1–7
CRQ dyspnea score	5–35

(42,46). Dyspnea ratings can be compared at similar time periods or at similar work intensities; alternatively, the slope and intercept of the power-dyspnea relationship can be calculated to summarize the magnitude of data obtained during a progressive incremental exercise test (46). For example, Silvestri et al. (47) showed that the slope of the power-dyspnea relationship was significantly greater in 20 patients with symptomatic moderate to severe COPD compared with 20 healthy subjects of similar age (Fig. 5), although there was no difference when power was calculated as a percentage of maximal exercise capacity.

Reliability and responsiveness of dyspnea ratings during exercise are important measurement criteria that require further investigation.

IV. Dyspnea as an Outcome in Pulmonary Rehabilitation

Although the results from observational studies have revealed improvements in the sensation of dyspnea in patients following participation in pulmonary rehabilitation (48–50), only a limited number of randomized controlled trials have examined effects of pulmonary rehabilitation on the severity of dyspnea in symptomatic patients with respiratory disease. In 1977 McGavin and colleagues (51) studied 24 men (12 in an exercise group and 12 in a control group) with chronic bronchitis in a 3-month trial of unsupervised progressive stair-climbing exercises at home. Those in the exercise group exhibited significant improvements in a 12-min walking test and a progressive cycle ergometer task, but comparable changes were not evidenced in the control group. Eight patients in the exercise condition reported that breathlessness "improved" after the study

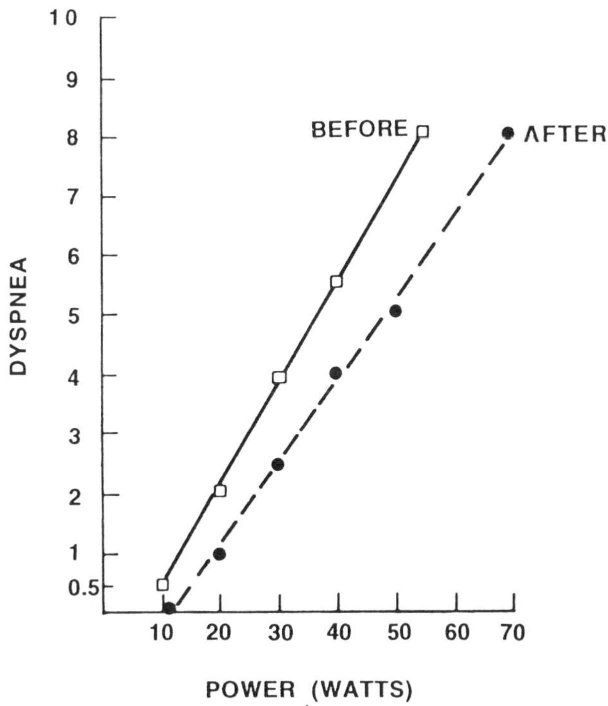

Figure 4 Values for power and dyspnea ratings during two progressive incremental exercise tests in a 67-year-old patient with COPD before (open squares with solid line) and after (closed circles with dashed line) an 8-week exercise training program. Although peak ratings for dyspnea are similar, dyspnea ratings after exercise training are lower at comparable power outputs.

period whereas all 12 patients in the control condition indicated that breathing difficulty had "not improved" (chi square = 9.2; $p < 0.01$). Unfortunately, these investigators did not measure or quantify the level of the patient's dyspnea so it is impossible to assess the actual magnitude of the change in reported breathlessness.

Strijbos et al. (52) randomly assigned patients with COPD to either a therapy group ($n = 30$; $FEV_1 = 49 \pm 5\%$ predicted) or a control group ($n = 15$; $FEV_1 = 9 \pm 9\%$ predicted) to investigate effects of a 12-week pulmonary rehabilitation program involving relaxation exercises, breathing retraining, and reconditioning on exercise tolerance and dyspnea. Subjects rated dyspnea using the CR-10 scale at each workload during incremental exercise testing on a cycle ergometer prior to and upon completion of the program. Significant improvements in exercise tolerance and exertional dyspnea were observed for the pa-

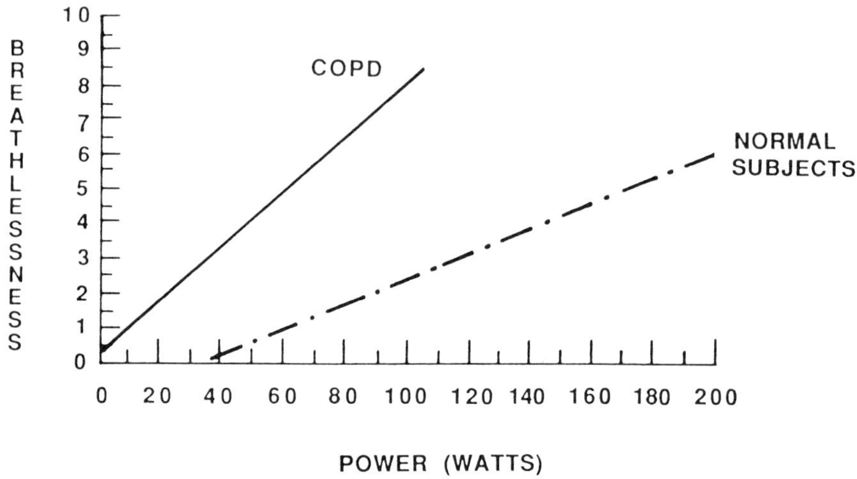

Figure 5 Mean values for breathlessness relative to power production during progressive incremental exercise on the cycle ergometer in 20 male patients with moderate to severe COPD (mean ± SD, age 72 ± 6 years; FEV_1, 35 ± 13% predicted) and 20 healthy male subjects (age 66 ± 7 years) with normal lung function.

tients in the therapy group but not for those in the control group. Specifically, exercise tolerance [maximal workload (Wmax) and 4-min walking distance] increased significantly and there was a marked and significant decrease (from 6.5 ± 1.3 to 4.6 ± 1.7 on the Borg CR-10 scale; $p<0.001$) in dyspnea scores at equivalent workloads (Wmax) before and after treatment (Fig. 6).

The benefits of an intensive (4–5 hr day for a period of 3 months) pulmonary rehabilitation program in patients with asthma or mild COPD were examined by Cox et al. (53). The rehabilitation group consisted of 44 subjects with an age of 43 ± 13 years and an FEV_1 of 68 ± 20% predicted; the control group was comprised of 43 subjects with an age of 44 ± 14 years and an FEV_1 of 69 ± 24% predicted. Physical training consisted of individual and team sports, swimming, walking, cycling, and skill exercises, as well as coordination and relaxation exercises. Patients in the control condition completed the same tests and questionnaires and visited the outpatient clinic as often as the rehabilitation group patients, but were otherwise not involved in the program. Dyspnea was graded from 1 (no complaints) to 5 (severe complaints) for dyspnea in general, at rest, during exercise, and at night (range, 4–20). After 3 months the rehabilitation group showed a slight, but significant, decrease in dyspnea [−1.6 ± 0.4 (mean ± SE) from baseline of 9.2 + 0.4; $p < 0.001$ by paired t-test]. The control group was not tested at this same time period. Covariate analyses showed

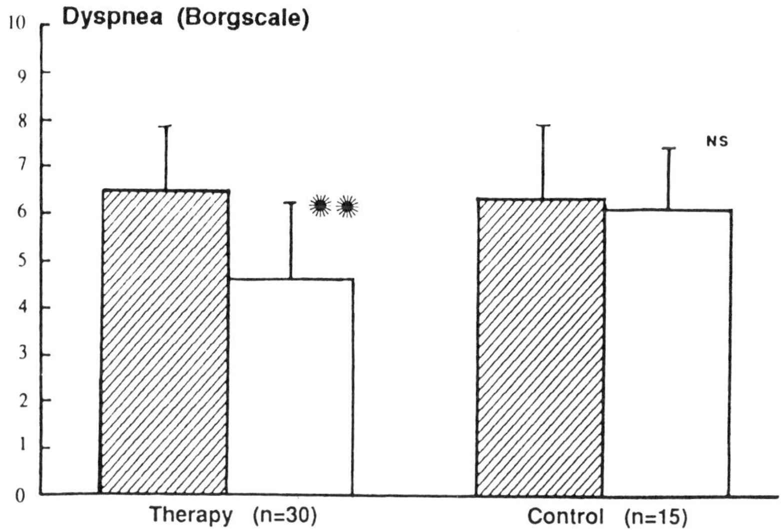

Figure 6 Ratings of dyspnea during submaximal cycle ergometry in patients with COPD before and after a 12-week period in therapy (exercise training) and control groups. There was a significant decrease in dyspnea ratings in the therapy group (noted by asterisks), but no change in the control group (p = NS). (From Ref. 52, with permission.)

a significant decrease ($p<0.05$) in dyspnea scores for the training group (-1.4 ± 0.4) compared to the control group (0.2 ± 0.5) at 6-month follow-up, but the changes in dyspnea were similar for each group at 12 (p=NS) and 24 (p=NS) months. On the other hand, the change in maximal load during cycle ergometry for the rehabilitation group was significantly improved compared to baseline at each measurement period.

O'Donnell et al. (54) reported the benefits of an 8-week multimodality exercise training program in 23 elderly patients with advanced COPD who had a FEV_1 of $38 \pm 10\%$ predicted and 13 age-matched controls who had a FEV_1 of $35 \pm 10\%$ predicted and did not participate in exercise training. The training group showed significant improvements in exercise performance, CR-10 ratings during exercise testing, and clinical rating scales (Table 5). The control group exhibited no significant changes in either exercise tolerance or dyspnea.

The effect of outpatient pulmonary rehabilitation on dyspnea intensity was reported most recently by Reardon and colleagues (55). They evaluated 20 patients assigned randomly to either a treatment group ($n=10$) or a control group ($n=10$). The treatment group evidenced a significant decrease in ratings of dyspnea on a VAS at peak exercise (-24 ± 25 versus 7 ± 19; $p<0.01$) and a higher score (i.e., less breathlessness) on the TDI focal score ($+2.3 \pm 1.1$

Table 5 Ratings of Dyspnea Before and After Exercise Training in Patients with COPD

	Training group ($n=23$, aged 66 ± 7 years)			Control group ($n=13$, aged 70 ± 7 years)		
Dyspnea rating	Before	After	p-value	Before	After	p-value
BDI	5.3 ± 2.5	8.0 ± 2.7	<0.001	4.6 ± 1.3	4.6 ± 1.3	NS
TDI	—	$+2.7 \pm 1.9$	<0.001	—	0 ± 0	NS
MRC scale	2.5 ± 1.1	1.4 ± 0.7	<0.001	2.2 ± 1.0	2.4 ± 1.0	NS
OCD (mm)	40 ± 14	51 ± 14	<0.001	52 ± 12	54 ± 14	NS

BDI = Baseline Dyspnea Index; TDI = Transition Dyspnea Index; MRC = Medical Research Council Scale; OCD = oxygen-cost diagram; NS = not significant.
p-value represents paired t-test comparison of individual values before and after exercise training in each group.
Source: Data obtained from O'Donnell DE (personal communication).

versus $+0.2 \pm 1.8$; $p=0.06$) compared to control subjects following participation in a 6-week rehabilitation program comprised of education, breathing retraining, and physical conditioning.

Recently, Ries et al. (55a) reported that exercise training reduced dyspnea ratings related to daily activities and during submaximal exercise in patients with COPD compared with a similar group randomized to education.

These collective investigations provide consistent demonstrations of both physiological and symptomatic improvements in patients with COPD (although improvements in the two dimensions are not always related) following participation in a pulmonary rehabilitation program that includes exercise reconditioning. What is not clear from these investigations is the possible mechanism(s) underlying the reduction in dyspnea intensity. The mechanisms contributing to improvements in dyspnea are most likely multifactorial and could include reductions in exercise ventilation due to physiological training or enhanced mechanical efficiency, desensitization, increased sense of well-being, or improved emotional state, as well as other cognitive and behavioral factors (56). A formidable challenge in pulmonary rehabilitation research will be the disassociation of the independent, as well as interactive, contributions of these variables to improvement in breathlessness.

V. Dyspnea Ratings for Prescribing Exercise Intensity

Recommendations for exercise training include guidelines for the mode as well as for the frequency, intensity, and duration of activity. In general, determining the appropriate intensity is the most difficult part of writing an exercise prescription for patients with respiratory disease. The usual guidelines for using a target heart rate in healthy individuals or in individuals with cardiac disease do not apply because exercise performance in patients with lung disease is usually limited not by cardiovascular factors, but by diminished ventilatory capacity and/or oxygen desaturation.

In healthy individuals as well as in patients with cardiac disease, ratings of perceived exertion (RPE) have been used as an alternative method for prescribing and regulating training intensity (57–60). Such ratings are closely related to heart rate responses during various kinds of activities (61,62). However, the effort or distress experienced by patients with cardiorespiratory disease during exercise, and reported as overall perceived exertion, may derive from a focus on a single symptom. For example, many patients with severe COPD report dyspnea as the major symptom that limits exercise performance.

Accordingly, it seems reasonable that dyspnea ratings can be used to prescribe exercise intensity for patients with COPD just as RPE are used to prescribe exercise intensity for healthy individuals (63). A preliminary investigation supports the approach of using dyspnea ratings for prescription of exercise intensity in patients with COPD. Horowitz and Mahler (64) studied 15 patients (68 ± 7 years) with moderate to severe COPD (FEV_1, 45 ± 8% predicted) who performed both estimation and production trials. In the estimation trial, patients performed symptom-limited incremental exercise on a cycle ergometer and rated breathlessness each minute using the CR-10 scale. Subsequently, two exercise production targets were selected based on dyspnea ratings corresponding to 50% and 80% of peak oxygen consumption (Vo_2) (Fig. 7). Following this, subjects performed two steady-state production trials based on the 50% peak Vo_2 dyspnea target (1.9 ± 0.9; range, 1–3) and the 80% peak Vo_2 dyspnea target (5.6 ± 1.5; range, 4–8). Using analysis of variance with repeat measures there were no significant differences in Vo_2 values at either intensity for production trials at 1 week and 1 month compared with the estimation trial (64).

There are several advantages to using dyspnea ratings as a target for monitoring the intensity of exercise training in patients with respiratory disease. First, self-monitoring of the intensity of dyspnea is simple and easy for most people. Second, this approach allows patients to continually monitor their breathing during exercise without the need to stop and "check the pulse." Many elderly individuals have difficulty palpating and counting their pulse rate even after instruction and practice. Third, the process of scaling the intensity of dyspnea provides the patient with a specific level of breathlessness that is considered safe and acceptable as part of reconditioning efforts. Finally, self-monitoring of dyspnea has greater application for patients in their performance of daily activities compared with self-monitoring pulse rate.

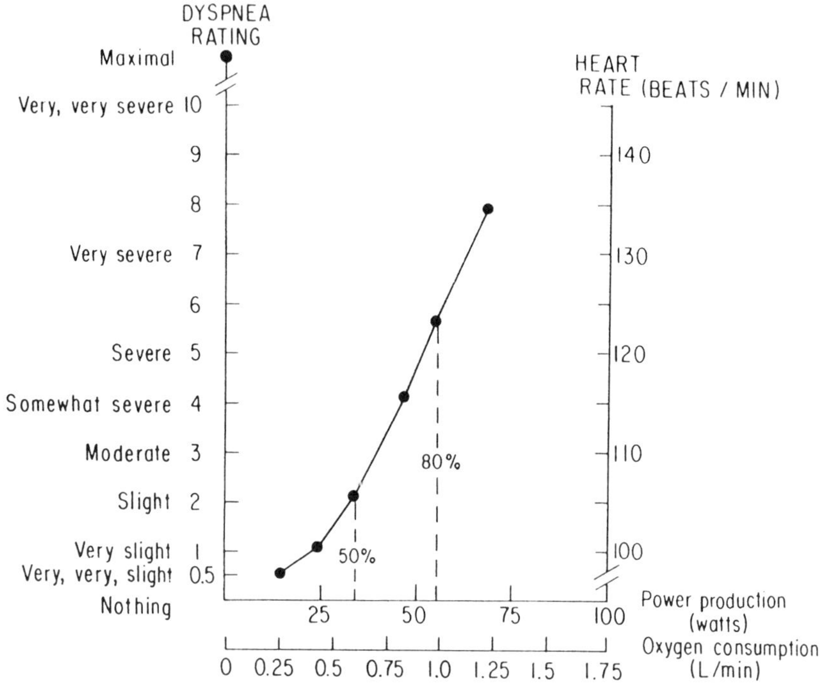

Figure 7 Ratings of dyspnea obtained during a progressive incremental exercise test on the cycle ergometer in a patient with COPD. In this example a dyspnea rating of 2 (slight) corresponded to 50% of peak oxygen consumption (Vo_2), and a dyspnea rating of 6 (severe to very severe) corresponded to 80% of peak Vo_2. These dyspnea ratings were used as targets for achieving an exercise intensity.

VI. Summary and Conclusions

Difficulty in breathing is a distressing experience for patients with chronic respiratory disease. Dyspnea impacts on the patient's ability to perform physical tasks and on quality of life. These circumstances may then direct the physician to recommend that the patient participate in a pulmonary rehabilitation program. In this chapter we have reviewed briefly the phenomenon of dyspnea and highlighted the shift in attention toward dyspnea as an important outcome in pulmonary rehabilitation. The routine measurement of dyspnea using available clinical instruments has been emphasized. Randomized controlled trials clearly demonstrate that pulmonary rehabilitation that incorporates exercise reconditioning reduced the severity of breathlessness in symptomatic patients with COPD (51–55). Furthermore, both clinical experience and preliminary data show that dyspnea ratings can be used as a target by the patient to regulate or monitor the intensity of exercise training.

Additional randomized investigations are needed to address more clearly the mechanisms underlying the subjective improvements in patients who participate in pulmonary rehabilitation programs as well as the relation between changes in dyspnea and changes in affect, cognition, and behavior. The independent contributions of the components of comprehensive programs to subjective improvement, and techniques to enhance the long-term benefits of such programs, should also be considered more fully. In all these efforts the selection of valid and reliable measures of dyspnea is critical. Although there is and will be a need for a variety of assessment tools, a more uniform approach to measuring dyspnea along with other variables could yield numerous benefits, including: providing for direct comparisons among the results of particular programs, establishing the validity of new tools, and specifying the sensitivity of both existing and new instruments.

References

1. Lertzman MM, Cherniack RM. Rehabilitation of patients with chronic obstructive pulmonary disease. Am Rev Respir Dis 1976; 114:1145–1165.
2. Fishman, AP, chairman. NIH workshop summary: pulmonary rehabilitation research. Am J Respir Crit Care Med 1994; 149:825–833.
3. Heim E, Blaser A, Waidelich E. Dyspnea: psychophysiologic relationships. Psychosom Med 1972; 34:405–423.
4. Altose MD. Assessment and management of breathlessness. Chest 1985; 88(Suppl):77S–83S.
5. Dudley DL, Sitzman J, Rugg M. Psychiatric aspects of patients with chronic obstructive pulmonary disease. In: Thompson WL, Thompson TL II, eds. Advances in Psychosomatic medicine. Vol 14. Basel, Switzerland: S Karger, 1985:64–77.
6. Pennebaker JW. The Psychology of Physical Symptoms. New York: Springer-Verlag, 1982.
7. Harver A, Mahler DA. The symptom of dyspnea. In: Mahler DA, ed. Dyspnea. Mt. Kisco, NY: Futura, 1990:1–53.
8. Turcotte H, Boulet LP. Perception of breathlessness during early and late asthmatic responses. Am Rev Respir Dis 1993; 148:514–518.
9. Kikuchi Y, Okabe S, Tamura G, et al. Chemosensitivity and perception of dyspnea in patients with a history of near-fatal asthma. N Engl J Med 1994; 330:1329–1334.
10. Rubinfeld AR, Pain MCF. Perception of asthma. Lancet 1976; 1:882–884.
11. Burdon JGW, Juniper EF, Killian KJ, et al. The perception of breathlessness in asthma. Am Rev Respir Dis 1982; 126:825–828.
12. Orehek J, Beaupre A, Badier M, et al. Perception of airway tone by asthmatic individuals. Bull Eur Physiopathol Respir 1982; 18:601–606.

13. Leventhal EA, Prohaska TR. Age, symptom interpretation, and health behavior. J Am Geriatr Soc 1986; 34:185–191.
14. Comroe JH Jr. Some theories on the mechanism of dyspnoea. In: Howell JBL, Campbell EJM, eds. Breathlessness. Philadelphia, PA: FA Davis, 1966:1–7.
15. Rosser R, Guz A. Psychological approaches to breathlessness and its treatment. J Psychosom Res 1981; 25:439–447.
16. Dudley DL, Martin CJ, Holmes TH. Dyspnea: psychologic and physiologic observations. J Psychosom Res 1968; 11:325–339.
17. Bass C, Gardner W. Emotional influences on breathing and breathlessness. J Psychosom Res 1985; 29:599–609.
18. Greenberg GD, Ryan JJ, Bourlier PF. Psychological and neuropsychological aspects of COPD. Psychosomatics 1985; 26:29–33.
19. Janson-Bjerklie S, Carrieri VK, Hudes M: The sensations of pulmonary dyspnea. Nurs Res 1986; 35:154–159.
20. Comroe JH Jr. Summing up. In: Howell JBL, Campbell EJM, eds. Breathlessness. Philadelphia, PA: FA Davis, 1966:233–238.
21. Guz A. Respiratory sensations in man. Br Med Bull 1977; 33:175–177.
22. Campbell EJM, Guz A. Breathlessness. In: Hornbein TF, ed. Regulation of Breathing. Part II. New York: Marcel Dekker, 1981:1181–1195.
23. Simon PM, Schwartzstein RM, Weiss JW, et al. Distinguishable sensations of breathlessness induced by normal volunteers. Am Rev Respir Dis 1989; 140:1021–1027.
24. Simon PM, Schwartzstein RM, Weiss JW, Fencl V, Teghtsoonian M, Weinberger SE. Distinguishable types of dyspnea in patients with shortness of breath. Am Rev Respir Dis 1990; 142:1009–1014.
25. Elliott MW, Adams L, Cockcroft A, Macrae KD, Murphy K, Guz A. The language of breathlessness. Am Rev Respir Dis 1991; 144:826–832.
26. Harver A, Mahler DA, Schwartzstein RM, Beck K, Chambers JB. The language of breathlessness: a prospective evaluation. Am J Respir Crit Care Med 1994; 149(Suppl):A1087.
27. Scott J, Mahler DA, Harver A, Beck K, Schwartzstein RM. Descriptors of breathlessness in interstitial lung disease. Chest 1994; 106(Suppl):156S.
28. Mahler DA, Rosiello RA, Harver A, Lentine T, McGovern JF, Daubenspect JA. Comparison of clinical dyspnea ratings and psychophysical measurements of respiratory sensation in obstructive airway disease. Am Rev Respir Dis 1987; 135:1229–1233.
29. Mahler DA, Harver A. A factor analysis of dyspnea ratings, respiratory muscle strength, and lung function in patients with chronic obstructive pulmonary disease. Am Rev Respir Dis 1992; 145:467–470.
30. Mahler DA, Harver A. Clinical measurement of dyspnea. In: Mahler DA, ed. Dyspnea. Mt Kisco, NY: Futura, 1990:75–126.
31. Eakin EG, Kaplan RM, Ries AL. Measurement of dyspnoea in chronic obstructive pulmonary disease. Qual Life Res 1993; 2:181–191.
32. Aitken RCB. Measurement of feelings using visual analogue scales. Proc Roy Soc Med 1969; 62:989–993.

33. Borg GAV. Psychophysical bases of perceived exertion. Med Sci Sports Exerc 1982; 14:377–381.
34. O'Donnell DE, Sanii R, Giesbrecht G, Younes M. Effect of continuous positive airway pressure on respiratory sensation in patients with chronic obstructive pulmonary disease during submaximal exercise. Am Rev Respir Dis 1988; 138.1185–1191.
35. Mahler DA, Weinberg DH, Wells CK, Feinstein AR. The measurement of dyspnea: contents, interobserver agreement, and physiologic correlates of two new clinical indexes. Chest 1984; 85:751–758.
36. Guyatt GH, Berman LB, Townsend M, Pugsley SO, Chambers LW. A measure of quality of life for clinical trials in chronic lung disease. Thorax 1987; 42:773–778.
37. Guyatt GH, Townsend M, Keller J, Singer J, Nogradi S. Measuring functional status in chronic lung disease: conclusions from a randomized control trial. Respir Med 1989; 83:293–297.
38. Mahler DA, Faryniarz K, Tomlinson D, et al. Impact of dyspnea and physiologic function on general health status in patients with chronic obstructive pulmonary disease. Chest 1992; 102:395–401.
39. Mahler DA, Tomlinson D, Olmstead EM, Tosteson ANA, O'Connor GT. Changes in dyspnea, health status, and lung function in chronic airway disease. Am J Respir Crit Care Med 1995; 151:61–65.
40. Killian KJ, LeBlanc P, Martin DH, Summers E, Jones NL, Campbell EJM. Exercise capacity and ventilatory, circulatory, and symptom limitation in patients with chronic airflow limitation. Am Rev Respir Dis 1992; 146:935–940.
41. LeBlanc P, Bowie DM, Summers E, Jones NL, Killian KJ. Breathlessness and exercise in patients with cardiorespiratory disease. Am Rev Respir Dis 1986; 133:21–25.
42. Mahler DA, Faryniarz K, Lentine TL, Ward J, Olmstead EM, O'Connor GT. Measurement of breathlessness during exercise in asthmatics: predictor variables, reliability, and responsiveness. Am Rev Respir Dis 1991; 144:39–44.
43. Dean NC, Brown JK, Himelman RB, Doherty JJ, Gold WM, Stulbarg MS. Oxygen may improve dyspnea and endurance in patients with chronic obstructive pulmonary disease and only mild hypoxemia. Am Rev Respir Dis 1992;146:941–945.
44. O'Donnell DE, Webb KA. Exertional breathlessness in patients with chronic airflow limitation: the role of lung hyperinflation. Am Rev Respir Dis 1993; 148:1351–1357.
45. Marciniuk DD, Watts RE, Gallagher CG. Reproducibility of incremental maximal cycle ergometer testing in patients with restrictive lung disease. Thorax 1993; 48:894–898.
46. Mahler DA. The measurement of dyspnea during exercise in patients with lung disease. Chest 1992; 101(Suppl.):242S–247S.
47. Silvestri GA, Mahler DA, Lentine T, Olmstead EM, O'Connor GT. Measurement of breathlessness during exercise in patients with COPD and age-matched controls. Am Rev Respir Dis 1993; 147(Suppl):A192.
48. Mall RW, Medeiros M. Objective evaluation of results of a pulmonary rehabilitation program in a community hospital. Chest 1988; 94:1156–1160.

49. Niederman MS, Clemente PH, Fein AM, et al. Benefits of a multidisciplinary pulmonary rehabilitation program: improvements are independent of lung function. Chest 1991; 99:798–804.
50. Reardon J, Patel K, ZuWallack RL. Improvement in quality of life is unrelated to improvement in exercise endurance after outpatient pulmonary rehabilitation. J Cardiopulm Rehab 1993; 13:51–54.
51. McGavin CR, Gupta SP, Lloyd EL, McHardy GJR. Physical rehabilitation for the chronic bronchitic: results of a controlled trial of exercises in the home. Thorax 1977; 32:307–311.
52. Strijbos JH, Sluiter HJ, Postma DS, Gimeno F, Koeter GH. Objective and subjective performance indicators in COPD. Eur Respir J 1989; 2:666–669.
53. Cox NJM, Hendricks JC, Binkhorst RA, van Herwaarden CLA. A pulmonary rehabilitation program for patients with asthma and mild chronic obstructive pulmonary diseases (COPD). Lung 1993; 171:235–244.
54. O'Donnell DE, Webb KA, McGuire MA. Older patients with COPD: benefits of exercise training. Geriatrics 1993; 48:59–66.
55. Reardon J, Awad E, Normandin E, Vale F, Clark B, ZuWallack RL. The effect of comprehensive outpatient pulmonary rehabilitation on dyspnea. Chest 1994; 105:1046–1052.
55a. Ries AL, Kaplan RM, Lindberg TM, Prewitt LM. Effects of pulmonary rehabilitation on physicologic and psychosocial outcomes in patients with chronic obstructive pulmonary disease. Ann Intern Med 1995; 122:823–832.
56. Carrieri-Kohlman V, Douglas MK, Gormley JM, Stulbarg MS. Desensitization and guided mastery: treatment approaches for the management of dyspnea. Heart Lung 1993; 22:226–234.
57. American College of Sports Medicine. Position stand on the recommended quantity and quality of exercise for developing and maintaining cardiorespiratory and muscular fitness in healthy adults. Med Sci Sports Exerc 1990; 22:265–274.
58. Chow RJ, Wilmore JH. The regulation of exercise intensity by ratings of perceived exertion. J Cardiac Rehabil 1984; 4:382–387.
59. Dunbar CC, Robertson RJ, Baun R, et al. The validity of regulating exercise intensity by ratings of perceived exertion. Med Sci Sports Exerc 1992; 24:94–99.
60. Glass SC, Knowlton RG, Becque MD. Accuracy of RPE from graded exercise to establish exercise training intensity. Med Sci Sports Exerc 1992; 24:1303–1307.
61. Borg G. Perceived exertion as an indicator of somatic stress. Scand J Rehabil Med 1970; 2:92–98.
62. Robertson RJ. Central signals of perceived exertion during dynamic exercise. Med Sci Sports Exerc 1982; 14:390–396.
63. Faryniarz K, Mahler DA. Writing an exercise prescription for patients with COPD. J Respir Dis 1990; 11:638–644.
64. Horowitz MB, Mahler DA. Dyspnea ratings for prescribing exercise intensity in patients with chronic obstructive pulmonary disease (submitted for publication).

7

Respiratory Muscle Fatigue

STEVEN G. KELSEN and GERARD J. CRINER

Temple University School of Medicine
Philadelphia, Pennsylvania

The respiratory skeletal muscles, the thoracic ventilatory pump, are required, like the heart, to contract 24 hr a day over a lifetime without deterioration in performance. However, the inspiratory muscles, like skeletal muscle in other parts of the body, under some circumstances, fatigue and fail as pressure and flow generators. Evidence that human respiratory skeletal muscles fatigue was first provided in the late 1970s by Roussos and Macklem in normal subjects in a laboratory setting (1). These investigators demonstrated that strenuous, volitional diaphragm contractions led eventually to mechanical failure of the muscle and decreased ability to generate pressure.

Much has been accomplished since the seminal studies of Roussos and Macklem. A generally accepted definition of respiratory muscle fatigue in the intact human has been developed. The pathogenesis of human respiratory muscle fatigue is largely understood. And finally, the potential role of diaphragm fatigue as a cause of morbidity in the clinical setting has been appreciated.

In this chapter, we will discuss: (1) the definition of respiratory muscle fatigue and its distinction from muscle weakness; (2) techniques used to detect fatigue in humans; (3) the effects of fatigue on the intrinsic contractile properties of the diaphragm; (4) the pathogenetic factors underlying human respiratory muscle fatigue; (5) evidence that respiratory muscle fatigue may occur in a population at high risk, i.e., patients with chronic obstructive pulmonary disease (COPD); and (6) potentially useful approaches to treat respiratory muscle fatigue or prevent fatigue by training the respiratory muscles to enhance their strength and/or endurance.

I. Definitions

Definitions of respiratory muscle fatigue and weakness were developed during a National Institutes of Health workshop attended by leading investigators (2). After much discussion, respiratory muscle fatigue was defined as a loss in the capacity to develop force and/or shorten resulting from muscle fiber activity under load which was reversible by rest. A commonly accepted classification of fatigue based on presumed sites of impaired function within the neuromuscular system is given in Table 1.

In contrast to fatigue, respiratory muscle weakness was defined as impairment in the capacity of a fully rested muscle to generate force (2).

The important operational components of the definition of fatigue involve impaired mechanical output of the muscle and its reversibility with rest. In addition, fatigue-induced mechanical impairment of the muscle function is viewed as developing when the muscle is highly active and generating appreciable levels of force. Recovery from fatigue is generally observed over a short time scale, e.g., minutes to hours. Muscle weakness is commonly caused by muscle fiber atrophy, metabolic derrangements that impair the ability of cross-bridges to generate force (e.g., acidosis or electrolyte abnormalities that affect intracellular calcium flux), or chronic reductions in muscle precontraction length that impose a mechanical disadvantage (e.g., hyperinflation of the thorax and its effects on the inspiratory muscles). Implied in the definition of weakness is the idea that alterations in muscle function are secondary to alterations in muscle structure or lung volume and hence induce changes in muscle function that are more slowly reversible than fatigue, e.g., days to weeks.

In the clinical setting, the distinction between muscle weakness and fatigue is difficult and not easily accomplished. Moreover, as will become apparent in the remainder of this chapter, a close association exists between respiratory muscle weakness and respiratory muscle fatigue. In fact, weak muscles are predisposed to fatigue.

II. Effects of Fatigue on Respiratory Muscle Contractile Properties

Studies in isolated strips of the costal region of the diaphragm, stimulated electrically to contract in vitro, as well as a limited number of studies in intact animals and humans demonstrate the changes shown in Figure 1 (3–20a).

Table 1 Classification of Respiratory Muscle Fatique

I.	Central (i.e., decreases in phrenic motor output mediated by spinal or supraspinal mechanisms)
II.	Peripheral (i.e., fatigue occurring at the level of the muscle itself)
	a. Transmission: failure of mechanisms involved in muscle excitation (i.e., "high frequency" fatigue)
	b. Contractile: failure of mechanisms involved in excitation-contraction coupling or contractile protein function (i.e., "low frequency" fatique)

In both fresh and fatigued respiratory muscle, a single electrically or neuronally induced supramaximal depolarization of the sarcolemma (i.e., stimulus levels 1.2–1.5 times those that produce a maximum compound action potential or mechanical response) initiates the bell-shaped tension waveform shown in Figure 1 (i.e., a twitch). The time from tension development to its peak (i.e., the contraction time) is generally shorter than the time from peak back to baseline (i.e., the relaxation time). Fatigue prolongs the time course of the isometric tension waveform. Contraction and relaxation time are prolonged in the fatigued muscle (7,7a,11,12). Slowing of the tension waveform is thought to result from impaired calcium release from storage sites in the sarcoplasmic reticulum and in its rate of reuptake (13).

Isometric muscle force is a function of the frequency of neuronal firing or the rate of electrically induced depolarizations (7a,18). In both fresh and fatigued muscle, increasing stimulus frequency progressively increases diaphragmatic tension in isolated muscles or transdiaphragmatic pressure in intact subjects (3,7a,8,9,14–17). In contrast to a twitch, the force-frequency curve is

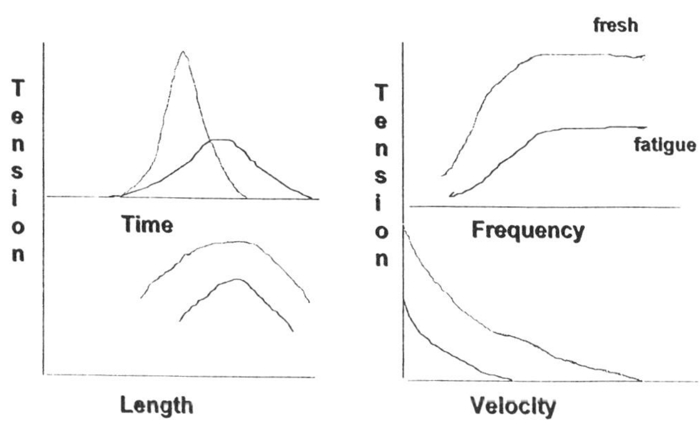

Figure 1 Effects of fatigue on the twitch-tension waveform (upper left), the length-tension relationship (lower left), the force-frequency relationship (upper right), and the isotonic force-velocity relationship (lower right). Responses of fatigued muscle are indicated by lower tracing in each panel.

generated by applying a train of stimuli for approximately 1–2 sec. Instantaneous impulse frequency is steadily increased and the curve generated in Figure I is developed. At stimulus frequencies in excess of 50 Hz, a fully fused tetanic contraction is developed and muscle mechanical output is maximum. Fatigue depresses the force generated at a given frequency. Depending on the nature of the fatigue-inducing regimen, depression of force output can occur at primarily subtetanizing frequencies (e.g., <15–20 Hz), a condition termed low-frequency fatigue, or at frequencies associated with a fully fused tetanus, (i.e., >50 Hz), a condition called high-frequency fatigue. The biochemical and biophysical processes that underlie low-frequency and high-frequency fatigue appear to differ (13,18). At subtetanizing frequencies (i.e., generally <15–20 Hz) muscle mechanical output is primarily determined by the processes of excitation-contraction coupling (e.g., calcium release from the sarcoplasmic reticulum, calcium-troponin interactions). In contrast, muscle force responses to tetanizing frequencies of stimulation (i.e., >50 Hz) are primarily determined by the processes of neuromuscular transmission (e.g., acetylcholine release, sarcolemmal excitability, T-tubular conduction). Accordingly, low-frequency fatigue is thought to reflect impairments in muscle excitation-contraction coupling at the level of either the sarcoplasmic reticulum or binding of activator calcium to troponin. High frequency, on the other hand, is thought to reflect impairment of muscle excitation at the level of the neuromuscular junction or sarcolemma. Of interest, recovery from high-frequency fatigue appears to be shorter (i.e., minutes) than from low-frequency fatigue (i.e., hours) (7a). The two forms of fatigue have different physiological consequences. High-frequency fatigue impairs muscle force output under conditions in which the muscle is maximally driven by the central nervous system (CNS), i.e., when muscle strength is being evaluated. Low-frequency fatigue, on the other hand, impairs force generation during eupneic breathing when phrenic motor unit discharge rates are typically 15–20 Hz (19).

Active isometric force of the respiratory muscles is a function of the extent of actin-myosin contractile filament overlap as reflected in muscle fiber length (i.e., the active length-tension relationship) (14,17,20). That is, active tension increases progressively as fiber length is increased up to an optimum length (i.e., Lo) beyond which active force falls. Fatigue is associated with a downward displacement of the isometric, length-tension relationship (14). At a given fiber length, tension is diminished in fatigued muscles. There is some evidence that low-frequency fatigue may produce preferentially greater reductions in the tension developed at shorter fiber lengths when the activation process in general appears to be submaximal (21). Of note, reduction in the rate of muscle relaxation during fatigue affects the tendency of the muscle to form a fused contraction at a given stimulus frequency. Slowing of the twitch contraction waveform in the fatigued muscle, especially the prolonged rate of muscle relaxation, may displace the force-frequency curve leftward (18). That is, the stimulation frequency required to achieve a fully fused contraction may be lower following fatigue if relaxation time is markedly prolonged. In vivo, changes in the rate of relaxation of fatigued muscle seem to be sensed by the CNS and elicit a slowing in neuronal firing rates in limb muscles during maximal isometric voluntary contractions (18).

Finally, the respiratory muscles do not contract isometrically but rather shorten while contracting against a load. Application of afterloads against which the respiratory muscles contract diminishes the velocity of shortening and converts the energy of cross-bridge cycling into force (i.e., the isotonic force-velocity relationship). The shape of the isotonic force-velocity curve is hyperbolic (22,23). Fatigue diminishes the velocity of muscle fiber shortening against a given load thereby displacing the force-velocity relationship downward (22). However, in general, fatigue produces relatively greater effects on maximum force than on maximum unloaded shortening such that the force-velocity relationship is not symmetrically displaced on the force axis than the velocity axis. These changes indicate that fatigue not only diminishes the load-bearing capacity of the respiratory muscles (i.e., maximum force output), but also slows the velocity of shortening at a given force or load. In the respiratory system, the load against which the inspiratory muscles contract is represented by the inspiratory impedance, a function of respiratory resistance and compliance. Inspiratory impedance changes throughout inspiration in complex fashion. The resistive load progressively decreases while the elastic load progressively increases. Consequently, the inspiratory muscles contract auxotonically in vivo, that is, against a load that increases throughout inspiration as the muscle shortens. The analog of the isotonic force-velocity relationship in the intact organism, i.e., the maximum inspiratory pressure-flow curve, is nearly linear rather than hyperbolic (24,25,25a).

III. Detection of Diaphragm Muscle Fatigue in Humans

Diaphragm muscle fatigue has been diagnosed in the intact human from changes in: (1) the force-frequency relationship of the muscle, (2) the power spectral content of the electromyogram (EMG), and (3) the maximal static inspiratory and expiratory pressures (MIP and MEP, respectively) (9,26–44). These indices used to detect respiratory muscle fatigue and grade its severity are analogous to approaches used to assess limb skeletal muscle fatigue (45,46). As will be seen, the force-frequency relationship and EMG power spectrum analyses are complex and require sophisticated electronics and instrumentation. Consequently, their use has been confined to the research laboratory. On the other hand, the MIP is convenient and easily performed at the bedside but suffers from being relatively nonspecific.

A. The Force-Frequency Relationship

Fatigue decreases the ability of muscle to develop tension at a given stimulus level. Accordingly, the force-frequency relationship represents a way of assessing the mechanical output of a muscle over a wide range of stimulus intensities and, hence, levels of activation. In the force-frequency relationship, the muscle of interest is electrically stimulated and the isometric tension or the mechanical analog, pressure, is assessed. In intact animals and humans, quasi-isometric contractions have been accomplished for the diaphragm by occluding the airway at end-expiration. Since the diaphragm may still shorten considerably despite airway occlusion because of collapse of the ribcage, diaphragm shortening may be minimized by casting the abdomen at functional residual capacity to prevent outward movement of the anterior abdominal wall (21,47,48). (In the case of the sternomastoid muscle, the head and neck are immobilized in a rigid frame and the airway remains open.)

In intact animals or humans, the diaphragm is stimulated electrically via the cervical phrenic nerves using electrodes placed either transcutaneously or percutaneously. Transcutaneous stimulation has the advantage of being noninvasive but requires larger, more easily felt voltage to overcome the high resistance of the skin. Percutaneous stimulation is more comfortable. The evoked diaphragmatic muscle compound action potential may be recorded from electrodes on the anterior rib cage at the 6th or 7th intercostal space in the midclavicular line or endoesophageally. It is considered essential to achieve supramaximal conditions of current or voltage to prevent small changes in electrode resistance or impedance at the electrode-muscle interface from affecting muscle activation.

Since fatigue shifts the force-frequency downward (and possibly to the left), the magnitude of the shift in the force-frequency relationship can be used to assess the severity of fatigue and the time course of recovery. Of interest, depending on the nature of the fatigue paradigm, tension responses may be depressed in response to subtetanizing frequencies (e.g., <15–20 Hz), a process called low-frequency fatigue, to tetanizing frequencies (i.e., >50 Hz), so-called high-frequency fatigue, or to the entire range of stimulus frequencies (7a–10,49). High-frequency fatigue appears to reflect impairment in neuromuscular transmission and muscle excitation at the level of the neuromuscular junction, neurotransmitter release, sarcolemma propagation of an action potential, or charge transfer within the T-tubular system (3,8,13,49,49a). Low-frequency fatigue, on the other hand, appears to reflect impairments in excitation-contraction coupling at the level of the dihydropyridine-sensitive charge sensor in the T-tubular system, the ryanodine-sensitive calcium channel in the sarcoplasmic reticulum, or the binding affinity of activator calcium to tropomyosin (13).

In the respiratory muscles, low- and high-frequency fatigue recover at different rates. In general, full recovery from high-frequency fatigue is generally rapid and requires minutes to 1–2 hr (7a). In contrast, full recovery from low-frequency fatigue in normal subjects, at least, is considerably slower and may require as long as 24 hr (50). The nature of the contraction appears to dictate whether high- or low-frequency fatigue will develop (18).

Electrical stimulation of the muscle of interest has several advantages. It allows the muscle to be activated in response to a standard stimulus without the cooperation of the subject. Hence, alterations in CNS function or decreased effort that may diminish muscle activation, i..e., "central fatigue," are circumvented (10,33,33a,51–53a). Second, electrical stimulation allows muscle mechanical output to be examined over a range of subtetanizing and tetanizing stimulus frequencies and, hence, sheds light on the diverse biophysical/biochemical processes that determine muscle function over a range of activation levels.

Unfortunately, tetanizing stimuli are painful, making this an unpalatable option in unanesthetized subjects. Moreover, current spread of the stimulus activates adjacent muscles in the neck and shoulder girdle. Activation of other respiratory muscles that insert on the chest wall may change chest wall compliance, or the activation of agonist and/or antagonist muscles capable of changing intrathoracic pressure, and hence affect the pressure generated.

A recent development that shows considerable promise is electrophrenic, twitch contraction of the diaphragm (7,33,47,48,54,55). This approach has the advantage over tetanizing stimuli needed to construct the force-frequency relationship in being less painful and well tolerated. In addition, it affords the opportunity of assessing muscle responses to low frequencies of stimulation and hence in theory should be highly sensitive to the presence of low-frequency fatigue. In this method, a single supramaximal pulse of 0.1 msec is applied to the phrenic nerves bilaterally during breath holding at end expiration (Fig. 2). The twitch waveform shown in Figure 1 is used to examine peak diaphragm pressure output and the time course (i.e., contraction and relaxation times) of the transdiaphragmatic pressure (Pdi) waveform. (As is the case with skeletal muscles, prior contraction of the diaphragm to >33% of maximum Pdi elicits contraction-intensity, postcontraction "twitch potentiation" (i.e., 16–70% augmentation of peak twitch height) (56,57). Twitch potentiation is relatively short-lived, however, and generally dissipates within 3 min.)

By combining twitch contraction during breath holding at end-expiration with superimposed twitches applied during the performance of graded inspiratory efforts, the twitch occlusion technique, maximum transdiaphragmatic pressure can be calculated (32,33,47,58). The rationale behind the twitch occlusion pressure is as follows. As a muscle is activated to a progressively greater extent, progressively more motor units are recruited and individual motor units

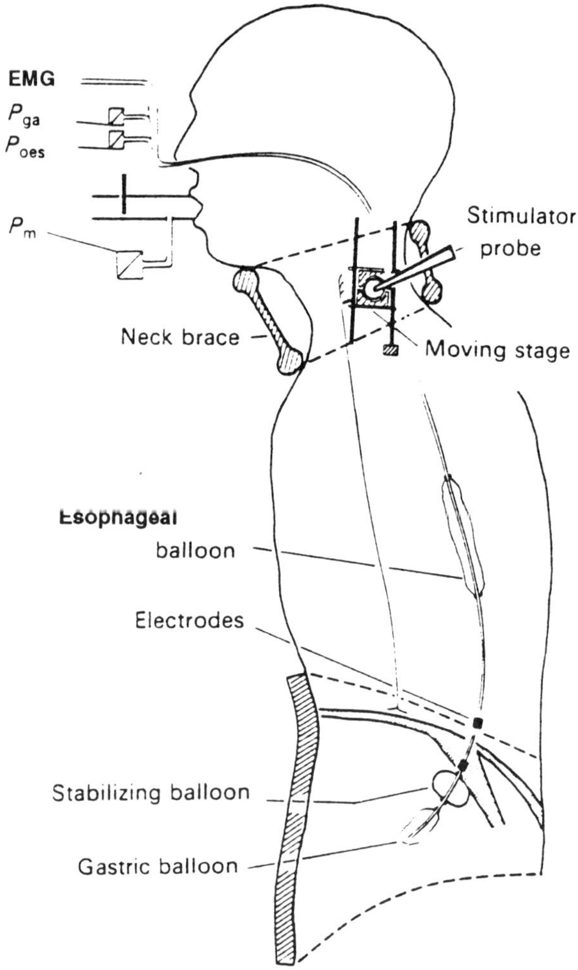

Figure 2 Experimental approach used to perform bilateral electrophrenic stimulation in human subjects. Head and neck are immobilized with a stiff neck collar. Phrenic stimulation is here performed transcutaneously with electrodes held in place with moving stage secured to a neck brace. Diaphragm EMG activity is recorded with an endo-esophageal electrode positioned at the esophageal hiatus. Transdiaphragmatic pressure is measured with balloon-tipped catheters positioned in the esophagus and stomach. Diaphragm descent is minimized by casting the abdomen. (From Ref. 47.)

move up their force-frequency curve toward the plateau. Consequently, the magnitude of the superimposed twitch is inversely proportional to the extent of muscle activation (Fig. 3). When the muscle is maximally activated, that is, all motor units are recruited and on the flat portion of their force-frequency curve, the superimposed twitch will be undetectable or zero. The twitch occlusion technique is analyzed quantitatively by plotting the magnitude of the volitional contraction on the X axis against the magnitude of the superimposed twitch on the Y axis (Fig. 4). The relationship is inversely linear and when extrapolated to the X axis, that is, to zero superimposed twitch, the maximum pressure output of the muscle is determined.

The twitch occlusion technique has been used to assess the intensity of CNS output to the contracting diaphragm during volitional contractions against large external inspiratory resistive loads to exhaustion and during maximum volitional contractions of the rested muscle (32,33,47,58). The data demonstrate that the fresh diaphragm can be maximally activated volitionally but that task performance during prolonged ventilatory loading to exhaustion, that is, the ability to generate a targeted transdiaphragmatic pressure, is in part limited

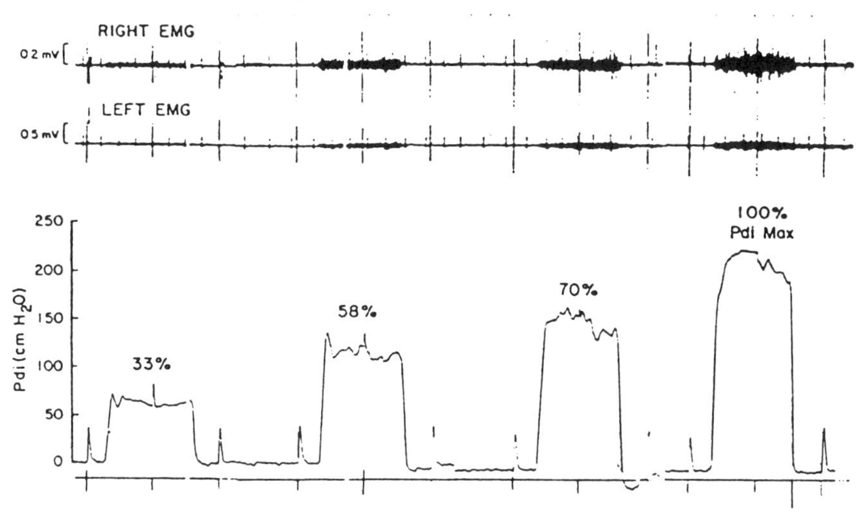

Figure 3 Effect of diaphragm contraction intensity as reflected in the transdiaphragmatic pressure (Pdi) on the diaphragm EMG (top) and magnitude of the superimposed twitch contraction (bottom). Subject is seated and performing progressively more intense combined Mueller-expulsive maneuvers. Vertical dotted lines (top and bottom) mark the time at which stimulus is applied to the phrenic nerves. Note that the superimposed twitch Pdi is greatest when the diaphragm is relaxed at FRC and decreases progressively with increasingly intense volitional efforts from 33% to 100% of maximum. (From Ref. 32.)

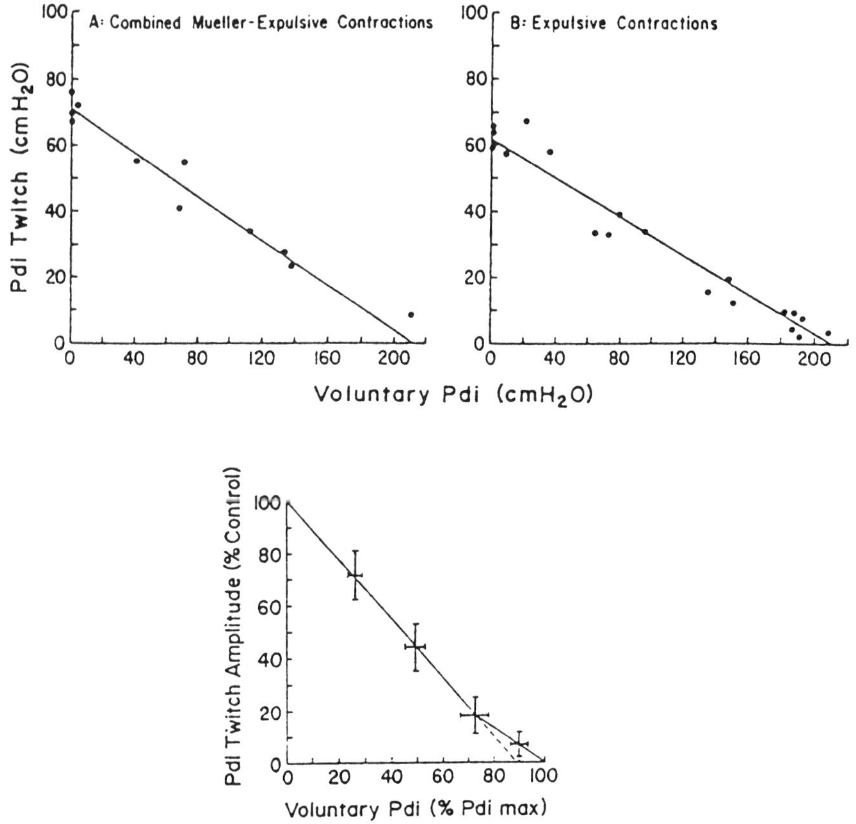

Figure 4 (Bottom) Relationship between the amplitude of the voluntary Pdi and the superimposed twitch contraction during a combined Mueller-expulsive maneuver (A) or expulsive contraction (B) in a single subject. (Top) Pooled data from a group of subjects with voluntary Pdi and twitch Pdi normalized as percentages. Note the inverse linear relationship. Maximum static Pdi is reflected in the X intercept (32).

by a failure of CNS mechanisms to fully activate the muscle, i.e., central fatigue (33).

Reductions in Pdi generated in response to electrical stimulation indicate a decrease in the capacity of the diaphragm to generate force. However, extrapolation of impairments in force output during electrically stimulated contractions to the behavior of the muscle during spontaneous breathing when the muscle is activated by the CNS is problematic. As stressed above, supramaximal electrical stimulation activates the entire motor neuron pool—that is, motoneurons made up of slow- and fast-twitch fibers. In contrast, motor unit recruitment when the diaphragm is activated endogenously during volitional or reflexly driven contractions demonstrates a stereotypic hierarchy (59). During eupneic breathing, only motor units made up of slow-twitch, fatigue-resistant (i.e., type I) muscle fibers are activated (20a,59). As efforts of greater magnitude are made, populations of fast-twitch, oxidative (i.e., type IIa) fibers are recruited followed ultimately by recruitment of fast-twitch, glycolytic (i.e., type IIb) fibers. Of note, the susceptibility to fatigue of the three fiber types demonstrates the following rank order: IIb>IIa>I. Accordingly, eupneic breathing is accomplished by highly fatigue-resistant type I fibers while strenuous efforts approaching maximum involve more easily fatigable types IIa and IIb fibers. The rank order of muscle fiber activation likely accounts for the fact that the diaphragm contracts rhythmically, 24 hr a day for a lifetime and only undergoes fatigue above a critical threshold of activation, i.e., with inspiratory efforts exceeding 40–50% of maximum (see below).

The force and pressure output of the respiratory muscles depends on muscle length and alignment with their origins and insertions on the rigid structures of the chest wall. These, in turn, depend on thoracic volume and, to a lesser extent, thoracic configuration (58,60–69). For the inspiratory muscles, increases in thoracic volume above functional residual capacity (FRC) shorten their precontraction length and unfavorably affect their alignment with their origins and insertions. Consequently, hyperinflation decreases their ability to generate force as well as convert force into changes in intrathoracic pressure. Accordingly, increases in lung volume above FRC impose a mechanical disadvantage on the inspiratory muscles. Conversely, increases in lung volume favorably alter the mechanical advantage of the expiratory muscles and their ability to generate changes in pressure. Changes in thoracic configuration can affect muscle length at iso lung volume, but these effects are relatively small compared to the lung volume effect (64). Accordingly, interpretation of respiratory muscle mechanical output requires knowledge of and, better yet, control of lung volume and thoracoabdominal configuration.

B. The Maximum Static Inspiratory Pressure (MIP)

The MIP performed at residual volume or functional residual capacity against an occluded airway has been used to assess the mechanical output of the inspiratory muscles (26,27,70–75). The MIP provides a global assessment of inspiratory muscle function and is relatively easy to perform. However, this index of inspiratory muscle fatigue has a number of significant limitations. First, since the measurement is volitional and requires maximal activation of the respiratory muscles, MIP depends on subject cooperation and, accordingly, may be reduced simply because of submaximal subject effort (75). Second, MIP reflects the response to a high-frequency stimulus. That is, the muscle must be activated on the flat portion of the force-frequency curve. Because the MIP refects muscle mechanical output in response to "high frequency" stimulation, it cannot detect the presence of low-frequency fatigue, which is believed to be the most important form of fatigue in humans. Finally, MIP depends on the strength and mechanical advantage of the inspiratory muscles and may be similarly reduced in conditions of respiratory muscle weakness or fatigue. Hence, MIP may be diminished in the presence of electrolyte disturbances (e.g., hypocalcemia, hypokalemia, hypomagnesemia, hypophosphatemia), marked undernutrition, or hyperinflation of the chest) (76–79). Nonetheless, a number of studies have helped to elucidate respiratory muscle fatigability using this approach (26,27).

C. The Power Spectral Density

The power spectral content of the amplified, rectified, raw EMG of a muscle can be analyzed by fast Fourier transform to generate the curvilinear relationship shown in Figure 5. In the fresh diaphragm, the power (or voltage) contained in the EMG waveform reaches a maximum between approximately 85 and 105 Hz and thereafter declines (31a,39,52,80,81a). (Maximum power in the EMG of the diaphragm, parasternal intercostal, and sternocleidomastoid occurs at somewhat different frequencies, however.) Fatigue causes a leftward

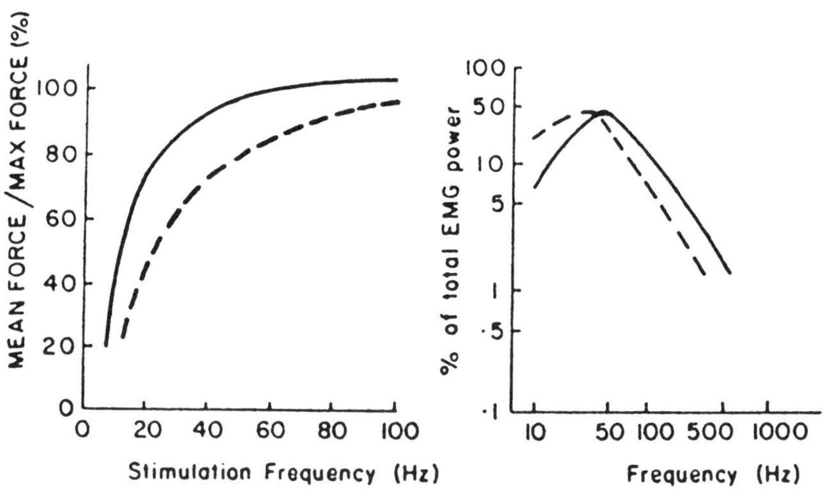

Figure 5 Schematic representation of the power spectral density of a respiratory muscle electromyogram determined by fast Fourier transform. Note the concave appearance of the relationship. Note that fatigue decreases and increases power in the high- and low-frequency domains, respectively, thereby shifting the relationship toward the left. (From Ref. 41.)

shift of the power spectral density of a contracting muscle such that more of the power in the EMG is contained in a lower-frequency domain (9,31a,39,41,52,80). Of note, the power spectral density of the contracting diaphragm changes almost immediately in the setting of fatiguing contractions and considerably before the mechanical output of the muscle fails (9,31,35,41). The diaphragmatic EMG power spectrum can be obtained from the raw EMG of the muscle recorded from surface electrodes on the chest wall or within the esophagus. It is, therefore, relatively noninvasive and well tolerated. Moreover, the EMG power spectrum, unlike maximal static pressure, can be measured continuously, i.e., breath by breath, and does not require subject cooperation.

The effect of fatigue on the spectral content of the respiratory muscles has been assessed in several ways. Initial studies assessed leftward shifts in the power spectrum using band pass filters to partition the raw signal into high-frequency (>125–150 Hz) and low-frequency domains (<50 Hz) (9,35,39,41,43,43a). The integrated activity in the high- and low-frequency domains was taken as a reflection of the position of the spectrum. Since leftward shifts in the spectrum induced by fatigue decrease the EMG power in a high-frequency domain, i.e., >150 Hz, and increase the power in a low-frequency domain, i.e., <50 Hz, the ratio of activity in the >150-Hz range over activity in the <50-Hz range was taken as a reflection of this phenomenon and termed the "high/low ratio." Twenty to 30% reductions in the high/low ratio were taken as evidence of fatigue. This method obviates the need for fast Fourier analysis and, hence, sophisticated computational analysis of the EMG waveform. It can also be assessed real time with relatively inexpensive equipment.

Another method of assessing the spectral content of an EMG signal is via the centroid (or median) frequency, i.e., the frequency at which the power below and above are equal (31,31a,39,43a,44,45,80,81a). The centroid frequency requires sophisticated computational analysis to construct the fast Fourier transform and at present cannot be performed real time. The centroid frequency, unlike the high/low ratio, is a concept based on sound principles of signal analysis, has a lower signal-to-noise ratio, and is more stable than the high/low ratio (33a,43a,45). Changes in the two indices appear to correlate reasonably well, however (31,33a,44).

A significant caveat in the use of the power spectrum is the suggestion that it may be insensitive to the presence of low frequency or peripheral fatigue (41,45). In addition, differences in the power spectrum of the several respiratory muscles introduce the possibility that signal contamination by activity from adjacent muscles may produce false negative or false positive results in the power spectrum recorded from surface electrodes. Bellemare and Grassino found significant variability in the spectrum of the human diaphragm EMG while simultaneously recording with esophageal and skin surface electrodes (35,35a). Recording the diaphragm EMG with surface electrodes on the chest wall produced false positive reductions in the power spectrum of the diaphragm high/low ratio due to inspiratory activity of the overlying abdominal muscles. More recently, Sharp and colleagues have shown that diaphragm centroid frequencies recorded from surface electrodes are consistently lower than simultaneously measured EMG recordings obtained from an esophageal electrode and may fail to reflect reductions in the centroid frequency detected with an esophageal electrode (81,81a). Moreover, although it was initially believed that the EMG signal was unaffected by thoracic volume, a distinct disadvantage of all mechanical indices of respiratory muscle function, it is now clear that the EMG is muscle-length-dependent and, hence, changes with thoracic volume (82,83).

The physiological basis for shifts in the power spectral density of the muscle is not well understood (45,46,51–53,80,84,85). Possibilities include: slowing in action potential conduction velocity along the sarcolemma membrane; reduction in the activity of upper and/or lower respiratory motor neurons with consequent reductions in motor unit firing rate; and greater synchronization of firing of activated motor units. There is strong evidence that the EMG power spectrum may depend primarily on the firing pattern of the bulbospinal respiratory motor neurons in the medulla, which project to the spinal phrenic motor neuron pool (43a,51–53). In fact, the power spectrum may change when central respiratory motor output is heightened even in the absence of fatigue (e.g., hypercapnia in the absence of load) (43a). Moreover, the power spectrum of the diaphragm may increase in response to centrally acting drugs (e.g., the endogenous opiate antagonist naloxone) even when the muscle is fatigued by severe inspiratory ventilatory loads (51–53).

IV. Pathophysiology

A. The Experimental Model

Studies in intact humans designed to examine the pathogenetic mechanisms that lead to respiratory muscle fatigue have largely focused on the diaphragm and have used the experimental approach shown schematically in Figure 6 (1,7a,35,35a). The diaphragm has been the primary focus of attention for several reasons. First, the diaphragm is the major respiratory muscle. Second, anatomical considerations allow the mechanical output of the diaphragm (i.e., transdiaphragmatic pressure) to be assessed easily from measurements of esophageal and gastric pressure. Third, the diaphragm EMG, an index of phrenic motor outflow and fatigue state, can be recorded easily from surface electrodes on the chest wall or within the esophagus. Finally, the cervical phrenic nerves can be electrically stimulated, thereby allowing the mechanical output

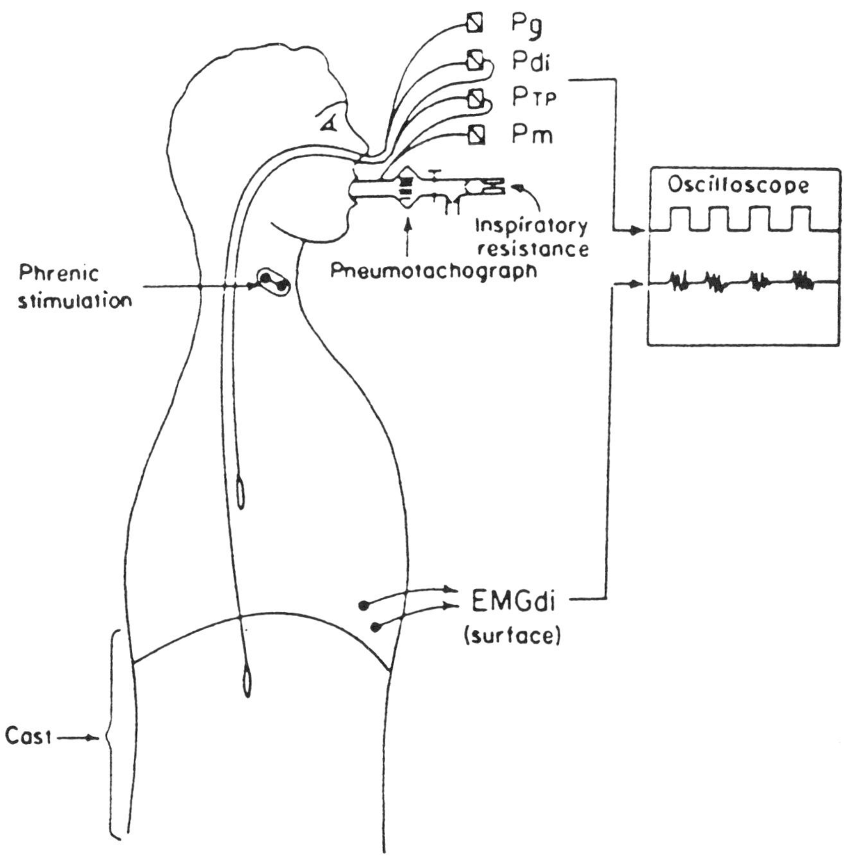

Figure 6 Schematic representation of the experimental approach used to assess diaphragmatic endurance in humans. Subjects inspire through ventilatory loads to produce predetermined Pdi. Pdi generated is measured by catheters in the esophagus and stomach and displayed on an oscilloscope for visual feedback to the subject. Phrenic nerves are stimulated in the neck transcutaneously. Diaphragm EMG is recorded with surface electrode on the lower ribcage. Constancy of lung volume and thoracoabdominal configuration is achieved by monitoring end expiratory transpulmonary pressure (Ptp) and by placing a cast around the abdomen and lower one-quarter of the ribcage. (From Ref. 7a.)

of the muscle to be assessed under standard conditions as well as during volitional contractions.

In most experiments examining diaphragm fatigue, subjects inspire against resistive or threshold ventilatory loads of great magnitude and are instructed to generate target levels of transdiaphragmatic pressure until exhaustion. The level of transdiaphragmatic pressure generated on each breath may be varied by varying the magnitude of the load. Fatigue has been defined as the time point at which mechanical failure of the muscle develops, i.e., the point at which the subject can no longer generate the targeted level of pressure or the power spectrum of the diaphragm EMG changes to a predominance of lower spectral frequency. Similar sorts of studies have been performed with the sternocleidomastoid muscle, which also lends itself to electrical stimulation (29,38).

B. Pattern of Muscle Use

In their seminal studies, Roussos and Macklem (1) observed that the time of onset of task failure for the diaphragm was *not* related either to the magnitude of the phasic inspiratory swings in transdiaphragmatic pressure (Pdi) during loading alone or to maximum transdiaphragmatic pressure (i.e., Pdimax-diaphragm strength) alone. Rather the time of onset of mechanical failure of the diaphragm was a unique curvilinear function of the ratio of Pdi generated on each breath over Pdimax (i.e., Pdi/Pdimax) (Figs. 7, 8). Values of Pdi/Pdimax less than 40–50% could be maintained indefinitely; values greater than this threshold were associated with progressively more rapid ventilatory muscle exhaustion. These results made several important points. First, diaphragm fatigue depended on the relative intensity of contraction, i.e., muscle force output as a percentage of its strength. Second, contractions below some critical threshold could be sustained indefinitely and did not lead to fatigue.

Subsequent studies demonstrated that the experimental end-point, i.e., failure to maintain target Pdi values, did, in fact, reflect mechanical failure of the muscle and was not simply a behavioral phenomenon. Aubier et al. (7a) demonstrated in highly motivated normal subjects that the force-frequency relationship of the diaphragm was depressed over the entire range of tetanizing and subtetanizing stimulus frequencies at the point of task failure signifying the presence of both high- and low-frequency fatigue. Of interest, high-frequency fatigue (i.e., Pdi at 50-Hz stimulation) disappeared within minutes after cessation of loaded breathing, but low-frequency fatigue (Pdi at 20-Hz stimulation) recovered much more slower.

Subsequent studies by Bellemare and Grassino (35,35a) demonstrated that the timing as well as the intensity of diaphragmatic contractions determined the time of onset of mechanical failure of that muscle. Increases in the ratio of the time of contraction of the diaphragm (Ti) over the duration of the total respiratory cycle (Ttot), Ti/Ttot, increased the rapidity of onset of fatigue at any given Pdi/Pdi max ratio (Fig. 9). That is, increasing the duration of diaphragm contraction relative to the period during which the diaphragm is relaxed, the so-called duty cycle of breathing, predisposes the diaphragm to fatigue. In fact, diaphragm fatigue was a unique function of the product of Pdi/

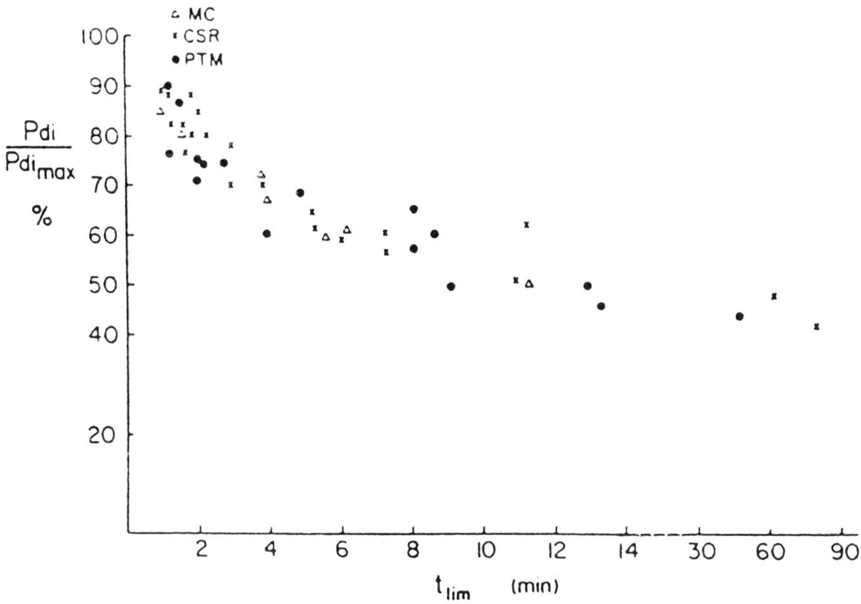

Figure 7 Relationship between the ratio of Pdi during inspiratory resistive ventilatory loading over maximum static Pdi (i.e., Pdi/Pdimax (ordinate) and the time of onset of mechanical failure of the diaphragm, t_{lim} (abscissa) in three normal subjects. Data from individual subjects are shown as separate symbols. Note the curilinear nature of the relationship with apparent asymtote between 40 to 50% Pdi/Pdimax. Note also the break in the abscissa at 14 min. (From Ref. 1.)

Pdimax times Ti/Ttot, which has been termed the diaphragm pressure-time (PTI) or tension-time (TTI) index, and is, in essence, the integrated area under the pressure waveform over time (Fig. 10). This representation of the pressure-time relationship correlated closely with: (1) the time of onset of mechanical failure of the diaphragm; (2) respiratory muscle oxygen consumption (86,86a); and (3) the rate of change in the power spectral density of the diaphragm. That is, the greater the diaphragm PTI, the greater the oxygen uptake and the greater the fall in the power spectral density. A threshold was noted for the PTI of approximately 15–20% of maximum (Fig. 10). Above 15–20% of maximum, the diaphragm fatigued. Below this value, fatigue did not ensue (Fig. 11). These results are qualitatively similar to those observed in limb muscles and indicate that the intensity of contraction assessed from both the magnitude *and* duration of pressure swings determines muscle energy utilization. Of interest, contracting at 70–80% maximum isometric tension, the rate of fall of isometric tension and changes in muscle ATP, phosphocreatine, glycogen, and lactate

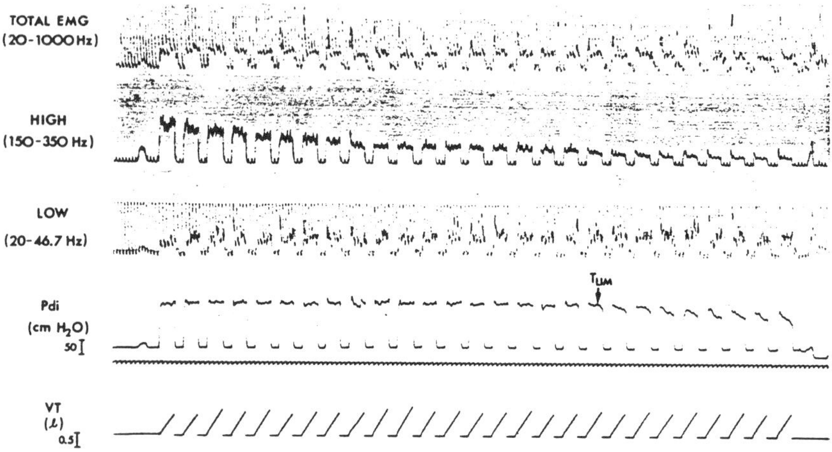

Figure 8 Polygraph record of a fatigue run at 75% Pdimax and a Ti/Ttot of 60% produced during inspiratory resistive ventilatory loading. Total integrated diaphragm EMG signal in bandwidth 20–1000 Hz; high integrated EMG signal in bandwidth 150–350 Hz; low integrated EMG signal in bandwidth 20–46.7 Hz. Time markers on the X axis are 1 sec. T_{Lim} indicates the time that the breathing effort could be sustained. Note that the EMG power in the high- and low-frequency domain changes on the first several breaths and well before T_{Lim}. (From Refs. 35, 35a.)

during electrically stimulated contracted in isolated rodent diaphragmatic muscle strips depend on Ti/Ttot but not the absolute duration of Ti or Ttot (3,87). These latter results indicate that muscle contractile performance and energy utilization depend on the tension-time index expressed in relative rather than absolute terms.

Subsequent studies by Clanton et al. (88) and McCool et al. (24) in normal subjects demonstrated that mechanical failure of the inspiratory muscles as pressure generators could be accelerated at a given PTI by increasing the rate of inspiratory airflow rate as reflected in the ratio of the tidal volume (Vt) over Ti (Vt/Ti). Increases in Vt/Ti reflect an increase in the velocity of inspiratory muscle shortening. Moreover, Collett et al. (86a) have shown that while respiratory muscle oxygen consumption is linearly related to the PTI, the slope of the relationship is increased by increasing Vt/Ti. Recent studies in diaphragmatic muscle strips in vitro and in vivo have supported the observation of Clanton (4,89,90). That is, at a given tension-time index, shortening contractions cause more rapid onset of fatigue than isometric contractions. This is not surprising since shortening contractions have long been known to consume more energy because of greater external work performed and greater ATP split-

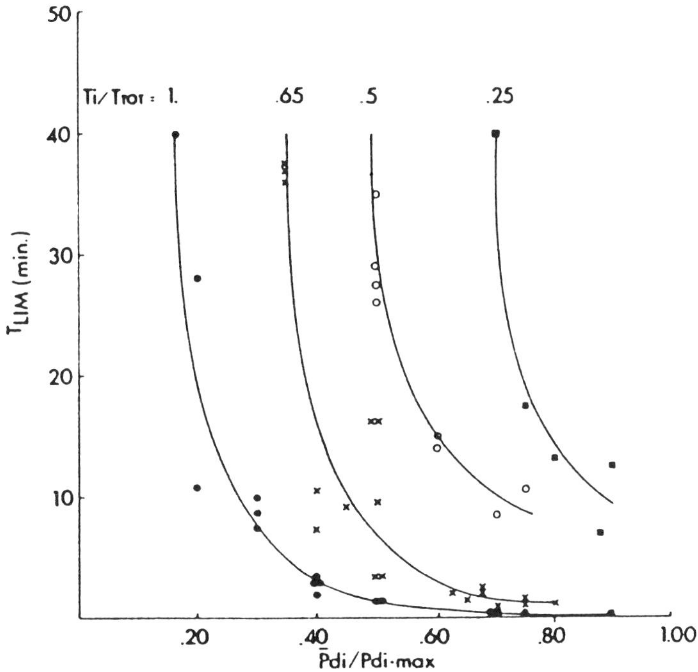

Figure 9 Effect of the breathing duty cycle, Ti/Ttot, on the time of mechanical failure of the diaphragm, T_{LIM}, over a range of Pdi/Pdimax values obtained during inspiratory flow-resistive loading in normal subjects. Each symbol represents a separate Ti/Ttot isopleth. Note that increases in Ti/Ttot from 0.25 to 1.0 shift the relationship to the left. That is, increases in Ti/Ttot decrease the onset of T_{LIM} at any given Pdi/Pdimax. (From Refs. 35, 35a.)

ting by the requirement for more rapid cross-bridge cycling during isotonic than isometric contractions (i.e., the Fenn effect).

McCool et al. (25) have shown, in addition, that in normal subjects the fatigue paradigm, i.e., the nature of the respiratory manuever used to induce fatigue, determines subsequent muscle function. McCool et al. induced inspiratory muscle fatigue by requiring subjects either to generate high levels of inspiratory pressure and relatively low inspiratory flow rates during inspiratory resistive loading (i.e., an esophageal pressure time product of 40–50 cmH_2O and inspiratory flow < 1 L/sec) or, conversely, to generate high levels of inspiratory flow and low levels of pressure (i.e., inspiratory flow rate ~ 5 L/sec and esophageal pressure time product of 20–30 cmH_2O) until exhaustion. The nature of the muscle groups used to generate these tasks was not controlled. Subjects

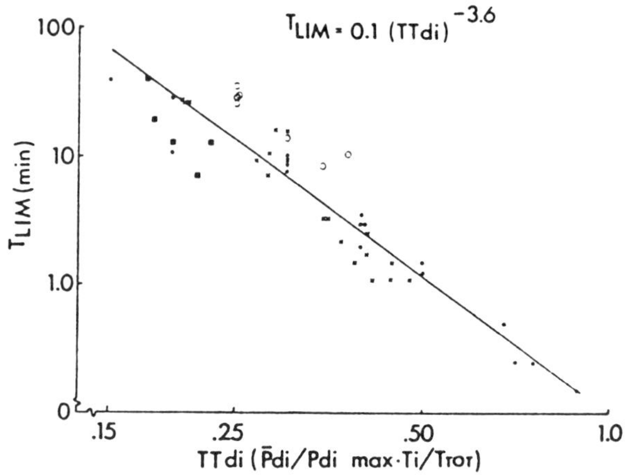

Figure 10 Relationship of the time of mechanical failure of the diaphragm, T_{LIM}, and TTdi, the diaphragm PTI, i.e., the product of Pdi/Pdimax × Ti/Ttot. Data were obtained in four normal subjects during strenuous volitional contractions performed in the setting of inspiratory resistive ventilatory loading. The two scales are logarithmic. Note that above approximately 15% TTdi, T_{LIM} decreases progressively with increasing TTdi. These data indicate that the effects of the magnitude and timing of diaphragm contractions on diaphragm endurance collapse into the primary factor, the TTdi. (From Refs. 35, 35a.)

were free to carry out the task ad lib. McCool found that the the time to exhaustion, T_{Lim}, was similar with the two forms of loading. However, "pressure loading" markedly reduced the maximum static Pes (−25%) but produced only negligible reductions in maximum inspiratory airflow (−2%). On the other hand, "flow loading" caused only small reductions in maximum static Pes (−8%) but large reductions in the velocity of maximum inspiratory airflow (−16%). Consequently, the different contraction paradigms differentially affected the slope and intercept of the active pressure-flow relationship of the respiratory system, the analog of the force-velocity relationship of the inspiratory muscles. Pressure loading caused large reductions in the slope of the pressure-flow relationship while flow loading caused relatively parallel downward shifts in the relationship. maximum static Pdi. Of interest, the two forms of loading also affected maximum static Pdi differently. Pressure loading had no significant effect on Pdi max while flow loading decreased Pdimax by 11%.

The mechanisms underlying the differing effects of breathing pattern on respiratory muscle performance are unclear. However, it seems possible that the different respiratory maneuvers may involve the use of different respiratory muscles and selectively fatigue some, but not other, respiratory muscles. Prece-

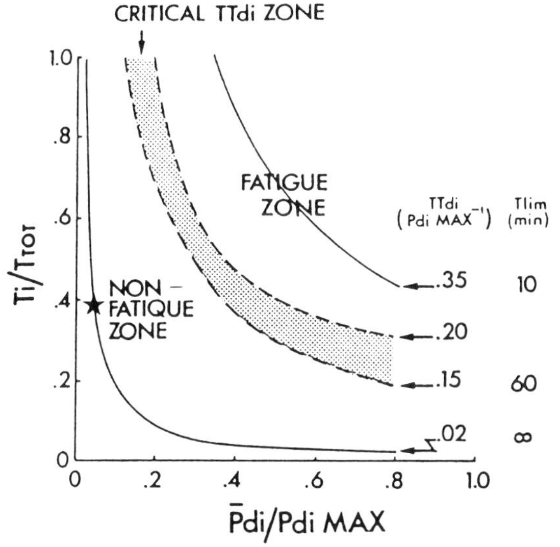

Figure 11 Schematic isodiaphragm tension time index (TTdi). Relationship between breathing duty cycle, Ti/Ttot, and Pdi/Pdimax for different TTdi isopleths: 2%, 15%, 20%, and 35%. Each TTdi, the product of Pdi/Pdimax × Ti/Ttot, indicates an isoendurance time, i.e., T_{LIM} in normal subjects. Note that below a critical TTdi zone of 15–20%, breathing efforts can be sustained indefinitely. Above this zone increases in TTdi are associated with progressively smaller values of T_{LIM}. (From Ref. 36.)

dent exists for this possibility (91). High-pressure efforts may involve greater activation of ribcage and neck accessory muscles than diaphragm. Conversely, efforts involving high flow rates may produce relatively greater activation of the diaphragm than the ribcage and neck accessory muscles. This latter possibility is supported by the observation that pressure loading is associated with smaller reductions in maximum Pdi than flow fatigue. Alternatively, the two fatigue paradigms may affect energy consumption of the respiratory muscles differently. Efforts generating high flow rates may require greater power output and energy utilization than efforts involving high levels of pressure. Regardless, these interesting data suggest that respiratory maneuvers associated with high levels of ventilation are likely to fatigue the diaphragm and impair the shortening capacity of the inspiratory musculature in aggregate. Conversely, maneuvers that produce high levels of pressure may primarily impair the ability of the inspiratory musculature to reduce intrathoracic pressure, i.e., Pes.

Finally, fatigue differentially affects the mechanical output of the diaphragm at long and short precontraction lengths (14,21). Following a fatigue trial performed at functional residual capacity (FRC), Pdi generated at high lung volume (i.e., shorter muscle length) falls to a greater extent than Pdi generated at lower lung volumes (i.e., FRC) (21). Conversely, Pdi recovers more quickly at high compared to low lung volumes (Fig. 12). These data suggest that fatiguing maneuvers performed at FRC disproportionately impair diaphragm function at short compared to long muscle lengths perhaps by exaggerating the length dependency of activation (14). Even in fresh muscle, calcium release from the sarcoplasmic reticulum is less at fiber lengths below Lo than above Lo (13).

C. Muscle Blood Flow

Experiments in the intact dog diaphragm in vivo as well as isolated, perfused strips of costal diaphram contracting isometrically indicate that diaphragm blood flow increases with increasing muscle activity (92–100). However, the relationship of diaphram blood flow to muscle contractile activity is complex

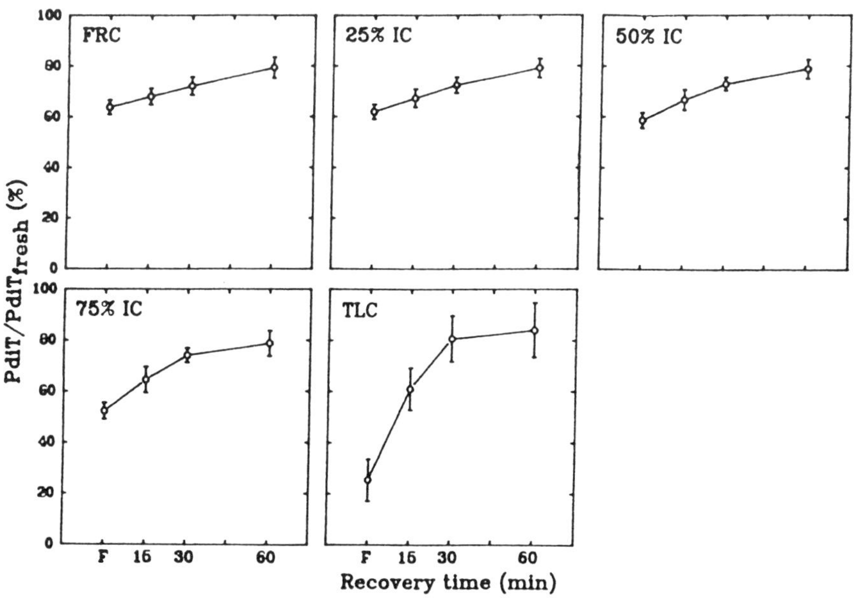

Figure 12 Effect of lung volume on the decrease in twitch Pdi during electrophrenic stimulation following inspiratory resistive ventilatory loading to the point of diaphragm fatigue in normal subjects. Fatigue trials were performed at resting lung volume. Increasing lung volume from functional residual capacity (FRC) to total lung capacity (TLC) is expressed as % inspiratory capacity (i.e., 25–75% IC). Time F corresponds to time of first postfatigue determination. Note that fatigue is associated with greater falls in twitch Pdi at higher lung volume than at FRC. (From Ref. 21.)

and depends on both the intensity and timing of contractions (93–95). The level and pattern of diaphragm activation, therefore, determine not only muscle energy utilization, but also the availability of metabolic fuel needed for energy generation, i.e., oxygen, glucose, free fatty acids, lactate, and so forth, as a result of effects on muscle blood flow.

During 30-sec, sustained, nonrhythmical contractions, diaphragm blood flow increases as the intensity of contractions increases (93,94). However, contractions in excess of 20–30% of Pdimax mechanically compromise blood flow and cause postcontraction hyperemia (Fig. 13). The presence of a postcontraction hyperemia indicates the presence of an oxygen debt. Contractions in excess of 75% of Pdimax completely eliminate blood flow. The effect of contraction intensity may be explained by the fact that phrenic arterial blood flow is mechanically impeded by increases in intramuscular pressure that act as an increase in vascular back pressure. When downstream vascular pressure equals upstream vascular pressure, the driving pressure for flow is reduced to zero. Of interest, the increase in intramuscular pressure produced by a given increase in muscle tension is less in the costal region of the dog diaphragm than in a more pennate muscle, the vastus lateralis (101). Since mechanical limitation of blood

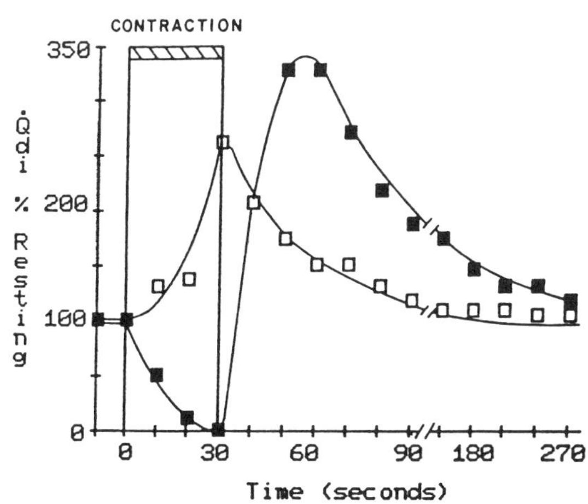

Figure 13 Effect of a single sustained contraction (30 sec) on diaphragm muscle blood flow in the anesthetized dog. Blood flow to the perfused costal diaphragm muscle strip preparation was measured by collecting the phrenic venous effluent. Muscle contraction was induced by electrical stimulation of the phrenic nerve. Contraction period is followed by 4 min. of rest. (Open squares) Tension = 10% maximum; (closed squares) tension = 80% of maximum. Note that 80% contraction mechanically impedes blood flow during the period of contraction and elicits a postcontraction hyperemia lasting several minutes. (From Ref. 94.)

flow during contraction depends on the increase in intramuscular pressure relative to vascular pressure, blood flow is less likely to be compromised in the costal diaphragm than in the vastus lateralis. In addition, increases in muscle fiber length above Lo decrease diaphragm blood flow probably secondary to changes in intramuscular pressure (102). In addition, the ratio of Pes to Pab at any given value of Pdi affects diaphragm blood flow (103). At a given value of Pdi, the higher the ratio of Pab to Pes, the lower the diaphragm blood flow. The adverse effect of increases in Pes on diaphragm may be a result of decreases in venous return and cardiac output.

When the diaphragm contracts rhythmically, the Ti/Ttot also affects diaphragm blood flow (Fig. 14) (93,94,96). At Pdi/Pdimax values that compromise blood flow during contraction (i.e., >20–30%), increases in the Ti/Ttot ratio decrease overall blood flow by encroaching on the time available for blood flow. Diaphragm blood flow, at least in the open-chested dog in which the diaphragm is made to contract isometrically, is therefore a function of the PTI rather than Pdi/Pdi max or the Ti/Ttot alone. Blood flow increases up to a PTI of 20–30% and thereafter falls progressively with further increases in PTI. Of

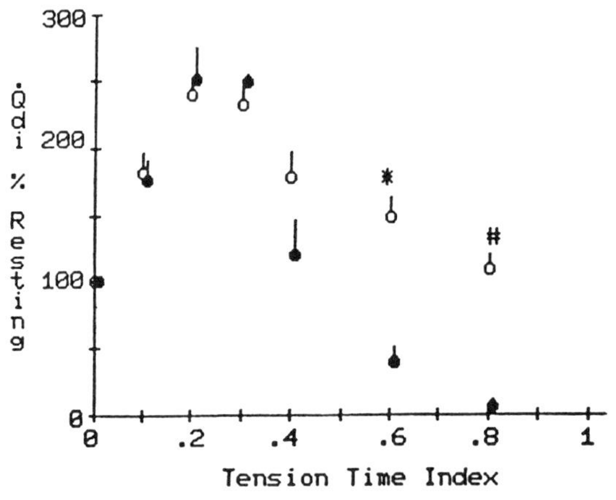

Figure 14 Relationship of diaphragm blood flow to diaphragm contractile activity as reflected in the tension time index of the rhythmically contracting dog diaphragm. Same preparation as in Figure 13. Note the curvilinear relationship of blood flow and contractile activity during 30 sec. of contraction. (Closed circles) Ti/Ttot of 100%; (open circles) tension 100% of maximum. Blood flow reaches a maximum at a tension time index of approximately 20% of maximum and thereafter falls progressively with increasing activity. Note, however, that above the critical tension time index of 20%, duty cycle of 100% produces greater reductions in blood flow than tension 100%. These data suggest that at any given tension time index above 20%, increases in duty cycle exert relatively greater effects than increases in tension. (From Ref. 94.)

interest, above a PTI of 20–30%, the pattern of the contraction affects blood flow. Specifically, contractions in which Ti/Ttot is relatively greater and Pdi/Pdimax is relatively lower are associated with lower levels of blood flow than when the same PTI is achieved by lower Ti/Ttot ratios and higher Pdi/Pdi max ratios (94). In fact, at PTI greater than 30%, diaphragm blood flow is inversely, linearly related to Ti/Ttot.

These studies indicate that intense contractions of the diaphragm mechanically limit diaphragmatic blood flow and explain, in part, the onset of diaphragmatic fatigue. Compromise of diaphragm blood flow when PTI is greater than 20–30% of maximum may lead to a condition in which the metabolic needs of the muscle outstrip the availability of energy supply. Alternatively, the importance of blood flow may lie in washing out toxic metabolites (i.e., hydrogen ions, lactate, phosphate ions) from the muscle. For example, at the same O_2 delivery rate, increasing the rate of blood flow slows the rate of fatigue in the pump-perfused, electrically stimulated dog diaphragm (104).

The diaphragmatic PTI associated with limitation of blood flow is also a complex function of the level of systemic arterial pressure (95,96). Reductions in arterial pressure produced in the dog by bleeding decrease blood flow at any given level of PTI and reduce the PDI value at which blood flow is mechanically impeded. For example, with arterial hypotension (mean blood pressure 50 mmHg), phrenic and internal mammary blood flow is mechanically limited and oxygen uptake falls at 10% Pdi/Pdimax and Ti/Ttot of 50% (95).

The importance of blood flow in the pathogenesis of diaphragm fatigue is supported by a number of studies (97,100,105–108). First, diaphragm blood flow is autoregulated over the normal range of systemic arterial pressure in the dog (i.e., mean 90–120 mmHg) but decreases when blood pressure falls below this range (94). Second, the tension generated by the fatiguing diaphragm can be augmented by increasing blood flow mechanically using a roller pump or pharmacologically by infusing norepinephrine (98,99). Third, in animal models of low cardiac output state (i.e., ~50% reduction in cardiac output and systemic blood pressure by saline percardial tamponade or infusion of endotoxin) progressive respiratory failure and death occur in spontaneously breathing dogs but not mechanically ventilated, tamponaded animals (105). In endotoxemic animals, Pdi fell despite progressive increases in peak integrated diaphragm and external intercostal EMG (106,108). These latter data suggest that extreme reductions in cardiac output and blood pressure may compromise respiratory muscle blood flow and lead to mechanical failure of the inspiratory muscles and lethal ventilatory failure. Of note, spontaneously breathing animals in low cardiac output states divert blood flow from essential visceral organs (e.g., heart, kidneys, brain, etc.) to the actively contracting diaphragm (97,106). These data suggest that in shock states diversion of blood flow to the metabolically active respiratory muscles may comprise organ function.

Recent studies by Supinski et al. (100) have shown that congestive heart failure produced in dogs by 6 weeks of pacing the ventricles at a rate of 250/min impairs diaphragm contractile function and the diaphragm blood flow response to changes in muscle activity. For example, the in situ perfused diaphragms of dogs in congestive heart failure generated 10–15% less tension at any given stimulus frequency than diaphragms from control animals. Moreover, animals in congestive failure manifested lower levels of diaphragm blood flow at a given level of muscle activity (i.e., tension) and less endurance during repeated contraction than control animals.

The importance of diaphragm blood flow as a determinant of steady-state contractile function in the human diaphragm was suggested recently by Aubier et al. (109). These authors demonstrated that diaphragm blood flow could be increased by 30–50% using intravenous dopamine (8 μg/kg/min) to increase cardiac output in patients with COPD in acute respiratory failure. Increases in diaphragm blood flow were associated with approximately 40% increases in twitch Pdi, which returned to baseline after cessation of dopamine infusion. These data suggest that diaphragm blood flow may limit diaphragm function in patients severe lung disease in whom the intensity of diaphragm contractions is high. Furthermore, pharmacologically mediated increases in diaphragm blood flow may augment diaphragm function in selected COPD patients in this setting.

D. Oxygen-Derived Free Radicals

Oxygen-derived free radicals are formed by a wide range of mitochondrial and microsomal electron transport activities or as a result of the xanthine oxidase reaction, which converts hypoxanthine to xanthine during reperfusion following ischemia (110). When the balance of oxygen-derived free radical activity exceeds the capacity of the cells' endogenous antioxidant defenses (e.g, glutathione, superoxide dismutase, catalase, vitamin E, and vitamin C), cell injury ensues. In limb skeletal muscles with depletion of glutathione, superoxide dismutase, catalase, vitamin E, and vitamin C, cell injury ensues. In limb skeletal muscles, depletion of glutathione impairs limb muscle endurance and increases free radical–mediated biochemical effects in the exercising muscle (111).

The mechanism by which reactive oxygen species (ROS) impair contractile function of strenuously contracting muscle is not entirely clear (110,111). However, ROS produce a variety of destructive intracellular chain reactions. Free radicals attack polyunsaturated fatty acids present in membrane lipids to initiate the process of lipid peroxidation. In turn, lipid peroxides are powerful inhibitors of many cellular enzymes and decompose to yield other toxic by-products damaging to proteins and membranes. Accordingly, ROS may damage the sarcolemma and/or T tubules and impair their ability to propagate an action potential and charge into the interior of the cell. Free radicals may also impair sarcoplasm reticulum, mitochondria, or contractile protein function.

Recently, a number of studies suggest that ROS contribute to respiratory muscle dysfunction during fatiguing contractions (110,112–118). First, several studies have found evidence of superoxide and hydrogen peroxide generation in strenuously contracting isolated strips of diaphragmatic muscle, which is diminished in the presence of the ROS scavengers, superoxide dismutase, DMSO, or catalase (117,118). Second, administration of ferric chloride–ADP to generate hydroxyl and superoxide anions into the phrenic artery worsens the fatigue process, an effect that can be attenuated by infusion of zinc-copper SOD (119). Third, strenuous diaphragmatic contractions produced by breathing against severe inspiratory resistive loads in vivo decrease the ratio of GSH/GSSH and increase lipid peroxidation (112,115). Fourth, depletion of antioxidant defenses either by reduction of diaphragm GSH or by dietary-induced vitamin E deficiency impairs respiratory muscle performance and predisposes to ventilatory failure during inspiratory resistive loading (110). Finally, administration of antioxidants (i.e., *n*-acetyl cysteine, superoxide dismutase, DMSO, or catalase) slows the rate of fall of diaphragmatic tension during fatiguing contractions in vivo and in vitro (113,114,117).

Anzueto et al. (112) have demonstrated in anesthestized spontaneously breathing rats that inspiratory resistive loads applied to the point of near apnea reduce the level of diaphragm GSH, the major cellular antioxidant, increase glutathione disulfide (GSSH), the oxidized form of GSH, and form lipid peroxides. Moreover, inhibition of GSH synthesis using the γ-glutamyl-cysteine transferase inhibitor, buthionine sulfoximine, or diethyl malate in anesthestized rats breathing against inspiratory resistive loads impairs diaphragm force output, increases lipid peroxidation, and produces greater reductions in the ratio of GSH/GSSH than occurs in control animals (110). Similarly, vitamin E–deficient rats demonstrate greater impairment in in vitro contractile properties of the diaphragm than control animals (110).

More recent studies by Borzone et al. (115) have used the same model as that of Anzueto et al. (112) with the exception that severe hypoxemia and shock were prevented by administering 70% O_2. In Borzone's experiments animals could sustain breathing on the load for 2.5 hr rather than the 6–10 min reported by Anzueto. In contrast to Anzueto et al. (112), Borzone et al. reported negligible (~15%) decreases in diaphragm GSH with no changes in intercostal GSH or diaphragm and intercostal GSSH following 2.5 hr of inspiratory resistive loading. The lack of change in GSSH levels and correlation of changes in GSH with increase in $Paco_2$ suggest that reductions in GSH were not caused by free radical–induced oxidation, but rather reflected decreases in GSH synthesis perhaps due to acidemia.

Shindoh et al. (113,114) have demonstrated in animal models that pretreatment with the free radical scavengers *N*-acetyly cysteine (NAC), polyethyleneglycol-superoxide dismutase (PEG-SOD), or dimethylsulfoxide (DMSO) attenuates the rate of diaphragm fatigue. For example, the rate of diaphragm fatigue in the vivo, perfused diaphragm strip preparation was greater in saline-treated control animals than in animals pretreated with either NAC (Fig. 15). Free radical scavengers do not appear to protect the diaphragm simply by changing muscle blood flow or its distribution in the microvasculature. For example, Reid et al. (117), using SOD, catalase, or DMSO, and Diaz et al. (116), using NAC, found that these antioxidants slowed the rate of diaphragm fatigue in electrically stimulated muscle strips in vitro in the absence of a blood supply. Moreover, the effects of antioxidants appear to be exerted directly on the muscle rather than on the neuromuscular junction since the NAC effects in isolated diaphragm strips were similar in muscle strips stimulated directly and via the phrenic nerve (116). Of interest, SOD and DMSO minimize the rate of fatigue in muscles electrically stimulated in response to 20-Hz shocks but have no protective effect when muscles are stimulated at higher frequencies, i.e.,

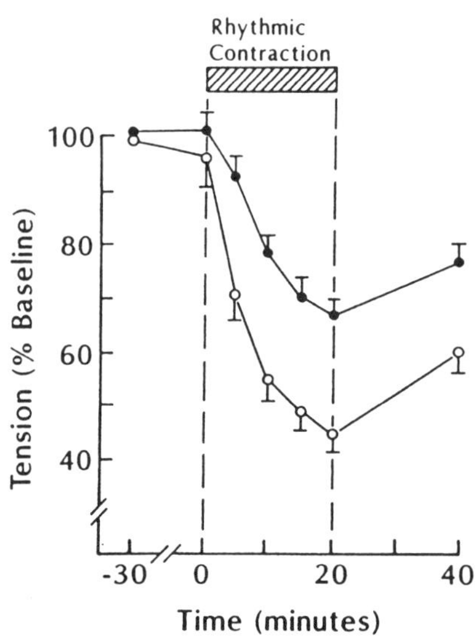

Figure 15 Effect of infusion of *N*-acetyl cysteine into the phrenic artery in anesthetized rabbits. Note that *N*-acetyl cysteine slowed the rate of fall in diaphragm tension during the 20-min period of rhythmical electrically stimulated contractions. (Solid circles) *N*-acetyl cysteine–treated animals; (open circles) control animals. (From Ref. 113.)

200 Hz (117). The particular importance of oxidant injury on the long-lasting, low-frequency fatigue is suggested by the study of Nashawati et al. (119), who found the infusion of iron-ADP into the phrenic artery of the dog disproportionately impaired the diaphragmatic response to 20 Hz relative to 100-Hz stimuli.

The possibility that the diaphragm may sustain ischemia/reperfusion injury as a result of strenuous contractions was suggested by Supinski et al. (98), who perfused the in vivo isolated perfused diaphragm strip at low arterial pressures followed by a period of reperfusion. Reperfusion caused significant impairments in contractile function compared to control animals in which blood flow was not increased. Administration of the hydroxyl radical scavenger DMSO prevented all deleterious effects of ischemia/reperfusion. Of interest, the concentration of glutathione, the major cellular antioxidant, is 60% greater in the rat diaphragm than in the intercostal muscles (115). In contrast, levels of SOD are similar in the primary respiratory muscles of the dog (i.e., costal and crural diaphragm, parasternal intercostal muscles, and triangularis sterni) and greater than in the secondary respiratory muscles (120). Greater levels of glutathione suggest that the diaphragm may be more resistant to the formation of ROS than the other primary respiratory muscles.

At present, studies demonstrating ROS formation and the beneficial effects of free radical scavengers on respiratory muscle fatigue are largely limited to animal models in which fatigue is produced in extreme and somewhat artificial circumstances. Moreover, antioxidants (i.e., NAC) decrease twitch amplitude but increase maximum tetanic diaphragm tension even in the fresh muscle, raising the possibility that they may affect excitation-contraction coupling or even contractile protein function directly (116). Consequently, the potential importance of ROS injury on human respiratory muscle fatigue remains unclear at this point. Moreover, the fatigue process is highly complex and involves multiple biochemical and biophysical processes involved in muscle excitation and contraction (113). Almost certainly, free radical formation will not entirely explain muscle fatigue.

E. Muscle Fiber Composition/Myosin Heavy-Chain Phenotype

Skeletal muscle fatigability depends on fiber composition and, more precisely, on the pattern of myosin heavy-chain expression (121). Muscle fibers predominantly expressing slow myosin are less susceptible to fatigue than fibers expressing fast myosin (85). Conversely, fast fibers generate greater force per unit cross-sectional area than slow fibers (85). Each of the respiratory muscles is a mosaic of slow and all three types of fast fibers (20,122–130). The precise mix of fibers varies across muscles and even regionally within a given muscle (20,122–130). In a given muscle, fiber composition is highly plastic and changes dramatically during growth, development, aging, changes in nutrition, hormonal milieu (e.g., hyper- and hypothyroidism), and activity (124,125,131–146). Moreover, fast fibers in the diaphragm are more susceptible to chronic changes in nutrition and corticosteroid hormone levels than slow fibers (138,147–149).

In the developing diaphragm of rats and baboons, the percentage of slow and IIb fibers increases while type IIc and IIb myosins decrease reciprocally from newborn life to adulthood (6,15,140). In both the rat and baboon diaphragm, in vitro fatigability in response to electrically stimulated contractions increases progressively with postnatal age through to adulthood (6,140). That is, diaphragms from animals in the first week of life are least fatigable while diaphragms from adults are most fatigable. All things being equal, similarity of results in these two widely differing species (rodent and primate) suggest that the adult human diaphragm is likely to be more fatigable than that of the neonate. In addition, diaphragm contractile function in neonatal animals may be more resistant to the effects of hypoxemia than in older animals (150).

In rodent models, aging is associated with preferential type II fiber atrophy, a general effect of aging on skeletal muscle in all parts of the body, replacement of type IIx/d myosin with more fatigable type IIb myosin, and an increase in collagen content in the diaphragm (15,131,139,144). Moreover, aging and senility decrease diaphragm force output by 20–30% (15,151) and increase the fatigability of the costal diaphragm from the hamster during electrically stimulated contractions in vitro (151). Of interest, changes in diaphragm force generation and fatigability are not continuous over the adult life span but rather occur only in the extreme elderly (151).

Fiber atrophy in the aged rodent diaphragm does not entirely explain the reductions in tension-generating capacity, since tension is reduced out of proportion to reductions in muscle mass (i.e., cross-sectional area). Rather, reductions in tension per unit cross-sectional area require: (1) an increase in the relative mass of slow fibers whose tension-generating capacity is less than that of fast fibers; (2) a reduction in the force-generating capacity of residual fast and slow myofibrillar material; (3) an increase in the mass of nonmuscle material (e.g., collagen, water, etc.); or (4) some combination of the first three mechanisms. Moreover, the greater fatigability of the aged diaphragm is not easily explained by preferential fast-fiber atrophy or a switch from IIb to IIx/d myosin, which should, if anything, increase the relative mass of fatigue-resistant fibers and, hence, increase endurance during electrical stimulation. Rather, the data suggest that aging may impair the endurance of residual slow and fast fibers.

Of note, diaphragm performance assessed during electrical stimulation may not reflect performance during physiological tasks in vivo. Supramaximal electrical stimulation activates all motor units simultaneously. Consequently, muscle performance during electrical stimulation is associated with progressive reductions in force as fibers fatigue in reverse sequence to their endurance properties (i.e., IIb, then IIx/d, then IIa, then I). In contrast, contractions performed under CNS control involve a typical hierarchy of recruitment in which type I fibers are recruited first followed by IIa, then II x/d, then IIb. In vivo, diaphragm contractions involving low levels of activation (e.g., during eupneic breathing) usually involve only type I fibers and can be maintained indefinitely. Consequently, diaphragm performance in vivo may not be affected during low-level contractions by conditions that produce preferential fast-fiber atrophy. On the other hand, diaphragm contractions of high intensity in which fast fatigable fibers are activated (e.g., during strenuous exercise) may not be sustained in the setting of preferential fast-fiber atrophy and decreased Pmax. Nonetheless, it seems likely that developmental and aging-related changes in diaphragm structure and function observed in the rodent can be extrapolated to humans.

In fact, it is clear that aging impairs overall human respiratory muscle strength as reflected in the MIP and MEP and produces intercostal muscle fiber atrophy (70,141,142). These changes may also affect the human diaphragm. Tolep et al. (152) found that in healthy elderly humans, aging (age > 65 years) decreases Pdimax generated during maximum volitional efforts by approximately 25% at all lung volumes (Fig. 16). Reductions in diaphragm strength likely reflect preferential atrophy of fast fibers. As pointed out above, selective atrophy of fast fibers with aging may not affect diaphragm performance during eupneic breathing when only motor units comprised of slow fibers are active.

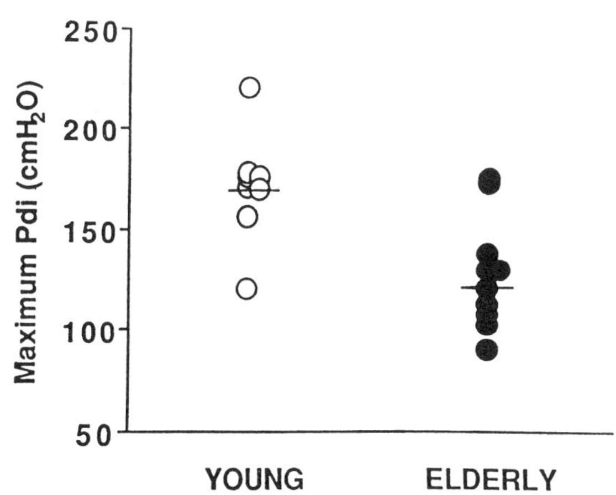

Figure 16 Effect of aging on maximum static transdiaphragmatic pressure (Pdimax) in normal young and elderly men. Pdimax was measured during the performance of an expulsive Mueller maneuver with visual feedback of the Pdi signal. Note that Pdimax is ~25% lower in the healthy elderly group. (From Ref. 152.)

However, when more strenuous inspiratory efforts are made and progressively more fast-twitch motor units are recruited, the diaphragm is likely to be more susceptible to fatigue because the PTI required to perform that breathing task will be increased.

In summary, while the intensity and timing of contractions are important determinants of respiratory muscle fatigue, the nature of the contraction, the age of the subject, and muscle fiber length and fiber composition likely affect the susceptibility of the diaphragm fatigue.

F. Clinical Conditions That Predispose to Diaphragm Muscle Fatigue

The clinical conditions that predispose to inspiratory muscle fatigue are shown in Table 2. In overview, breathing conditions that increase the level of phasic inspiratory muscle activity (i.e., the numerator of the Pdi/Pdimax ratio), or the duty cycle of breathing, or decrease the maximal pressure generating capacity of the muscle (i.e., the denominator of the Pdi/Pdimax ratio) increase the pressure-time product and make fatigue more likely.

For example, derrangements in the mechanical properties of the lung or chest wall (i.e., increases in airway resistance, or decreases in compliance) and increases in ventilatory drive (i.e., hypoxia, hypercapnia, or acidosis, lung inflammation, or exercise) all increase the PTI. Of note, Increases in ventilatory drive increase both the Pdi/Pdimax and Ti/Ttot ratio, the latter by causing greater reductions in the duration of expiration than inspiration.

Decreases in inspiratory muscle strength predispose to fatigue at any given level of inspiratory impedance or ventilation by increasing the Pdi/Pdimax. Aging, protein-calorie malnutrition, and electrolyte imbalances all act to decrease the Pdimax.

Table 2 Clinical Conditions Predisposing to Respiratory Muscle Fatigue

1. Abnormal lung or chest wall mechanics—hyperinflation, increased airway resistance, decreased compliance (e.g., COPD, asthma, interstitial pulmonary fibrosis, kyphoscoliosis, ARDS)
2. High ventilatory drive—hypoxemia, hypercapnia, fever, acidosis, lung injury inflammation (e.g., sepsis, ARDS, pneumonia, pulmonary embolus, postthoractomy)
3. Low cardiac output state—cardiogenic, hypovolemic or septic shock, congestive heart failure
4. Metabolic abnormalities—hypercapnia, metabolic acidosis, hypoxemia, electrolyte disturbances
5. Nutritional depletion—chronic protein-calorie malnutrition, hypoglycemia, starvation
6. Aging

Finally, based on data in animal models, reductions in diaphragm blood flow are likely to decrease the critical PTI, which leads to fatigue. For example, reductions in cardiac output (i.e., congestive heart failure, sepsis, or hypovolemic shock) diminish diaphragm blood flow at any given PTI and slow the protective postcontraction hyperemic response to ischemic contractions.

Severe obstructive lung disease (i.e., COPD and asthma) is an example of the interacting effects of several of these variables and arguably the clinical conditions most likely to cause inspiratory muscle fatigue. In obstructive lung disease, increases in airway resistance and hyperinflation require considerably greater-than-normal swings in intrathoracic pressure to generate normal levels of airflow and tidal volume. Moreover, abnormalities in lung gas exchange for O_2 and CO_2 (i.e., increased dead space volume and alveolar-arterial oxygen gradient) require greater-than-normal levels of ventilation to maintain eucapnia and euoxia. Consequently, in subjects with advanced COPD or asthma, minute ventilation is typically 2–3 times the normal value of 5 L/min. Since increases in ventilation require increases in airflow rate, tidal volume, and the duty cycle of breathing, the respiratory neuromuscular drive to breathe, peak inspiratory intrathoracic pressure, and the pressure-time index are increased considerably in subjects with advanced obstructive lung disease (153). (Hypoxemia and/or hypercapnia would tend to drive ventilation to still higher levels.)

In subjects with severe COPD and asthma, hyperinflation-induced reductions in inspiratory muscle mechanical advantage decrease the capacity of the inspiratory muscles to generate pressure (Pmax) to values one-third to one-half that of age-matched normal subjects (81). Of interest, recent studies suggest that adaptations in sarcomere number in the diaphragm and other chronically foreshortened respiratory muscles favorably affect the length-tension relationship in chronically hyperinflated animals and humans with COPD (i.e., reestablish Lo at shorter fiber lengths) (58,154–156). Anatomical reductions in the fiber length at which Lo occurs allow greater-than-normal levels of Pdi at high lung volume (58,157). However, these adaptive changes in Lo have no effect on the mechanical disadvantage imposed by changes in diaphragm shape (i.e., flattening) and alignment with the rib cage (i.e., more horizontal).

Moreover, aging- and malnutrition-associated changes in the diaphragm further impair Pdimax in subjects with COPD (152,158). Both slow and fast fibers in respiratory muscle (e.g., the diaphragm and intercostals) appear to atrophy in subjects with advanced COPD (158,159). COPD typically becomes disabling in the 6th and 7th decades of life, a period of life at which Pdi falls normally. Accordingly, aging may further decrease Pdimax by ~25%, at least in elderly COPD subjects.

The combined effects of increases in inspiratory muscle activity and decreases in muscle strength in severe obstructive lung disease increase the PTI during eupneic breathing in elderly COPD patients considerably above the normal value of 1–2% (36). The PTI may in fact approach or exceed the fatigue threshold (i.e., 15–20%) in patients with COPD (36). Finally, subjects with COPD and congestive heart failure may manifest disturbances in respiratory muscle blood flow, an unfavorable ratio of blood flow for a given level of tension, and hence a lower PTI fatigue threshold (100).

An important factor offsetting these factors that predispose to fatigue are alterations in the pattern of breathing that decrease PTI. Subjects with severe COPD breathe shallowly and rapidly at rest and during exercise due to a reduction in the duty cycle of breathing, Ti/Ttot (160,161). The Ti/Ttot ratio is reduced in subjects with COPD because Ti is reduced out of proportion to the duration of expiration (Te). The mechanism(s) underlying changes in the Ti/Ttot ratio and the shallow, rapid pattern of breathing in subjects with COPD are unclear. However, reductions in breathing duty cycle are greatest when lung mechanics are most derranged and return toward normal as lung function improves. Regardless, reductions in the Ti/Ttot ratio, which tend to reduce the PTI toward normal values, appear to be an important adaptive mechanism minimizing the tendency for fatigue to develop in patients with COPD.

V. Respiratory Muscle Fatigue in Patients with COPD

As mentioned above, several of the pathophysiological factors that cause inspiratory muscle fatigue are present in subjects with advanced COPD. The following section will summarize data indicating the presence of respiratory muscle fatigue in spontaneously breathing subjects. In fact, available data suggest that most subjects with severe but stable COPD rarely develop diaphragm fatigue unless ventilatory efforts above the eupneic levels are required (162).

In an attempt to determine whether fatigue occurs during spontaneous breathing in stable outpatients with advanced COPD, Bellemare and Grassino (36) examined the the diaphragm PTI and EMG power spectrum in 20 middle-aged patients with severe COPD (mean $FEV_1/FVC = 43\%$) and hyperinflation. COPD patients breathing spontaneously at rest had a diaphragm PTI, on average, 33% of the critical PTI that leads to diaphragm fatigue, i.e., 2.5 times greater than that of normal subjects (Fig. 17). Furthermore, five COPD subjects who were instructed to increase the diaphragm PTI from 8% to 17% of maximum by increasing either tidal volume or the Ti/Ttot ratio from 0.33 to 0.49 demonstrated reductions in the diaphragm EMG high/low ratio (Fig. 18). (Similar results were obtained by Pardy and Roussos (162a), who examined the effect on diaphragm activity of decreasing the resting $Paco_2$ in hypercapnic patients with COPD by voluntary hyperventilation. A twofold increase in ventilation resulted in a more than doubling of the Pdi/Pdimax ratio (from 0.17 to 0.44) and resulted in inspiratory muscle fatigue in four of six subjects.) These

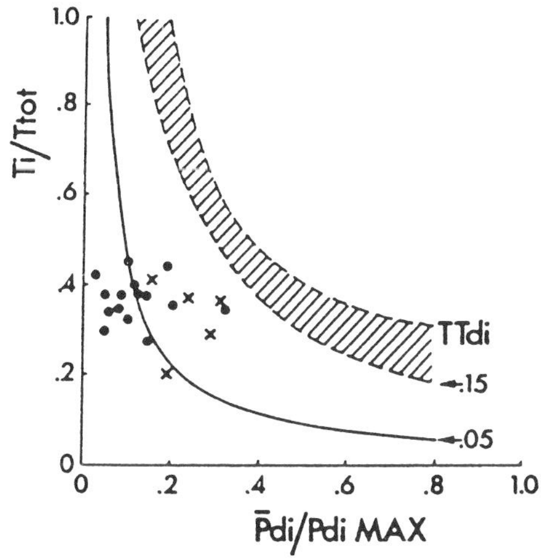

Figure 17 Relationship between the Pdi/Pdimax and the Ti/Ttot in 20 subjects with COPD while breathing room air at rest. Note that all points are below the critical TTdi fatigue threshold. However, TTdi values of ~5% are considerably higher than values obtained in normal subjects (~2% or less). (From Ref. 36.)

authors concluded that the "force reserve" of the diaphragm is markedly decreased in subjects with advanced COPD because of a reduction in Pdimax and that even minor increases in tidal volume or Ti/TOT can lead to diaphragm fatigue.

Begin and Grassino (162) subsequently evaluated the relationship between CO_2 retention, lung mechanics, and inspiratory muscle strength in 311 clinically stable subjects with COPD studied as outpatients. As expected, subjects with the most severe hypercapnia had the most impaired airway function. That is, mean FEV_1 was 0.79 L in subjects with mean $Paco_2=62$ mmHg, 1.13 L in subjects with mean $Paco_2=46$ mmHg, and 1.73 L in eucapnic subjects with $Paco_2$eq38 mmHG. $Paco_2$ was inversely related to the FEV_1 ($r=0.53$) and directly related to lung resistance (RL) ($r = 0.53$). The diaphragm PTI was higher in hypercapnic than eucapnic subjects. However, even in hypercapnic subjects, the PTI did not exceed the fatigue threshold. Mean PTI for the group of hypercapnic subjects was 9.8%. This study shows that hypercapnia per se is probably not a reflection of respiratory muscle fatigue even in severely obstructed patients with COPD. Rather, the authors postulated that hypercapnia may be a manifestation of a breathing strategy (i.e., rapid, shallow breathing) that minimizes inspiratory muscle activity and hence the susceptibility to fatigue (see below).

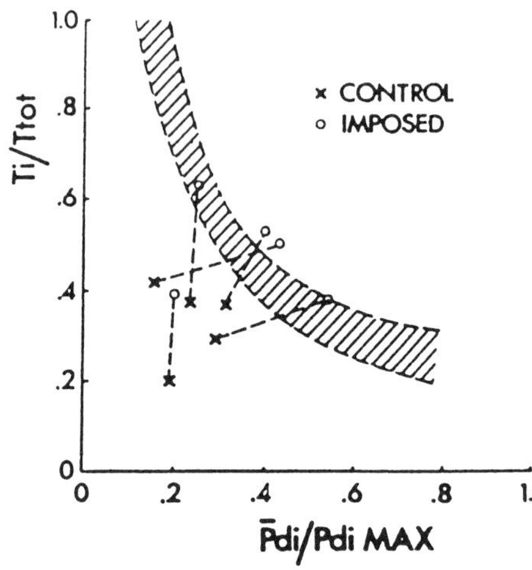

Figure 18 Effect of increasing tidal volume on TTdi in five subjects with COPD. (x) Control spontaneous breathing. (o) Imposed pattern of breathing. In four of five subjects, the imposed pattern of breathing brought the diaphragm within or above the fatigue threshold (cross-hatched area). (From Ref. 36.)

Pardy et al. (43) studied 12 subjects with moderate to severe COPD (mean FEV_1 $33 \pm 7\%$ and FRC $159 \pm 18\%$ predicted) during endurance exercise to a symptom-limited maximum on a bicycle ergometer at two-thirds maximal workload. Subjects were recruited to participate in a study examining the effectiveness of inspiratory resistive load training on respiratory muscle endurance and exercise performance. Six of the subjects demonstrated a >20% fall in the high/low ratio of either the scalene or diaphragm EMG (or both) recorded with surface electrodes prior to the termination of exercise. Of interest, the six subjects with EMG evidence of fatigue achieved considerable improvement in excerise performance and elimination of the EMG spectral shifts indicative of fatigue following a 2-month period of inspiratory resistance training at the reference workload. This study suggested that inspiratory muscle fatigue may be a common occurrence in COPD subjects during exercise and could contribute to exercise limitation in these subjects.

Subsequently, Levine and Gillen (44) examined the diaphragm EMG power spectrum and Pdi waveform during spontaneous breathing in the course of a progressive incremental work test on a treadmill to a symptom-limited maximum in 11 eucapnic, euoxic subjects with COPD and eight age-matched normal subjects. All 11 COPD subjects stopped excercising because of breathlessness. However, only three of the 11 COPD subjects demonstrated diaphragm EMG changes compatible with fatigue (i.e., decreases in the centroid frequency, mean frequency, and high/low ratio of the EMG greater than two standard deviations from the resting values). COPD subjects who developed EMG signs of diaphragm fatigue could not be distinguished from those who did not on the basis of airway function, Pa_{O_2}, and Pa_{CO_2}. Of interest, the shape of the Pdi waveform during exercise differed considerably in normals and subjects with COPD. COPD subjects developed peak Pdi at 25–50% of inspiration in contrast to normal subjects, who developed peak Pdi much later in inspiration, i.e., >90% Ti. Of note, the three COPD subjects who manifested EMG evidence of diaphragm fatigue during exercise showed the greatest reduction in Pdi late in inspiration. These data indicate that diaphragm fatigue is present in at least a subset of subjects who spontaneously increase ventilation during strenuous total body exercise. Moreover, those subjects who fatigued could not be distinguished from those who did not on the basis of respiratory or resting blood gas tensions. Finally, fatigue was associated with an alteration in the Pdi waveform and loss of pressure late in inspiration.

The uncommon occurrence of respiratory muscle fatigue in stable COPD subjects breathing at rest may reflect changes in the pattern of breathing that minimize the PTI. In fact, normal human subjects and animal models fatigued by inspiratory resistive loads in the laboratory adopt a shallow, rapid pattern of breathing post fatigue that minimizes the diaphragm PTI (10,163). In animal models, decreases in tidal volume with fatigue result from reductions in diaphragm and external intercostal electrical activity as well as decreases in the transduction of muscle electrical activity into pressure (Figs. 19,20) (10,49a). Moreover, animal models demonstrate reductions in integrated minute electrical

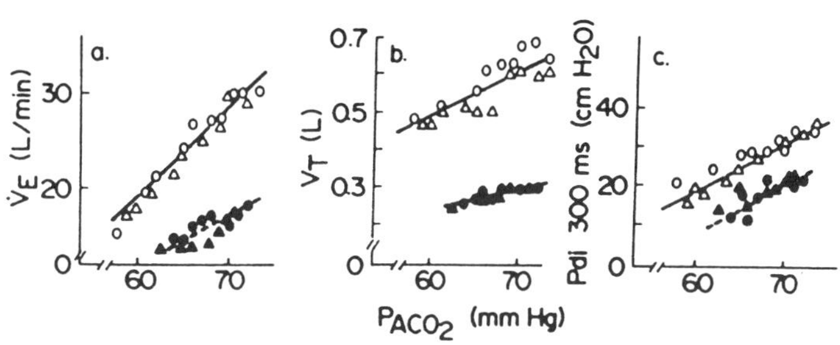

Figure 19 Effect of a prolonged period (82 min) of inspiratory resistive loading (135 $cmH_2O/L/sec$) on ventilatory and trandiaphragmatic pressure responses to hypercapnia in a single unanesthetized goat. (Open symbols) Data from two separate rebreathing trials performed prior to ventilatory loading. (Closed symbols) Data from two rebreath ing trials performed 10–30 min post loading. Pdi at 300 msec equals transdiaphragmatic pressure 300 msec after the onset of inspiration against an occluded airway. Note the decrease in ventilation, tidal volume, and Pdi at 300 msec following the fatigue trial at any given level of Pco_2. (From Ref. 10.)

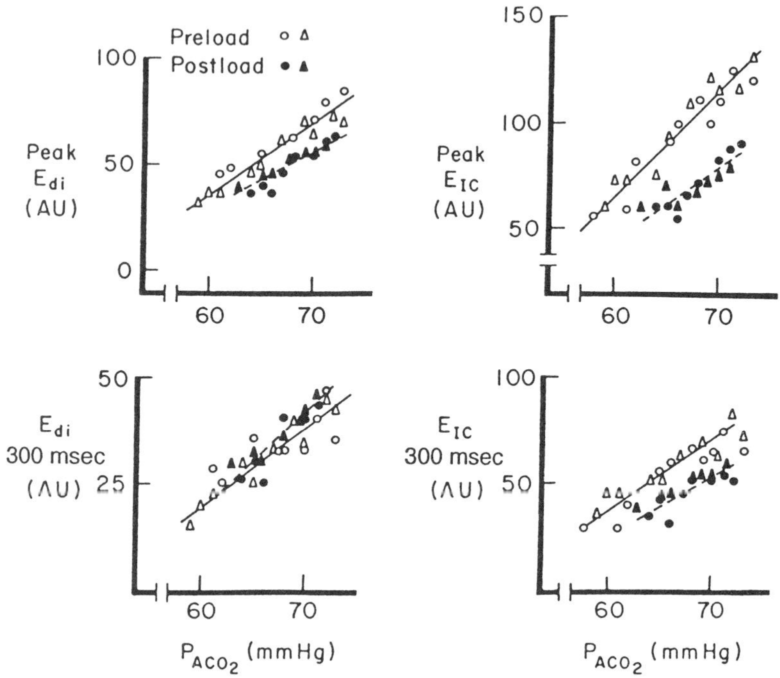

Figure 20 Effect of prolonged inspiratory resistive loading on diaphragm and external intercostal muscle EMG responses to hypercapnia in the unanesthetized goat. (Top) Peak integrated diaphragm electrical activity (left) and peak integrated external intercostal electrical activity (right). (Bottom) Electrical activity at 300 msec of inspiration, a reflection of the rate of rise of electrical activity. (Open symbols) Data prior to loading; (closed symbols) data post load. Note that post loading, Edi and Eic differ in some respects. Peak Edi and Eic are both decreased at a given level of P_{CO_2}. However, the rate of rise of diaphragm electrical activity is unaffected post load while intercostal electrical activity at 300 msec is decreased. These data indicate the presence of central fatigue of the diaphragm and external intercostal muscles after strenuous loading. (From Ref. 10.)

activity, the electrical analog of the PTI (10). Of course, reductions in tidal volume tend to increase the dead space/tidal volume ratio and predispose to hypercapnea. A rapid shallow breathing pattern would tend to increase Pa_{CO_2}.

The neurophysiological mechanism(s) driving the altered pattern of breathing are unclear. Moreover, whether changes in breathing pattern in animal models and humans with fatigue are reflexly induced, behaviorally mediated, or reflect changes in brain neurotransmittor levels (e.g., endorphins) is unclear (51–53,163–165). Of interest, afferent information arising in diaphragm Golgi tendon organs and type III and type IV endings and spindle organs in the intercostal muscles reflexly modify the intensity and timing of phrenic motor activity in deeply anesthetized animals (166–168).

In fact, the intensity of the sense of breathlessness is minimized at a given level of ventilation by breathing shallowly and rapidly (169). The intensity of the sense of dyspnea is chiefly a function of the central motor command to the inspiratory muscles as reflected in the peak diaphragm electrical activity and peak inspiratory esophageal pressure (169,170). In contrast to the effects of peak inspiratory motor activity, increases in the frequency of breathing have quantitatively trivial effects on the sense of dyspnea. Accordingly, at a given level of ventilation, a shallow, rapid pattern of breathing tends to minimize the sense of breathlessness. In fact, those COPD subjects with the greatest sensory acuity for changes in inspiratory pressure show the greatest reductions in tidal volume while breathing against severe inspiratory flow resistive loads (171). Of interest, the sense of respiratory effort (i.e., dyspnea) is increased in the setting of inspiratory muscle fatigue probably because a greater motor command is required to generate a given level of muscle force (40,172–174).

Subjects with COPD in acute respiratory failure requiring mechanical ventilation are more likely to show evidence of inspiratory muscle fatigue (42,175). For example, Cohen and colleagues (175) studied 12 patients with a variety of cardiopulmonary diseases in acute respiratory failure during weaning from mechanical ventilation. In seven patients, the high/low ratio of the diaphragm EMG decreased to less than 80% of the control value, tachypnea occurred, and the $Paco_2$ levels increased during spontaneous breathing with no ventilatory support. These authors hypothesized that diaphragm fatigue contributed to ventilator dependence after the onset of hypercapnic respiratory failure in at least some critically ill subjects.

Similar findings were reported by Murciano et al. (42) in 16 COPD patients weaning from mechanical ventilation during a bout of acute respiratory failure. Diaphragm fatigue was detected by reductions in the high/low ratio of the diaphragm EMG obtained via an endoesophageal catheter. In addition, these authors assessed the neuromuscular drive to breathe from the airway occlusion pressure developed at the trachea 0.1 sec after the onset of an occluded inspiration (P150.1). After 24 hr of mechanical ventilation, all patients with a $P_{0.}1$ greater than 6 cmH_2O had a high/low ratio $< 50\%$ of control during a 15-min period of spontaneous breathing. Eleven patients who showed a decrease in tracheal occlusion pressure ($\leq$4 cmH_2O) within 5–9 days were successfully extubated. The remaining five patients who had persistently elevated Po.ɪ (> 6 cmH_20) values and persistent reductions in the diaphragm high/low ratio continued to require mechanical ventilation. These data suggest that a high neuromuscular drive to breathe secondary to marked abnormalities in lung mechanics or blood gas tensions accompanies diaphragm fatigue and distinguishes those who fail weaning from those who succeed.

Finally, Pourriat and colleagues (176) studied 15 mechanically ventilated COPD patients in respiratory failure breathing spontaneously during 40 weaning attempts. Pdi/Pdimax was greater (mean 46% versus 33%) and Pga was significantly lower in COPD patients who failed weaning and were reintubated within 12 hr compared to subjects who were successfully weaned. However, Ti/Ttot was less in the subjects who were not weaned (29% versus 35%). The diaphragm PTI was therefore similar in those who were not weaned and those who were (13% and 11%, respectively). These data show that some patients with COPD in respiratory failure generate extremely high Pdi/Pdimax values during spontaneous breathing.

Although Pourriat, Cohen, and Murciano demonstrated that diaphragm fatigue may contribute to the need for mechanical ventilation in COPD patients in respiratory failure, the number of subjects studied was small and may represent a highly select population. In fact, Efthimiou et al. (176a) found evidence of respiratory muscle fatigue in less than 10% of COPD patients hospitalized for worsening respiratory distress. These authors studied the force-frequency curve of the sternomastoid muscle in 34 patients admitted to hospital for worsening respiratory symptoms. Only three of 34 subjects had evidence of low-frequency fatigue of the sternomastoid muscle (i.e., greater than 15% reduction in the ratio of force at 20 Hz over force at 50 Hz).

In summary, several studies have demonstrated that inspiratory muscle fatigue contributes to the morbidity of a subgroup of patients with chronic obstructive lung disease by preventing weaning from mechanical ventilation, and possibly by impairing exercise capability. However, the majority of stable subjects with COPD appear to adopt a pattern of breathing that minimizes the diaphragm PTI and prevents development of inspiratory muscle fatigue. Behavioral mechanisms activated in response to the sense of dyspnea may be operative in an attempt to minimize the sensation. However, further work is required to determine the neurophysiological mechanisms that alter breathing pattern and the acute situations in which these defense mechanisms are insufficient to prevent fatigue from ensuing.

VI. Treatment of Respiratory Muscle Fatigue

The treatment of respiratory muscle fatigue has not been systematically studied. Rather, treatment is based on theoretical principles derived from an understanding of the pathophysiological mechanisms that caused fatigue in the first place (see Tables 3 and 4). First and foremost, therapy should be directed at correcting the abnormalities that increased the PTI, decreased diaphragm blood flow,

Table 3 Principles of Therapy of Respiratory Muscle Fatigue

I. Decrease inspiratory swings in transdiaphragmatic pressure (Pdi)
  a. Improve the mechanics of breathing, i.e., decrease airway resistance, improve thoracic compliance and static lung volume
  b. Decrease ventilatory drive, i.e., relieve hypoxemia, hypercapnia, metabolic acidosis, fever, pulmonary congestion/inflammation, ARDS

II. Increase Pdimax
  a. Correct hyperinflation
  b. Correct muscle atrophy induced by protein-calorie deficiency
  c. Correct electrolyte and blood gas abnormalities (i.e., hypoxemia, hypercapnia, hypophosphatemia, hypokalemia, hypocalcemia, hypomagnesemia

III. Optimize muscle blood flow and substrate availability
  a. Correct low cardiac output state (e.g., cardiogenic shock, hypovolemic shock)
  b. Correct hypoxemia, anemia, hypoglycemia

or derranged both to critical levels associated with fatigue. In many clinical settings respiratory muscle activity is considerably increased because of abnormalities in lung or chest wall mechanics, hypoxemia, or hypercapnia (e.g., patients with severe COPD or asthma). In these settings, bronchodilators to decrease airway resistance and supplemental oxygen to eliminate hypoxemia-mediated increases in ventilatory drive may be sufficient to reduce the phasic swings in Pdi to subfatiguing levels. In addition, bronchodilators may reverse hyperinflation-induced decreases in Pdimax. In contrast, many clinical settings are associated with reductions in diaphragm blood flow because of reductions in cardiac output (e.g., patients with cardiogenic shock or advanced sepsis). In these settings, treatment should be directed at optimizing circulatory function with volume expansion, vasopressors, and cardiac ionotropes as appropriate. In addition, elimination of hypoxemia and hypercapnia may reverse diaphragm fatigue by improving muscle metabolism (177) or enhancing Pdimax (178,179).

Table 4 Overview of Therapeutic Approaches to the Treatment of Respiratory Muscle Fatigue

Well accepted	Experimental
1. Decrease PTI	1. Vasoactive drugs (e.g., dopamine)
2. Optimize blood flow	2. Antioxidants (e.g., glutathione, vitamin E, *n*-acetylcysteine)
3. Training, adrenergic	3. Muscle ionotropic agents (e.g., digitalis, methylxanthines, β-agonists)

Treatment of a fatigued skeletal muscle involves rest. However, complete rest of the respiratory skeletal muscles (i.e., mechanically assisted ventilation) is usually not necessary to allow full recovery of the muscle. In fact, the weight of available evidence suggests that reducing ventilatory work (i.e., the PTI) to subfatiguing levels does indeed allow full recovery of the muscle and the ability to successfully accomplish even strenuous respiratory tasks within a short period of time. First, diaphragmatic fatigue in elite athletes at the end of a period of strenuous exertion (i.e., marathon running) or normal subjects fatigued by external ventilatory loading resolves when eupneic breathing is resumed (7a,37,74). In fact, Eastwood et al. (37) found that following inspiratory muscle fatigue induced by incremental threshold ventilatory loading, the inspiratory muscles in normal young adults can sustain pressure loads of 70% MIP without difficulty for 15 min. Furthermore, immediately following this 15-min period of generating 70% MIP, subjects could subsequently achieve the level of maximum ventilatory performance observed prior to the fatigue trial. Second, long experience with patients in acute respiratory failure secondary to acute exacerbations of COPD supports this approach. Most patients (~80–90%) in this situation recover in response to bronchodilators and supplemental oxygen (180,181).

Pharmacological approaches to prevent or reverse respiratory muscle fatigue are in their infancy. A number of drugs have been tested for their ability to augment respiratory muscle contractility, including methylxanthines, β-adrenergic agonists, digitalis glycosides, and vasoactive drugs (12,16,30,38,182–196). Methylxanthines (theophylline, caffeine, enprofylline) have been most intensely studied.

Most (12,16,30,40,182,183,185,189,190,193,194,196), but not all (38,188,195), studies indicate that methylxanthines augment respiratory muscle contractility in vivo and in vitro in animals and human subjects. Methylxanthines appear to act by enhancing calcium influx from the extracellular space and/or by facilitating release of calcium sequestered in the sarcoplasmic reticulum and not by antagonism of adenosine receptors. While theophylline and caffeine given in therapeutically relevant doses augment diaphragm contractility in fresh and fatigued muscle in normal subjects and patients with chronic obstructive lung disease (40,189,190,193), the exact role of inotropic agents in the treatment of respiratory muscle fatigue is unclear. Theoretical concerns exist about the use of ionotropic agents to augment the force output of a fatiguing muscle. Since muscle energy consumption is proportional to tension development, augmenting tension would be expected to enhance energy consumption. The consequences of "driving" a fatiguing muscle to generate heightened tension and consume greater levels of energy on muscle structure and function are unclear. Generation of high levels of force causes structural damage in diaphragm muscle fibers (129).

The use of therapeutic agents that act on the circulatory system to increase respiratory muscle blood flow has a more rational basis. Under conditions of strenuous contractions when blood flow is mechanically impeded by contraction of the muscle, the balance between energy utilization and availability is unfavorable. It seems possible that augmenting diaphragm blood flow

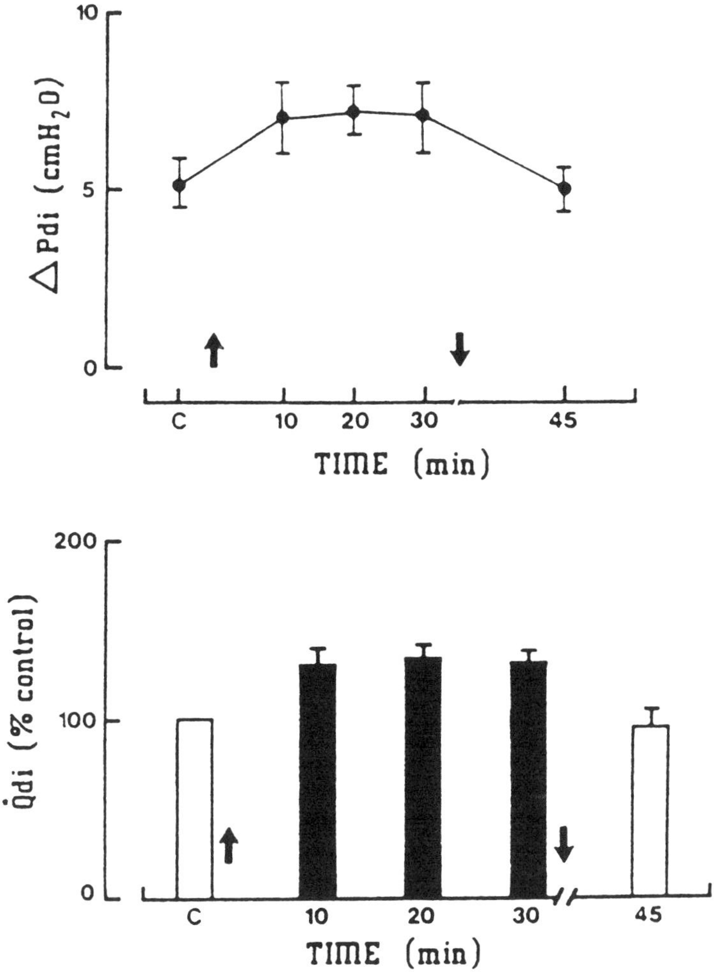

Figure 21 Time course of changes in twitch Pdi during (top) electrophrenic stimulation and (bottom) diaphragm blood flow in eight COPD subjects in acute respiratory failure. Arrows indicate the point at which dopamine infusion (8μg/kg/min) started and stopped. Note that dopamine infusion increased Pdi and diaphragm blood flow. (From Ref. 109.)

may improve steady-state muscle function. The limited study by Aubier et al. mentioned above (109) indicates that increasing diaphragm blood flow increases twitch Pdi in patients with chronic obstructive lung disease (Fig. 21).

The potential role of oxidant injury in the pathogenesis of long-lasting fatigue suggests the possible therapeutic role of antioxidant agents such as vitamin E or *n*-acetyl cysteine which have little toxicity. However, free radical scavengers have been used only in animal models either to prevent or to partially reverse muscle dysfunction associated with fatigue. To date, no studies have tested the effectiveness and safety of antioxidant agents in human respiratory muscles. In fact, fatigue is generally thought to be a protective mechanism employed by the body to prevent muscle injury (13,18). Therefore, the use of approaches that bypass this normal protective mechanism must be examined very carefully and the balance between potential long-term consequences and short-term benefits needs to be assessed in considerable detail. At this time, drug therapy is not recommended for routine use in the treatment of respiratory muscle fatigue.

VII. Prevention of Respiratory Muscle Fatigue/Muscle Training

Since the landmark studies of Bradley and Leith in the mid-1970s (72,197), it is clear that the respiratory skeletal muscles, like skeletal muscles in other parts of the body, can be trained to increase their strength and/or endurance. In addition, ventilatory muscle training appears to be successful in human subjects over 65 years of age (198). In animal models, inspiratory muscle overload produced by a strenuous regime of treadmill running, swimming, or inspiratory resistive loading increased diaphragm oxidative enzyme activity (i.e., citrate synthase, succinic dehydrogenase, β-hydroxyacyl-CoA dehydrogenase) in most (120,132,135,136,143,199–201), but not all, studies (22). Increases in diaphragm oxidative enzyme activity induced by strenuous total body exercise training (i.e., treadmill running, swimming) were modest (20–30%), quantitatively similar in young and senescent animals, and confined to the costal region (120,201). Increases in oxidative ennzyme activity induced by severe inspiratory resistive ventilatory loading may be slightly greater than those achieved by total body exercise (~30–50) perhaps because the level of muscle activation is greater (199). In humans, respiratory muscle training induced by sustained hyperpnea increases maximal respiratory muscle oxygen uptake and oxygen uptake at a given level of ventilation (197,202). Accordingly, strenuous training of the respiratory muscles by exercise-induced hyperpnea or ventilatory loading enhances muscle aerobic capacity and does not appear to have an upper age limit. [Conversely, exercise capacity on a treadmill or bicycle ergometer may be impaired following induction of respiratory muscle fatigue even in normal subjects (54,180).]

Training the respiratory muscles produces results in keeping with well-described principles for training of other skeletal muscles. That is, to achieve a training response, respiratory muscle fibers must be overloaded at regular intervals over a period of weeks to months. In turn, the effects on muscle task performance are specific to the training maneuver and, in particular, to the pattern of contractile activity used for training (203–205). In general, training to improve muscle strength requires contractions of high intensity and low frequency. In animal models strength training regimes generally elicit hypertrophy of diaphragm muscle fibers with little or no change in muscle aerobic capacity (206,207). Similar findings have been obtained with the respiratory muscles (129,136,199,205a).

A. Respiratory Muscle Strength Training

Since the studies of Bradley and Leith, the conventional method of training to enhance respiratory muscle strength involves the performance of maximum static efforts against an occluded airway at functional residual capacity or over a range of vital capacity. Inspiratory efforts (Mueller maneuvers) train the inspiratory muscles while expiratory efforts (Valsalva maneuvers) train the expiratory muscles. In addition, specific respiratory muscle groups (e.g., the sternomastoid muscles, pectoralis major) may be trained by performing forceful contractions against resistance using the stereotyped direction of motion of that muscle, i.e., opposed head flexion and rotation or arm abduction, respectively, in the case of the sternomastoid or pectoralis. Maximum static efforts produced every 3–5 min for periods of 20–30 min a day produce considerable increases in inspiratory muscle strength assessed from the MIP. Response is time-dependent and increases progressively over a 10-week period in normal subjects (72).

Inspiratory muscle strength can also be increased by loading protocols involving inspiration against flow-resistive or threshold loads to generate targeted levels of peak inspiratory mouth pressure in excess of 33% of MIP for 30–60 min daily for 5–7 days a week (71,73,208–210). This approach has been commonly employed in subjects with COPD (71,73,208–210).

As mentioned previously, enhancements in respiratory muscle strength per se should translate into enhanced task performance, that is, the ability to sustain increased levels of inspiratory pressure without developing fatigue. In effect, increases in strength decrease the ratio of P/Pmax and the PTI.

B. Respiratory Muscle Endurance Training

In highly motivated athletes, the endurance of the respiratory muscles can be enhanced by nonspecific training (e.g., swimming, running, or canoeing) that produces high levels of minute ventilation (72a,74). In contrast, subjects with COPD do not seem to achieve enhancements in respiratory muscle endurance by training the limb muscles probably because the levels of ventilation achieved may be too low (211).

Specific training of the respiratory muscles has been accomplished in several ways. The first approach involves voluntary isocapnic hyperpnea to generate levels of ventilation greater than those achieved except during extremely intense total-body exercise. The other approach involves inspiring against an external resistive or threshold ventilatory load. The nature of the contractions performed by the respiratory muscles and hence the training responses achieved with these two approaches are quite different.

Voluntary isocapnic hyperpnea involves generating extremely high inspiratory flows with the subjects' internal impedance as the load opposing the inspiratory muscles. In contrast, resistive or threshold loads require the muscles to contract considerably more forcefully with slower rates of shortening and at much lower respiratory frequencies.

Voluntary Hyperpnea

In this approach subjects generate predetermined levels of ventilation that represent a high percentage of their 12-sec maximum voluntary ventilation, i.e., 70–90%. The subject is given a visual target so that the predetermined level of ventilation is achieved. Isocapnia is accomplished by rebreathing through a dead space or by bleeding supplemental carbon dioxide into the circuit. The usual duration of a single voluntary isocapnic hyperpnea run is 15–20 min, which is typically performed two to three times each day, four to seven times each week.

This form of training has been used successfully in some (72,202), but not all, studies (212) in normal subjects and patients with chronic obstructive disease to enhance the ability to sustain high levels of ventilation (72,202). In addition, Belman and Mittman have show that the oxygen consumption of the respiratory muscles at a given level of ventilation is enhanced in patients with COPD, suggesting a favorable alteration in the aerobic capacity of the respiratory muscles (202). It is believed that this form of training may exert beneficial clinical effects by allowing COPD subjects to sustain high levels of ventilation and hence improve exercise capacity (202).

Inspiratory Flow Resistive Loading

Ventilatory flow resistive loading is accomplished by inspiring through a narrow orifice to increase inspiratory pressure. With flow-resistive devices, phasic swings in inspiratory pressure depend on the inspiratory flow rate. Inspiring slowly through a small orifice allows subjects to generate lower inspiratory pressure than when a rapid inspiration is made through the same orifice. In fact, left to themselves, subjects with COPD tend to inspire slowly to reduce peak inspiratory pressure and presumably minimize the sense of dyspnea (208). As a consequence, peak inspiratory pressures may not be sufficiently great to overload the muscle and achieve a training effect. Accordingly, it is essential that pressure and specifically inspiratory flow must be targeted when using flow-resistive devices. Most studies using targeted inspiratory resistive loads have demonstrated increases in MIP and the ability to breathe against a given level of resistance for longer periods (71,73,213). In the spontaneously breathing sheep model, Akabas et al. (199) have shown that after 3 weeks of breathing against inspiratory resistive loads of 50–100 $cmH_2O/L/sec$ for 40 min daily, 5 days a week, task performance during ventilatory loading is enhanced. That is, Pdi and ventilation are preserved for longer periods on the same load. In pilot studies, Criner et al. (215) performed a 10-week period of inspiratory resistive-load training (30 min a day, 5 days a week, while maintaining the PTI at 25%—P/Pmax 50% and Ti/Ttot 50%) in three highly motivated, normal subjects. Diaphragm strength and endurance were assessed using the twitch occlusion technique and time to exhaustion during inspiratory resistive loading before and after the 10-week training period. After training, Pdi twitch and calculated Pdi max increased by ~40%. Moreover, the time to exhaustion during resistive loading increased by ~300% (Fig. 22).

There is some evidence in a small number of subjects with COPD that a combined training program involving breathing on resistance loads at high respiratory rate increases inspiratory muscle strength and the ability to sustain high levels of ventilation (209). For example, subjects with COPD breathing on targeted resistive loads at respiratory rates of 15–30 times a minute to generate high levels of ventilation and inspiratory muscle shortening as well as inspiratory mouth pressures in excess of 50% of the maximum demonstrate increases in sustainable ventilation as well as increases in inspiratory muscle strength. These data suggest that loads designed to produce both high levels of ventilation and high inspiratory pressure may increase ventilatory capacity as well as strength.

Inspiratory Threshold Loading

Threshold loads, usually a weighted plunger or adjustable spring loaded valve, require a preset level of inspiratory pressure to initiate and maintain inspiratory airflow (40). Once the valve is open, inspiratory pressure is relatively independent of changes in inspiratory airflow rates. Accordingly, inspiratory threshold loads have the advantage over resistive loads in that the nature of the load targets pressure to a predetermined level. However, alterations in the timing of

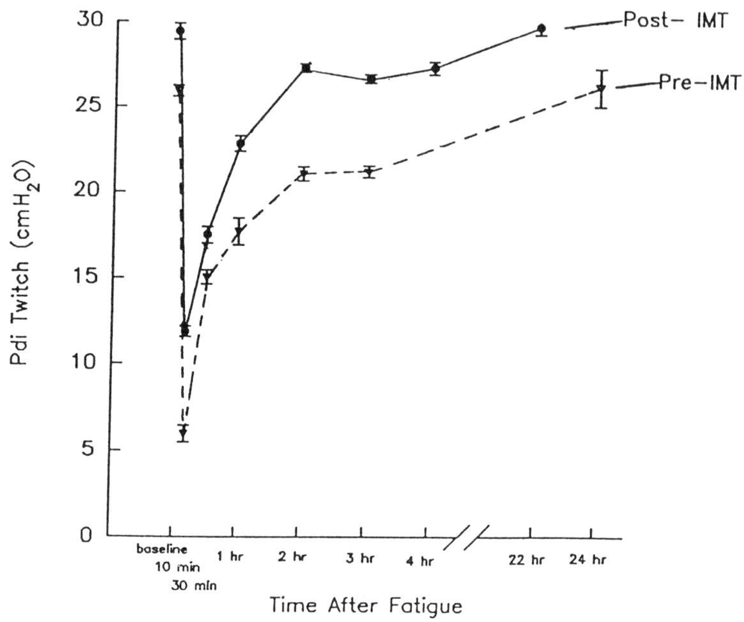

Figure 22 Peak Pdi twitch amplitude as a function of time following a period of prolonged inspiratory resistive loading in a single subject before and after a 10-week period of inspiratory resistive load draining. (From Ref. 215.)

breathing efforts, especially at high loads, may affect the PTI, which may be the most important training variable. For example, subjects tend to breathe with high tidal volumes, short inspiratory time, very high flow rates, and a short duty cycle on severe threshold loads. Thus, the PTI could vary widely on a given level of pressure. Hence, it is important to target the breathing pattern even on a threshold load.

VIII. Conclusions

It is now clear that the respiratory muscles, like skeletal muscles in the limbs, can fatigue under extreme conditions in which the mechanics of breathing are derranged and the level of muscle activation markedly increased. That diaphragm fatigue occurs in the clinical arena in at least a subset of subjects with severe lung disease breathing spontaneously is now reasonably well established. Furthermore, the pathophysiological mechanisms that underlie diaphragm fatigue in the clinical setting are relatively well understood. However, a number of important issues still remain to be addressed. For example, the prevalence of respiratory muscle fatigue in subjects at risk (e.g., patients with COPD, neuromuscular disease, severe kyphoscoliosis, etc.) is unknown. Lack of information on the prevalance of diaphragm fatigue in subjects at risk can be attributed to the lack of sensitive, specific, easy-to-use methods of diagnosing respiratory muscle weakness or fatigue in the clinical setting. The twitch occlusion technique is promising as an investigational tool to detect respiratory muscle weakness and low-frequency fatigue as well as to assess the level of diaphragm activation during spontaneous inspiratory efforts. However, sophisticated electronics and recording equipment are required to perform this test. Moreover, basic aspects of the technique have not been standardized (e.g., the location and nature of electrodes used to stimulate the phrenic nerves and record the diaphragm compound action potential, methods to minimize diaphragm shortening, etc.).

Finally, approaches to the treatment of diaphragm fatigue are in their infancy. There is general consensus that reductions in the level of diaphragm activation (by improving lung mechanics, diminishing ventilatory drive) and correction of disturbances in diaphragm blood flow are essential in reversing diaphragm fatigue. However, the role of respiratory muscle inotropes (i.e., digoxin, β-adrenergic agonists, theophylline), antioxidants, and agents to augment diaphragmatic blood flow (dopamine, norepinephrine) in the treatment of diaphragm fatigue currently awaits further study. Likewise, the value of respiratory muscle training in subjects at high risk (e.g., those with COPD, neuromuscular disease, etc.) and the method(s) of training most efficacious in this regard remain to be determined. In particular, the consequences of ventilatory muscle training on exercise capacity, the sense of breathlessness, and the susceptibility of patients with lung disease to develop respiratory failure have not been well studied.

References

1. Roussos CS, Macklem PT. Diaphragmatic fatigue in man. J Appl Physiol 1977; 43(2):189–197.
2. NHLBI Workshop Summary. Respiratory muscle fatigue. Am Rev Respir Dis 1990; 142:474–480.
3. Kelsen SG, Nochomovitz ML. Fatigue of the mammalian diaphragm in vitro. J Appl Physiol 1982; 53(2):440–447.
4. Seow CY, Stephens NL. Fatigue of mouse diaphragm muscle in isometric and isotonic contractions. J Appl Physiol 1988; 64(6):2388–2393.
5. Road J, Vahi R, Del Rio P, Grassino A. In vivo contractile properties of fatigued diaphragm. J Appl Physiol 1987; 63(2):471–478.
6. Sieck GC, Fournier M, Blanco CE. Diaphragm muscle fatigue resistance during postnatal development. J Appl Physiol 1991; 71(2):458–464.

7. Aubier M, Murciano D, Lecocguic Y, Viires N, Pariente R. Bilateral phrenic stimulation: a simple technique to assess diaphragmatic fatigue in humans. J Appl Physiol 1985; 58(1):58–64.
7a. Aubier M, Farkas G, DeTroyer A, Mozes, Roussos C. Detection of diaphragmatic fatigue in man by phrenic stimulation. J Appl Physiol Respir Environ Exerc Physiol 1981; 50(3):538–544.
8. Aldrich TK. Transmission fatigue of the rabbit diaphragm. Respir Physiol 1987; 69:307–319.
9. Gross D, Grassino A, Ross WRD, Macklem PT. Electromyogram pattern of diaphragmatic fatigue. J Appl Physiol Respir Environ Exerc Physiol 1979; 46(1): 1–7.
10. Oliven A, Lohda S, Adams ME, Simhai B, Kelsen SG. Effect of fatiguing resistive loads on the level and pattern of respiratory activity in awake goats. Respir Physiol 1988; 73:311–324.
11. Esau SA, Bellemare F, Grassino A, Permutt S, Roussos C, Pardy RL. Changes in relaxation rate with diaphragmatic fatigue in humans. J Appl Physiol Respir Environ Exerc Physiol 1983; 54(5):1353–1360.
12. Esau SA. Slowing of relaxation in the fatiguing hamster diaphragm is enhanced by theophylline. J Appl Physiol 1988; 65(3):1307–1313.
12a. Enad JG, Fournier M, Sieck GC. Oxidative capacity and capillary density of diaphragm motor units. J Appl Physiol 1989; 67(2):620–627.
13. Fitts RH. Cellular mechanisms of muscle fatigue. Physiol Rev 1994; 74(1):49–94.
14. Farkas GA, Rousso C. Acute diaphragmatic shortening: in vitro mechanics and fatigue. Am Rev Respir Dis 1984; 130:434–438.
15. Gosselin LE, Johnson BD, Sieck GC. Age-related changes in diaphragm muscle contractile properties and myosin heavy chain isoforms. Am J Respir Crit Care Med 1994; 150:174–178.
15a. Jardim J, Farkas G, Prefaut C, Thomas D, Macklem PT, Roussos CH. The failing inspiratory muscles under normoxic and hypoxic conditions. Am Rev Respir Dis 1981; 124:274–279.
16. Howell S, Roussos C. Isoproterenol and aminophylline improve contractility of fatigued canine diaphragm. Am Rev Respir Dis 1984; 129:118–124.
17. Road J, Newman S, Derenne JP, Grassino A. In vivo length-force relationship of canine diaphragm. J Appl Physiol 1986; 60(1):63–70.
18. Enoka RM, Stuart DG. Neurobiology of muscle fatigue. J Appl Physiol 1992; 72:1631–1648.
19. Iscoe S, Dankoff J, Migicousky R, Polosa C. Recruitment and discharge frequency of phrenic motoneurons during inspiration. Respir Physiol 1976; 26:113–128.
20. Arnold JS, Thomas AJ, Kelsen SG. Length-tension relationship of abdominal expiratory muscles: effect of emphysema. J Appl Physiol 1987; 62(2):739–745.
20a. Sieck GC, Cheung TS, Blanco CE. Diaphragm capillarity and oxidative capacity during postnatal development. J Appl Physiol 1991; 70(1):103–111.
21. Yan S, Similowski T, Gauthier AP, Macklem PT, Bellemare F. Effect of fatigue on diaphragmatic function at different lung volumes. J Appl Physiol 1992; 72:1064–1067.

22. Metzger JM, Fitts RH. Contractile and biochemical properties of diaphragm: effects of exercise training and fatigue. J Appl Physiol 1986; 60(5):1725–1758.
23. Kelsen SG, Sexauer WP, Mardini IA, Criner GJ. The comparative effects of elastase induced emphysema on costal and crural diaphragm and parasternal intercostal muscle contractility. Am J Respir Crit Care Med 1994; 140:168–173.
24. McCool FC, Hershenson MB, Tzelephis GE, Kikuchi Y, Leith DE. Effect of fatigue on maximal inspiratory pressure-flow capacity. J Appl Physiol 1992; 73(1):36–43.
25. McCool FD, McCann DR, Leith DE, Hoppin FG. Pressure-flow effects on endurance of inspiratory muscles. J Appl Physiol 1986; 60(1):299–303.
25a. Topulos GP, Reid MB, Leith DE. Pliometric activity of inspiratory muscles: maximal pressure-flow curves. J Appl Physiol 1987; 62(1):322–327.
26. McKenzie DK, Gandevia SC. Strength and endurance of inspiratory, expiratory, and limb muscles in asthma. Am Rev Respir Dis 1986; 134:999–1004.
27. McKenzie DK, Gandevia SC. Recovery from fatigue of human diaphragm and limb muscles. Respir Physiol 1991; 84:49–60.
28. Tzelepis G, McCool FD, Leith DE, Hoppin FG. Increased lung volume limits endurance on inspiratory muscles. J Appl Physiol 1988; 64(5):1796–1802.
29. Wilson SH, Cooke NT, Moxham J, Spiro SG. Sternomastoid muscle function and fatigue in normal subjects and in patients with chronic obstructive pulmonary disease. Am Rev Respir Dis 1984; 129:460–464.
30. Aubier M, De Troyer A, Sampson M, Macklem PT, Roussos C. Aminophylline improves diaphragmatic contractility. N Engl J Med 1981; 305:249–252.
31. Badier M, Guillot C, Lagier-Tessonnier F, Burnet H, Jammes Y. EMG power spectrum of respiratory and skeletal muscles during static contraction in healthy man. Muscle Nerve 1993; 16:1–8.
31a. Aldrich TK, Adams JM, Arora NS, Rochester DF. Power spectral analysis of the diaphragm electromyogram. J Appl Physiol 1983; 54(6):1579–1584.
32. Bellemare F, Bigland-Ritchie B. Assessment of human diaphragm strength and activation using phrenic nerve stimulation. Respir Physiol 1984; 58:263–277.
33. Bellemare F, Bigland-Ritchie B. Central components of diaphragmatic fatigue assessed by phrenic nerve stimulation. J Appl Physiol 1987; 62(3):1307–1316.
33a. Aldrich TK. Central fatigue of the rabbit diaphragm. Lung 1988; 166:233–241.
34. Bellemare F, Bigland-Ritchie B, Woods JJ. Contractile properties of the human diaphragm in vivo. J Appl Physiol 1986; 61(3):1153–1161.
35. Bellemare F, Grassino A. Effect of pressure and timing of contraction on human diaphragm fatigue. J Appl Physiol Respir Environ Exerc Physiol 1982; 53(5):1190–1195.
35a. Bellemare F, Grassino A. Evaluation of human diaphragm fatigue. J Appl Physiol Respir Environ Exerc Physiol 1982; 53(5):1196–1206.
36. Bellemare F, Grassino A. Force reserve of the diaphragm in patients with chronic obstructive pulmonary disease. J Appl Physiol Respir Environ Exerc Physiol 1983; 55(1):8–15.
37. Eastwood PR, Hillman DR, Finucane KE. Ventilatory responses to inspiratory threshold loading and role of muscle fatigue in task failure. J Appl Physiol 1994; 76(1):185–195.

38. Efthimiou J, Fleming J, Edwards RHT, Spiro SG. Effect of aminophylline on fatigue of the sternomastoid muscle in man. Thorax 1986; 41:122–127.
39. Hary D, Belman MJ, Propst J, Lewis S. A statistical analysis of the spectral moments used in EMG tests of endurance. J Apply Physiol Respir Environ Exerc Physiol 1982; 53(3):779–783.
40. Supinski GS, Levin S, Kelsen SG. Caffeine effect on respiratory muscle endurance and sense of effort during loaded breathing. J Appl Physiol 1986; 60(6):2040–2047.
41. Moxham J, Edwards RHT, Aubier M, et al. Changes in EMG power spectrum (high-to-low ratio) with force fatigue in humans. J Appl Physiol Respir Environ Exerc Physiol 1982; 53(5):1094–1099.
42. Murciano D, Boczkowski J, Lecocguic Y, Emili M, Pariente R, Aubier M. Tracheal occlusion pressure: a simple index to monitor respiratory muscle fatigue during acute respiratory failure in patients with chronic obstructive pulmonary disease. Ann Intern Med 1988; 108:800–805.
43. Pardy R, Rivington R, Despas P. The effects of inspiratory muscle training on exercise performance in chronic airflow limitation. Am Rev Respir Dis 1981; 123:426–433
43a. Sieck GC, Mazar A, Belman MJ. Changes in diaphragmatic EMG spectra during hypercapnic loads. Respir Physiol 1985; 61:137–152.
44. Levine S, Gillen M. Diaphragmatic pressure waveform can predict electromyographic signs of diaphragmatic fatigue. J Appl Physiol 1987; 62(4):1681–1689.
44a. Levine S, Henson D. Low-frequency diaphragmatic fatigue in spontaneously breathing humans. J Appl Physiol 1988; 64(2):672–680.
45. Hagg GM. Interpretation of EMG spectral alterations and alteration indexes at sustained contraction. J Appl Physiol 1992; 73(4):1211–1217.
46. Bigland-Ritchie B, Donovan EF, Rousso CS. Conduction velocity and EMG power spectrum changes in fatigue of sustained maximal efforts. J Appl Physiol 1981; 51(5):1300–1305.
47. Gandevia SC, Killian KJ, Campbell EJM. The effect of respiratory muscle fatigue on respiratory sensations. Clin Sci 1980; 60:463–466.
48. McKenzie DK, Gandevia SC. Phrenic nerve conduction times and twitch pressures of the human diaphragm. J Appl Physiol 1985; 58(5):1496–1504.
49. Bark H, Scharf SM. Effect of phrenic nerve stimulation on neural transmission and diaphragmatic force generation in the dog. Respir Physiol 1986; 63:187–199.
49a. Bazzy AR, Donnelly DF. Diaphragmatic failure during loaded breathing: role of neuromuscular transmission. J Appl Physiol 1993; 74:1679–1683.
50. Travaline JM, Criner CJ, Sudarshan S. Recovery of Pdi twitch following the induction of diaphragm fatigue in normal subjects. Am J Crit Care Med 1995 (in press).
51. Scardella AT, Parisi RA, Phair DK, Santiago TV, Edelman NH. The role of endogenous opiods in the ventilatory response to acute flow-resistive loads. Am Rev Respir Dis 1986; 133:26–31.

52. Petrozzino JJ, Scardella AT, Li JKJ, Krawciw N. Effect of naloxone on spectral shifts of the diaphragm EMG during inspiratory loading. J Appl Physiol 1990; 68(4):1376–1385.
52a. Sadoul N, Baxxy AR, Akabas SR, Haddad GG. Ventilatory response to fatiguing and nonfatiguing resistive loads in awake sleep. J Appl Physiol 1985; 59(3):969–978.
53. Petrozzino JJ, Scardella AT, Santiago TV, Edelman NH. Dichloroacetate blocks endogenous opioid effects during inspiratory flow-resistive loading. J Appl Physiol 1992; 72(2):590–596.
53a. Bazzy AR, Haddad GG. Diaphragmatic fatigue in unanesthetized adult sleep. J Appl Physiol 1984; 57:182–190.
54. Mador M, Acevedo F. Effect of respiratory muscle fatigue on breathing pattern during incremental exercise. Am Rev Respir Dis 1991; 143:462–468.
55. Mador MJ, Magalang UJ, Rodis A, Kufel TJ. Diaphragmatic fatigue after exercise in healthy human subjects. Am Rev Respir Dis 1993; 148:1571–1575.
56. Mador MJ, Magalang UG, Jufel TJ. Twitch potentiation following voluntary diaphragmatic contraction. Am J Respir Crit Care Med 1994; 149:739–743.
57. Ferguson GT. Use of twitch pressures to assess diaphragmatic function and central drive. J Appl Physiol 1994; 77(4):1705–1715.
58. Similowski T, Yan S, Gauthier AP, Macklem PT, Bellemare F. Contractile properties of the human diaphragm during chronic hyperinflation. N Engl J Med 1991; 325:917–923.
59. Sieck GC, Fournier M. Diaphragm motor unit recruitment during ventilatory and nonventilatory behaviors. J Appl Physiol 1989; 66:2539–2545.
60. Braun NMT, Arora NS, Rochester DF. Force-length relationship of the normal human diaphragm. J Appl Physiol Respir Environ Exerc Physiol 1982; 53(2):402–412.
61. Druz WS, Sharp JT. Electrical and mechanical activity of the diaphragm accompanying body position in severe chronic obstructive pulmonary disease. Am Rev Respir Dis 1982; 125:275–280.
62. Evanich MJ, Franco MJ, Lourenco RV. Force output of the diaphragm as a function of phrenic nerve firing rate and lung volume. J Appl Physiol 1973; 35(2):208–212.
63. Grassino A, Goldman MD, Mead J, Sears TA. Mechanics of the human diaphragm during voluntary contraction: statics. J Appl Physiol 1978; 44(6):829–839.
64. Hubmayr RD, Litchy WJ, Gay PC, Nelson SB. Transdiaphragmatic twitch pressure: effects of lung volume and chest wall shape. Am Rev Respir Dis 1989; 1139:647–652.
65. Loring SH, Mead J, Griscom NT. Dependence of diaphragmatic length on lung volume and thoracoabdominal configuration. J Appl Physiol 1985; 59(6):1961–1970.
66. Pengelly LD, Alderson AM, Miclic-Emili J. Mechanics of the diaphragm. J Appl Physiol 1971; 30(6):797–805.
67. Ninane V, Gorini M. Adverse effect of hyperinflation on parasternal intercostals. J Appl Physiol 1994; 77(5):2201–2206.

68. Paiva M, Verbanck S, Estenne M, Poncelet B, Segebarth C, Macklem PT. Mechanical implications of in vivo human diaphragm shape. J Appl Physiol 1992; 72(4):1407–1412.
69. Whitelaw WA, Hajdo LE, Wallace JA. Relationships among pressure, tension, and shape of the diaphragm. J Appl Physiol 1983; 55(6):1899–1905.
70. Enright PL, Kronmal RA, Manolio TA, Schenker MB, Hyatt RE. Respiratory muscle strength in the elderly: correlates and reference values. Am J Respir Crit Care Med 1994; 149:430–438.
71. Harver A, Mahler DA, Daubenspeck JA. Targeted inspiratory muscle training improves respiratory muscle function and reduces dyspnea in patients with chronic obstructive pulmonary disease. Ann Intern Med 1989; 111:117–124.
72. Leith DE, Bradley M. Ventilatory muscle strength and endurance training. J Appl Physiol 1976; 41(4):508–516.
72a. Clanton TL, Dixon GF, Drake J, Gadek JE. Effects of swim training on lung volumes and inspiratory muscle conditioning. J Appl Physiol 1987; 62(1):39–46.
73. Larson JL, Kim MJ, Sharp JT, Larson DA. Inspiratory muscle training with a pressure threshold breathing device in patients with chronic obstructive pulmonary disease. Am Rev Respir Dis 1988; 138:689–696.
74. Loke J, Mahler DA, Virgulto JA. Respiratory muscle fatigue after marathon running. J Appl Physiol 1982; 52(4):821–824.
75. Multz AS, Aldrich TK, Prezant DJ, Karpel JP, Hendler JM. Maximal inspiratory pressure is not a reliable test of inspiratory muscle strength in mechanically ventilated patients. Am Rev Respir Dis 1990; 142:529–532.
76. Aubier M, Viires N, Piquet J, et al. Effects of hypocalcemia on diaphragmatic strength generation. J Appl Physiol 1985; 58(6):2054–2061.
77. Aubier M, Murciano D, Lecocguic Y, et al. Effect of hypophosphatemia on diaphragmatic contractility in patients with acute respiratory failure. N Engl J Med 1985; 313:420–424.
78. Arora NS, Rochester DF. Respiratory muscle strength and maximal voluntary ventilation in undernourished patients. Am Rev Respir Dis 1982; 126:5–8.
79. Dhingra S, Solven F, Wilson A, McCarthy DS. Hypomagnesemia and respiratory muscle power. Am Rev Respir Dis 1984; 129:497–498.
80. Schweitzer TW, Fitzgerald JW, Bowden JA, Lynne-Davies P. Spectral analysis of human inspiratory diaphragmatic electromyograms. J Appl Physiol 1979; 46(1):152–165.
81. Sharp JT, Van Lith P, Nuchprayoon CV, Briney R, Johnson FN. The thorax in chronic obstructive lung disease. Am J Med 1968; 44:39–46.
81a. Sharp JT, Hammond MD, Aranda AU, Rocha RD. Comparison of diaphragm EMG centroid frequencies: esophageal versus chest surface leads. Am Rev Respir Dis 1993; 147:764–767.
82. Grassino A, Whitelaw WA, Milic-Emili J. Influence of lung volume and electrode position on electromyography of the diaphragm. J Appl Physiol 1976; 40(6):971–975.
83. Gandevia SC, McKenzie DK. Human diaphragmatic EMG: changes with lung volume and posture during supramaximal phrenic stimulation. J Appl Physiol 1986; 60(4):1420–1428.

84. Brody LR, Pollock MT, Roy SH, De Luca CJ, Celli B. pH-induced effects on median frequency and conduction velocity of the myoelectric signal. J Appl Physiol 1991; 71(5):1878–1885.
85. Sieck GC, Fournier M. Changes in diaphragm motor unit EMG during fatigue. J Appl Physiol 1990; 68(5):1917–1926.
86. Field S, Sanci S, Grassino A. Respiratory muscle oxygen consumption estimated by the diaphragm pressure-time index. J Appl Physiol Respir Environ Exerc Physiol 1984; 57(1):44–51.
86a. Collett PW, Perry C, Engel LA. Pressure-time product, flow, and oxygen cost of resistive breathing in humans. J Appl Physiol 1985; 58(4):1263–1272.
87. Massarelli PS, Green HJ, Hughson RL, Sharratt MT. Mechanical and metabolic alterations in rat diaphragm during electrical stimulation. J Appl Physiol 1989; 67(1):210–220.
88. Clanton TL, Dixon GF, Drake J, Gadek JE. Effects of breathing pattern on inspiratory muscle endurance in humans. J Appl Physiol 1985; 59(6):1834–1841.
89. Ameredes BT, Clanton TL. Increased fatigue of isovelocity vs. isometric contractions of canine diaphragm. J Appl Physiol 1990; 69(2):740–746.
90. Ameredes BT, Julian MW, Clanton TL. Muscle shortening increases sensitivity of fatigue to severe hypoxia in canine diaphragm. J Appl Physiol 1991; 71(6):2309–2316.
91. Fitting JW, Bradley TD, Easton PA, Lincoln MJ, Goldman MD, Grassino A. Disociation between diaphragmatic and rib cage muscle fatigue. J Appl Physiol 1988; 64(3):959–965.
92. Robertson CH, Foster GH, Johnson RL. The relationship of respiratory failure to the oxygen consumption of, lactate production by, and distribution of blood flow among respiratory muscles during increasing inspiratory resistance. J Clin Invest 1977; 59:31–42.
93. Bellemare F, Wight D, Lavigne CM, Grassino A. Effect of tension and timing of contraction on the blood flow of the diaphragm. J Appl Physiol 1983; 54(6):1597–1606.
94. Bark H, Supinski GS, Lamanna JC, Kelsen SG. Relationship of changes in diaphragmatic muscle blood flow to muscle contractile activity. J Appl Physiol 1987; 62(1):291–299.
95. Hussain SNA, Roussos C, Magder S. Autoregulation of diaphragmatic blood flow in dogs. J Appl Physiol 1988; 64(1):329–336.
96. Hussain SNA, Roussos C, Magder S. Effects of tension, duty cycle, and arterial pressure on diaphragmatic blood flow in dogs. J Appl Physiol 1989; 66(2):968–976.
97. Madger S, Lockhat D, Luo BJ, Roussos C. Respiratory muscle and organ blood flow with inspiratory elastic loading and shock. J Appl Physiol 1985; 58(4):1148–1156.
98. Supinski G, DiMarco A, Ketai L, Hussein F, Altose M. Reversibility of diaphragm fatigue by mechanical hyperperfusion. Am Rev Respir Dis 1988; 138:604–609.
99. Supinski GS, DiMarco AF, Gonzalez J, Altose MD. Effect of norepinephrine on diaphragm contractility and blood flow. J Appl Physiol 1990; 69(6):2019–2038.

100. Supinski G, DiMarco A, Dibner-Dunlap M. Alterations in diaphragm strength and fatiguability in congestive heart failure. J Appl Physiol 1994; 76(6):2707–2713.
101. Supinski GS, DiMarco AF, Altose MD. Effect of diaphragmatic contraction on intramuscular pressure and vascular impedance. J Appl Physiol 1990; 68(4):1486–1493.
102. Supinski GS, Bark H, Guanciale A, Kelsen SG. Effect of alterations in muscle fiber length on diaphragm blood flow. J Appl Physiol 1986; 60(5):1789–1796.
103. Buchler B, Magder S, Katsardia H, Jammes Y, Roussos C. Effects of pleural pressure and abdominal pressure on diaphragmatic blood flow. J Appl Physiol 58(3):691–697.
104. Ward ME, Magder SA, Hussain SHA. Oxygen delivery-independent effect of blood flow on diaphragm fatigue. Am Rev Respir Dis 1992; 145:1058–1063.
105. Aubier M, Trippenbach T, Roussos C. Respiratory muscle fatigue during cardiogenic shock. J Appl Physiol 1981; 51(2):499–508.
106. Hussain SNA, Roussos C. Distribution of respiratory muscle and organ blood flow during endotoxic shock in dogs. J Appl Physiol 1985; 59(6):1802–1808.
107. Hussain SNA, Rutledge F, Graham R, Magder S, Roussos C. Effects of norepinephrine and fluid administration on diaphragmatic O_2 consumption in septic shock. J Appl Physiol 1987;62(4):1368–1376.
108. Hussain SNA, Simkus G, Roussos C. Respiratory muscle fatigue: a cause of ventilatory failure in septic shock. J Appl Physiol 1985; 58(6):2033–2040.
109. Aubier M, Murciano D, Menu Y. Dopamine effects on diaphragmatic strength during acute respiratory failure in chronic obstructive pulmonary disease. Ann Intern Med 1989; 110:17–23.
110. Anzueto A, Supinsik GS, Levine SM, Jenkinson SG. Mechanisms of disease: are oxygen-derived free radicals involved in diaphragmatic dysfunction? Am J Respir Crit Care Med 1994;149:1048–1052.
110a. Morales CF, Anzueto A, Andrade F, et al. Buthionine sulfoximine treatment impairs rat diaphragm function. Am J Respir Crit Care Med 1994; 149:915–919.
111. Sen CK, Atalay M, Hanninen O. Exercise-induced oxidative stress: glutathione supplementation and deficiency. J Appl Physiol 1994; 77(5):2177–2187.
112. Anzueto, A, Andrade FH, Maxwell LC, et al. Resistive breathing activates the glutathione redox cycle and impairs performance of rat diaphragm. J Appl Physiol 1992; 72(2):529–534.
113. Shindoh C, Dimarco A, Thomas A, Manubay P, Supinski G. Effect of *N*-acetylcysteine on diaphragm fatigue. J Appl Physiol 1990; 68(5):2107–2113.
114. Shindoh A, Dimarco A, Nethery D. Effect of PEG-superoxide dismutase on the diaphragmatic response to endotoxin. Am Rev Respir Dis 1992; 145:1350–1354.
115. Borzone G, Julian MW, Merola AJ, Clanton TL. Loss of diaphragm glutathione is associated with respiratory failure induced by resistive breathing. J Appl Physiol 1994; 76(6):2825–2831.
116. Dekhuijzen PNR, Gayan-Ramirez G, de Bock V, Dom R, Decramer M. Triamcinolone and prednisolone affect contractile properties and histopathology of rat diaphragm differently. J Clin Invest 1993; 92:1534–1542.

117. Reid MB, Haack KE, Francik KM, Volberg PA, Kabzik L, Wes MS. Reactive oxygen in skeletal muscle. I. Intracellular oxygen kinetics and fatigue in vitro. J Appl Physiol 1992; 73:1797–1804.
118. Reid MB, Shoji T, Moody MR, Entman ML. Reactive oxygen in skeletal muscle. II. Extracellular release of free radicals. J Appl Physiol 1992; 73:1805–1809.
119. Nashawati E, Dimarco A, Supinski G. Effects produced by infusion of a free radical-generating solution into the diaphragm. Am Rev Respir Dis 1993; 147:60–65.
120. Powers SK, Lawler J, Criswell D, et al. Endurance-training-induced cellular adaptations in respiratory muscles. J Appl Physiol 1990; 68(5):2114–2118.
121. Swynghedauw B. Developmental and functional adaptation of contractile proteins in cardiac and skeletal muscles. Physiol Rev 1986;66(3):710–772.
122. Sieck GC, Sacks RD, Blanco CE, Edgerton VR. SDH activity and cross-sectional area of muscle fibers in cat diaphragm. J Appl Physiol 1986; 60(4):1284–1292.
123. Kelsen SG, Wolanski T, Supinski GS, Roessmann U. The effect of elastase-induced emphysema on diaphragmatic muscle structure in hamsters. Am Rev Respir Dis 1983; 127:330–334.
124. LaFramboise WA, Daood MJ, Guthrie RD, Butler-Browne GS, Whalen RG, Ontell M. Myosin isoforms in neonatal rat extensor digitorum longus, diaphragm and soleus muscles. Am J Physiol 1990; 259 (Lung Cell Mol Physiol. 3):L116–L122.
125. LaFramboise WA, Daood MJ, Guthrie RD, et al. Emergence of the mature myosin phenotype in the rat diaphragm muscle. Dev Biol 1991; 144:1–15.
126. Lieberman DA, Faulkner JA, Craig AB, Maxwell LC. Performance and histochemical composition of guinea pig and human diaphragm. J Appl Physiol 1973; 34(2):233–237.
127. Kelsen SG, Shanhui B, Thomas AJ, Issam AM, Criner GJ. Structure of parasternal intercostal muscles in the adult hamster: topographic effects. J Appl Physiol 1993; 75(3):1150–1154.
128. Reid WD, Wiggs BR, Pare PD, Pardy RL. Fiber type and regional differences in oxidative capacity and glycogen content in the hamster diaphragm. Am Rev Respir Dis 1992; 146:1266–1271.
129. Reid WD, Huang J, Bryson S, Walker DC, Belcastro AN. Diaphragm injury and myofibrillar structure induced by resistive loading. J Appl Physiol 1994; 76(1):176–184.
130. Powers SK, Farkas GA, Criswell D, Herb RA, Zambito K, Dodd S. Metabolic characteristics of primary inspiratory and expiratory muscles in the dog. J Appl Physiol 1994; 77(5):2188–2193.
131. Eddinger TJ, Moss RL, Cassens RG. Fiber number and type composition in extensor digitorum longus, soleus, and diaphragm muscles with aging in fisher 344 rats. J Histochem Cytochem 1985; 33(10):1033–1041.
132. Green HJ, Plyley MJ, Smith DM, Kile JG. Extreme endurance training and fiber type adaptation in rat diaphragm. J Appl Physiol 1989;66(4):1914–1920.

133. Ianuzzo CD, Hamilton N, Li B. Competitive control of myosin expression: hypertrophy vs hyperthyroidism. J Appl Physiol 1991; 70(5):2328–2330.
134. Ianuzzo CD, Chen V, O'Brien P, Keens TG. Effect of experimental dysthyroidism on the enzymatic character of the diaphragm. J Appl Physiol Respir Environ Exerc Physiol 1984; 56(1):117–121.
135. Ianuzzo CD, Nobel EG, Hamilton N, Dabrowski B. Effects of streptozotocin diabetes, insulin treatment, and training on the diaphragm. J Appl Physiol Respir Environ Exerc Physiol 1982; 52(6):1471–1475.
136. Keens TG, Chen V, Patel P, O'Brien P, Levison H, Ianuzzo CD. Cellular adaptations of the ventilatory muscles to a chronic increased respiratory load. J Appl Physiol Respir Environ Exerc Physiol 1978; 44(6):905–908.
137. Kelly AM, Rosser BWC, Hoffman R, et al. Metabolic and contractile protein expression in developing rat diaphragm muscle. J Neurol 1991; 11(5):1231–1242.
138. Kelsen SG, Ference M, Kappor S. Effects of prolonged undernutrition on structure and function of the diaphragm. J Appl Physiol 1985; 58(4):1354–1359.
139. Maltin CA, Duncan L, Wilson AB. Rat diaphragm: changes in muscle fiber type frequency with age. Muscle Nerve 1985; 8:211–216.
140. Maxwell LC, McCarter RJM, Kuehl TJ, Robotham JL. Development of histochemical and functional properties of baboon respiratory muscles. J Appl Physiol 1983; 4(2):551–561.
141. Mizuno M, Secher NH. Histochemical characteristics of human expiratory and inspiratory intercostal muscles. J Appl Physiol 1989; 67(2):592–598.
142. Mizuno M. Human respiratory muscles: fibre morphology and capillary supply. Eur Respir J 1991; 4:587–601.
143. Sugiura T, Morimoto A, Sakata Y, Watanabe T, Murakami N. Myosin heavy chain isoform changes in rat diaphragm are induced by endurance training. Jpn J Physiol 1990; 40:759–763.
144. Tamaki T. Effect of growth on muscle capillarity and fiber type composition in rat diaphragm. Eur J Appl Physiol 1985; 54:24–29.
145. Thomas AJ, Arnold JS, Simhai B, Kelsen SG. Structure of abdominal muscles in the hamster: effect of elastase-induced emphysema. J Appl Physiol 1987; 63(4):1665–1670.
146. Zhan W, Sieck GC. Adaptations of diaphragm and medial gastrocnemius muscles to inactivity. J Appl Physiol 1992; 72(4):1445–1453.
147. Ferguson GT, Irvin CG, Cherniack RM. Effect of corticosteroids on respiratory muscle histopathology. Am Rev Respir Dis 1990; 142:11047–11052.
148. Dekhuijzen PNR, Gayan-Ramirez G, de Bock V, Dom R, Decramer M. Triamcinolone and prednisolone affect contractile properties and histopathology of rat diaphragm differently. J Clin Invest 1993; 92:1534–1542.
149. Viires N, Pavlovic D, Pariente R, Aubier M. Effects of steroids on diaphragmatic function in rats. Am Rev Respir Dis 1990; 142:34–38.
150. Watchko JF, LaFramboise WA, Standaert TA, Woodrum DE. Diaphragmatic function during hypoxemia: neonatal and developmental aspects. J Appl Physiol 1986; 60(5):1599–1604.

151. Zhang Y, Kelsen S. Effects of aging on diaphragm contractile function in golden hamsters. Am Rev Respir Dis 1990; 142:1396–1401.
152. Tolep K, Higgins H, Muza S, Criner G, Kelsen SG. Comparison of diaphragm strength between healthy adult elderly and young men. Am J Respir Crit Care Med 1995 (in press).
153. Altose MD, McCauley WC, Kelsen SG, Cherniack NS. Effects of hypercapnia and inspiratory flow-resistive loading on respiratory activity in chronic airways obstruction. J Clin Invest 1977; 59:500–507.
154. Supinski GS, Kelsen SG. Effect of elastase-induced emphysema on the force-generating ability of the diaphragm. J Clin Invest 1982; 70(5):978–988.
155. Farkas GA, Roussos C. Adaptability of the hamster diaphragm to exercise and/or emphysema. J Appl Physiol Respir Environ Exerc Physiol 1982; 53(5):1263–1272.
156. Farkas GA, Roussos C. Diaphragm in emphysematous hamsters: sarcomere adaptability. J Appl Physiol Respir Environ Exerc Physiol 1983; 54(6):1635–1640.
157. Oliven A, Supinski GS, Kelsen SG. Functional adaptation of diaphragm to chronic hyperinflation in emphysematous hamsters. J Appl Physiol 1986; 60(1):225–231.
158. Sanchez J, Brunet A, Medrano G, Debesse B, Derenne J.Ph. Metabolic enzymatic activities in the intercostal and serratus muscles and in the latissimus dorsi of middle-aged normal men and patients with moderate obstructive pulmonary disease. Eur Respir J 1988; 1:376–383.
159. Arora NS, Rochester DF. COPD and human diaphragm muscle dimensions. Chest 1987; 91:719–724.
160. Sorli J, Grassino A, Lorange G, Milic-Emili J. Control of breathing in patients with chronic obstructive lung disease. Clin Sci Mol Med 1978; 54:295–304.
161. Murciano D, Aubier M, Vian F. Effects of airway anesthesia on pattern of breathing and blood gases in patients with chronic obstructive pulmonary disease in acute respiratory failure. Am Rev Respir Dis 1982; 126:113–117.
162. Begin P, Grassino A. Inspiratory muscle dysfunction and chronic hypercapnia in chronic obstructive pulmonary disease. Am Rev Respir Dis 1991; 143:905–912.
162a. Pardy RL, Roussos C. Endurance of hyperventilation in chronic airflow obstruction. Chest 1983; 83:744–750.
163. Supinski G, DiMarco A, Hussein F. Alterations in respiratory muscle activation in the ischemic fatigued canine diaphragm. J Appl Physiol 1989; 67:720–729.
163a. Gallagher CG, Im Hof, V, Younes M. Effect of inspiratory muscle fatigue on breathing pattern. J Appl Physiol 1985; 59(4):1152–1158.
164. Hussain SNA, Magder S, Chatillon A, Roussos C. Chemical activation of thin-fiber phrenic afferents: respiratory responses. J Appl Physiol 1990; 69(3):1002–1011.
165. Jammes Y, Buchler B, Delpierre S, Rasidakis A, Grimaud C, Roussos C. Phrenic afferents and their role in inspiratory control. J Appl Physiol 1986; 60:(3):854–860.
165a. Revelette WR, Jewell LA, Frazier DT. Effect of diaphragm small-fiber afferent stimulation on ventilation in dogs. J Appl Physiol 1988; 65(5):2097–2106.

166. Shannon R. Reflexes from respiratory muscles and costovertebral joints. in: Handbook of Physiology. The Respiratory System. Control of Breathing. Bethesda, MD: Am Physiol Soc sect. 3, vol II, part 1, chap 13, 1986:431–447.
167. Bolser DC, Lindsey BG, Shannon R. Medullary inspiratory activity: influence of intercostal tendon organs and muscle spindle endings. J Appl Physiol 1987; 62(3):1046–1056.
168. Frazier DT, Revelette WR. Role of phrenic nerve afferents in the control of breathing. J Appl Physiol 1991; 70(2):491–496.
169. Killian KJ, Bucens DD, Campbell EJM. Effect of breathing patterns on the perceived magnitude of added loads to breathing. J Appl Physiol 1982; 52:578–584.
170. Altose MD, Dimarco AF, Gottfried SB, Strohl KP. The sensation of respiratory muscle force. Am Rev Respir Dis 1982; 126:807–811.
171. Oliven A, Kelsen SG, Deal EC, Cherniack NS. Respiratory pressure sensation: relationship to changes in breathing pattern and P_{CO_2} during acute increase in airway resistance in patients with chronic obstructive pulmonary disease. Am Rev Respir Dis 1985; 132:1214–1218.
172. Gandevia SC, McKenzie DK. Activation of the human diaphragm during maximal static efforts. J Physiol 1985; 367:45–56.
173. Ward ME, Eidelman D, Stubbing DG, Bellemare F, Macklem PT. Respiratory sensation and pattern of respiratory muscle activation during diaphragm fatigue. J Appl Physiol 1988; 65(5):2181–2189.
174. Bradley TD, Chartrand DA, Fitting JW, Killian KJ, Grassino A. The relation of inspiratory effort sensation to fatiguing patterns of the diaphragm. Am Rev Respir Dis 1986; 134:1119–1124.
175. Cohen CA, Zagelbaum G, Gross D, Rousso CH, Macklem PT. Clinical manifestations of inspiratory muscle fatigue. Am J Med 1982; 73:308–316.
176. Pourriat JL, Camberto C, Hoang P. Diaphragmatic fatigue and breathing pattern during weaning from mechanical ventilation in COPD patients. Chest 1986; 90:703–707.
176a. Efthimiou J, Fleming J, Spiro SG. Sternomastoid muscle function and fatigue in breathless patients with severe respiratory disease. Am Rev Respir Dis 1987; 136:1099–1105.
177. Bye PTP, Esau SA, Walley KR, Macklem PT, Pardy RL. Ventilatory muscles during exercise in air and oxygen in normal men. J Appl Physiol Respir Environ Exerc Physiol 1984; 56(2):464–471.
178. Juan G, Calverley P, Talamo C, Schnader J, Roussos C. Effect of carbon dioxide on diaphragmatic function in human beings. N Engl J Med 1984; 310:874–879.
179. Schnader J, Howell S, Fitzgerald RS, Roussos C. Interaction of fatigue and hypercapnia in the canine diaphragm. J Appl Physiol 1988; 64(4):1636–1643.
180. Campbell EJM. The management of acute respiratory failure in chronic bronchitis and emphysema. Am Rev Respir Dis 1967; 96:626–639.
181. Weiner P, Suo J, Fernandez E, Cherniack RM. The effect of hyperinflation on respiratory muscle strength and efficiency in healthy subjects and patients with asthma. Am Rev Respir Dis 1990; 141:1501–1505.

182. Wittmann TA, Kelsen SG. The effect of caffeine on diaphragmatic muscle force in normal hamsters. Am Rev Respir Dis 1982; 126:499–504.
183. Viires N, Aubier M, Murciano D, Fleury B, Talamo C, Pariente R. Effects of aminophylline on diaphragmatic fatigue during acute respiratory failure. Am Rev Respir Dis 1984; 129:396–402.
184. Aubier M, Viires N, Murciano D, Medrano G, Lecocguic Y, Pariente R. Effects and mechanism of action of terbutaline on diaphragmatic contractility and fatigue. J Appl Physiol Respir Environ Exerc Physiol 1984; 56(4):922–929.
185. Aubier M, Murciano D, Viires N, Lecocguic Y, Palacios S, Pariente R. Increased ventilation caused by improved diaphragmatic efficiency during aminophylline infusion. Am Rev Respir Dis 1983; 127:148–154.
186. DiMarco AF, Nochomovitz M, DiMarco MS, Altose MD, Kelsen SG. Comparative effects of aminophylline on diaphragm and cardiac contractility. Am Rev Respir Dis 1985; 132:800–805.
187. Howell S, Fitzgerald RS, Roussos C. Effects of neostigmine and salbutamol on diaphragmatic fatigue. Respir Physiol 1985; 62:15–29.
188. Lewis MI, Belman MJ, Sieck GC. Aminophylline and fatigue of the sternomastoid muscle. Am Rev Respir Dis 1986; 133:672–675.
189. Murciano D, Auclair MH, Pariente R, Aubier M. A randomized, controlled trial of theophylline in patients with severe chronic obstructive pulmonary disease. N Engl J Med 1989; 320:1521–1525.
190. Murciano D, Aubier M, Lecocguic Y, Pariente R. Effects of theophylline on diaphragmatic strength and fatigue in patients with chronic obstructive pulmonary disease. N Engl J Med 1984; 311:349–353.
191. Nava S, Crotti P, Gurrieri G, Fracchia C, Rampulla C. Effect of a β_2-agonist (broxaterol) on respiratory muscle strength and endurance in patients with COPD with irreversible airway obstruction. Chest 1992; 101:133–140.
191a. Aubier M, Viires N, Murciano D, Seta JP, Pariente R. Effects of digoxin on diaphragmatic strength generation. J Appl Physiol 1986; 61(5):1767–1774.
192. Suzuki S, Numata H, Sano F, Yoshiike Y, Mitashita A, Okubo T. Effects and mechanism of fenoterol on fatigued canine diaphragm. Am Rev Respir Dis 1988; 137:1048–1054.
193. Supinski GS, Deal EC, Kelsen SG. The effects of caffeine and theophylline on diaphragm contractility. Am Rev Respir Dis 1984; 130:429–433.
194. Sigrist S. Thomas D, Howell S, Roussos C. The effect of aminophylline on inspiratory muscle contractility. Am Rev Respir Dis 1982; 126:46–50.
195. Foxworth JW, Reisz GR, Knudson SM, Cuddy PG, Pyszczynski DR, Emory CE. Theophylline and diaphragmatic contractility. Am Rev Respir Dis 1988; 138:1532–1534.
196. Supinski GS, Arnold JS, Kelsen SG. Effect of theophylline on the velocity of diaphragmatic muscle shortening. J Appl Physiol 65(3):1410–1415.
197. Bradley ME, Leith DE. Ventilatory muscle training and the oxygen cost of sustained hyperpnea. J Appl Physiol 1973; 45(6):885–892.
198. Belman MJ, Gaesser GA. Ventilatory muscle training in the elderly. J Appl Physiol 1988; 64(3):899–905.

199. Akabas SR, Bazzy AR, DiMauro S, Haddad GG. Metabolic and functional adaptation of the diaphragm to training with resistive loads. J Appl Physiol 1989; 66(2):529–535.
200. Moore RL, Gollnick PD. Response of ventilatory muscles of the rat to endurance training. Eur J Physiol 1982; 392:268–271.
201. Gosselin LE, Betlach M, Vailas AC, Thomas DP. Training-induced alterations in young and senescent rat diaphragm muscle. J Appl Physiol 1992; 72(4):1506–1511.
202. Belman MJ, Mittman C. Ventilatory muscle training improves exercise capacity in chronic obstructive pulmonary disease patients. Am Rev Respir Dis 1980; 121:273–280.
203. Duchateau J, Hainaut K. Isometric or dynamic training: differential effects on mechanical properties of a human muscle. J Appl Physiol Respir Environ Exerc Physiol 1984; 56(2):296–301.
204. Dudley GA, Djamil R. Incompatibility of endurance—and strength—training modes of exercise. J Appl Physiol 1985; 59(5):1446–1451.
205. Tarasiuk A, Scharf SM, Miller MJ. Effect of chronic resistive loading on inspiratory muscles in rats. J Appl Physiol 1991; 70(1):216–222.
205a. Fanta CH, Leith DE, Brown R. Maximal shortening of inspiratory muscles: effect of training. J Appl Physiol 1983; 54(6):1618–1623.
206. Booth FW, Thomason DB. Molecular and cellular adaptation of muscle in response to exercise: perspectives of various models. Physiol Rev 1981; 71(2):541–585.
207. Holloszy JO, Coyle EF. Adaptations of skeletal muscle to endurance exercise and their metabolic consequences. J Appl Physiol 1984; 56(4):831–838.
208. Belman MJ, Shadmehr R. Targeted resistive ventilatory muscle training in chronic obstructive pulmonary disease. J Appl Physiol 1988; 65(6):2726–2735.
209. Belman MJ, Botnick WC, Nathan SD, Chon KH. Ventilatory load characteristics during ventilatory muscle training. Am J Respir Crit Care Med 1994; 149:925–929.
210. Chen H, Dukes R, Martin BJ. Inspiratory muscle training in patients with chronic obstructive pulmonary disease. Am Rev Respir Dis 1985; 131:251–255.
211. Belman MJ, Kendregan BA. Physical training fails to improve ventilatory muscle endurance in patients with chronic obstructive pulmonary disease. Chest 1982; 81(4):440–443.
212. Levine S, Weiser P, Gillen J. Evaluation of a ventilatory muscle endurance training program in the rehabilitation of patients with chronic obstructive pulmonary disease. Am Rev Respir Dis 1986; 133:4000–4406.
213. Smith K, Cook D, Guyatt GH, Madhavan J, Oxman AD. Respiratory muscle training in chronic airflow limitation: a meta-analysis. Am Rev Respir Dis 1992; 145:533–539.
214. Sonne LJ, Davis JA. Increased exercise performance in patients with severe COPD following inspiratory resistive training. Chest 1982; 81:432–439.
215. Criner GJ, Travaline JM, Sudarshan S, Leyenson V. Effect of inspiratory muscle training on diaphragm strength and fatiguability. Am J Respir Crit Care Med 1995 (in press).

8

Neuromuscular Disorders

ANDRÉ DE TROYER and MARC ESTENNE

Erasme University Hospital
and Brussels School of Medicine
Brussels, Belgium

Ventilatory failure, often associated with pneumonia, is a frequent cause of death in many neuromuscular disorders. It may appear at the onset of the disease, as in the acute inflammatory stage of poliomyelitis, in the Guillain-Barré syndrome, or during an episode of myasthenia gravis. The acute clinical syndrome in these conditions is relatively stereotyped and may be summarized as: (1) involvement of inspiratory and expiratory muscles; (2) rapidly progressive decrease in vital capacity; and (3) rapidly progressive alveolar hypoventilation with hypercapnia and hypoxemia. However, in many diseases, such as muscular dystrophy and amyotrophic lateral sclerosis, respiratory insufficiency develops slowly over the years. Chronic respiratory insufficiency also occurs in many patients with poliomyelitis after recovery from the acute illness. Respiratory failure in these patients is not simply due to the direct effect of weakness of the respiratory muscles leading to inability to inflate the lungs and alveolar hypoventilation. A variety of additional pathogenic mechanisms, such as alterations in the mechanical properties of the lungs and of the chest wall and dysfunction of the "respiratory centers," are important.

The first two sections of this chapter discuss the mechanisms leading to respiratory insufficiency in patients with chronic neuromuscular disorders. The general pattern of clinical and pathophysiological abnormalities is common to a range of disorders, although the detailed changes are influenced by the distribution and rate of progression of respiratory muscle weakness and, of course, by the severity and chronicity of the disease. The first section provides a general account of the abnormalities when severe, chronic muscle weakness involves both inspiratory and expiratory muscles; this account is based largely on studies in patients with muscular dystrophies, which have been more extensively studied than other disorders. The second section deals with certain individual disorders, such as quadriplegia and diaphragmatic paralysis, in which this general pattern is modified by the particular distribution of muscle weakness. The last section focuses on recent developments in the management of these disorders.

I. Pathophysiology of Respiratory Muscle Weakness

A. Lung Volumes

The severe poliomyelitis epidemics in the early 1950s made it necessary to have objective criteria for starting treatment with a respirator during the acute illness and for guiding subsequent weaning from the respirator (1,2). The increasing success of treatment during the acute stages of respiratory failure also rapidly emphasized the need for more knowledge of the changes in pulmonary function during recovery from the acute illness and stimulated interest in the pathophysiology of respiratory muscle weakness. Early studies on poliomyelitis patients reported decreases in vital capacity (VC) and its two components, inspiratory capacity (IC) and expiratory reserve volume (ERV) (3–5). A number of studies on various neuromuscular disorders have since amply confirmed that VC is reduced as a consequence of respiratory muscle weakness, and that it decreases consistently with progression of the disease (6–10).

The decrease in VC was initially attributed to the direct effect of weakness of inspiratory and expiratory muscles. As early as 1952, however, Ferris et al. (11) showed reductions in lung and chest wall compliance in convalescent patients with poliomyelitis, while Spencer and Vallbona (12), in 1959, noted that the inspiratory capacity obtained with a positive-pressure breathing device in similar patients was regularly smaller than the one obtained in comparable healthy subjects. More recent work has confirmed that factors other than the reduced ability to inflate and to deflate the lungs completely are acting to decrease the VC in patients with chronic respiratory muscle weakness. Because of the sigmoid shape of the pressure-volume curve of the normal relaxed respiratory system, so that at the extremes of the VC large changes in pressure produce only small changes in volume (13), VC would be expected to be relatively well preserved until muscle weakness became very severe. However, in practice, even though VC is highly correlated with respiratory muscle strength in patients with chronic respiratory muscle weakness, reductions in VC are greater than anticipated for the degree of muscle weakness (Fig. 1) (14–16). Scoliosis, heart failure, or bronchopneumonia may contribute to the loss of VC in some patients, but a disproportionate loss of VC may be present without any of these complications. As discussed in the following two sections, this is essentially related to alterations in the mechanical properties of the lungs and chest wall.

Although it is clearly established that VC is decreased as a consequence of respiratory muscle weakness, data on the resting end-expiratory position (functional residual capacity, FRC) and the residual volume (RV) are conflicting. The FRC has been alternatively reported to be unchanged (4,8,10,17,18), decreased (7,15,19–22), or slightly increased (23). Similarly, some investiga-

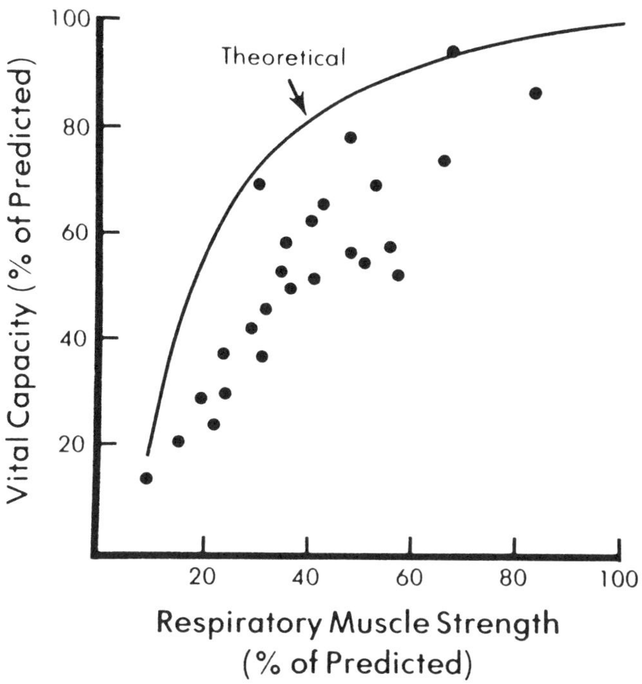

Figure 1 Relationship between respiratory muscle strength and vital capacity in 25 patients with long-standing neuromuscular disorders. The solid curve indicates the theoretical effect of respiratory muscle weakness (with proportionate effects on inspiratory and expiratory muscles) on vital capacity. This relationship is calculated from the standard maximal pressure-volume curve, assuming that respiratory system recoil in such patients is the same as that measured in normal subjects. Note that the reductions in vital capacity are disproportionate to the degree of muscle weakness. (From Ref. 15.)

tors have reported no change in RV (7,15,18,21), while others found it to be increased (4,5,8,10,17,23). These differences are, in part, due to differences in the patients studied, in the extent and the distribution of muscular involvement, and in the body position in which the studies were made.

B. Pulmonary Mechanics

Since the position of full inflation (TLC) is set by a balance between the lung recoil pressure (Pst, L) and the most negative pleural pressure that can be generated by the inspiratory muscles (Ppl min) (24,25), weakness of the inspiratory muscles prevents a normal Pst, L from being developed in the lung at full inflation and so truncates the upper part of the static pressure-volume (PV) curve of the lung. Simple truncation of the upper part of the PV curve without alteration in the remainder of the curve is found when moderate respiratory muscle weakness and reduction in VC are produced acutely in normal subjects

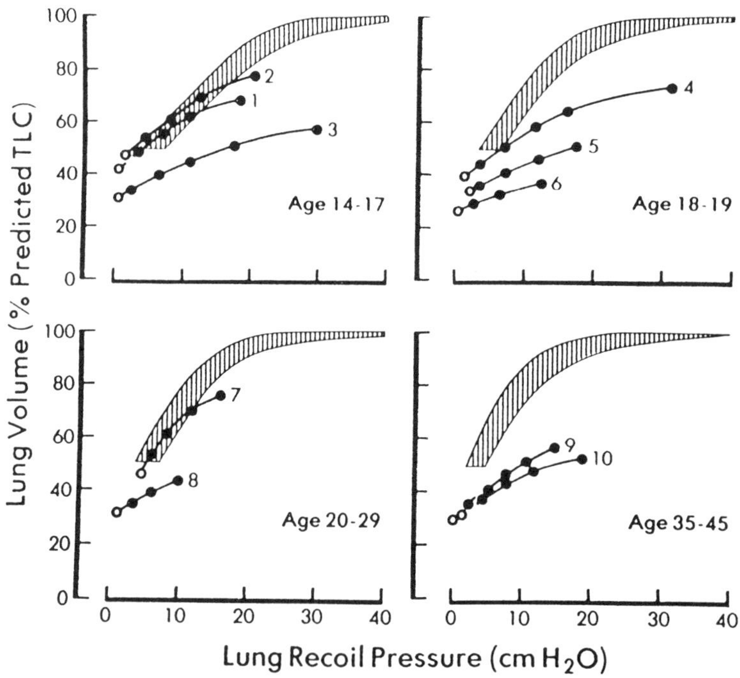

Figure 2 Static expiratory pressure-volume curves of the lungs in 10 patients with chronic respiratory muscle weakness. (Open circles) The position of functional residual capacity. The hatched area represents ± 1 SD of normal values. Volume is expressed as percent of predicted TLC to allow for differences in patient size. (From Ref. 19.)

by partial curarization (26–28). Similarly, no change in pulmonary compliance is seen in patients with myasthenia gravis and moderate muscle weakness who show a good acute response to pyridostigmine (29). However, in patients with long-standing and severe respiratory muscle weakness, the inability to expand the lungs fully is associated with further changes in the lung PV curve, apart from truncation of its upper part (15,19,21). Static expiratory PV curves from 10 patients with chronic respiratory muscle weakness due to muscular dystrophy are shown in Figure 2. In most patients, not only is the Pst, L at TLC low in relation to the normal value, but Pst, L is increased at any absolute lung volume and pulmonary compliance is reduced.

Because of the normal hysteresis of the lung PV curve, a reduction in the Pst, L achieved on full inspiration alters the position of the expiratory curve and tends to reduce the static expiratory compliance. However, this effect is small and cannot account for reductions in pulmonary compliance of the magnitude observed in patients with long-standing respiratory muscle weakness. Moreover, values of compliance obtained during inspiration are also markedly reduced (15,19,21), indicating that the elastic properties of the lung are themselves altered in these patients. This decrease in lung distensibility is an important determinant of the loss of lung volume in these patients, as shown by the clear relationship between TLC and the compliance at FRC (15,16,19).

The cause of this reduced lung distensibility is uncertain, but in most cases, this alteration is present without any radiographic changes suggesting parenchymal disease. Since most patients with muscular dystrophy develop signs and symptoms of the disease in early childhood, failure of development of a normal complement of alveoli might account for these changes. Similar alterations in the lung PV curve are found, however, in patients who develop disease in adult life, such as patients with spinal cord injury or poliomyelitis (11,15,21,30). When expressed as specific compliance, which relates static expiratory compliance to actual TLC, pulmonary compliance measured at FRC is in the normal range in almost all patients (15,19,21). This finding has been interpreted as indicating that the majority of ventilated alveoli in these lungs retain relatively normal elastic properties and that most of the changes in the lung PV curve are therefore due to dispersed alveolar collapse (15,21). As a matter of fact, patchy atelectasis has been reported to be a frequent finding at necropsy in ventilator-dependent patients with poliomyelitis (31–33). Atelectasis, however, was not found in all patients. In addition, using a high-resolution computerized tomographic (CT) scanner, Estenne et al. (34) have been unable to confirm the presence of atelectasis in a group of eight patients with traumatic tetraplegia and six patients with muscular dystrophy. Yet, these patients had a clear-cut restrictive ventilatory impairment and a 30% reduction in static expiratory pulmonary compliance.

Two factors are theoretically capable of reducing lung distensibility in otherwise normal lungs when the respiratory muscles are weak. As suggested by Young et al. (35), one mechanism is a generalized increase in the surface tension of the alveolar lining layer, due to breathing at low lung volume. Indeed, there is ample physiological evidence from acute experiments, beginning with the work in dogs by Mead and Collier (36), that breathing at a small, constant tidal volume is associated with a decrease in the compliance of the lungs (37–39). To the extent that patients with respiratory muscle weakness breathe faster and with a smaller tidal volume than healthy subjects (21,40–44), this disturbance might be a determining factor. In laboratory animals and in human subjects, the alteration produced by rapid, shallow breathing can be rapidly corrected by a few deep breaths (36–38). In contrast, the decreased pulmonary compliance of patients with chronic respiratory muscle weakness is not reversed by short periods of positive-pressure, mechanical hyperinflation of the lungs (19,45), suggesting that alterations in surface forces are not the primary determinant of the reduced pulmonary distensibility in these patients.

The second mechanism is an alteration in lung tissue elasticity. The elastic properties of a system are, in part, determined by the stresses to which the system is subjected. Therefore, the elastic properties of lung tissue might change in patients with chronic respiratory muscle weakness because of their chronically limited range of activity. The normal appearance of the lung parenchyma on the CT scanner (34), the absence of improvement after mechanical hyperinflation of the lungs (19,45), and the preservation of normal gas exchange in most patients (34,40,42,46), are all compatible with such an alteration. It must be emphasized, however, that we know of no data to show that such patients do have abnormal stiffening of the elastic fibers within the lungs.

C. Chest Wall Mechanics

Patients with chronic neuromuscular disorders also show abnormalities in chest wall compliance. Direct measurements of chest wall compliance have been performed in patients with respiratory muscle weakness due to poliomyelitis, muscular dystrophy, or tetraplegia. Two methods have been used: (1) the cycling tidal volume method, which requires that the subject relax the respiratory muscles and allow the lungs to be expanded passively by the cyclical negative pressures imposed by the tank respirator (11); and (2) the midposition shift method of Heaf and Prime (47), in which a weight-loaded spirometer induces an airway pressure that causes an increment in thoracic volume (45,48,49). Assuming relaxation of the respiratory muscles, both methods relate an imposed pressure change to an induced thoracic volume change, and measurements of esophageal pressure permit separation of lung, chest wall, and total respiratory system compliance. The two methods have yielded virtually identical results and demonstrated that in patients with long-standing neuromuscular disorders, chest wall compliance is decreased to about two-thirds of normal values.

These measurements of chest wall compliance apply to the entire chest wall, but Estenne and De Troyer (49), using pairs of respiratory magnetometers, have partitioned chest wall compliance into its ribcage and abdominal components in 20 patients in the late stages of quadriplegia. Ribcage compliance, on average, was decreased to 55% of normal, whereas abdominal compliance was increased to 170% of normal (Fig. 3). Thus, if the chest wall is stiffer in quadriplegic patients than in healthy subjects, it is because the ribcage is abnormally stiff. Although similar measurements have not been reported in patients with muscular dystrophies, it seems reasonable to speculate that the reduced chest wall compliance in such patients is also related primarily to increased stiffness of the ribcage. The chronically decreased physical activity of these patients diminishes the need for large respiratory excursions. The movements of the cage may be further reduced because of the small tidal volume and possibly because of the weakness of the ribcage muscles. These factors

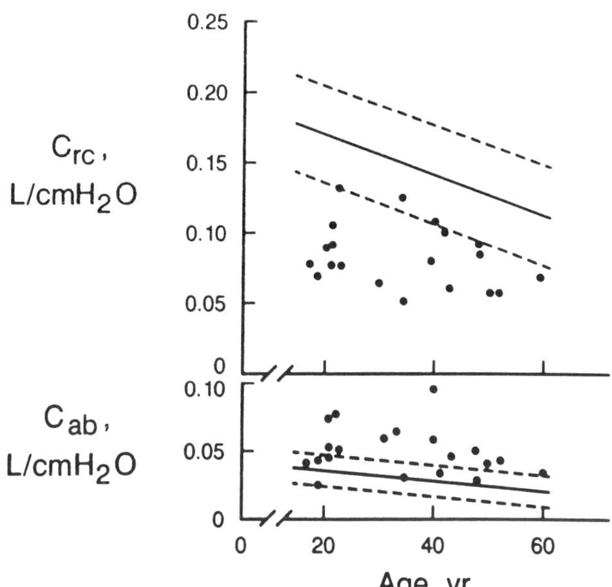

Figure 3 Values of ribcage (C_{rc}) and abdominal (C_{ab}) compliance obtained in 20 seated quadriplegic patients. Solid and dashed lines represent regression equations ± 1 SEM in 61 healthy adults. Ribcage compliance is below the normal range and abdominal compliance is above the normal range in most patients. (From Refs. 49 and 144.)

should lead to ankylosis in the costosternal and costovertebral joints and to gradual stiffening of ribcage tissues (tendons and ligaments). A further contributory factor may be the development of scoliosis, particularly in patients in the latter stages of muscular dystrophy.

D. Airway Mechanics—Mechanics of Cough

Although the intrinsic properties of the airways are normal in patients with neuromuscular disorders, the configuration of the maximal expiratory flow-volume curve is abnormal in many patients (15,19,21,23,29,50,51). Indeed, because maximum expiratory flow rates at large and small lung volumes are closely dependent on the force and velocity of expiratory muscle contraction, a weakness of expiratory muscles will frequently induce a reduction in the slope of the ascending limb of the curve with peak expiratory flow occurring at a lower percent VC than in normal subjects, a decrease in peak expiratory flow, and an abrupt vertical drop of expiratory flow near residual volume. However, maximum expiratory flow can be achieved over most of the VC with rather low driving pressures and is assisted by the increased lung recoil. Hence, the rate of forced lung emptying is usually well preserved in these patients, and the FEV_1/VC ratio (FEV_1 = forced expiratory volume in 1 sec) is normal or even supranormal.

On the other hand, the effectiveness of cough is markedly reduced. In healthy subjects, vigorous contraction of the expiratory muscles elicited by coughing produces large positive pleural pressures. These pressures result in dynamic compression of the central intrathoracic airways, which induces high flow velocities so as to suspend and to accelerate mouthward the secretions adherent to the airway walls. The physiological correlate of this dynamic airway compression is a peak flow transient, i.e., a brief spike of airflow that adds to the sustained flow coming from the lungs. However, as expiratory muscle weakness develops, the pleural pressures generated during coughing efforts are decreased. Hence, the dynamic airway compression is reduced in magnitude. A gradual reduction in peak flow transients has been observed in healthy subjects during partial curarization (52), and a complete disappearance has been observed in patients with muscular dystrophy (53) and in patients with traumatic tetraplegia (Estenne and De Troyer, unpublished observations). The impaired clearance of secretions associated with such a defective cough presumably contributes to the high prevalence of bronchopulmonary infections in these patients.

E. Ventilatory Drive

Pattern of Breathing

Patients with respiratory muscle weakness breathe faster and with a smaller tidal volume than do healthy subjects (21,40–44). This altered breathing pattern is not necessarily associated with abnormal blood gases and is similar to that described in patients with a restrictive ventilatory defect of intrapulmonary origin. In interstitial lung disease, the tachypnea is believed to be caused by the stimulation of the juxtacapillary receptors, pulmonary stretch receptors, and irritant receptors. When stimulated, these receptors produce vagally mediated reflexes that terminate inspiration and thereby control the respiratory frequency. Similar reflexes may operate as well in patients with respiratory muscle weakness in whom pulmonary compliance is also decreased. Alternatively, the tachypnea in these patients could be related to afferent signals from the weakened respiratory muscles themselves. In keeping with this suggestion is the observation that partial curarization in healthy subjects elicits a similar rapid, shallow breathing pattern (41,54).

Control of Breathing

Specific dysfunction of the respiratory centers undoubtedly occurs in bulbar poliomyelitis, in which there is gross irregularity in the rate of respiration and incoordination of the respiratory muscles in the absence of anterior horn cell disease (55). Plum and Swanson (56) initially emphasized that the ventilatory response to inhalation of carbon dioxide mixtures was abnormally low in convalescing poliomyelitis patients without bulbar symptoms. Similarly, Kilburn et al. (18) found a decreased ventilatory response to CO_2 inhalation in nine patients with myotonic dystrophy and an apparently mild muscle weakness. Hypoventilation with blunted responses to CO_2 and/or hypoxia has also been reported in occasional cases of acid maltase deficiency (57), nonspecific congenital myopathy (58,59), and in patients with oculocraniosomatic neuromuscular disease (60). These alterations have repeatedly been interpreted as indicating intrinsic abnormalities of the central control mechanisms of respiration. However, reductions in the ventilatory response can be accepted as evidence of damaged medullary respiratory centers only if there are no accompanying abnormalities of lower motor neurons, respiratory muscles, or lung mechanics. In practice, therefore, in patients with weakness of the respiratory muscles, it is exceedingly difficult to determine the precise contribution of specific dysfunction of medullary respiratory centers to a reduction in ventilatory response.

Because the pressure developed at the onset of inspiration is only a small fraction of the maximum pressure that the inspiratory muscles can generate, the possibility exists that measurements of mouth occlusion pressure (Pm 0.1) might provide a more reliable estimate of central respiratory drive in patients with respiratory muscle weakness. In a study of eight normal volunteers undergoing CO_2 rebreathing during progressive curarization, Holle et al. (61) found that despite increasing muscle weakness and decreasing ventilation, Pm 0.1 was maintained or increased. Similarly, normal or elevated Pm 0.1 values have been reported in patients with various chronic neuromuscular disorders who had normal or slightly elevated arterial Pco_2 (40–42), and in patients with traumatic tetraplegia (62). These observations suggest that the central respiratory drive is, in general, well preserved in these patients.

F. Ventilation "Sleep" Muscle Fatigue

As discussed in the previous section, many patients with respiratory muscle weakness have a rapid, shallow breathing pattern, possibly related to the reduced pulmonary compliance. In the early stages of the disease, this pattern usually causes an increase in minute ventilation. Hence, although the dead space ventilation is greater than normal, there is also an increase in alveolar ventilation, resulting in alveolar and arterial hypocapnia (7,42,63). At this stage, the arterial Po_2 is usually normal. However, as weakness progresses, the bellows action of the chest decreases and tidal volume decreases further. As tidal volume falls, an increasing proportion of total ventilation is wasted in

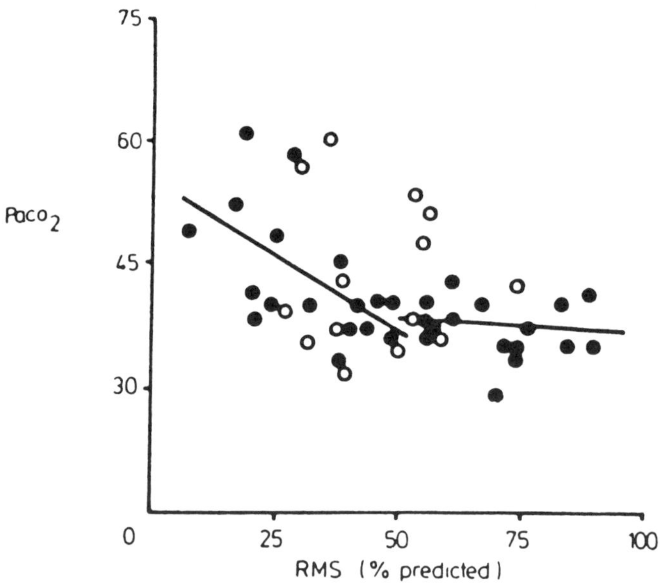

Figure 4 Relationship between respiratory muscle strength (RMS) and arterial Pco_2 (mmHg) in 33 patients with uncomplicated myopathy (closed circles, regression line) and 14 patients with myopathy plus chronic lung disease (open circles). Respiratory muscle strength is the arithmetic sum of maximum static inspiratory and expiratory mouth pressure expressed as percentage of normal and divided by 2. Note that Pco_2 increases as respiratory muscle weakness is more severe; there is, however, a considerable variability between patients. (From Ref. 46.)

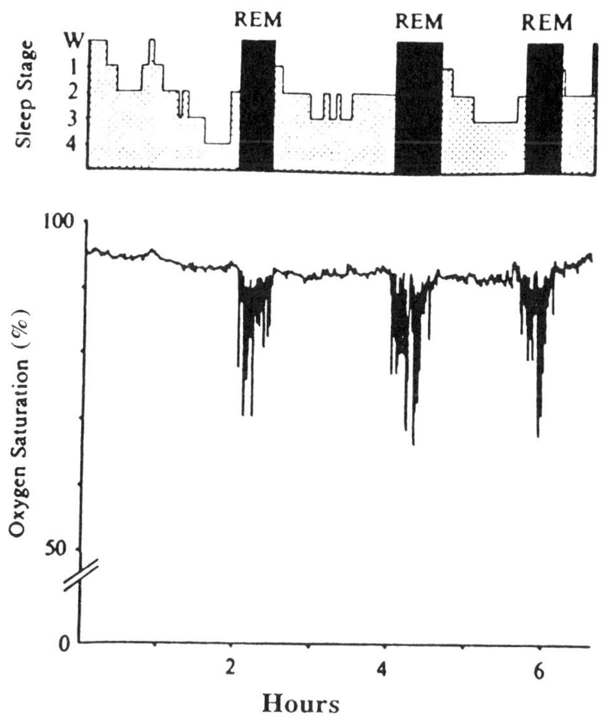

Figure 5 Overnight sleep record and oxygen saturation in a 17-year-old patient with Duchenne's muscular dystrophy. REM, rapid-eye-movement sleep; W, awake. Note the recurrent severe desaturation during REM sleep. (From Ref. 100.)

dead space ventilation, and consequently, alveolar ventilation is reduced first to normal and then to low levels. This results in hypercapnia and arterial hypoxemia.

In a study of 37 patients with respiratory muscle weakness due to polymyositis and various chronic myopathies without lung disease, Braun et al. (46) confirmed that the development of hypercapnia is usually related to the severity of muscle weakness (Fig. 4). In fact, hypercapnia was a frequent finding in patients whose values of maximum respiratory pressures were less than 30–40% of normal and in whom VC was below 55% of predicted. Similar observations were reported by Gibson et al. (64). In several patients, however, despite values of respiratory muscle strength that were less than 20% of predicted, values for Pa_{CO_2} were normal. Conversely, hypercapnia was present in some patients with moderate respiratory muscle weakness. In addition, many hypercapnic patients with chronic neuromuscular diseases can decrease their values for Pa_{CO_2} to normal levels by voluntary hyperventilation (43,65), indicating that muscle weakness is not the only factor responsible for the development of ventilatory failure.

A number of studies have suggested that sleep may be a key determinant of the development of hypercapnia in these patients. As a matter of fact, breathing during sleep is altered in many patients with chronic neuromuscular disorders, even in patients who retain normal gas exchange during the daytime: specifically, their pattern of breathing during sleep is fragmented by frequent episodes of hypopnea and apnea that are associated with hypercapnia and hypoxemia (65–71). As shown in Figure 5, these nocturnal episodes of hypoventilation and arterial desaturation are particularly frequent during rapid eye movement (REM) sleep, due apparently to a combination of factors. First, alveolar ventilation is reduced during sleep because of the loss of the stimulatory effects of wakefulness on the ventilatory drive. Second, intercostal and accessory muscle inspiratory activity is inhibited during REM sleep; this may further reduce alveolar ventilation, particularly in patients in whom the diaphragm is weakened and unable to increase its contribution to ventilation. Third, when the rapid, shallow breathing pattern typical of REM sleep is superimposed on the rapid, shallow breathing associated with respiratory muscle weakness, dead space ventilation increases inordinately, leading to further reduction in alveolar ventilation. Finally, the decrease in tone of the muscles of the upper airways associated with REM sleep may produce an increase in airway resistance; this mechanism may become prominent in patients whose pharyngeal muscles are affected by the disease process.

Although the reason why nocturnal hypoventilation might predispose to the development of ventilatory failure during the daytime is uncertain, the following observations strongly suggest that this relationship does exist. First, sleep hypoventilation is usually present well before daytime hypoventilation appears (66,67,71). Second, daytime hypercapnia is uncommon in patients who have normal gas exchange during sleep, as in patients with traumatic quadriplegia. Third, patients with chronic neuromuscular disorders show a relationship between the lowest Sa_{O_2} during REM sleep and Pa_{CO_2} during daytime, such that a more severe desaturation during sleep is associated with a more severe hypercapnia during the day (66). Finally, correction of nocturnal hypoventilation in these patients using either negative- (cuirass, tank) or positive-pressure ventilation improves arterial blood gas tensions (increased Pa_{O_2} and decreased Pa_{CO_2}) during the daytime; this improvement can be maintained for several years in the face of progressing muscle weakness (67,68,72–78). Perhaps the alterations in gas exchange during sleep progressively decrease the sensitivity of central and peripheral chemoreceptors.

Respiratory muscle fatigue could be another factor leading to persistent hypercapnia in patients with chronic neuromuscular disorders. The weak inspiratory muscles of these patients work chronically against an increased elastic load due to the reduced distensibility of the lungs and chest wall. These muscles are thus closer to their fatigue threshold than they are in healthy subjects. In patients with severe respiratory muscle weakness, the inspiratory muscles may even operate persistently beyond their fatigue threshold. Therefore, they could become fatigued and lead to CO_2 retention. Alternatively, the central nervous system might set a lower level of ventilation to avoid overt muscle fatigue. This would also lead to alveolar hypoventilation. It is important to stress, however, that none of these mechanisms has as yet been proved. Indeed, it is very difficult to test for respiratory muscle fatigue, in particular for low-frequency fatigue.

II. Features of Specific Disorders

A. Quadriplegia

Patients with traumatic transection of the lower cervical cord have a particular pattern of chronic respiratory muscle weakness, in that the intercostal and abdominal muscles are completely paralyzed while the diaphragm is intact. This particular distribution of muscle paralysis causes distinct abnormalities in the pattern of thoracoabdominal motion during breathing, as shown in Figure 6. Thus, in contrast to healthy subjects, the inspiratory expansion of the abdomen is usually associated with an inspiratory decrease (paradoxical motion) of the anteroposterior diameter of the upper ribcage (79–81). Yet, the alterations in the mechanical properties of the respiratory system in these patients resemble those observed in patients with generalized neuromuscular disorders. In the chronic stage of the disease, inspiratory muscle strength is decreased to 60% of normal, the static PV curve of the lung shows a 30% reduction in static expiratory compliance (30,45,48,49), and the chest wall compliance in the tidal breathing range is reduced to approximately 70% of predicted values, due to the abnormal stiffness of the ribcage (48,49,82). As a result of these alterations, VC and TLC are reduced to 50–80% of predicted normal values (30,45,48,83–87).

The particular distribution of muscle paralysis in quadriplegic subjects also induces profound alterations in expiratory maneuvers. In fact, because all the well-recognized muscles of expiration (abdominal muscles, expiratory intercostals, triangularis sterni) receive their motor supply from the dorsal and lumbar segments of the spinal cord, expiratory muscle function in these patients has conventionally been considered as totally lost (88). Studies in our laboratory, however, have demonstrated that these patients have residual expiratory muscle function, related to the clavicular portion of the pectoralis major (89,90). In patients with transection of the lower segments of the cervical cord,

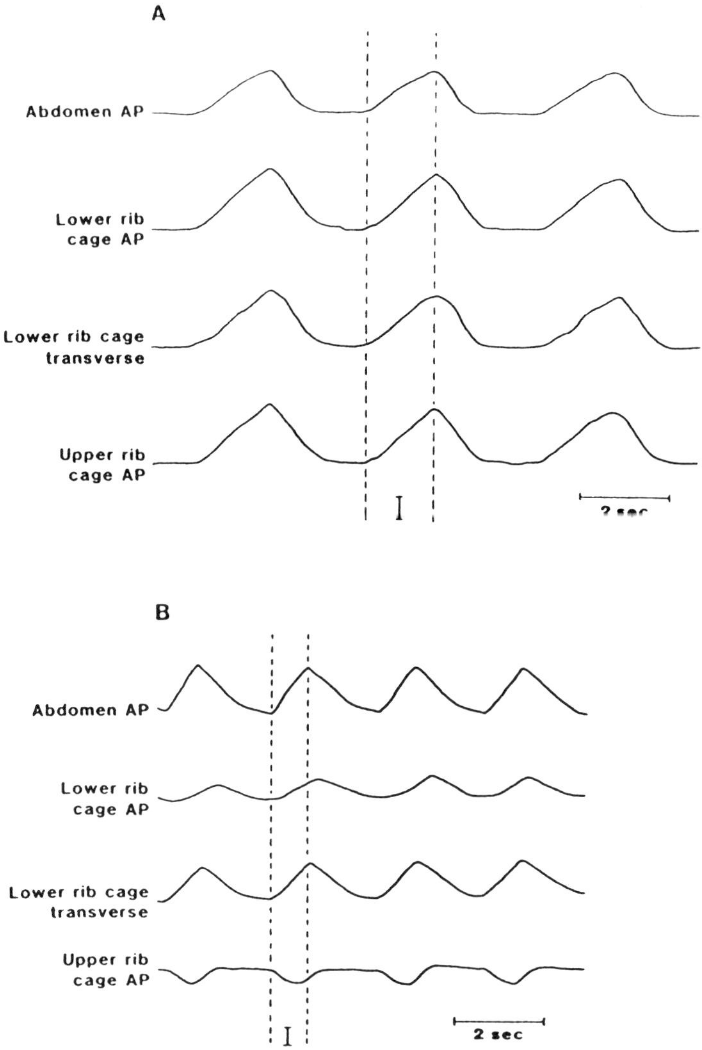

Figure 6 Pattern of chest wall motion in (A) a healthy subject and (B) a C5 quadriplegic patient breathing at rest in the seated posture. The respiratory changes in anteroposterior (AP) diameter of the abdomen, lower ribcage (5th costal cartilage), and upper rib cage (manubrium sterni) are shown, as well as the changes in transverse diameter of the lower ribcage. In all traces, an upward deflection corresponds to an increase in diameter, and a downward deflection corresponds to a decrease in diameter. I indicates the duration of inspiration. Note that during inspiration in the normal subject, the abdomen and the ribcage diameters increase uniformly and synchronously. In the quadriplegic patient, however, the AP diameter of the upper ribcage decreases rather than increases.

this muscle bundle invariably contracts during voluntary expiration (Fig. 7) and during cough; its insertions on the humerus and the medial half of the clavicle make it pull the manubrium sterni and upper ribs caudally so as to produce collapse of the upper ribcage and emptying of the lungs.

The clavicular portion of the pectoralis major does not compensate for the paralysis of the abdominal and expiratory intercostal muscles. ERV in quadriplegic subjects is thus markedly reduced, so that RV is greater than normal, and the increments in pleural pressure during cough are low. In contrast to normal subjects, who develop peak pleural pressures above 100 cmH_2O during cough, values between 8 and 36 cmH_2O have recently been obtained in a group of 12 quadriplegic patients (91). Consequently, despite the contraction of the pectoralis major, the efficiency of cough and the clearance of bronchial secretions are severely impaired. However, isovolume pressure flow (IVPF)

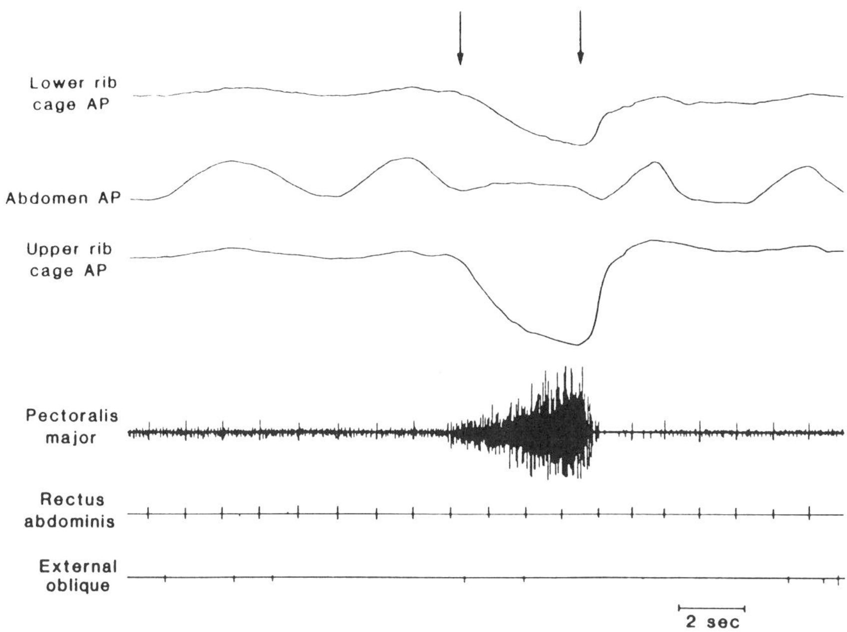

Figure 7 Pattern of chest wall motion and respiratory muscle use during slow expiration from functional residual capacity in a C6 quadriplegic patient. The changes in anteroposterior (AP) diameter of the abdomen, lower ribcage, and upper ribcage are shown (increase upward). Arrows mark the onset and the end of the expiratory effort. Voluntary expiration elicits a large amount of EMG activity in the pectoralis major and causes a clear-cut decrease in the AP diameter of the upper ribcage. The abdominal muscles show no activity. (From Ref. 89.)

curves have shown plateaus of flow at all lung volumes between 60 and 80 and 20% of the VC in six of nine patients in whom the curves could be interpreted with certainty (91). Video endoscopic recordings have also demonstrated collapse of the trachea and main bronchi during cough in three of five patients. Thus, in contrast to conventional thinking, cough in quadriplegic patients is not a passive phenomenon that results entirely from the (inward) recoil of the respiratory system. Instead, cough in these patients is an active, muscular process that may even induce dynamic compression of the intrathoracic airways.

B. Diaphragm Paralysis

Although paralysis or severe weakness of both hemidiaphragms is seen usually in the context of generalized respiratory muscle weakness, in occasional patients the diaphragm is specifically or disproportionately affected. Conditions most often associated with bilateral diaphragmatic paralysis include amyotrophic lateral sclerosis, spinal muscular atrophy, limb girdle dystrophy, and acid maltase deficiency. Bilateral diaphragmatic paralysis may also occur after surgery, in particular after open heart surgery as a result of cold injury to the phrenic nerves. Such patients demonstrate severe restrictive ventilatory impairment, the VC in the erect posture frequently being less than 50% of predicted. The TLC and static pulmonary compliance are reduced as well (43,65,92–96).

In healthy subjects breathing at rest, the diaphragm and the inspiratory muscles of the ribcage contract in concert. As a result, abdominal pressure (Pab) rises and pleural pressure (Ppl) falls. However, when the diaphragm is paralyzed, the inspiratory muscles of the ribcage are the only muscles that are active during inspiration. Hence, as the ribcage expands, the fall in Ppl is transmitted through the flaccid diaphragm so that ΔPab remains equal to ΔPpl. As a result, the abdomen moves paradoxically inward, opposing the inflation of the lung (Fig. 8) (43,65,93,97,98). In the erect posture, some patients partially compensate for diaphragm paralysis by contracting the abdominal muscles during expiration, displacing the abdomen inward and the diaphragm cranially into the thorax. Relaxation of the abdominal muscles at the start of the following inspiration may then cause outward abdominal motion and (passive) descent of the diaphragm (43,93,98). However, in the supine posture, the abdominal muscles usually remain relaxed during the entire respiratory cycle, causing an obvious inward motion of the abdominal wall during inspiration.

Adoption of the supine posture has another effect in patients with diaphragm paralysis, in that the restrictive ventilatory impairment deteriorates further. The marked (>25%) decrease in VC that occurs when the patient changes from the erect to the supine position is, in fact, characteristic of severe diaphragmatic weakness. The mechanism of this deterioration is related to the

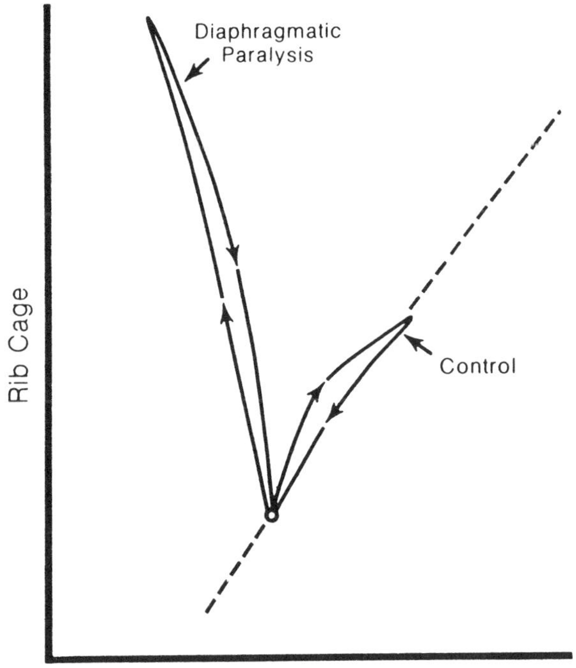

Figure 8 Pattern of chest wall motion during resting breathing in a supine anesthetized dog before (control) and after bilateral section of the phrenic nerves in the neck (diaphragmatic paralysis). The broken line represents the relaxation curve of the thoracoabdominal system, and the solid loops represent tidal volume cycles; arrows indicate the direction of the loops, and the open circle corresponds to end-expiration. Note that during breathing in the control condition, the chest wall moves on its relaxed configuration. After induction of diaphragmatic paralysis, however, the ribcage expansion during inspiration is markedly increased, but the abdomen moves paradoxically. (From Ref. 145.)

action of gravitational forces on the abdominal visceral mass. In the upright position, the hydrostatic pressure exerted by the abdominal contents tends to displace the passive diaphragm caudally at end-expiration and to oppose the tendency of the ribcage inspiratory muscles to suck the diaphragm into the thorax; in contrast, in the supine position, the hydrostatic forces displace the paralyzed diaphragm cranially and aid, rather than oppose, the action of the ribcage inspiratory muscles in sucking the diaphragm. As a result, FRC and VC are further reduced, and dyspnea is increased.

Newsom Davis et al. (43) first drew attention to the frequent elevation of Pa_{CO_2} in patients with bilateral diaphragm paralysis and to the further deterioration of arterial blood gases during sleep (68,76). Similar findings were subsequently reported by Skatrud et al. (65) in a patient with limb girdle dystrophy who had considerable hypoventilation during REM sleep. In normal subjects, inactivity of the intercostal and neck muscles during REM sleep causes ventilation to depend heavily on the diaphragm. Accordingly, it was suggested that patients with paralysis of the diaphragm would be unusually vulnerable to sleep. However, Laroche et al. (94) were unable to find hypercapnia, night or day, in six patients with severe and apparently isolated bilateral diaphragmatic weakness whom they studied in a stable state. They argued that the nocturnal hypoventilation reported in previous studies was related to the presence of generalized respiratory muscle weakness and concluded that bilateral diaphragm paralysis alone does not lead to significant nocturnal hypoventilation or chronic ventilatory failure. However, this issue is not completely resolved since there are other well-documented reports of apparently isolated diaphragm paralysis with nocturnal hypercapnia, with or without daytime hypercapnia (71,93).

C. Muscular Dystrophies

Duchenne Dystrophy

Respiratory failure, often in association with pneumonia, is a major factor in the death of more than 75% of patients with Duchenne dystrophy (8,99,100). Respiratory muscle weakness appears at a relatively early stage of the disease (6,7) and progresses until death, which invariably occurs by the second or third decade. Despite the importance of eventual respiratory failure, chronic hypercapnia appears to be rare, suggesting that the development of a raised Pa_{CO_2} is usually rapidly fatal. In two studies of 41 patients with Duchenne dystrophy, some of whom had major respiratory muscle weakness and severe reductions in lung volume, hypercapnia was found in only one case; the majority of patients had hypocapnia (7,8). Newsom Davis (101) has suggested that this might be due to relative preservation of diaphragmatic function until late in the illness.

Limb-Girdle Dystrophy

Neustadt and coworkers (102) first drew attention to the development of chronic hypercapnia in limb-girdle dystrophy. Their patient was a 41-year-old man in whom the diagnosis had been made at 32 years of age. Symptoms of chronic hypercapnia were evident some months before hospitalization; while in the hospital, the patient became comatose from CO_2 narcosis. Contamin et al. (103) described the same syndrome in a 44-year-old man and commented on the possible significance of the total diaphragm paralysis in the development of chronic hypercapnia. In three patients with limb-girdle dystrophy, Newson Davis and Loh (68) demonstrated severe diaphragm weakness in one and total paralysis in the two others; two of their patients had chronic hypercapnia. More recently, Skatrud et al. (65) also reported a patient with limb-girdle dystrophy and complete paralysis of the diaphragm; the patient had hypercapnia and hypoxemia while awake and deteriorated substantially during sleep. Patients with limb-girdle dystrophy thus seem much more likely to develop chronic hypercapnia than do those with Duchenne dystrophy, apparently because of relatively early and severe involvement of the diaphragm. Nevertheless, not all patients with limb-girdle dystrophy develop this problem. Many of them have only moderate respiratory muscle weakness and normal arterial blood gases (18).

Myotonic Dystrophy

A number of earlier reports have emphasized the occurrence of chronic hypercapnia in patients with myotonic dystrophy (18,104–107). For example, Kilburn et al. (18) found chronic hypercapnia in seven of nine patients even though the respiratory muscles appeared to be only moderately involved. Since these patients also had a poor ventilatory response to inhaled CO_2, these investigators suggested that central respiratory control mechanisms were abnormal and contributed to hypoventilation. A similar suggestion was made by Carroll et al. (108), who reported that patients with myotonic dystrophy often have a decreased ventilatory response to hypoxia. In addition, many patients with myotonic dystrophy have a grossly disordered (chaotic) pattern of ventilation, as shown in Figure 9 (18,107,109,110); these irregularities have been taken as further evidence that a primary abnormality of central respiratory control is present in the disease.

On the other hand, only one of 10 patients studied by Gillam et al. (109) and none of the 20 patients studied by Bégin et al. (41) and by Jammes et al. (111) had hypercapnia. The Pm 0.1 values measured in these patients were also normal or supranormal (41,42). Furthermore, although five of the 19 patients studied by Serisier et al. (110) had hypercapnia and a reduced ventilatory response to inhaled CO_2, the relationships between VC or respiratory muscle strength and Pa_{CO_2} found in these patients were similar to those observed in patients with other nonmyotonic neuromuscular diseases (64,110). These investigators, therefore, concluded that hypercapnia in myotonic dystrophy may be attributable simply to the effects of respiratory muscle weakness, and they suggested that the "unexpected" hypercapnia reported in earlier studies was probably due to inadequate recognition of respiratory muscle weakness.

To understand the mechanism of the irregular breathing pattern seen in these patients, Gibson et al. (64) have also performed detailed sleep studies. They paid particular attention to the breathing pattern during slow-wave (stages

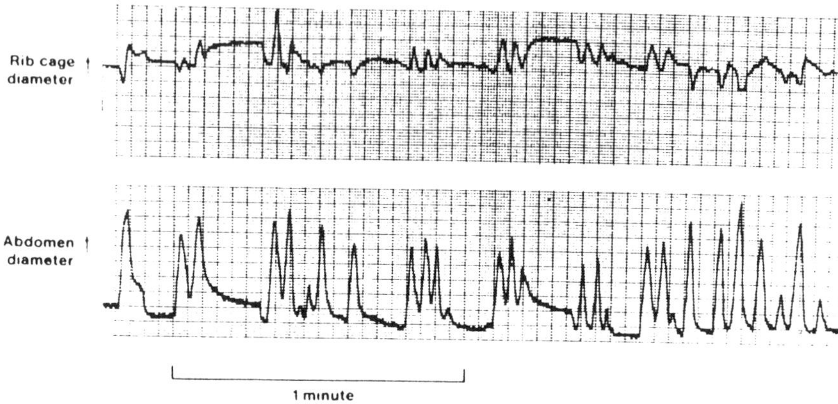

Figure 9 Pattern of breathing in a patient with myotonic dystrophy. The patient was awake and breathing at rest in the supine posture, and the respiratory changes in ribcage (upper trace) and abdomen (lower trace) anteroposterior diameter were measured with pairs of magnetometers (increase upward). The pattern was grossly disorganized ("chaotic") with respect to both the rate and depth of breathing. (From Ref. 110.)

3 and 4) sleep, when ventilation is most dependent on the metabolic pathway of respiratory control and behavioral influences are minimized. They found that during these stages of sleep, patients with myotonic dystrophy do not behave differently from normal subjects or patients with nonmyotonic respiratory muscle weakness, thus suggesting that patients with myotonic dystrophy indeed do not have any peculiar abnormality of central rhythm generation. The explanation of the "chaotic" breathing observed in many of these patients is uncertain, but Gibson et al. (64) suggested that it might be related to disordered afferent information from muscle spindles, which are known to be structurally abnormal in this condition (112).

D. Amyotrophic Lateral Sclerosis

Weakness of the respiratory muscles is an obligatory component of amyotrophic lateral sclerosis (ALS). However, the pattern of respiratory muscle dysfunction in the early stages of the disease is usually characterized by preferential involvement of the abdominal muscles and a relative preservation of the intercostal and diaphragm muscles; this explains why in these patients, unlike most patients with other neuromuscular disorders, the residual volume (RV) is increased (10,23). Moreover, progression in ALS is faster than in most other chronic neuromuscular disorders, explaining why respiratory failure is the most common cause of death. Some ALS patients develop hypercapnia at a relatively early stage of the disease, probably related to the early involvement of the diaphragm (110,113). However, in general, hypercapnia occurs as a preterminal event as in Duchenne dystrophy.

III. Principles of Management

Because of the predictable unhappy sequence of events (progressive respiratory muscle weakness followed by ventilatory failure and terminal pulmonary infection) and the absence of any specific treatment of the primary neuromuscular disease, most physicians have long had a pessimistic "nontreatment" approach to the management of respiratory insufficiency in patients with neuromuscular disorders. Indeed, providing ventilatory support to such patients was usually synonymous with continuous, intermittent positive-pressure ventilation (IPPV) via a tracheostomy; to the observer, this practice ethically seemed to seriously compromise the patient's quality of life. However, surveys of such patients have shown that the patient's perception of the quality of life was greatly underestimated (114,115). Furthermore, many reports have shown that assisted ventilation only at night could bring about a substantial improvement in many patients, and several noninvasive methods of ventilatory support have been introduced as an alternative to tracheostomy. As a result, health care professionals have developed more positive attitudes toward these patients.

A. Nocturnal Assisted Ventilation

The efficacy of assisted ventilation at night in patients with severe neuromuscular disorders and chronic hypercapnia was first noted by Neustadt et al. (102) in a patient with limb-girdle dystrophy who, after having developed CO_2 narcosis on several occasions, was later able to resume his previous life pattern after nocturnal ventilation had been instituted. Even though no controlled prospective trials have been done, the value of this type of treatment has since been confirmed in a number of studies (67,72–75,78,116,117). Virtually all patients report a marked improvement in their clinical status and quality of life within a few weeks after initiation of this treatment; morning headaches, daytime hypersomnolence, and mood disorders disappear, and intellectual performance is improved. The signs and symptoms of systemic venous congestion disappear as well. The physiological counterpart is an improvement of arterial blood gas values during the daytime. There is an increase in Pa_{O_2} and a decrease in Pa_{CO_2}, and in some patients, the values eventually fall within the normal range.

Vianello et al. (118) have also compared the clinical course of five patients with Duchenne muscular dystrophy and hypercapnia who accepted nocturnal assisted ventilation to that of five comparable patients who refused it. After 2 years of follow-up all ventilated patients were alive. However, four of five nonventilated patients had died, thus suggesting that in addition to alleviating the symptoms related to chronic hypercapnia and hypoxemia, this treatment may prolong life.

Negative-pressure body ventilators (the so-called "iron lungs") were widely used to support ventilation in patients with poliomyelitis and other neuromuscular disorders until the late 1950s. However, use of these ventilators is cumbersome. In addition, negative-pressure ventilation is frequently associated with upper airways obstruction, particularly during REM sleep when there is a loss of tone in the dilating muscles of the upper airways (119). Therefore, in some patients, these ventilators cannot achieve adequate ventilation; consequently, positive-pressure ventilation is required. Tracheostomy used to be the treatment of choice for delivering IPPV; it is effective not only in achieving adequate ventilation, but also in managing airway secretions. However, because numerous complications have been associated with the use of IPPV delivered via tracheostomy, several noninvasive methods of positive-pressure ventilation have been developed in recent years (120). Although molded nasal interfaces are now widely used, positive-pressure ventilation can also be provided via mouthpieces, oral interfaces, and oronasal interfaces (121). These methods are as effective as IPPV via tracheostomy in achieving adequate overnight ventilation. In addition, they optimize patient mobility, comfort, safety, and possibilities for discharge to the community. Adequate ventilation can also be achieved in some patients by using an abdominal positive-pressure ventilator (122); this method of ventilation, however, is not appropriate for patients with obesity or severe scoliosis.

There is no ideal method of IPPV, and selection for an individual patient has to be based on efficiency, the patient's personal choice, and the physician's expertise with a particular device. As a rule, however, nasal ventilation seems to be the most appropriate method of nocturnal assisted ventilation. When patients need to be ventilated for long periods of time, ventilation through a tracheostomy is often preferred in Europe. But good results have also been obtained in North America with mouth IPPV up to 24 hr a day (121). Preliminary results of a French multicenter prospective trial in patients with Duchenne muscular dystrophy suggest that the 4-year survival may be better in patients ventilated through a tracheostomy than in patients receiving nasal IPPV (123); this study, however, was not randomized, and the final results have yet to be published.

Who should be given nocturnal assisted ventilation? Although definite criteria have not been established, this treatment should clearly be considered in patients with severe respiratory muscle weakness and chronic ventilatory failure. Nocturnal assisted ventilation should thus be given to these patients who, when in a stable clinical condition, meet at least one of the following criteria: daytime $P_{CO_2} > 45$ mmHg, Pimax < 25–30 cmH_2O, VC $< 25\%$ predicted, MVV $< 25\%$ predicted, daytime $P_{O_2} < 60$ mmHg (123,124). Mechanical ventilation should also be considered in patients who have developed one (or two) episodes of acute ventilatory failure and have received endotracheal intubation.

The mechanism by which nocturnal assisted ventilation reverses ventilatory failure during the daytime remains uncertain, but several possibilities must be considered. By inflating the respiratory system with larger tidal volumes, assisted ventilation might reduce the abnormal stiffening of lung and ribcage tissues so as to produce an increase in lung and chest wall compliance and a decrease in the elastic work of breathing. In agreement with this idea, several studies have reported an increase in VC in the weeks following initiation of nocturnal assisted ventilation in patients with severe neuromuscular disorders (74,92,125). Other studies, however, have reported a decrease or no change in VC after treatment (67,72,75,77). Alternatively, nocturnal assisted ventilation may improve inspiratory muscle function by rest. Indeed, Marino and Braun (78) and others (67,74,92) have reported increases in inspiratory muscle strength and endurance as a result of this treatment. However, other studies have failed to confirm these improvements in inspiratory muscle function (75,77). Although it is possible that the improved blood gases at night elicit a resetting of the central control mechanisms, there has been no direct evidence to support this possibility.

B. Respiratory Muscle Training

As outlined in the previous sections of this chapter, in patients with generalized neuromuscular disorders, pulmonary and chest wall compliance are reduced. These alterations increase the work of breathing, which is increased further by the distortions of the chest wall that may occur during breathing. Yet, because the respiratory muscles are weak, the functional abilities of these patients are profoundly altered. As a result, even a minor insult to the respiratory system, such as an acute infection of the respiratory tract, which increases the work of breathing still further, may precipitate acute respiratory failure. One could argue, therefore, that increasing the strength and endurance of the inspiratory muscles in such patients might protect them against the development of respiratory failure. On the other hand, it has also been suggested that inspiratory muscle training, by adding to the burden of breathing on weak and already overloaded muscles, may, by itself, precipitate muscle fatigue (126).

Six studies have investigated the effects of strength and/or endurance training of the inspiratory muscles in patients with chronic neuromuscular disorders, primarily Duchenne muscular dystrophy (127–132). The training programs consisted of one or two daily sessions of either 10 static maximal inspiratory efforts or 10–15 min of breathing through a fixed inspiratory resistance; training duration ranged from 18 days to 6 months. Three studies have failed to show any beneficial effect of training (128–130), whereas three studies have reported significant increases in inspiratory muscle strength (132) and endurance (127,131,132).

These discrepant results may be attributed to several factors. First, most of these studies did not include appropriate control groups. Second, the design of the study did not always ensure that the patients did actually adhere to the prescribed training program; the amount of work performed, therefore, may have been too weak in several studies. Third, repeated baseline measurements were not performed systematically, which would have reduced the learning effect. Finally, to the extent that muscle training is likely to act predominantly, if not exclusively, on relatively preserved muscle fibers, the effects of training could vary depending on the stage of the disease, as recently suggested by Wanke et al. (132). Indeed, although these investigators reported substantial increases in diaphragmatic and global inspiratory muscle strength and endurance after 6 months of training in a group of patients with Duchenne muscular dystrophy, they were unable to find any changes in a subgroup of patients with Pco_2 values greater than 45 mmHg and/or VC values smaller than 25% of predicted. This suggests that muscle training programs should be instituted in the early stages of the disease, at a time when the patients still have a significant mass of functional respiratory muscles (127,132).

Patients with traumatic transection of the cervical cord would thus appear to be good candidates for muscle training; indeed, the respiratory muscles that survive the transection are essentially normal. Two studies have investigated the effects of resistive breathing exercises on the strength and endurance of the inspiratory muscles in quadriplegic patients (133,134); in both studies, the strength and endurance of the muscles were found to be significantly increased after 6–16 weeks of training. Similarly, the effect of strength training of the pectoralis major, the primary muscle of expiration in such subjects, has been investigated in a group of six patients. After 6 weeks of training, the patients had developed marked increases in the maximal isometric strength of the muscle and significant reductions in RV (135). Although maximal intrathoracic pressures were not measured in this study, these changes suggest that dynamic airway collapse during cough may occur more readily and at lower lung volumes. If so, the effectiveness of cough and the clearance of bronchial secretions could be improved. However, the effects of such training programs on the prevalence of bronchopulmonary infections and on the patient's ability to sustain infectious episodes have yet to be assessed.

C. Assisted Cough

Improving the clearance of airway secretions is a priority in the management of patients with chronic neuromuscular disorders and severe expiratory muscle weakness, particularly during intercurrent respiratory tract infections. Although tracheal and airway suctioning is easy to perform via an endotracheal or a tracheostomy tube, it is difficult and poorly tolerated otherwise.

Many patients can benefit from manually assisted coughing techniques, such as anterior chest compression and abdominal thrust. Indeed, when delivered during the expiratory phase of the coughing effort, anterior chest compression and/or abdominal thrust has been shown to produce significant increases in peak expiratory flow rates (136). However, to be effective, these techniques require experienced physiotherapists and precise coordination between the patient and the physiotherapist. These techniques are also most effective when the expiratory phase of cough is preceded by a large inflation of the lung, so that the (increased) elastic recoil of the respiratory system can be used to assist exsufflation. In these patients who have very severe reductions in inspiratory capacity, such large insufflations can be achieved with a ventilator or by glossopharyngeal breathing. However, a significant proportion of patients cannot be insufflated. In addition, manually assisted coughing techniques are inadequate for patients with poor coordination or severe scoliosis. In such patients, the use of a mechanical exsufflator has been recommended (136–138). This device consists of a two-stage axial compressor that delivers, via a tracheostomy or an anesthesia mask, a deep insufflation followed by a sudden drop in pressure of about 80 cmH_2O, resulting in a forced exsufflation. Mechanical exsufflation appears to be currently the most effective noninvasive technique to clear airway secretions and to prevent lobar atelectasis in patients with advanced disease (136).

D. Nutrition

The limited range of physical activity and the misguided desire to increase muscle mass by overeating lead many patients with chronic neuromuscular disorders to obesity. Obesity, however, is associated with a decrease in chest wall compliance and an increase in the mechanical work of breathing (139). Consequently, it should have a deleterious effect in patients whose respiratory muscles are already weak. It is important that these patients be given a weight-reducing diet.

More specific dietary therapy might also play a role in the treatment of some patients. Specifically, Slonim et al. (140) and Margolis and Hill (141) have reported substantial increments in peripheral and respiratory muscle strength and endurance after several months of a high-protein diet (>80 g/day) in patients with acid maltase deficiency. This beneficial effect is consistent with the fact that increased muscle protein catabolism is a prominent feature of this disorder. Such improvements in muscle strength, however, have not been confirmed in other studies (142,143), so no firm conclusion can be drawn at present.

References

1. Dail CW, Affeldt JE. Vital capacity as an index of respiratory muscle function. Arch Phys Med Rehab 1957; 38:383–391.
2. Ferris BG, Warren A, Beals CA. The vital capacity as a measure of the spontaneous breathing ability in poliomyelitis. N Engl J Med 1955; 252:618–621.
3. Affeldt JE. Neuromotor paralysis. In: Fenn WO, Rahn H, eds. Handbook of Physiology, section 3: Respiration, vol 2. Washington, DC: American Physiological Society, 1965:1509–1518.
4. Ferris BG, Whittenberger JL, Affeldt JE. Pulmonary function in convalescent poliomyelitic patients. I. Pulmonary subdivisions and maximum breathing capacity. N Engl J Med. 1952; 246:919–923.
5. Lukas DS, Plum F. Pulmonary function in patients convalescing from acute poliomyelitis with respiratory paralysis. Am J Med 1952; 12:388–396.
6. Burke SS, Grove NM, Houser CR, Johnson DM. Respiratory aspects of pseudohypertrophic muscular dystrophy. Am J Dis Child 1977; 121:230–234.
7. Hapke EJ, Meek JC, Jacobs J. Pulmonary function in progressive muscular dystrophy. Chest 1972; 61:41–47.
8. Inkley SR, Oldenburg FC, Vignos PJ. Pulmonary function in Duchenne muscular dystrophy related to stage of disease. Am J Med 1974; 56:297–306.
9. Keltz H. The effect of respiratory muscle dysfunction on pulmonary function. Studies in patients with neuromuscular disease. Am Rev Respir Dis 1965; 91:934–938.
10. Nakano KK, Bass H, Tyler RH, Carmel RJ. Amyotrophic lateral sclerosis: a study of pulmonary function. Dis Nerv Syst 1976; 37:32–35.
11. Ferris BG, Mead J, Whittenberger JL, Saxton GA. Pulmonary function in convalescent poliomyelitic patients. III. Compliance of the lungs and thorax. N Engl J Med 1952; 247:390–393.
12. Spencer WA, Vallbona C. Estimation of inspiratory capacity in health and in subjects with respiratory muscle paralysis. J Appl Physiol 1959; 14:279–283.
13. Rahn H, Otis AB, Chadwick LE, Fenn WO. The pressure-volume diagram of the thorax and lung. Am J Physiol 1946; 146:161–178.
14. Braun NMT, Rochester DF. Muscular weakness and respiratory failure. Am Rev Respir Dis 1979; 119(2):123–125.
15. De Troyer A, Borenstein S, Cordier R. Analysis of lung volume restriction in patients with respiratory muscle weakness. Thorax 1980; 35:603–610.
16. Gibson GJ, Pride NB. Lung mechanics in diaphragmatic paralysis. Am Rev Respir Dis 1979; 119(2):119–120.
17. Affeldt JE, Whittenberger JL Mead J, Ferris, BG Jr. Pulmonary function in convalescent poliomyelitic patients. II. The pressure-volume relations of the thorax and lungs of chronic respiratory patients. N Engl J Med 1952; 247:43–47.
18. Kilburn KH, Eagan JT, Sieker HO, Heyman A. Cardiopulmonary insufficiency in myotonic and progressive muscular dystrophy. N Engl J Med 1959; 261:1089–1096.

19. De Troyer A, Deisser P. The effects of intermittent positive pressure breathing on patients with respiratory muscle weakness. Am Rev Respir Dis 1981; 124:132–137.
20. Faerber I, Liebert PB, Suskind M. Loss of functional residual capacity in poliomyelitis. J Appl Physiol 1962; 17:289–292.
21. Gibson GJ, Pride NB, Newsom Davis J, Loh LC. Pulmonary mechanics in patients with respiratory muscle weakness. Am Rev Respir Dis 1977; 115:389–395.
22. Vallbona C, Spencer WA. The total lung capacity and its subdivisions in respiratory poliomyelitis. J Chronic Dis 1959; 9:617–635.
23. Kreitzer SM, Saunders NA, Tyler HR, Ingram RH. Respiratory muscle function in amyotrophic lateral sclerosis. Am Rev Respir Dis 1978; 117:437–447.
24. Gibson GJ, Pride NB, O'Cain C, Quagliato R. Sex and age differences in pulmonary mechanics in normal non-smoking subjects. J Appl Physiol 1976; 41:20–25.
25. De Troyer A, Estenne M, Yernault JC. Disturbance of respiratory muscle function in patients with mitral valve disease. Am J Med 1980; 69:867–873.
26. De Troyer A, Bastenier-Geens J. Effects of neuromuscular blockade on respiratory mechanics in conscious man. J Appl Physiol 1979; 47:1162–1168.
27. Gal TJ, Arora NS. Respiratory mechanics in supine subjects during progressive partial curarization. J Appl Physiol 1982; 52:57–63.
28. Gal TJ, Goldberg SK. Relationship between respiratory muscle strength and vital capacity during partial curarization in awake subjects. Anesthesiology 1981; 54:141–147.
29. De Troyer A., Borenstein S. Acute changes in respiratory mechanics after pyridostigmine injection in patients with myasthenia gravis. Am Rev Respir Dis 1980; 121:629–638.
30. De Troyer A, Heilporn A. Respiratory mechanics in quadriplegia. The respiratory function of the intercostal muscles. Am Rev Respir Dis 1980; 122:591–600.
31. Blossom RA, Affeldt JE. Chronic poliomyelitic respirator deaths. Am J Med 1956; 20:77–87.
32. Landon JF. Analysis of 88 cases of poliomyelitis treated in Drinker respirator, with control series of 68 cases: clinical studies in poliomyelitis. J Pediatr 1934; 5:1–8.
33. Nordenstam H. Patho-anatomical findings in 26 fatal cases of poliomyelitis. Acta Med Scand 1956; 316(Suppl):114–121.
34. Estenne M, Gevenois PA, Kinnear W, Soudon P, Heilporn A, De Troyer A. Lung volume restriction in patients with chronic respiratory muscle weakness: the role of microatelectasis. Thorax 1993; 48:698–701.
35. Young SL, Tierney DF, Clements JA. Mechanism of compliance change in excised rat lungs at low transpulmonary pressure. J Appl Physiol 1970; 29:780–785.
36. Mead J, Collier C. Relation of volume history of lungs to respiratory mechanics in anesthetized dogs. J Appl Physiol 1959; 14:669–678.
37. Egbert LD, Laver MB, Bendixen HH. Intermittent deep breaths and compliance during anesthesia in man. Anesthesiology 1963; 24:57–59.
38. Ferris BG, Pollard DS. Effect of deep and quiet breathing on pulmonary compliance in man. J Clin Invest 1960; 39:143–149.

39. Williams JV, Tierney DF, Parker HR. Surface forces in the lung, atelectasis, and transpulmonary pressure. J Appl Physiol 1966; 21:819–827.
40. Baydur A. Respiratory muscle strength and control of ventilation in patients with neuromuscular disease. Chest 1991; 99:330–338.
41. Bégin R, Bureau MA, Lupien L, Lemieux B. Control and modulation of respiration in Steinert's myotonic dystrophy. Am Rev Respir Dis 1980; 121:281–289.
42. Bégin R, Bureau MA, Lupien L, Bernier JP, Lemieux L. Pathogenesis of respiratory insufficiency in myotonic dystrophy. Am Rev Respir Dis 1982; 125:312–318.
43. Newsom Davis J, Goldman M, Loh L, Casson M. Diaphragm function and alveolar hypoventialtion. Q J Med 1976; 45:87–100.
44. Newsom Davis J, Stagg D, Loh L, Casson M. The effects of respiratory muscle weakness on some features of the breathing pattern. Clin Sci 1976; 50:10P–11P.
45. McCool FD, Mayewski RF, Shayne DS, Gibson CJ, Griggs RC, Hyde RW. Intermittent positive pressure breathing in patients with respiratory muscle weakness. Alterations in total respiratory system compliance. Chest 1986; 90:546–552.
46. Braun NMT, Arora NS, Rochester DF. Respiratory muscle and pulmonary function in polymyositis and other proximal myopathies. Thorax 1983; 38:616–623.
47. Heaf PDJ, Prime FJ. Compliance of the thorax in normal human subjects. Clin Sci 1956; 15:319–327.
48. Estenne M, Heilporn A, Delhez L, Yernault JC, De Troyer A. Chest wall stiffness in patients with chronic respiratory muscle weakness. Am Rev Respir Dis 1983; 128:1002–1007.
49. Estenne M, De Troyer A. The effect of tetraplegia on chest wall statics. Am Rev Respir Dis 1986; 134:121–124.
50. Black LF, Hyatt RE. Maximal static respiratory pressures in generalized neuromuscular disease. Am Rev Respir Dis 1971; 103:641–650.
51. Vincken WG, Elleker MG, Cosio MG. Flow-volume loop changes reflecting respiratory muscle weakness in chronic neuromuscular disorders. Am J Med 1987; 83:673–680.
52. Arora NS, Gal TJ. Cough dynamics during progressive expiratory muscle weakness in healthy curarized subjects. J Appl Physiol 1981; 51:494–498.
53. Szeinberg A, Tabachnik E, Rashed N, et al. Cough capacity in patients with muscular dystrophy. Chest 1988; 94:1232–1235.
54. Gal TJ, Smith TC. Partial paralysis with d-tubocurarine and the ventilatory response to CO_2. Anesthesiology 1976; 45:22–29.
55. Whittenberger JL, Sarnoff SJ. Physiologic principles in the treatment of respiratory failure. Med Clin North Am 1950; 34:1335–1362.
56. Plum F, Swanson AG. Abnormalities in central regulation of respiration in acute and convalescent poliomyelitis. Arch Neurol Psychiatry 1958; 80:267–285.
57. Rosenow EC, Engel AG. Acid maltase deficiency in adults presenting as respiratory failure. Am J Med 1978; 64:485–491.
58. Bellamy D, Newsom Davis JM, Hickey BP, Benatar SR, Clark TJH. A case of primary alveolar hypoventilation associated with mild proximal myopathy. Am Rev Respir Dis 1975; 112:867–873.

59. Riley DJ, Santiago TV, Daniele RP, Schall B, Edelman NH. Blunted respiratory drive in congenital myopathy. Am J Med 1977; 63:459–466.
60. Carroll JE, Zwillich C, Weil JV, Brooke MH. Depressed ventilatory response in oculocraniosomatic neuromuscular disease. Neurology 1976; 26:140–146.
61. Holle RHO, Schoene RB, Pavlin EJ. Effect of respiratory muscle weakness on PO.1 induced by partial curarization. J Appl Physiol 1984; 57:1150–1157.
62. McCool FD, Brown R, Mayewski RJ, Hyde RW. Effects of posture on stimulated ventilation in quadriplegia. Am Rev Respir Dis 1988; 138:101–105.
63. Harrison BDW, Collins JV, Brown KGE, Clark TJH. Respiratory failure in neuromuscular diseases. Thorax 1971; 26:579–584.
64. Gibson GJ, Gilmartin JJ, Veale D, Walls TJ, Serisier DE. Respiratory muscle function in neuromuscular disease. In: Jones NL, Killian KJ, eds. Breathlessness. The Campbell Symposium, Hamilton, Canada, Boehringer Ingelheim (Canada), Inc., 1992:66–73.
65. Skatrud J, Iber C, McHugh W, Rasmussen H, Nichols D. Determinants of hypoventilation during wakefulness and sleep in diaphragmatic paralysis. Am Rev Respir Dis 1980; 121:587–593.
66. Bye PTP, Ellis ER, Issa FG, Donnelly PM, Sullivan CE. Respiratory failure and sleep in neuromuscular disease. Thorax 1990; 45:241–247.
67. Goldstein RS, Molotiu N, Skrastins R, et al. Reversal of sleep-induced hypoventilation and chronic respiratory failure by nocturnal negative pressure ventilation in patients with restrictive ventilatory impairment. Am Rev Respir Dis 1987; 135:1049–1055.
68. Newsom Davis J, Loh L. Alveolar hypoventilation and respiratory muscle weakness. Bull Eur Physiopathol Respir 1979; 15:45–51.
69. Smith PEM, Calverley PMA, Edwards RHT. Hypoxemia during sleep in Duchenne muscular dystrophy. Am Rev Respir Dis 1988; 137:884–888.
70. Smith PEM, Edwards RHT, Calverley PMA. Ventilation and breathing pattern during sleep in Duchenne muscular dystrophy. Chest 1989; 96:1346–1351.
71. Stradling JR, Warley ARH. Bilateral diaphragm paralysis and sleep apnea without diurnal respiratory failure. Thorax 1988; 43:75–77.
72. Curran FJ. Night ventilation by body respirators for patients in chronic respiratory failure due to late stage Duchenne muscular dystrophy. Arch Phys Med Rehabil 1981; 82:270–274.
73. Ellis ER, Bye PTP, Bruderer JW, Sullivan CE. Treatment of respiratory failure during sleep in patients with neuromuscular disease. Positive-pressure ventilation through a nose mask. Am Rev Respir Dis 1987; 135:148–152.
74. Kerby GR, Mayer LS, Pingleton SK. Nocturnal positive pressure ventilation via nasal mask. Am Rev Respir Dis 1987; 135:738–740.
75. Kinnear W, Hockley S, Harvey J, Shneerson J. The effects of one year of nocturnal cuirass-assisted ventilation in chest wall disease. Eur Respir J 1988; 1:204–208.
76. Loh L, Hughes JMB, Newsom Davis J. Gas exchange problems in bilateral diaphragm paralysis. Bull Eur Physiopathol Respir 1979; 15:137–141.
77. Mohr CH, Hill NS. Long-term follow-up of nocturnal ventilatory assistance in patients with respiratory failure due to Duchenne-type muscular dystrophy. Chest 1990; 97:91–96.

78. Marino W, Braun NMT. Reversal of the clinical sequelae of respiratory muscle fatigue by intermittent mechanical ventilation. Am Rev Respir Dis 1982; 125(2):85.
79. Estenne M, De Troyer A. Relationship between respiratory muscle electromyogram and rib cage motion in tetraplegia. Am Rev Respir Dis 1985; 132:53–59.
80. Mortola JP, Sant'Ambrogio G. Motion of the rib cage and the abdomen in tetraplegic patients. Clin Sci 1978; 54:25–32.
81. Urmey W, Loring S, Mead J, et al. Upper and lower rib cage deformation during breathing in quadriplegics. J Appl Physiol 1986; 60:618–622.
82. Goldman JM, Williams SJ, Denison DM. The rib cage and abdominal components of respiratory system compliance in tetraplegic patients. Eur Respir J 1988; 1:242–247.
83. Bergofsky EH. Mechanism for respiratory insufficiency after cervical cord injury. A source of alveolar hypoventilation. Ann Intern Med 1964; 61:435–447.
84. Fugl-Meyer AR. Effects of respiratory muscle paralysis in tetraplegic and paraplegic patients. Scand J Rehabil Med 1971; 3:141–150.
85. McKinley AC, Auchincloss JH, Gilbert R, Nicholas JJ. Pulmonary function, ventilatory control, and respiratory complications in quadriplegic subjects. Am Rev Respir Dis 1969; 100:526–532.
86. McMichan JC, Michel L, Westbrook PR. Pulmonary dysfunction following traumatic quadriplegia. Recognition, prevention, and treatment. JAMA 1980; 243:528–531.
87. Stone DG, Keltz H. The effect of respiratory muscle dysfunction on pulmonary function. Studies in patients with spinal cord injuries. Am Rev Respir Dis 1963; 88:621–629.
88. Siebens AA, Kirby NA, Poulos DA. Cough following transection of spinal cord at C6. Arch Phys Med Rehabil 1964; 45:1–8.
89. De Troyer A, Estenne M, Heilporn A. Mechanism of active expiration in tetraplegic subjects. N Engl J Med 1986; 314:740–744.
90. Estenne M, De Troyer A. Cough in tetraplegic subjects: an active process. Ann Intern Med 1990; 112:22–28.
91. Estenne M, Van Muylem A, Gorini M, Kinnear W, Heilporn A, De Troyer A. Evidence of dynamic airway compression during cough in tetraplegic subjects. Am J Respir Crit Care Med 1994; 150:1081–1085.
92. Celli BR, Rassulo J, Corral R. Ventilatory muscle dysfunction in patients with bilateral idiopathic diaphragmatic paralysis: reversal by intermittent external negative pressure ventilation. Am Rev Respir Dis 1987; 136:1276–1278.
93. Kreitzer SM, Feldman NT, Saunders NA, Ingram RH. Bilateral diaphragmatic paralysis with hypercapnic respiratory failure. A physiologic assessment. Am J Med 1978; 65:89–95.
94. Laroche CM, Carroll N, Moxham J, Green M. Clinical significance of severe isolated diaphragm weakness. Am Rev Respir Dis 1988; 138:862–866.
95. McCredie M, Lovejoy FW, Kaltreider NL. Pulmonary function in diaphragmatic paralysis. Thorax 1962; 17:213–217.
96. Sandham JD, Shaw DT, Guenter CA. Acute supine respiratory failure due to bilateral diaphragmatic paralysis. Chest 1977; 72:96–98.

97. Higenbottam T, Allen D, Loh L, Clark TJH. Abdominal wall movement in normals and patients with hemidiaphragmatic and bilateral diaphragmatic palsy. Thorax 1977; 32:589–595.
98. Hillman DR, Finucane KE. Respiratory pressure partitioning during quiet inspiration in unilateral and bilateral diaphragmatic weakness. Am Rev Respir Dis 1988; 137:1401–1405.
99. Gilroy J, Cahalan JL, Berman R, Newman M. Cardiac and pulmonary complications in Duchenne's progressive muscular dystrophy. Circulation 1963; 27:484–493.
100. Smith PEM, Calverley PMA, Edwards RHT, Evans GA, Campbell EJM. Practical problems in the respiratory care of patients with muscular dystrophy. N Engl J Med 1987; 316:1197–1205.
101. Newsom Davis J. The respiratory system in muscular dystrophy. Br Med Bull 1980; 36:135–138.
102. Neustadt JE, Levy RC, Spiegel IJ. Carbon dioxide narcosis in association with muscular dystrophy. JAMA 1964; 187:616–617.
103. Contamin F, Lissac J, Nick J. Myopathie tardive avec hypoventilation alvéolaire par paralysie complète du diaphragme. Presse Méd 1966; 74:1939–1942.
104. Bashour F, Winchell P, Reddington J. Myotonia atrophica and cyanosis. N Engl J Med 1955; 252:768–770.
105. Benaim S, Worster-Drought C. Dystrophia myotonica with myotonia of the diaphragm causing pulmonary hypoventilation with anoxaemia and secondary polycythaemia. Med Illustr 1954; 8:221–226.
106. Cannon PJ. The heart and lungs in myotonic muscular dystrophy. Am J Med 1962; 32:765–775.
107. Coccagna G, Mantovadi M, Parchi C, Mironi F, Lugaresi E. Alveolar hypoventilation and hypersomnia in myotonic dystrophy. J Neurol Neurosurg Psych 1975; 38:977–984.
108. Carroll JE, Zwillich C, Weil JV. Ventilatory response in myotonic dystrophy. Neurology 1977; 27:1125–1128.
109. Gillam PMS, Heaf PJD, Kaufman L, Lucas BGB. Respiration in dystrophia myotonica. Thorax 1964; 19:112–120.
110. Serisier DE, Mastaglia FL, Gibson GJ. Respiratory muscle function and ventilatory control. I. In patients with motor neuron disease. II. In patients with myotonic dystrophy. Q J Med 1982; 51:205–226.
111. Jammes Y, Ponget J, Grimaud C, Serratrice G. Pulmonary function and electromyographic study of respiratory muscles in myotonic dystrophy. Muscle Nerve 1985; 8:586–594.
112. Stranock SD, Newsom Davis J. Ultrastructure of the muscle spindle in dystrophia myotonica. I. The intrafusal muscle fibers. Neuropathol Appl Neurobiol 1978; 4:393–406.
113. Parhad IM, Clark AW, Barron KD, Stauton SB. Diaphragmatic paralysis in motor neuron disease. Neurology 1978; 28:18–22.
114. Bach JR, Campagnolo D, Hoeman S. Life satisfaction of individuals with Duchenne muscular dystrophy using long-term mechanical ventilatory support. Am J Phys Med Rehabil 1991; 70:129–135.

115. Bach JR, Campagnolo D. Psychosocial adjustment of post-poliomyelitis ventilator-assisted individuals. Arch Phys Med Rehabil 1992; 73:934–939.
116. Bach JR, Alba AS, Bohatiuk G, Saporito L, Lee M. Mouth intermittent positive ventilation in the management of postpolio respiratory insufficiency. Chest 1987; 91:859–864.
117. Garay SH, Turino GM, Goldring RM. Sustained reversal of chronic hypercapnia in patients with alveolar hypoventilation syndromes. Long-term maintenance with noninvasive nocturnal mechanical ventilation. Am J Med 1981; 70:269–274.
118. Vianello A, Bevilacqua M, Salvador V, Cardaioli C, Vincenti E. Long-term nasal intermittent positive pressure ventilation in advanced Duchenne's muscular dystrophy. Chest 1994; 105:445–448.
119. Hill NS, Redline S, Carskadon MA, Curran FJ, Millman RP. Sleep-disordered breathing in patients with Duchenne muscular dystrophy using negative pressure ventilators. Chest 1992; 102:1656–1662.
120. Willig TN, Robert D, Paulus J, Leger P, eds. International conference on nasal ventilation in neuromuscular disorders. Eur Respir Rev 1993; 3:243–307.
121. Bach JR, Sortor SM, Saporito LR. Interfaces for non-invasive intermittent positive pressure ventilatory support in North America. Eur Respir Rev 1993; 3:254–259.
122. Bach JR, Alba AS. Intermittent abdominal pressure ventilator in a regimen of noninvasive ventilatory support. Chest 1991; 99:630–636.
123. Raphaël JC, Chevret S, Chastany C, Bouvet F. Home mechanical ventilation in Duchenne's muscular dystrophy: in search of a therapeutic strategy. Eur Respir Rev 1993; 3:270–274.
124. Rochester DF, Martin LL. Respiratory muscle rest. In: Roussos C, Macklem PT, eds. The Thorax, part B. New York: Marcel Dekker, 1986:1303–1328.
125. Sawicka EH, Loh L, Branthwaite MA. Domiciliary ventilatory support: an analysis of outcome. Thorax 1988; 43:31–35.
126. Schiffman PL, Belsh JM. Effect of inspiratory resistance and theophylline on respiratory muscle strength in patients with amyotrophic lateral sclerosis. Am Rev Respir Dis 1989; 139:1418–1423.
127. DiMarco AF, Kelling JS, DiMarco MS, Jacobs I, Shields R, Altose MD. The effects of inspiratory resistive training on respiratory muscle function in patients with muscular dystrophy. Muscle Nerve 1985; 8:284–290.
128. Rodillo E, Noble-Jamieson CM, Aber V, Heckmatt JZ, Muntoni F, Dubowitz V. Respiratory muscle training in Duchenne muscular dystrophy. Arch Dis Child 1989; 64:736–738.
129. Smith PEM, Coakley JM, Edwards RHT. Respiratory muscle training in Duchenne muscular dystrophy. Muscle Nerve 1988; 11:784–785.
130. Stern LM, Martin AJ, Jones N, Garett R, Yeates J. Training inspiratory resistance in Duchenne dystrophy using adapted computer games. Dev Med Child Neurol 1989; 31:494–500.
131. Martin AJ, Stern L, Yeates J, Lepp D, Little J. Respiratory muscle training in Duchenne dystrophy. Dev Med Child Neurol 1986; 28:314–318.

132. Wanke T, Toifl K, Merkle M, Formanek D, Lahrmann H, Zwick H. Inspiratory muscle training in patients with Duchenne muscular dystrophy. Chest 1994; 105:475–482.
133. Gross D, Ladd HW, Riley EJ, Macklem PT, Grassino A. The effect of training on strength and endurance of the diaphragm in quadriplegia. Am J Med 1980; 68.27–35.
134. Huldtgren AC, Fugl-Meyer AR, Jonasson E, Bake B. Ventilatory dysfunction and respiratory rehabilitation in post-traumatic quadriplegia. Eur J Respir Dis 1980; 61:347–356.
135. Estenne M, Knoop C, Vanvaerenbergh J, Heilporn A, De Troyer A. The effect of pectoralis muscle training in tetraplegic subjects. Am Rev Respir Dis 1989; 139:1218–1222.
136. Bach JR. Management of neuromuscular ventilatory failure by 24-hour noninvasive intermittent positive pressure ventilation. Eur Respir Rev 1993; 3:284–291.
137. Barach AL, Beck GJ, Bickerman HA, Seanor HE. Physical methods simulating cough mechanisms. JAMA 1952; 150:1380–1385.
138. Bickerman HA, Itkin S. Exsufflation with negative pressure. Arch Intern Med 1954; 93:698–704.
139. Naimark A, Cherniack RM. Compliance of the respiratory system and its components in health and obesity. J Appl Physiol 1960; 15:377–382.
140. Slonim AE, Coleman RA, McElligot MA, et al. Improvement of muscle function in acid maltase deficiency by high-protein therapy. Neurology 1983; 33:34–38.
141. Margolis ML, Hill AR. Acid maltase deficiency in an adult. Evidence for improvement in respiratory function with high-protein dietary therapy. Am Rev Respir Dis 1986; 134:328–331.
142. Umpleby AM, Trend PS, Chubb D, et al. The effect of a high protein diet on leucine and alanine turnover in acid maltase deficiency. J Neurol Neurosurg Psych 1989; 52:954–961.
143. Padberg GW, Wintzen AR, Giesberts MAH, Sterk PJ, Molenaar AJ, Hermans J. Effect of a high-protein diet in acid-maltase deficiency. J Neurol Sci 1989; 90:111–117.
144. Estenne M, Yernault JC, De Troyer A. Rib cage and diaphragm-abdomen compliance in humans: effects of age and posture. J Appl Physiol 1985; 59:1842–1848.
145. De Troyer A, Kelly S. Chest wall mechanics in dogs with acute diaphragm paralysis. J Appl Physiol 1982; 53:373–379.

9

Deconditioning

RICHARD CASABURI

Harbor–UCLA Medical Center
Torrance, California

Exercise intolerance is a prominent complaint of the patient with lung disease. The common conception is that these patients reach a ventilatory limitation dictated by the severity of their lung disease (1,2). Yet it has been repeatedly demonstrated that resting measures of lung mechanics or gas exchange deficits correlate poorly with exercise tolerance (3). Further, programs of pulmonary rehabilitation have been conclusively shown to improve exercise tolerance in the majority of participants without changes in lung function (4). It is a common experience to observe two patients with severe chronic obstructive pulmonary disease, one of whom is homebound because of poor exercise tolerance and the other capable of living a near-normal life. How can we explain this difference?

One factor is that some individuals are in some way more "sensitive" to dyspnea than others. This seems to be more of a psychological than a physiological phenomenon since techniques for desensitization to dyspnea on exertion are often effective (5). In particular, group exercise programs are often an effective setting for inducing desensitization to dyspnea; theories have been advanced to explain the mechanisms by which these programs are effective (5).

The second factor that exacerbates exercise intolerance in patients with lung disease is deconditioning. There is a tendency for most individuals to decrease their accustomed level of activity as they get older (6). In patients with lung disease this tendency is accentuated. Patients become sedentary to avoid the dyspneic sensation that activity brings. This is unfortunate since dyspnea, unlike, for example, anginal pain from coronary artery disease, is not a sign that the body is being damaged. Lung disease and deconditioning appear to be synergistic in decreasing exercise tolerance.

Because the lung disease of most patients who present for rehabilitation is essentially irreversible, it is an arguable proposition that pulmonary rehabilitation is aimed at optimizing the function of all of the body's organ systems *except* the lungs. [This includes the brain; the psychological adjustments that rehabilitation engenders are of great importance (7).] Reversing the deconditioned state is a practical and achievable aim (4). This chapter's goal is to describe the consequences of deconditioning. There is a large literature that describes the physiological effects of decreased activity in healthy subjects. There is also a growing body of knowledge concerning the severity of deconditioning in patients with lung disease. Finally, an "experiment of man" is relevant to the assessment of the consequences of deconditioning in patients with lung disease: the exercise intolerance experienced by patients who have undergone lung or heart-lung transplantation.

I. Pathophysiology of Inactivity

If we define deconditioning as the physiological changes that occur in the body as a result of inactivity, three lines of evidence become relevant. First, a series of experiments have studied the effects of confining healthy subjects to bed. Many of these studies were performed in an attempt to predict the effect of space flight (an environment in which work against gravity is not required) on the body's organ systems. Most of these studies were of 2–4 weeks' duration, which might cast doubt on their relevance to patients who have experienced years of inactivity. Yet it is well established that many of the cellular changes that result from the abrupt decrease in activity have a half-time of 1–2 weeks (8,9). Therefore, the physiological changes seen after bed rest provide a relevant model of deconditioning.

Second, a series of investigations have studied the response to abrupt cessation of a program of exercise training and the assumption of a sedentary life-style. Labeled "deconditioning" studies, these investigations follow the physiological consequences of relative inactivity for weeks to months.

Third, epidemiological studies have cataloged the differences between populations of active and sedentary individuals. The ability to characterize large groups of individuals often means that small differences may become manifest. Also, epidemiological studies are usually the only practical method to define long-term consequences of inactivity. However, care must be taken to isolate the effects of inactivity in such investigations. For example, since obesity often accompanies inactivity, it is important not to ascribe the consequences of obesity to inactivity.

A. Skeletal Muscle Function

Biochemical and structural changes occur in skeletal muscle that is inactive (10). Muscle mass declines. The concentration of enzymes involved in aerobic energy production decreases (8–10). The number and density of mitochondria, the organelles where most of the cell's ATP is generated, decreases. Though it seems unlikely that the number of myocytes decreases, the diameter of muscle cells decreases. The number of capillaries surrounding each muscle fiber decreases, increasing the diffusion distance for oxygen transport. Skeletal muscles are composed of two major fiber types. Type I fibers, classified as "slow twitch," have a high capacity for aerobic, endurance activities. Type II fibers, classified as "fast twitch," (as a group) have a lower capacity for aerobic activities. While deconditioning apparently yields no change in the proportion of these two fiber types, there is a distinct transformation of subtypes of type II fibers: type IIa fibers convert to type IIb fibers (8) and type IIa fibers have a higher aerobic capacity. All these changes conspire to decrease the potential of muscle to perform exercise aerobically.

B. Cardiovascular Function

Resting heart rate increases modestly after a period of bed rest (11–14). The cardiovascular response to exercise is dramatically altered. Saltin et al. (15) studied the effects of 20 days of bed rest in healthy young men. During maximal exercise, cardiac output was 26% lower and stroke volume was 29% lower, though maximum heart rate changed very little. In response to equal submaximal exercise tasks, heart rate was higher and stroke volume was lower. The net result was a mild decrease in cardiac output and increase in arteriovenous oxygen content. Other investigators have confirmed these findings (11,12,16,17). Blood pressure at rest is changed little by bed rest or inactivity (16) and has alternatively been reported to be mildly increased (17) or decreased (16) at submaximal work rates.

Plasma volume falls modestly (6–17%) after deconditioning or bed rest (14,15,18). Echocardiographic techniques demonstrate that left ventricular end-diastolic volume at rest is decreased (11,17), though ejection fraction changes little (11,17). At a given level of exercise, the end-diastolic size of the left ventricle decreases, with little change in end-systolic dimension. Both Martin et al. (16) and Ehsani et al. (17) found that very fit subjects who stopped training had substantial decreases in left ventricular mass (20–30%) within 2–3 weeks.

After bed rest, the ability of the cardiovascular system to adjust to abruptly assuming an upright posture is impaired (14,19). In tilt table studies, bed-rested subjects often fainted when tilted upward; despite an accentuated pulse rate response, a marked fall in blood pressure was seen.

C. Body Composition

The Skylab astronauts lost 4 g of body calcium per month during prolonged weightlessness (20). Bed rest is accompanied by a similar calcium deficit (14). Clinically significant bone demineralization can result. Protein wastage is marked by an increased urinary nitrogen excretion (14). Total body water decreases and there is a decrease in total body sodium as well (6). There is generally a loss of body weight (11) and an increase in the percentage of body fat.

D. Central Nervous System Function

Standing and walking balance is impaired by bed rest periods as short as 2 weeks (21). Although postural muscle weakness and orthostatic blood pressure changes likely contribute to this impairment, there seems to be a prominent component of apraxia in the integration of visual, kinesthetic, and other sensory information by the postural control centers in the brain.

Psychomotor tasks, such as reaction times, deteriorate after a period of inactivity (22,23). Total immobilization yields decreases in performance in tests of intellectual function (24) and may lead to disorientation (25,26). Further, alterations in the electroencephalogram are seen (6,24). During sleep, there is an increase in state 3 and 4 (deep) sleep, without a change in REM sleep (27).

E. Endocrine Function

Inactivity causes a deterioration in several of the body's hormonal mechanisms. Bed rest and inactivity result in substantial intolerance to glucose loads (28–30). In response to an oral glucose load, there is exaggerated increase in blood insulin level, often accompanied by elevated glucose levels (28,29). Sophisticated glucose clamp methods have demonstrated that insulin is less effective in stimulating cellular uptake of glucose after a period of inactivity (30). Further, pancreatic β cells secrete more insulin in response to hyperglycemia in the inactive subject (30).

Immobilization has been found to cause decreased spermatogenesis in subhuman primates (31). Androgen levels are low in immobilized ill male patients (32). Shetty et al. (33) found that insulin-like growth factor 1 (IgF1) levels are reduced in otherwise healthy quadriplegic men, suggesting that inactivity may reduce 1gF1 levels. IgF1 is thought to be the major mediator of the actions of growth hormone (34). It is at present unclear whether low IgF1 levels result from reduced secretion of growth hormone by the pituitary or resistance to the action of growth hormone on IgF1-secreting tissues.

F. Blood Composition

Blood cellular composition is altered by inactivity. Red cell mass decreases (15), probably as a result of decreased erythropoiesis. Decreased fibrinolytic activity yields an increased risk of thrombosis (6). Decreased peripheral lymphocyte counts have been reported after space flight (6). This may be part of a generalized impairment in immune system function that occurs with inactivity (6); immune function is distinctly improved by a moderate program of exercise training (35).

Serum lipids, including both triglycerides and cholesterol, are higher in those with a chronically sedentary or immobilized life-style (36,37) or after an extended period of bed rest (28). Making matters worse, high-density-lipoprotein cholesterol ("good cholesterol") is lower (28,36,37).

G. Other Physiological Effects

Inactivity produces no apparent deterioration in the pulmonary system, as assessed by resting spirometry and other resting pulmonary function measures (14,15,38). Nor is there evidence that renal function is impacted. Thermoregulation during exercise is impaired after bed rest; there is an excessive increase in body temperature, which might be related to inhibition of sweating or to decreased skin heat conductance (39). Finally, there is some evidence that drug metabolism may be altered by bed rest (40) leading to changed dose-response relationships.

H. Alteration of Exercise Tolerance

In response to incremental exercise tests, deconditioning has widely been found to result in a decreased maximum work rate and a decreased maximum oxygen uptake (11–13,15–18). Further, blood lactate starts to increase (lactate threshold (41)) at a lower work rate in less fit than in more fit individuals (42). The deconditioned subject will have a decreased endurance for constant work rate exercise as well, if the work rate is above his or her lactate threshold (LT). It has also been shown that the kinetics of oxygen uptake are slower for above-LT work rates (43).

Muscle strength is distinctly reduced by immobilization (14,26); strength changes are most marked in the leg muscles (14).

I. Predisposition to Disease

The risk of several types of cancer has been associated with a sedentary lifestyle (44). This association seems most certain for colon cancer (44,45) and is clearer for men than for women. The decreased bowel motility seen in sedentary individuals is hypothesized to increase colonic exposure to carcinogenic substances (44). The risks of breast and endometrial cancers are thought to be mildly increased in sedentary women (44,46).

Epidemiological studies have suggested that the risk of coronary artery disease is elevated in inactive individuals, likely related to unfavorable lipid profiles (36,47). Similar, the risk of non-insulin-dependent diabetes mellitus is felt to be increased in sedentary individuals in association with the observed impairment in glucose tolerance (36,47).

II. Contribution of Deconditioning to Exercise Intolerance in COPD

Much more is known about the determinants of exercise intolerance in chronic obstructive pulmonary disease (COPD) than in other chronic respiratory disorders (48). However, it seems reasonable to suppose that the information gleaned from study of COPD patients has at least qualitative relevance to patients with other pulmonary disorders.

Figure 1 quantitates the degree of exercise intolerance of 62 patients with COPD. These data are from studies of patients presenting for pulmonary rehabilitation in either Torrance, California, in the United States or in Veruno, Italy. Each performed an incremental exercise test on a cycle ergometer. It can be seen that the peak oxygen uptake is below predicted levels in *all* these patients; on average, peak $\dot{V}O_2$ is 62 ± 14% predicted. The source of the exercise intolerance is multifactorial, and although the contributions of the factors listed below often cannot be precisely quantitated, it is worth briefly considering them in turn.

A. Abnormal Lung Mechanics

Figure 2 presents a conceptual scheme for defining the contribution of abnormal lung mechanics to exercise intolerance in COPD (4). As the level of exercise increases, so does the level of pulmonary ventilation ($\dot{V}_E$). In the patient with COPD, the required level of $\dot{V}_E$ often approaches the maximum achievable $\dot{V}_E$ (i.e., the levels of $\dot{V}_E$ at which mechanical constraints become limiting) and

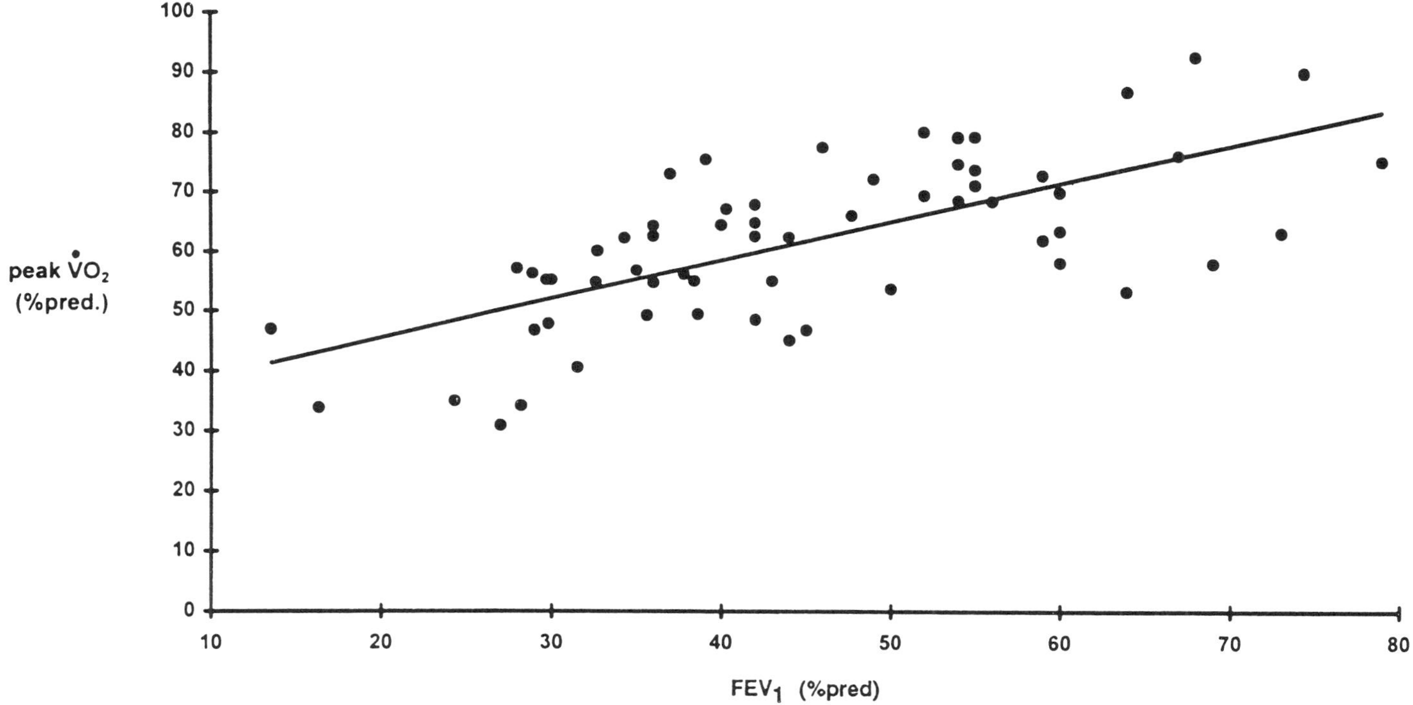

Figure 1 Exercise tolerance of 62 patients with COPD presenting for pulmonary rehabilitation, as a function of disease severity. (Abscissa) Percent of predicted forced expiratory volume in 1 sec (FEV_1); predicted values are those of Knudsen et al. (69). (Ordinate) Percent of predicted peak oxygen uptake measured in an incremental cycle ergometer exercise test; predicted values are those of Wasserman et al. (41). Equation of regression line: $y = 0.66x + 32.6$; $r^2 = 0.47$. (Data compiled from Refs. 55, 70, and 71.)

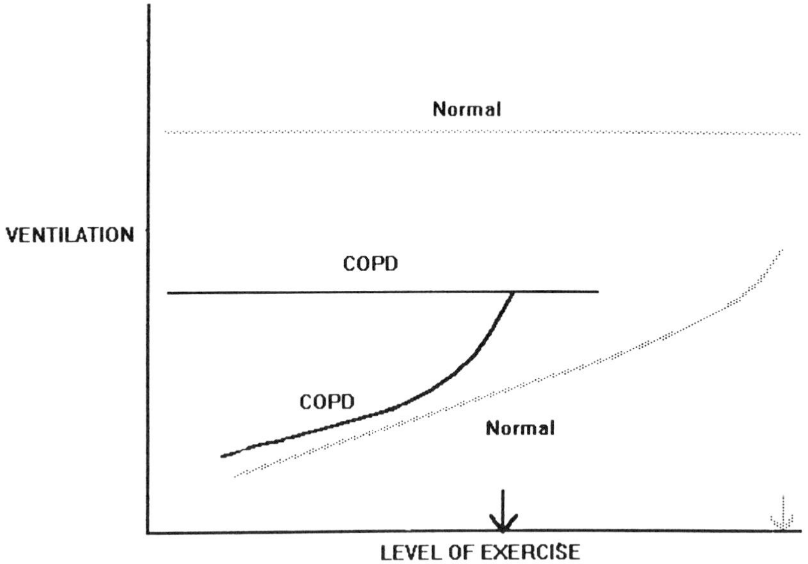

Figure 2 Schematic representation of the factors dictating exercise tolerance in patients with COPD and normal (i.e., healthy) subjects. Patients with COPD have a higher ventilatory requirement for a given level of activity. The maximum level of ventilation that can be sustained is lower in COPD patients than in healthy subjects. In contrast to healthy subjects, the maximum tolerable exercise level is achieved when the ventilatory requirement approaches the limiting ventilation. See text.

this mechanical limitation is the major factor defining exercise limitation. In the healthy subject, the limiting level of $\dot{V}_E$ is not approached; leg fatigue is likely dictated by intramuscular acidosis, which is the proximate cause of exercise limitation. Maximum achievable ventilation is limited by altered lung mechanics (49). This is due to increased airways resistance to expiratory airflow. This causes high work of breathing leading to respiratory muscle fatigue. Making matters worse, the expiratory airflow resistance leads to dynamic hyperinflation (50); end-expiratory lung volume increases, putting the respiratory muscles at a mechanical disadvantage.

As can be seen in Figure 1, there is a significant correlation between the degree of airflow obstruction (as measured by the percent predicted FEV_1) and the degree of exercise tolerance (as measured by the percent predicted peak $\dot{V}O_2$). However, as shown by the coefficient of determination (r^2) (51), only about half of the variation in exercise tolerance can be "explained" by the degree of airflow obstruction. Other factors must be in play.

B. Abnormal Pulmonary Gas Exchange

In COPD, the ability of the lung to oxygenate the blood and to excrete CO_2 is impaired. A higher level of pulmonary ventilation is required at a given level of exercise. This means that abnormal gas exchange contributes to the ventilatory limitation to exercise. In most patients, the extra ventilatory requirement is most clearly linked to deficits in CO_2 excretion. This is because ventilatory control is closely linked to the rate of CO_2 production (52,53). In the COPD patient, a larger fraction of the exhaled tidal volume is ineffective in excreting CO_2; this is quantitated by calculation of the dead space to tidal volume ratio (V_D/V_T). A second factor linking abnormal gas exchange to increased ventilatory requirement is hypoxemia. Poor matching of ventilation to perfusion yields a low enough arterial Po_2 to stimulate ventilation in some patients. Hypoxemia during exercise also contributes to pulmonary vasoconstriction and to reduced delivery of oxygen to the contracting muscles, which also limits exercise tolerance (see below).

C. Abnormal Pulmonary Vasculature

The pulmonary vasculature is required to vasodilate greatly to accommodate the increase in pulmonary blood flow that exercise demands. In COPD with a prominent emphysemic component, there is destruction of the pulmonary vasculature along with the alveolar architecture. Pulmonary vascular destruction means that pulmonary artery pressure rises and cardiac output increase may be limited. This is another mechanism by which oxygen flow to the exercising muscles may be compromised.

D. Deconditioning

As stated at the beginning of this chapter, many (almost certainly the majority) of patients with clinically significant chronic obstructive lung disease maintain a *very* sedentary life-style. The most profound influence on exercise tolerance of this life-style is its effect on the muscles of ambulation. The structural and biochemical changes induced by deconditioning yield a decreased ability of the muscles to utilize the oxygen delivered to them.

Three mechanisms that would tend to decrease the aerobic capacity of the exercising muscles in COPD were described above: hypoxemia, decreased muscle blood flow stemming from pulmonary vascular disease, and deconditioning. Decreased aerobic capacity implies early onset of lactic acidosis. Lactic acid is produced as a by-product of anaerobic metabolism, a backup scheme for continued production of high-energy phosphate compounds necessary for muscle contraction. Lactic acid production has, however, adverse affects. It is a strong acid that must be buffered and the main physiological buffering system is bicarbonate (41). This yields carbonic acid that dissociates to generate CO_2. Approximately 22 ml of CO_2 is generated for each milliequivalent of lactic acid produced. This is CO_2 *superimposed* on the CO_2 produced by aerobic metabolism. $\dot{V}_E$ must increase to accommodate this added CO_2 load or else CO_2 retention will occur. Further, lactic acid directly stimulates the carotid body chemoreceptors, which tends to introduce an additional increase in $\dot{V}_E$. The overall result of early onset of lactic acidosis in the COPD patient is an increase in the ventilatory requirement for exercise, which results in an earlier ventilatory limitation to exercise.

Figures 3 and 4 demonstrate that patients with COPD have a markedly early onset of lactic acidosis. These are data from 32 patients, a subset of those shown in Figure 1, who had arterial blood drawn every minute during incremental exercise testing. In each patient the lactate threshold was determined from a log-log plot of lactate versus $\dot{V}O_2$, as suggested by Beaver et al. (54). The acceleration of blood lactate concentration as $\dot{V}O_2$ increases defines the lactate threshold. Figure 3 demonstrates that the lactate threshold is below predicted levels in all patients studied (average = 58 ± 12% predicted). [It should be noted that predicted values were generated from the responses of a

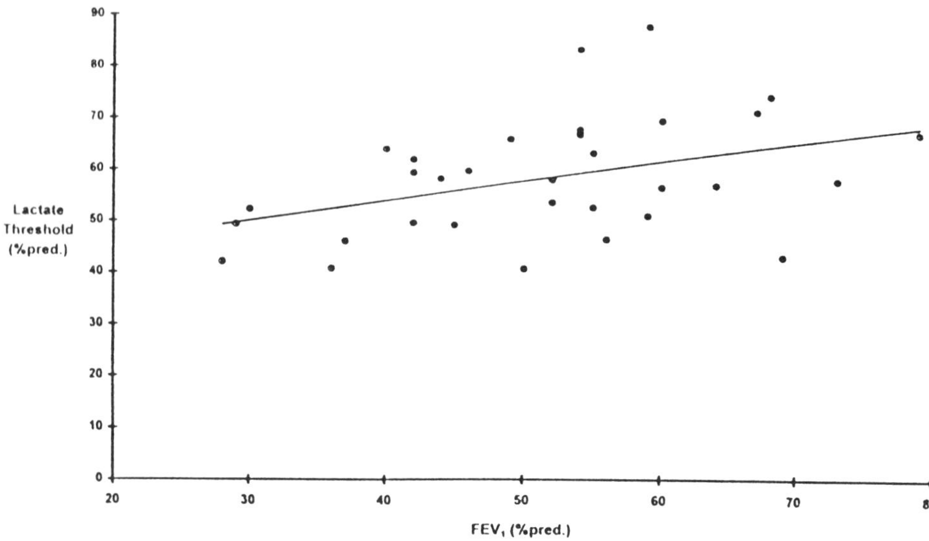

Figure 3 Oxygen uptake at which arterial blood lactic acid level increases during an incremental cycle ergometer test (lactate threshold) as a percent of the predicted level (41) as a function of % predicted FEV_1. Equation of the regression line is: $y = 0.38x + 38.5$; $r^2 = 0.18$. (Data compiled from Refs. 55 and 70.)

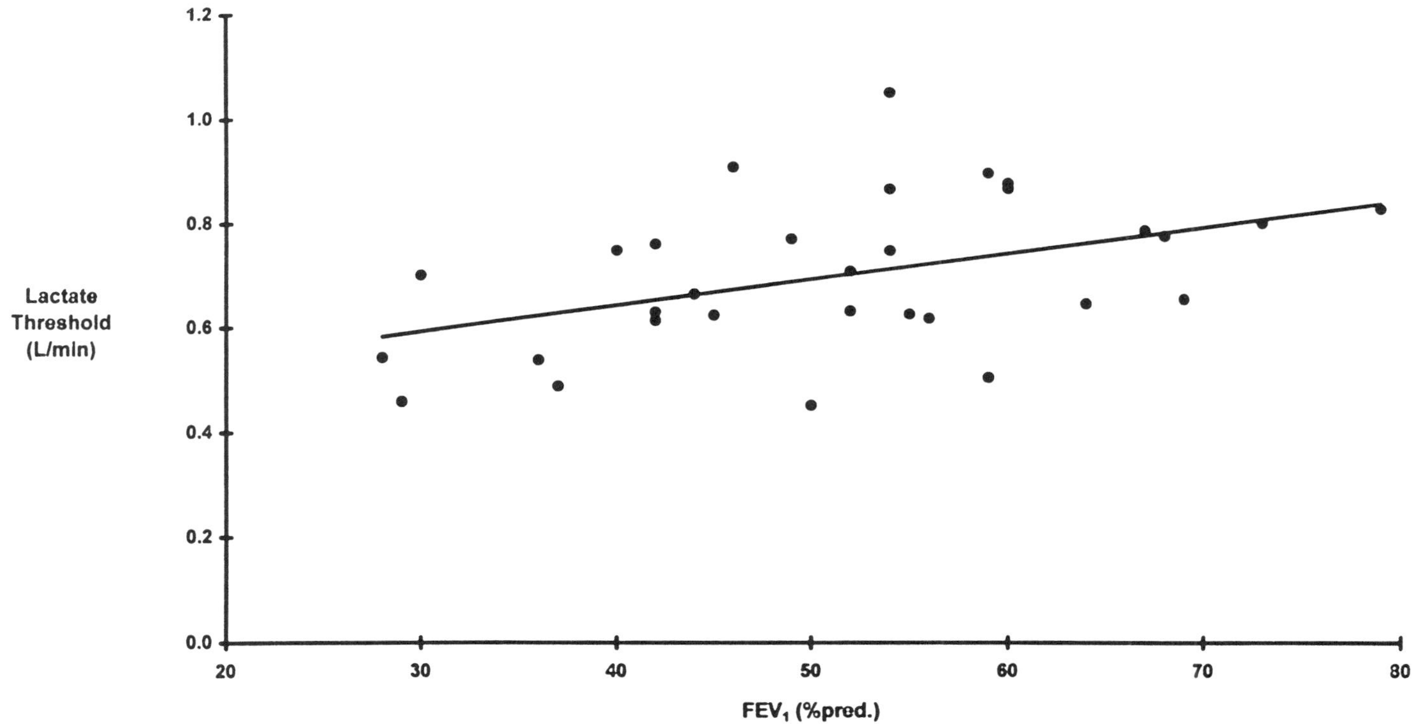

Figure 4 Lactate threshold as a function of % predicted FEV_1. Equation of the regression line is: $y = 0.0049x + 0.44$; $r^2 = 0.19$. See text. (Data compiled from Refs. 55 and 70.)

group of fairly *sedentary* healthy subjects! (41).] Also, it can be seen that the severity of airflow obstruction is a poor predictor of the impairment (r^2 = 0.18). Figure 4 makes a separate point. It is remarkable that the lactate threshold occurs at a *very* low $\dot{V}O_2$ in these patients (average = 0.70 ± 0.14 L/m). In most individuals, a brisk walking pace on level ground requires a $\dot{V}O_2$ of about 1 L/min. Unloaded pedaling on a cycle ergometer (i.e., moving the legs against no resistance) requires roughly 0.5 L/min. Therefore, most of these patients, even those with only mild to moderate airflow obstruction, experience lactic acidosis when engaging in activities that most of us would consider essential for everyday life.

What is not clear from these data is the predominant cause of the early onset of lactic acidosis in these patients. Circumstantial evidence suggests that deconditioning may play an appreciable role because a program of exercise training has been shown to appreciably increase (though not normalize) the lactate threshold (55).

III. Exercise Intolerance in the Lung Transplant Patient

Medical progress has allowed an observation relevant to the contribution of deconditioning to the exercise intolerance seen in patients with lung disease. Lung or heart-lung transplantation is intended to relieve gas exchange problems, restore pulmonary vascular adequacy, and normalize lung mechanics. In these patients, oxygen delivery problems resulting from hypoxemia and/or pulmonary blood flow insufficiency should no longer be a factor limiting exercise. Abnormal exercise tolerance, in particular an early onset of lactic acidosis, may well be a clear sign that muscle abnormalities are a significant determinant of exercise intolerance.

This is not to say that the exercise responses of patients who have undergone transplantation for the treatment of lung disease are pure measures of the effects of deconditioning. Patients who have undergone transplantation generally receive a chronic course of immunosuppressive therapy. Cyclosporine has been reported to engender skeletal muscle abnormalities (56). Myopathic changes from glucocorticoid therapy are well described (56). Patients on chronic immunosupressive therapy are often mildly anemic, and this will reduce O_2 delivery to the exercising muscles (57). In those patients who have undergone heart-lung transplantation, cardiac acceleration with exercise may be inadequate because the heart is denervated; this may impair cardiac output response (57–59). Finally, at least in patients who have undergone single-lung transplantation, pulmonary vascular capacitance may still not be adequate. To this point, Ross et al. (60) found that peak exercise mean pulmonary artery pressure in eight patients who underwent single-lung transplantation was 36

Table 1 Exercise Tolerance Following Lung Transplantation

Ref.	Operative procedure	Number of patients	Reason for transplant	Peak $\dot{V}O_2$	Peak $\dot{V}O_2$ (% pred.)	Lactate threshold	Lactate threshold (% pred. peak $\dot{V}O_2$)	Peak heart rate (beats/min)	Peak heart rate (% pred.)
Theodore et al. (1987) (58)	HLT	10	Pulm. hypertension Congenital heart disease	9.8 ml/min/kg	39	—	—	129	68
Sciurba et al. (1988) (59)	HLT	7	Pulm. hypertension (4)	1.03 L/min	57	0.78 L/min	43	134	73
Kimoff et al. (1990) (64)	HLT	2 2	Emphysema Pulm. vascular disease	0.92 L/min	53	0.62 L/min	36	145	78
Miyoshi et al.	SLT	6	Pulm. fibrosis	0.86 L/min	44	0.71 L/min	36	118	69
(1990) (66)	DLT	6	COPD (4)	0.88 L/min	49	0.79 L/min	44	126	71
Gibbons et al.	SLT	6	Pulm. fibrosis	0.99 L/min	41	0.74 L/min	30	142	85
(1992) (61)		6	COPD	0.76 L/min	43	0.61 L/min	35	129	76
Williams et al.	SLT	6	Pulm. fibrosis	1.24 L/min	53	1.10 L/min	47	133	75
(1992) (57)	DLT	7	COPD (4)	0.92 L/min	48	0.82 L/min	43	136	73
Ross et al. (1993) (60)	SLT	3 4	Pulm. fibrosis COPD	13.4 ml/min/kg	42	7.7 ml/min/kg	24	136	78
Levine et al. (1994) (63)	SLT	22	COPD	0.84 L/min	43	0.66 L/min	34	136	80

All values are the average of the subjects studied. HLT, heart-lung transplant; SLT, single-lung transplant; DLT, double-lung transplant; peak $\dot{V}O_2$, peak oxygen uptake; lactate threshold, oxygen uptake at which there is a sustained increase in blood lactate level. In the studies of Miyoshi et al. and Ross et al., the lactate threshold was measured directly; in the remainder of the studies, it was indirectly assessed from gas exchange responses (41).

torr, roughly 60% above predicted level. Nevertheless, the consensus is that the exercise intolerance seen in posttransplant patients is predominantly a manifestation of deconditioning (57,58,60–64). This opinion is given credence by the report of Biggar et al. (65) that lung transplant patients who participate in rigorous exercise training programs manifest progressive increases in exercise tolerance.

Table 1 presents the salient results from a series of reports of the exercise responses of posttransplant patients. Despite differences in operative procedure (heart-lung versus double-lung versus single-lung transplant) and in class of pulmonary disease (pulmonary vascular versus interstitial fibrosis versus COPD), the results are remarkably homogeneous. In each study it was determined that after transplantation, exercise was not limited by the ventilatory requirement (i.e., breathing reserve was adequate). Further, appreciable hypoxemia was not observed. Yet peak oxygen uptake remained severely reduced (averages ranged from 39 to 57% predicted). Because the maximum heart rate does not closely approximate the predicted level (averaging 76% predicted), the possibility exists that the low peak $\dot{V}O_2$ values are due to inadequate effort. However, the lactate threshold averaged approximately 0.75 L/min, not appreciably different from the values seen in Figure 4 in (untransplanted) COPD patients. These values are well lower than predicted; the lower limit of normal lactate threshold in these subjects would be in the range of 40–45% of predicted $\dot{V}O_2max$ (41). These results are consistent with the concept that deconditioning contributes to the substantial residual exercise intolerance in the posttransplant patient.

In summary, this chapter has reviewed the protean manifestations of deconditioning. A reasonable case has been made that patients with chronic obstructive lung disease are often severely deconditioned and that this is a cause of a portion of the exercise intolerance these patients manifest (67,68). Including rigorous programs of exercise training as an integral part of pulmonary rehabilitation is a practical method to reverse deconditioning (4).

Acknowledgments

The author wishes to thank Antonio Patessio, M.D., of the Medical Center for Rehabilitation in Veruno, Italy, and Mary Burns, R.N., of the Little Company of Mary Hospital in Torrance, California, for allowing the use of data utilized for Figures 1, 2, and 4. Mrs. Maclovia Wallace provided expert secretarial support.

References

1. Carter R, Peavler M, Zinkgraf S, Williams J, Fields S. Predicting maximal exercise ventilation in patients with chronic obstructive pulmonary disease. Chest 1987; 92:253–259.
2. Dillard TA, Piantadose S, Rayagopal R. Prediction of ventilation at maximal exercise in chronic air-flow obstruction. Am Rev Respir Dis 1985; 132:230–235.
3. Wasserman K. Exercise tolerance in the pulmonary patient. In: Casaburi R, Petty TL, eds. Principles and Practice of Pulmonary Rehabilitation. Philadelphia: WB Saunders, 1993:115–123.
4. Casaburi R. Exercise training in chronic obstructive lung disease. In: Casaburi R, Petty TL, eds. Principles and Practice of Pulmonary Rehabilitation. Philadelphia: WB Saunders, 1993:204–224.
5. Haas F, Salazar-Schicchi, Axen K. Desensitization to dyspnea in chronic obstructive pulmonary disease. In: Casaburi R, Petty TL, eds. Principles and Practice of Pulmonary Rehabilitation. Philadelphia: WB Saunders, 1993:241–251.
6. Bortz WM. Disuse and aging. JAMA 1982; 248:1203–1208.
7. Kaplan RM, Eakin EG, Ries AL. Psychosocial issues in the rehabilitation of patients with chronic obstructive pulmonary disease. In: Casaburi R, Petty TL, eds. Principles and Practice of Pulmonary Rehabilitation. Philadelphia: WB Saunders, 1993:351–365.
8. Coyle EF, Martin WH, Bloomfield SA, Lowry OH, Holloszy JO. Effects of detraining on responses to submaximal exercise. J Appl Physiol 1985; 59:853–859.
9. Coyle EF, Martin WH, Sinacore DR, Joyner MJ, Hagberg JM, Holloszy JO. Time course of loss of adaptations after stopping prolonged intense endurance training. J Appl Physiol Respir Environ Exerc Physiol 1984; 57:1857–1864.
10. Saltin B, Gollnick PD. Skeletal muscle adaptability: significance for metabolism and performance. In: Peachey LD, ed. Handbook of Physiology: Skeletal Muscle. Washington, DC: American Physiological Society, 1986:555–631.
11. DeBusk RF, Convertino VA, Hung J, Goldwater D. Exercise conditioning in middle-aged men after 10 days of bed rest. Circulation 1983; 68:245–250.
12. Hung J, Goldwater D, Convertino VA, McKillop JH, Goris ML, DeBusk RF. Mechanisms for decreased exercise capacity after bed rest in normal middle-aged men. Am J Cardiol 1983; 51:344–348.
13. Convertino V, Hung J, Goldwater D, DeBusk RF. Cardiovascular responses to exercise in middle-aged men after 10 days of bedrest. Circulation 1982; 65:134–140.
14. Deitrick JE, Whedon GD, Shorr E. Effects of immobilization upon various metabolic and physiologic functions of normal men. Am J Med 1948; 4:3–36.
15. Saltin B, Blomqvist G, Mitchell JH, Johnson RL, Wildenthal K, Chapman CB. Response to exercise after bed rest and after training. Circulation 1968; 38(Suppl 7):1–78.
16. Martin WH, Coyle EF, Bloomfield SA, Ehsani AA. Effects of physical deconditioning after intense endurance training on left ventricular dimensions and stroke volume. J Am Coll Cardiol 1986; 7:982–989.

17. Ehsani AA, Hagberg JM, Hickson RC. Rapid changes in left ventricular dimensions and mass in response to physical conditioning and deconditioning. Am J Cardiol 1978; 42:52–56.
18. Convertino VA, Sandler H, Webb P, Annis JF. Induced venous pooling and cardiorespiratory responses to exercise after bed rest. J Appl Physiol Respir Environ Exerc Physiol 1982; 52:1343–1348.
19. Fareeduddin K, Abelmann WH. Impaired orthostatic tolerance after bed rest in patients with myocardial infarction. N Engl J Med 1969; 280:345–350.
20. Rambaut PC, Leach CS, Whedon GD. A study of metabolic balance in crew members of Skylab IV. Acta Astronaut 1979; 6:1313–1321.
21. Haines RF. Effect of bed rest and exercise on body balance. J Appl Physiol 1974; 36:323–327.
22. Rikli R, Busch S. Motor performance of women as a function of age and physical activity level. J Gerontol 1986; 41:645–649.
23. Spirduso WW. Physical fitness, aging and psychomotor speed: a review. J Gerontol 1980; 35:850–865.
24. Zubek JP, Wilgosh L. Prolonged immobilization of the body: changes in performance and in the electroencephalogram. Science 1963; 140:306–308.
25. Downs F. Bed rest and sensory disturbances. Am J Nurs 1974; 74:434–438.
26. Siebens H. Deconditioning. In: Kemp B, Brummel-Smith K, Ramsdell JW, eds. Geriatric Rehabilitation. Boston: Little, Brown, 1990:177–191.
27. Ryback RS, Lewis OF. Effects of prolonged bed rest on EEG sleep patterns in young, healthy volunteers. Electroenceph Clin Neurophysiol 1971; 31:395–399.
28. Yanagibori R, Suzuki Y, Kawakubo K, Makita Y, Gunji A. Carbohydrate and lipid metabolism after 20 days of bed rest. Acta Physiol Scand 1994; 150(Suppl 616):51–57.
29. Rogers MA, King DS, Hagberg JM, Ehsani AA, Holloszy JO. Effect of 10 days of physical inactivity on glucose tolerance in master athletes. J Appl Physiol 1990; 68:1833–1837.
30. Mikines KJ. The influence of physical activity and inactivity on insulin action and secretion in man. Acta Physiol Scand 1992; 146(Suppl 609):1–43.
31. Cockett ATK, Elbadawi A, Zemjanis R, Adey WR. The effects of immobilization on spermatogenesis in subhuman primates. Fertil Steril 1970; 21:610–614.
32. Briggs MH, Garcia-Webb P, Cheung T. Androgens and exercise. Br Med J 1973; 3:49–50.
33. Shetty KR, Sutton CH, Mattson DE, Rudman D. Hyposomatomedinemia in quadriplegic men. Am J Med Sci 1993; 305:95–100.
34. Sara VR, Hall K. Insulin-like growth factors and their binding proteins. Physiol Rev 1990; 70:591–614.
35. Keast D, Morton AR. Long-term exercise and immune function. In: Watson RR, Eisinger M, eds. Exercise and Disease. Boca Raton, FL: CRC Press, 1992:89–120.
36. Raitakari OT, Porkka KVK, Taimela S, Telama R, Rasanen L, Viikari JSA. Effects of persistent physical activity and inactivity on coronary risk factors in children and young adults. Am J Epidemiol 1994; 140:195–205.

37. Shetty KR, Sutton CH, Rudman IW, Rudman D. Lipid and lipoprotein abnormalities in young quadriplegic men. Am J Med Sci 1992; 303:213–216.
38. Niinimaa V, Shephard RJ. Training and oxygen conductance in the elderly. J Gerontol 1978; 33:354–361.
39. Greenleaf JE, Reese RD. Exercise thermoregulation after 14 days of bed rest. J Appl Physiol Respir Environ Exerc Physiol 1980; 48:72–78.
40. Levy G. Effect of bed rest on distribution and elimination of drugs. J Pharmacol Sci 1967; 56:928–929.
41. Wasserman K, Hansen JE, Sue DY, Whipp BJ, Casaburi R. Principles of Exercise Testing and Interpretation. Philadelphia: Lea & Febiger, 1994.
42. Wasserman K, Whipp BJ. Exercise physiology in health and disease. Am Rev Respir Dis 1975; 112:219–249.
43. Convertino VA, Goldwater DJ, Sandler H. $\dot{V}O_2$ kinetics of constant-load exercise following bed-rest-induced deconditioning. J Appl Physiol Respir Environ Exerc Physiol 1984; 57:1545–1550.
44. Shephard RJ. Physical activity and cancer. Int J Sports Med 1990; 11:413–420.
45. Ballard-Barbash R, Schatzkin A, Albanes D, et al. Physical activity and risk of large bowel cancer in the Framingham study. Cancer Res 1990; 50:3610–3613.
46. Sturgeon SR, Brinton LA, Berman ML, et al. Past and present physical activity and endometrial cancer risk. Br J Cancer 1993; 68:584–589.
47. Paffenbarger RS, Wing AL, Hyde RT. Physical activity as an index of heart attack risk in college alumni. Am J Epidemiol 1978; 108:161–175.
48. Novitch RS, Thomas HM. Rehabilitation of patients with chronic ventilatory limitation from nonobstructive lung disease. In: Casaburi R, Petty TL, eds. Principles and Practice of Pulmonary Rehabilitation. Philadelphia: WB Saunders, 1993:416–423.
49. Whipp BJ, Pardy RL. Breathing during exercise. In: Macklem PT, Mead J, eds. Handbook of Physiology. The Respiratory System III. Bethesda, MD: American Physiological Society, 1986:605–629.
50. Detroyer A. Respiratory muscle function in chronic obstructive pulmonary disease. In: Casaburi R, Petty TL, eds. Principles and Practice of Pulmonary Rehabilitation. Philadelphia: WB Saunders, 1993:33–49.
51. Glantz SA. Primer of Biostatistics, 3rd ed. New York: McGraw-Hill, 1992.
52. Casaburi R, Whipp BJ, Beaver WL, Wasserman K, Koyal SN. Ventilatory and gas exchange dynamics in response to sinusoidal work. J Appl Physiol 1977; 42:300–311.
53. Wasserman K, Whipp BJ, Casaburi R. Respiratory control during exercise. In: Handbook of Physiology, Respiration II. Washington, DC: American Physiological Society, 1986:595–619.
54. Beaver WL, Wasserman K, Whipp BJ. Improved detection of lactate threshold during exercise using a log-log transformation. J Appl Physiol 1985; 59:1936–1940.
55. Casaburi R, Patessio A, Ioli F, Zanaboni S, Donner CF, Wasserman K. Reduction in exercise lactic acidosis and ventilation as a result of exercise training in obstructive lung disease. Am Rev Respir Dis 1991; 143:9–18.

56. Cameron DE, Traill TA. Complications of immunosupressive therapy. In: Baumgartner WA, Reitz BA, Achuff SC, eds. Heart and Heart-Lung Transplantation. Philadelphia: WB Saunders, 1990:237–248.
57. Williams TJ, Patterson GA, McClean PA, Zamel N, Maurer JR. Maximal exercise testing in single and double lung transplant recipients. Am Rev Respir Dis 1992; 145:101–105.
58. Theodore J, Morris AJ, Burke CM, et al. Cardiopulmonary function at maximum tolerable constant work rate exercise following human heart-lung transplantation. Chest 1987; 92:433–439.
59. Sciurba FC, Owens GR, Sanders MH, et al. Evidence of an altered pattern of breathing during exercise in recipients of heart-lung transplants. N Engl J Med 1988; 319:1186–1192.
60. Ross DJ, Waters PF, Mohsenifar Z, Belman JM, Kass RM, Koerner SK. Hemodynamic responses to exercise after lung transplantation. Chest 1993; 103:46–53.
61. Gibbons WJ, Levine SM, Bryan CL, et al. Cardiopulmonary exercise responses after single lung transplantation for severe obstructive lung disease. Chest 1991; 100:106–111.
62. Otulana BA, Higenbottam TW, Wallwork J. Causes of exercise limitation after heart-lung transplantation. J Heart Lung Transplant 1992; 11:S244–S251.
63. Levine SM, Anzueto A, Peters JI, et al. Medium term functional results of single-lung transplantation for endstage obstructive lung disease. Am J Respir Crit Care Med 1994; 150:398–402.
64. Kimoff RJ, Cheong TH, Cosio MG, Guerraty A, Levy RD. Pulmonary denervation in humans. Am Rev Respir Dis 1990; 142:1034–1040.
65. Biggar DG, Malen JF, Trulock EP, Cooper JD. Pulmonary rehabilitation before and after lung transplantation. In: Casaburi R, Petty TL, eds. Principles and Practice of Pulmonary Rehabilitation. Philadelphia: WB Saunders, 1993:459–467.
66. Miyoshi S, Trulock EP, Schaefers HJ, Hsieh CM, Patterson GA, Cooper JD. Cardiopulmonary exercise testing after single and double lung transplantation. Chest 1990; 97:1130–1136.
67. Carter R, Nicotra B, Blevins W, Holiday D. Altered exercise gas exchange and cardiac function in patients with mild chronic obstructive pulmonary disease. Chest 1993; 103:745–750.
68. Olopade CO, Beck KC, Viggiano RW, Staats BA. Exercise limitation and pulmonary rehabilitation in chronic obstructive pulmonary disease. Mayo Clin Proc 1992; 67:144–157.
69. Knudson RJ, Lebowitz MD, Holberg CJ, Burrows B. Changes in the normal maximal expiratory flow-volume curve with growth and aging. Am Rev Respir Dis 1983; 127:725–734.
70. Patessio A, Casaburi R, Carone M, Appendini L, Donner CF, Wasserman K. Comparison of gas exchange, lactate, and lactic acidosis thresholds in patients with chronic obstructive pulmonary disease. Am Rev Respir Dis 1993; 148:622–626.
71. Casaburi R, Burns M, Cooper C, Singer E, Chang R, Porszasz J. Physiological benefits of exercise training in severe COPD. Am J Respir Crit Care Med 1994; 149:A598.

10

Sleep Assessment in Pulmonary Rehabilitation

RICHARD P. MILLMAN

Brown University
and Rhode Island Hospital
Providence, Rhode Island

Over the last 15 years, there has been growing interest in sleep and breathing during sleep. Extensive work has been done on obstructive sleep apnea and breathing during sleep in various cardiopulmonary disorders. There has not been, however, any systematic approach to sleep assessment from the standpoint of its role in pulmonary rehabilitation. This chapter will attempt to provide this perspective.

I. Normal Sleep

Sleep consists of basically five stages: stages I and II (light sleep) and stages III and IV (deep or delta sleep) are classified as non-rapid-eye-movement (nREM) sleep. The remaining sleep stage is REM sleep. During the night, a normal individual will cycle through nREM and REM approximately every 2 hr. Thus, in an 8-hr period, there will be four such cycles. Typically, one does not reach the initial period of REM sleep for 70–100 min. There is a greater predominance of stage III–IV sleep in the first half of the night and REM sleep in the early-morning hours. Sleep need is highest in infancy and decreases until it reaches a stable plateau in the adult age range. There is a decrease in stage III–IV sleep with age, while REM sleep remains unchanged (1).

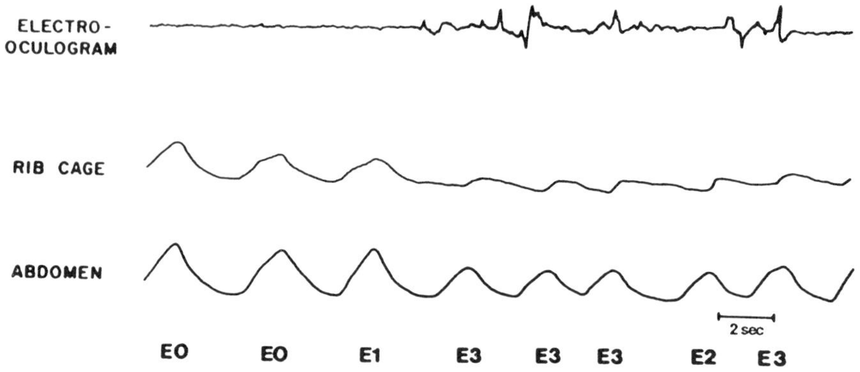

Figure 1 Relationship between eye movements and chest wall and abdominal movement. E0 breaths are not associated with eye movements. E1 breaths occur adjacent to eye movements, whereas E2 and E3 breaths are seen in association with increasing eye movement activity. Paradoxical rib cage and abdominal motion is seen in association with an eye movement burst. (Reprinted from Ref. 3 with permission.)

To better appreciate pathological changes during sleep in patients with chronic pulmonary disease, one needs a basic understanding of normal breathing patterns during sleep. Awake breathing is fairly irregular and one will observe intermittent sighing. When a healthy adult living at sea level enters stages I–II sleep, one observes an absence of sighs and periodic nonapneic breathing (2). Stage III–IV sleep is characterized by very regular breathing with an absence of periodicity (2).

Breathing during REM sleep can be very irregular and this appears to be related to intensity of REM activity (3). REM sleep can be classified into tonic and phasic components. Tonic REM is associated with pharyngeal muscle and intercostal muscle hypotonia. Phasic REM is associated with bursts of muscle activity including twitches of the extremities and rapid eye movements. This phasic activity also interferes with respiration. Chest wall and abdominal movement asynchrony and frank paradoxical breathing have been observed in association with increasing REM activity even in normals (3) (see Fig. 1).

II. Abnormal Sleep

One of the things lacking in medical school education is an understanding of how to take a sleep history. This is crucial in determining whether a patient is getting adequate or inadequate sleep, and whether the patient has a sleep disorder such as insomnia, obstructive sleep apnea, or narcolepsy.

Though a detailed discussion of the topic is out of the realm of this chapter, some basic questions are worthwhile to point out. It is important to establish how long the patient is actually sleeping. Specifically, one should ask, what time does the patient go to bed and how long does it take him or her to fall asleep? How often does the patient wake up in the middle of the night? How long does it take the patient to fall back to sleep each time in the middle of the night? What time does he or she get up in the morning? Does he or she feel refreshed? Does the patient have morning headaches? Does he snore and does his spouse observe apneic episodes while he is sleeping? Does the patient wake up gasping or choking during the course of the night or have orthopnea or paroxysmal nocturnal dyspnea? In addition, it is important to establish the adequacy of daytime function, including memory, concentrating ability, and tendency to be excessively sleepy. These questions become extremely important in assessing the need for further sleep evaluations in patients with chronic lung disease.

A. Effect of Sleep Deprivation

Sleep loss can occur in several situations. It can be voluntary, as typically seen in adolescents who basically are not getting enough sleep (4). Shift work can also cause significant sleep loss as can insomnia. Medical conditions, primary sleep disorders such as sleep apnea or periodic limb movements, and affective disorders, such as depression, can all cause insomnia. Behavioral psychophysiological insomnia is also common (5).

No matter what the cause of sleep loss, there are potential effects on musculoskeletal performance, respiratory muscle function, and cognitive capabilities. For example, several studies have examined the effect of 24–30 hr of sleep loss on respiratory function in normals. One study did demonstrate a small, but statistically significant, fall in forced vital capacity (FVC) and maximum voluntary ventilation (6). Ventilatory responsiveness decreases after sleep loss. There is approximately a 20% decrease in hypercapnic ventilatory responsiveness (6,7) and a 29% decrease in hypoxic ventilatory responsiveness (7) in normal subjects. Sleep deprivation has also been shown to selectively decrease genioglossal activity during hypercapnic rebreathing in subjects over 30 years of age (8). Respiratory muscle strength, as measured by maximal static inspiratory and expiratory pressures, has been shown to decrease at 30 hr of sleep loss (9). Inspiratory muscle endurance also decreased by 30% in these subjects (9).

Thirty hours of sleep loss has been demonstrated in normals to have some effect on exercise capabilities (10). Chen demonstrated a decrement in maximal exercise performance in 15 young, healthy male volunteers as indicated by a decrease in maximal heart rate, peak carbon dioxide production, peak oxygen consumption, and time to exhaustion (10). Other studies have not, however, shown an effect of sleep loss on cardiopulmonary responses to exercise levels of different intensity or on the aerobic or anaerobic performance capabilities of an individual (11). Electromechanical response times and muscle strength do not appear to be affected (12).

Chronic insomniacs have a greater tendency to be excessively sleepy and to have cognitive impairment, especially in the morning (13). Experimental sleep deprivation has been shown to increase sleepiness (14) and impair problem-solving capabilities (15).

B. Sleep Fragmentation and Its Effect on Performance

Sleep fragmentation in the presence of adequate hours of sleep has also been shown to affect daytime function. There have been studies examining the effect of experimentally induced sleep fragmentation. There are also several pathological states, such as obstructive sleep apnea, central sleep apnea, and periodic limb movements disorder, that can also fragment sleep.

Experimental Sleep Fragmentation

Sleep fragmentation has been induced in normal volunteers, generally using tones (16,17). These studies have resulted in excessive sleepiness (16,17) and some evidence of cognitive impairment (16). Minimal data are available on the effect of experimentally induced sleep fragmentation on respiratory function or exercise performance.

Obstructive Sleep Apnea

Obstructive sleep apnea is probably the most common cause of pathological sleep fragmentation. It is a condition associated with repetitive pharyngeal collapse during sleep. During sleep, the pharyngeal muscles relax. If there is structural narrowing, such as with retrognathia or adenotonsillar hypertrophy, or enhanced pharyngeal collapsibility, the pharynx may totally collapse. Thus, during obstructive apnea, there is continued respiratory effort against the closed airway with resultant hypoxemia and hypercapnia. Eventually, there is an arousal leading to pharyngeal muscle contraction and resumption of airflow. Spouses frequently note the apneic episodes and complain of loud snoring. Predisposing factors for the development of obstructive sleep apnea include male sex, obesity, nasal obstruction, retrognathia, enlarged tonsils and adenoids, excessive evening alcohol ingestion, hypothyroidism, and acromegaly (18). There is also evidence of family predisposition, though the mechanism is not well established (19,20).

The repetitive sleep fragmentation, as well as nocturnal oxygen desaturation, are associated with a myriad of daytime sequelae (18). Specifically, these include excessive sleepiness, problems with memory and attention-concentration (21), and personality changes including depression (22). The daytime sleepiness can be so severe that it can lead to uncontrollable sleepiness while driving an automobile. An increase in motor vehicle accidents (23) and even death (24) have been well documented.

With increasing respiratory efforts against a closed glottis, there is increased vagal tone with resultant bradycardia. With arousal the vagal tone is released with resultant tachycardia (25). Pulmonary artery pressures fluctuate in response to alveolar hypoxia (26), and either sustained or exercise-induced pulmonary hypertension can occur during the daytime (27). Some authors have demonstrated that sustained daytime pulmonary hypertension requires the presence of coexistent daytime hypoxia (28), often in association with chronic airflow obstruction (29,30). Pulmonary hypertension may also be related to individual differences in responsiveness of the pulmonary circulation to episodic alveolar hypoxia (31). In addition, sleep apnea has been associated with repetitive fluctuation in systemic blood pressure during sleep and daytime hypertension (32).

III. Sleep and Chronic Obstructive Pulmonary Disease

In assessing sleep pathology and its role in affecting pulmonary rehabilitation in patients with chronic obstructive pulmonary disease, one has to evaluate the patients in regard to sleep loss, the severity of oxygen desaturation in REM sleep, and whether there is coexistent obstructive sleep apnea.

A. Insomnia and Effect of Sleep Loss

In a large epidemiological study, patients with obstructive airway disease were found to have a high prevalence of insomnia, excessive daytime sleepiness, and nightmares compared to a general population (33). Fifty-three percent of the patients with chronic bronchitis and 55% of the patients with emphysema were found to have insomnia, while the prevalence of excessive daytime sleepiness was 26% and 29%, respectively, for each group. Though one could potentially implicate theophylline preparations or β agonists as a cause of this insomnia, most studies have failed to demonstrate any adverse effect of these medications on sleep efficiency or sleep staging (34,35).

It has been postulated, instead, that the symptoms of insomnia are probably related to the underlying obstructive airways disease. Arousals from sleep, for example, are common during episodes of oxygen desaturation (36,37). In addition, coughing, orthopnea, and shortness of breath during the night can cause insomnia. Insomnia and subsequent sleep loss may lead to daytime sleepiness. Though cognitive function abnormalities have been well described in patients with chronic obstructive lung disease, they have been attributed primarily to nocturnal hypoxemia rather than sleep loss (38–40).

The effects on respiratory function from chronic sleep loss are unknown in this population. Phillips and her colleagues measured the effect of one night of total sleep deprivation on pulmonary function in 15 male patients with chronic obstructive pulmonary disease (COPD) (41). As in normal subjects, there was a very small, but statistically significant, fall, in both the FVC and FEV_1. Though one night of total sleep deprivation may not have any major clinical consequences in patients with stable COPD, it is possible that total sleep deprivation during an acute exacerbation may have some profound effects. It is also not known whether chronic sleep loss could promote respiratory failure. In addition, no one has studied the effects of sleep loss in this population on exercise performance. There is no information available on whether chronic sleep loss adversely affects pulmonary rehabilitation potential.

To treat insomnia, it is important to maximize drug therapy to prevent coughing and dyspnea from disrupting sleep at night. If a patient has severe oxygen desaturation during sleep, then supplemental oxygen may help as well. The use of hypnotics is more controversial. A study using a short-acting sedative hypnotic such as triazolam and zolpidem in the presence of mild to moderate chronic obstructive lung disease has shown that in general, these agents can be safely tolerated without any worsening of oxygen saturation (42). Zolpidem has also been shown to have no effect on ventilatory responses in patients with severe chronic airflow obstruction (43). From a practical standpoint, these agents should probably be used only with caution, especially in those patients with carbon dioxide retention.

B. Oxygen Desaturation During Sleep in COPD

Oxygen desaturation during sleep, especially in REM sleep, has long been recognized in patients with significant chronic airflow obstruction (see Fig. 2). Daytime clinical parameters that have been associated with the presence of nocturnal oxygen desaturation include daytime hypoxemia ($Po_2 < 60$ mmHg) (44–46), blunted awake chemosensitivities (47,48), and chronic CO_2 retention (46,49).

There are several possible explanations for REM sleep–related oxygen desaturation (50,51). Though ventilation is reduced in all stages of sleep in these patients, there is marked alveolar hypoventilation during REM sleep, especially in association with periods of intense eye movement activity (52). It is probable that the hypoventilation results from REM sleep–induced hypotonia of the intercostal and accessory respiratory muscles. Since patients with chronic airflow obstruction often have mechanically disadvantaged flat diaphragms, the intercostal and accessory respiratory muscles play a key role in maintaining

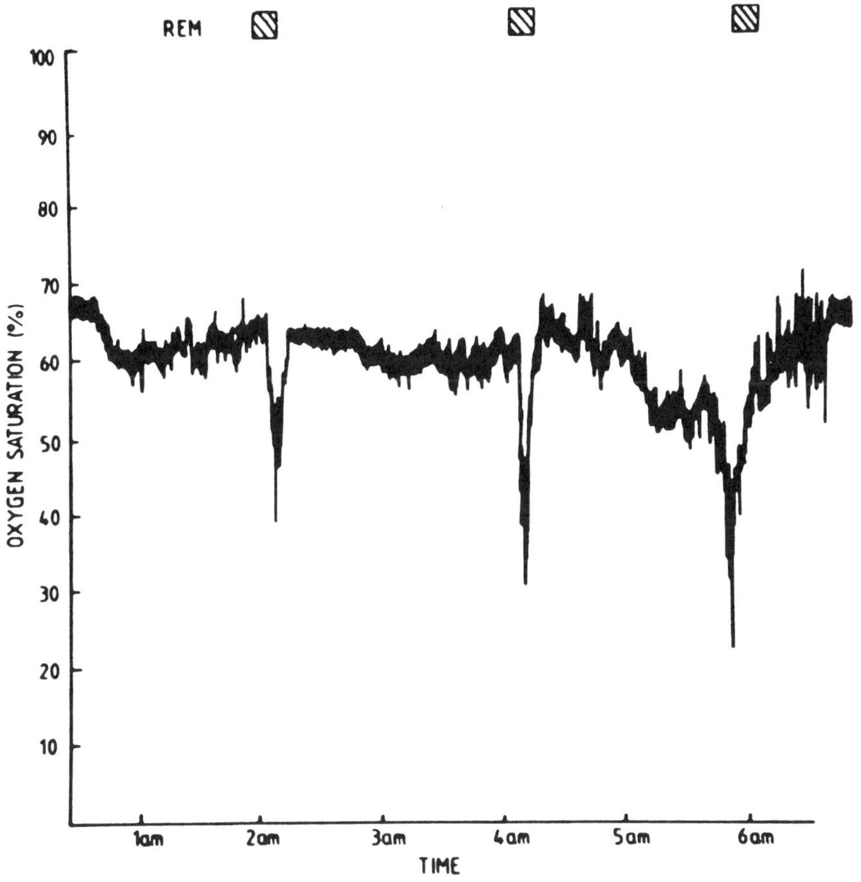

Figure 2 Oxygen saturation throughout the night in a typical patient with chronic obstructive pulmonary disease. The hatched areas represent rapid eye movement sleep. (Reprinted with permission from Ref. 55.)

normal ventilation. During REM sleep, contraction of a flattened diaphragm against a flaccid lower chest wall could result in an actual pulling in of the lower chest wall during inspiration, significantly reducing alveolar ventilation and causing oxygen desaturation. It has also been postulated that hypoxemia observed in REM sleep is related to ventilation-perfusion mismatching. This has been difficult to actually measure.

Oxygen desaturation during REM sleep is also associated with an increase in the pulmonary artery pressure (53,54). It is not totally clear whether isolated increases in pulmonary artery pressure at night in these patients can lead to sustained pulmonary hypertension during the day (55). Most of these patients who do have sustained pulmonary hypertension are also hypoxic during the daytime (55). There is recent evidence, however, that isolated nocturnal hypoxia may lead to daytime pulmonary hypertension. Studies of patients with nocturnal desaturation and daytime $Po_2 \geq 60$ mmHg have demonstrated higher daytime resting (56) and exercise-induced (57) pulmonary artery pressures than in similar patients without nocturnal oxygen desaturation at night.

There appears to be a relationship between mean nocturnal oxygen saturation and nocturnal oxygen saturation nadir and survival in patients with COPD (46). These authors, however, could not demonstrate that measurement of nocturnal oxygen levels improved the prediction of survival over measurements of vital capacity or awake oxygenation (46). Though survival is improved with nocturnal oxygen alone (58), 19 hr of continuous oxygen therapy has been shown to be superior to only 12 hr of nocturnal oxygen (59). Fletcher and his colleagues have found that there is even a decrement in survival in the subset of patients with chronic obstructive lung disease who have nocturnal oxygen desaturation and a daytime $Po_2 \geq 60$ mmHg (60). They could not demonstrate, however, a reduction in mortality with nocturnal oxygen supplementation in this subgroup of patients (61).

C. COPD and Coexistent Obstructive Sleep Apnea

Chronic airflow obstruction and obstructive sleep apnea may coexist in certain patients. There is no evidence, however, that this coexistence is more common than would be expected from the relative frequencies of the two conditions (55). Because of the sleep disruption from the obstructive sleep apnea, these patients may complain of daytime sleepiness and other related symptoms. They seem more likely to develop daytime hypertension, right-sided heart failure, and carbon dioxide retention than do patients who have only a single disorder (62). In fact, if one finds evidence of pulmonary hypertension or carbon dioxide retention at a level of lung function typically not associated with these findings (for example, an FEV_1 of 1.6 L), one should probably consider a coexistent process such as obstructive sleep apnea.

IV. Sleep and Interstitial Lung Disease

Compared to COPD, there is a paucity of data available about the prevalence of sleep complaints such as insomnia and daytime sleepiness in patients with interstitial lung disease. There are no studies examining the effect of sleep loss and daytime performance in these patients.

A few studies have examined sleep quality and arterial oxygen saturation during sleep (63–67). Sleep quality appears to be worse in patients with interstitial lung disease, with a greater percentage of light stage I sleep and more sleep fragmentation than in the controls (64). REM sleep has been associated with significant oxygen desaturation in some studies (63,64,67) but not others (65,66). Non-REM sleep desaturation has also been observed (63,67).

As in patients with chronic airflow obstruction, it has been postulated that alveolar hypoventilation and possible ventilation-perfusion mismatching in REM sleep secondary to respiratory muscle hypotonia may contribute to the development of oxygen desaturation in these patients (68). In non-REM sleep, oxygen desaturation may also occur because of episodes of obstructive apnea and hypopnea (67).

One study examined the relationship between snoring and oxygen desaturation (64). Snorers have an increased resistance to breathing as they attempt to breathe through a narrowed upper airway. Snoring was associated with falls in oxygen saturation during sleep in patients who had an awake oxygen saturation <90%. Full-blown relatively asymptomatic obstructive sleep apnea was observed in two of 13 patients in one study (63).

The magnitude of oxygen desaturation during sleep appears to be inversely correlated with the baseline oxygen saturation (67). Thus, patients whose oxygen saturation lies close to the steep portion of the oxyhemoglobin dissociation curve have a greater chance of having significant desaturation during sleep. There also appears to be an inverse relationship between awake hypercapnia ventilatory responsiveness and the degree of oxygen desaturation (67).

No data are available linking nocturnal oxygen desaturation during sleep in these patients and daytime performance, respiratory muscle function, cardiovascular sequelae, or the effect on pulmonary rehabilitation. It has also not been established whether nocturnal oxygen has any significant beneficial effect in decreasing mortality or morbidity.

V. Sleep and Kyphoscoliosis

REM sleep has been associated with severe oxygen desaturation in patients with kyphoscoliosis (66,69,70). Compared to patients with chronic obstructive lung disease or interstitial lung disease, scoliotics have been shown to demonstrate a greater degree of oxygen desaturation during sleep despite having similar baseline awake oxygen desaturation levels (69). It is possible that respiratory muscle hypotonia in the presence of chest wall deformity leads to marked alveolar hypoventilation and subsequent falls in oxygen saturation in these patients (68). Within scoliotic populations, there does not appear to be a relationship between the severity of nocturnal oxygen desaturation and the degree of thoracic deformity, pulmonary function, awake arterial carbon dioxide level, or

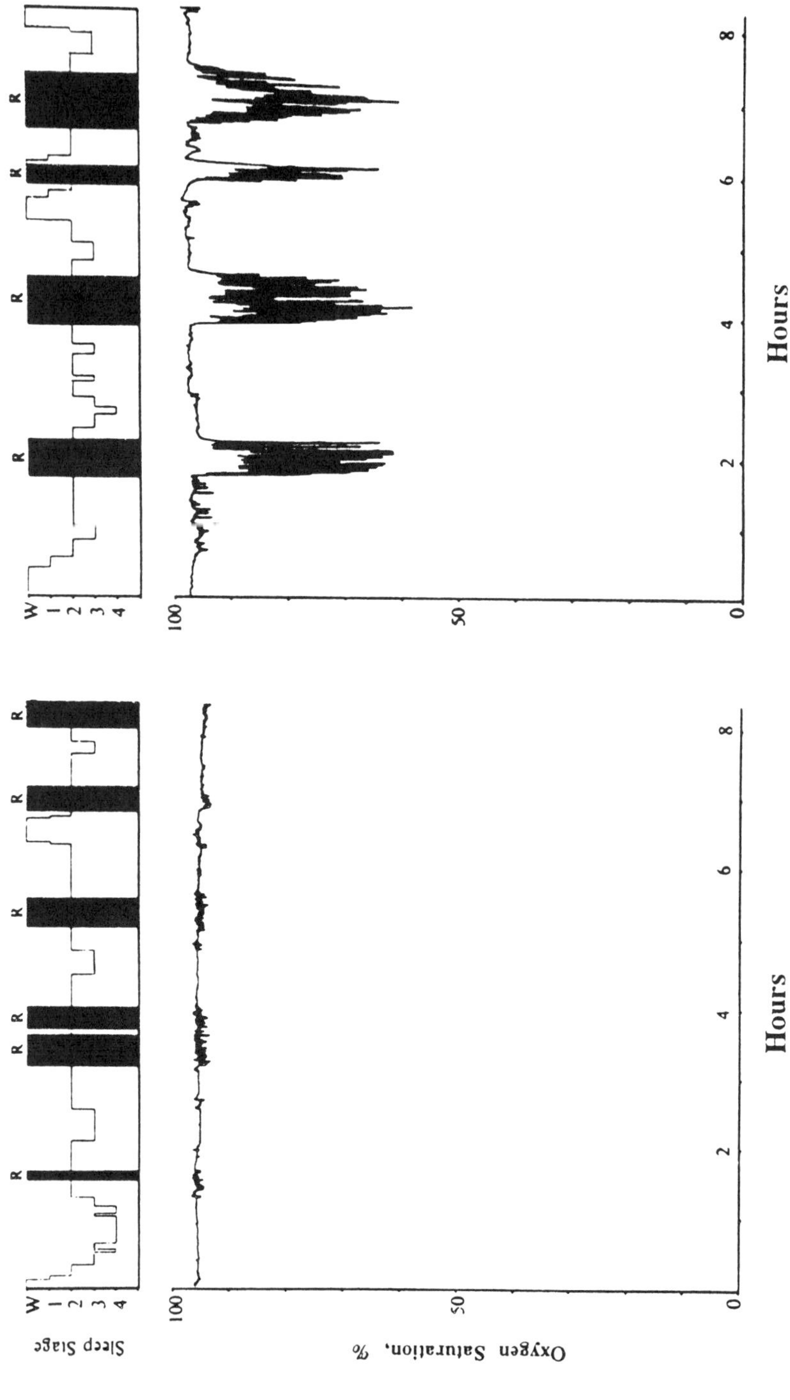

Figure 3

ventilatory responsiveness (69). However, those patients with evidence of daytime hypertension, polycythemia, and cor pulmonale demonstrated the most severe oxygen desaturation during sleep (69).

Untreated patients with chest wall deformity and chronic respiratory failure complain of morning headaches, feeling fairly less rested in the morning, and daytime sleepiness (71). Hill and his colleagues withdrew nocturnal nasal ventilation for 1 week in four patients with restrictive chest wall disease (71). Symptoms of nonrestorative sleep recurred without any change in daytime pulmonary function or gas exchange, suggesting that nocturnal hypoventilation in itself is sufficient to produce these symptoms (71). It is also probable that severe nocturnal hypoxemia contributes to the development of pulmonary hypertension and cor pulmonale (69) and eventual respiratory failure (72).

VI. Sleep and Neuromuscular Disorders

Disorders of respiratory muscle weakness have been demonstrated to be associated with sleep apnea and with nocturnal oxygen desaturation, especially in REM sleep (73). It has been postulated that the hypoventilation seen in REM sleep, as discussed above in the other chronic pulmonary disorders, is related to intercostal muscle inhibition in the presence of severe diaphragm weakness (73).

Each of the common neuromuscular disorders has been found to have a somewhat different pattern in regard to the respiratory findings during sleep. For example, several studies have examined respiration during sleep in myotonic dystrophy and have demonstrated that some patients with myotonic dystrophy have obstructive sleep apnea while sleeping (74–76). One author, however, found a predominance of central apneas (77). The development of sleep apnea does not appear to be directly related to respiratory muscle weakness (76). It is unknown, however, whether pharyngeal muscle weakness could contribute to the development of obstructive events during sleep. Patients with myotonic dystrophy frequently complain of daytime sleepiness. These studies could not demonstrate an association, however, with daytime sleepiness and the presence of sleep apnea. It is possible that daytime sleepiness in these patients may be related to some central mechanism.

Figure 3 Overnight oxygen saturation measurements in two patients with Duchenne muscular dystrophy demonstrating different severities of oxygen desaturation during REM sleep. The light shaded areas represent wakefulness (W) and stages I–IV sleep. REM is represented by solid bars labeled R. (Reprinted with permission from Ref. 79.)

Duchenne's muscular dystrophy has also been associated with a fall in tidal volume in non-REM sleep (78) and with obstructive apneas and hypopneas with significant oxygen desaturation in REM sleep (79) (see Fig. 3). These REM-related episodes could not be predicted from daytime pulmonary function parameters or arterial blood gases and were not associated with symptoms suggestive of a sleep disorder (78).

Survivors of previous polio tend to develop hypoventilation and hypoxemia during sleep in the presence of scoliosis or when there has been evidence of respiratory muscle involvement during the original illness (80). Obstructive sleep apnea is commonly associated with postpolio syndrome as well (81).

VII. The Need for Nocturnal Sleep Testing

Nocturnal sleep evaluation can be in the form of overnight oximetry, multichannel respiratory recording, or full polysomnography. It can be done in the home, in an inpatient setting, or in a sleep disorders laboratory. The complexity of testing really depends on the question that needs to be answered. For example, continuous pulse oximetry may be sufficient in assessing the need for supplemental oxygen in a patient with chronic obstructive airways disease. More extensive recording is necessary if one suspects coexistent obstructive sleep apnea or when assessing the degree of respiratory failure occurring during sleep.

The role of routine nocturnal oximetry in patients with chronic obstructive airways disease is controversial. The need for oxygen therapy can usually be predicted by measurement of daytime arterial blood gases (46). Clearly, there is a subset of patients, however, with an awake $Po_2 \geq 60$ mmHg, who do desaturate significantly during sleep (60). Since nocturnal oxygen supplementation has not been demonstrated to reduce mortality in this group of patients (61), it is difficult to justify the routine use of nocturnal oximetry in patients with a daytime $Po_2 \geq 60$ mmHg.

Nighttime desaturation, hypoventilation, and sleep disruption may represent early stages of respiratory failure in patients with kyphoscoliosis and neuromuscular disorder. It is also possible that nocturnal respiratory events may predispose these patients to the development of progressive respiratory failure. Possible mechanisms include blunting of hypoxic and hypercapnic ventilatory responses and respiratory muscle weakness. In addition, nocturnal hypoxemia may contribute to the development of pulmonary hypertension and cor pulmonale. It is often difficult to predict the severity of nocturnal oxygen desaturation or even the presence of obstructive sleep apnea in these latter patients. Thus, one could argue that there should be a lower threshold for sleep testing in

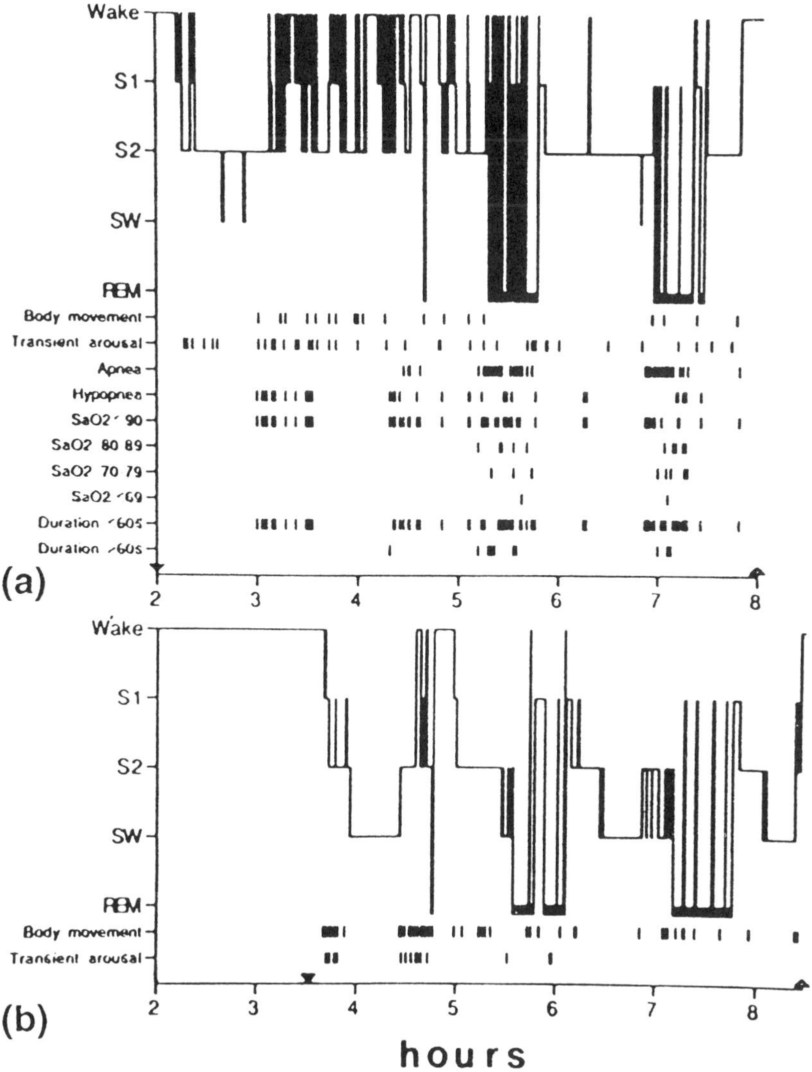

Figure 4 Nocturnal histograms in a patient with muscular dystrophy showing sleep-wake transition, transient arousals, apneas-hypopneas, oxygen desaturations, and duration of sleep-disordered breathing events. Hours indicate duration of monitoring. (a) Results during the use of negative-pressure ventilation, showing frequent apneas and hypopneas. (b) Many fewer awakenings and no apneas, hypopneas, or desaturations were noted during positive-pressure ventilation following tracheostomy. (Reproduced with permission from Ref. 84.)

this population. Several studies, in addition, have demonstrated the continued presence of sleep apnea despite supplemental oxygen (82), or sleep apnea and oxygen desaturation even with the use of a rocking bed (81), or negative-pressure ventilation (83,84) (see Fig. 4). Thus, without a sleep recording, one cannot even make the assumption that patients on some form of nocturnal ventilation are being adequately treated.

VIII. Conclusions

Patients with end-stage chronic pulmonary disorders should be assessed by careful sleep history to assess the presence of sleep loss or coexistent obstructive sleep apnea. Many of these patients will require nocturnal testing to assess the need and adequacy of supplemental oxygen or ventilatory support.

References

1. Carskadon MA, Dement WC. Normal human sleep: an overview. In: Krygen MK, Roth T, Dement WC, eds. Principles and Practice of Sleep Medicine, 2nd ed. Philadelphia: WB Saunders, 1994:16–25.
2. Shore ET, Millman RP, Silage DA, Chung DC, Pack AI. Ventilatory and arousal patterns during sleep in normal young and elderly subjects. J Appl Physiol 1985; 59(5):1607–1615.
3. Millman RP, Knight H, Kline LR, Shore ET, Chung DC, Pack AI. Changes in compartmental ventilation in association with eye movements during REM sleep. J Appl Physiol 1988; 65(3):1196–1202.
4. Strauch I, Meier B. Sleep need in adolescents: a longitudinal approach. Sleep 1988; 11(4):378–386.
5. Hauri P, Fisher J. Persistent psychophysiologic (learned) insomnia. Sleep 1986; 9(1):38–53.
6. Cooper KR, Phillips BA. Effect of short-term sleep loss on breathing. J Appl Physiol Respir Environ Exerc Physiol 1982; 53(4):855–858.
7. White DP, Douglas NJ, Pickett CK, Zwillich CW, Weil JV. Sleep deprivation and the control of ventilation. Am Rev Respir Dis 1983; 128:984–986.
8. Leiter JC, Knuth SL, Bartlett D Jr. The effect of sleep deprivation on activity of the genioglossus muscle. Am Rev Respir Dis 1985; 132:1242–1245.
9. Chen H, Tang Y. Sleep loss impairs inspiratory muscle endurance. Am Rev Respir Dis 1989; 140:907–909.
10. Chen H. Effects of 30-h sleep loss on cardiorespiratory functions at rest and in exercise. Med Sci Sports Exerc 1991; 23(2):193–198.
11. VanHelder T, Radomski MW. Sleep deprivation and the effect on exercise performance. Sports Med 1989; 7:235–247.

12. Symons JD, Bell DG, Pope J, VanHelder T, Myles WS. Electro-mechanical response times and muscle strength after sleep deprivation. Can J Sport Sci 1988; 13(4):225–230.
13. Schneider-Helmert D. Twenty-four-hour-sleep-wake function and personality patterns in chronic insomniacs and healthy controls. Sleep 1987; 10(5):452–462.
14. Carskadon MA, Dement WC. Cumulative effects of sleep restriction on daytime sleepiness. Psychophysiology 1981; 18(2):107–113.
15. Linde L, Bergstrom M. The effect of one night without sleep on problem-solving and immediate recall. Psychol Res 1992; 54:127–136.
16. Bonnet MH. Performance and sleepiness following moderate sleep disruption and slow wave sleep deprivation. Physiol Behav 1986; 37(6):915–918.
17. Magee J, Harsh J, Badia P. Effects of experimentally-induced sleep fragmentation on sleep and sleepiness. Psychophysiology 1987; 24:528–534.
18. Millman RP. Snoring and apnea. Clin Chest Med 1987; 8(2):253–264.
19. El Bayadi S, Millman RP, Tishler PV, et al. A family study of sleep apnea. Anatomic and physiologic interactions. Chest 1990; 98:554–559.
20. Redline S, Tosteson T, Tishler PV, Carskadon MA, Millman RP. Studies in the genetics of obstructive sleep apnea. Am Rev Respir Dis 1992; 145:440–444.
21. Cheshire K, Engleman H, Deary I, Shapiro C, Douglas NJ. Factors impairing daytime performance in patients with sleep apnea/hypopnea syndrome. Arch Intern Med 1992; 152:538–541.
22. Millman RP, Fogel BS, McNamara ME, Carlisle CC. Depression as a manifestation of obstructive sleep apnea: reversal with nasal continuous positive airway pressure. J Clin Psychiatry 1989; 50:348–351.
23. Findley LJ, Unverzagt ME, Suratt PM. Automobile accidents involving patients with obstructive sleep apnea. Am Rev Respir Dis 1988; 138:337–340.
24. Findley LJ, Weiss W, Jabour R. Drivers with untreated sleep apnea: a cause of death and serious injury. Arch Intern Med 1991; 151:1451–1452.
25. Zwillich C, Devlin T, White D, Douglas N, Weil J, Martin R. Bradycardia during sleep apnea: characteristics and mechanism. J Clin Invest 1982; 69:1286–1292.
26. Tilkian AG, Guilleminault C, Schroeder JS, Lehrman KL, Simmons FB, Dement WC. Hemodynamics in sleep-induced apnea. Ann Intern Med 1976; 85:714–719.
27. Podszus T, Bauer W, Mayer J, Penzel T, Peter JH, von Wichert P. Sleep apnea and pulmonary hypertension. Klin Wochenschr 1986; 64:131–134.
28. Bradley TD, Rutherford R, Grossman RF, et al. Role of daytime hypoxemia in the pathogenesis of right heart failure in the obstructive sleep apnea syndrome. Am Rev Respir Dis 1985; 131:835–839.
29. Weitzenblum E, Krieger J, Apprill M, et al. Daytime pulmonary hypertension in patients with obstructive sleep apnea syndrome. Am Rev Respir Dis 1988; 138:345–349.
30. Fletcher EC, Schaaf JW, Miller J, Fletcher JG. Long-term cardiopulmonary sequelae in patients with sleep apnea and chronic lung disease. Am Rev Respir Dis 1987; 135:525–533.
31. Sajkov D, Cowie RJ, Thorton AT, Espinoza HA, McEvoy RD. Pulmonary hypertension and hypoxemia in obstructive sleep apnea syndrome. Am J Respir Crit Care Med 1994; 149:416–422.

32. Levinson PD, Millman RP. Causes and consequences of blood pressure alterations in obstructive sleep apnea. Arch Intern Med 1991; 151:455–462.
33. Klink M, Quan SF. Prevalence of reported sleep disturbances in a general adult population and their relationship to obstructive airways diseases. Chest 1987; 91(4):540–546.
34. Berry RB, Desa MM, Branum JP, Light RW. Effect of theophylline on sleep and sleep-disordered breathing in patients with chronic obstructive pulmonary disease. Am Rev Respir Dis 1991; 143:245–250.
35. Martin RJ, Pak J. Overnight theophylline concentrations and effects on sleep and lung function in chronic obstructive pulmonary disease. Am Rev Respir Dis 1992; 145:540–544.
36. Fleetham J, West P, Mezon B, Conway W, Roth T, Kryger M. Sleep, arousals, and oxygen desaturation in chronic obstructive pulmonary disease. The effect of oxygen therapy. Am Rev Respir Dis 1982; 126:429–433.
37. Calverley PMA, Brezinova V, Douglas NJ, Catterall JR, Flenley DC. The effect of oxygenation on sleep quality in chronic bronchitis and emphysema. Am Rev Respir Dis 1982; 126:206–210.
38. Grant I, Prigatano GP, Heaton RK, McSweeny AJ, Wright EC, Adams KM. Progressive neuropsychologic impairment and hypoxemia. Relationship in chronic obstructive pulmonary disease. Arch Gen Psychiatry 1987; 44:999–1006.
39. Heaton RK, Grant I, McSweeny AJ, Adams KM, Petty TL. Psychologic effects of continuous and nocturnal oxygen therapy in hypoxemic chronic obstructive pulmonary disease. Arch Intern Med 1983; 143:1941–1947.
40. Prigatano GP, Parsons O, Wright E, Levin DC, Hawryluk G. Neuropsychological test performance in mildly hypoxemic patients with chronic obstructive pulmonary disease. J Consult Clin Psychol 1983; 51(1):108–116.
41. Phillips BA, Cooper KR, Burke TV. The effect of sleep loss on breathing in chronic obstructive pulmonary disease. Chest 1987; 91(1):29–32.
42. Steens RD, Pouliot Z, Millar TW, Kryger MH, George CF. Effects of zolpidem and triazolam on sleep and respiration in mild to moderate chronic obstructive pulmonary disease. Sleep 1993; 16(4):318–326.
43. Murciano D, Armengaud MH, Cramer PH, et al. Acute effects of zolpidem, triazolam and flunitrazepam on arterial blood gases and control of breathing in severe COPD. Eur Respir J 1993; 6:625–629.
44. Catterall JR, Douglas NJ, Calverley PMA, et al. Transient hypoxemia during sleep in chronic obstructive pulmonary disease is not a sleep apnea syndrome. Am Rev Respir Dis 1983; 128:24–29.
45. McKeon JL, Murree-Allan K, Saunders NA. Prediction of oxygenation during sleep in patients with chronic obstructive lung disease. Thorax 1988; 43:312–317.
46. Connaughton JJ, Catterall JR, Elton RA, Stradling JR, Douglas NJ. Do sleep studies contribute to the management of patients with severe chronic obstructive pulmonary disease? Am Rev Respir Dis 1988; 138:341–344.
47. Tatsumi K, Kimura H, Kunitomo F, Kuriyama T, Watanabe S, Honda Y. Sleep arterial oxygen desaturation and chemical control of breathing during wakefulness in COPD. Chest 1986; 90(1):68–72.

48. Littner MR, McGinty DJ, Arand DL. Determinants of oxygen desaturation in the course of ventilation during sleep in chronic obstructive pulmonary disease. Am Rev Respir Dis 1980; 122:849–857.
49. Perez-Padilla R, Conway W, Roth T, Anthonisen N, George C, Kryger M. Hypercapnia and sleep O_2 desaturation in chronic obstructive pulmonary disease. Sleep 1987; 10(3):216–223.
50. Catterall JR, Calverley PMA, MacNee W, et al. Mechanism of transient nocturnal hypoxemia in hypoxic chronic bronchitis and emphysema. J Appl Physiol 1985; 59(6):1698–1703.
51. Johnson MW, Remmers JE. Accessory muscle activity during sleep in chronic obstructive pulmonary disease. J Appl Physiol Respir Environ Exerc Physiol 1984; 57(4):1011–1017.
52. George CF, West P, Kryger MH. Oxygenation and breathing pattern during phasic and tonic REM in patients with chronic obstructive pulmonary disease. Sleep 1987; 10(3):234–243.
53. Boysen PG, Block AJ, Wynne JW, Hunt LA, Flick MR. Nocturnal pulmonary hypertension in patients with chronic obstructive pulmonary disease. Chest 1979; 76(5):536–542.
54. Fletcher EC, Levin DC. Cardiopulmonary hemodynamics during sleep in subjects with chronic obstructive pulmonary disease. The effect of short- and long-term oxygen. Chest 1984; 86(1):6–14.
55. Douglas NJ, Flenley DC. Breathing during sleep in patients with obstructive lung disease. Am Rev Respir Dis 1990; 141:1055–1070.
56. Levi-Valensi P, Weitzenblum E, Rida Z, et al. Sleep-related oxygen desaturation and daytime pulmonary haemodynamics in COPD patients. Eur Respir J 1992; 5:301–307.
57. Fletcher EC, Luckett RA, Miller T, Fletcher JG. Exercise hemodynamics and gas exchange in patients with chronic obstruction pulmonary disease, sleep desaturation, and a daytime Pao_2 above 60 mm Hg. Am Rev Respir Dis 1989; 140:1237–1245.
58. Medical Research Council Working Party. Long term domiciliary oxygen therapy in chronic hypoxic cor pulmonale complicating chronic bronchitis and emphysema. Lancet 1981; 1:681–686.
59. Nocturnal Oxygen Therapy Trial Group. Continuous or nocturnal oxygen therapy in hypoxemic chronic obstructive lung disease: a clinical trial. Ann Intern Med 1980; 93:391–398.
60. Fletcher EC, Donner CF, Midgren B, et al. Survival in COPD patients with a daytime $Pao_2 > 60$ mm Hg with and without nocturnal oxyhemoglobin desaturation. Chest 1992; 101:649–655.
61. Fletcher EC, Luckett RA, Goodnight-White S, Miller CC, Qian W, Costarangos-Galarza C. A double-blind trial of nocturnal supplemental oxygen for sleep desaturation in patients with chronic obstructive pulmonary disease and a daytime Pao_2 above 60 mm Hg. Am Rev Respir Dis 1992; 145:1070–1076.
62. Weitzemblum E, Krieger J, Oswald M, Chaouat A, Bachez P, Kessler R. Chronic obstructive pulmonary disease and sleep anpea syndrome. Sleep 1992; 15:S33–S35.

63. Bye PTP, Issa F, Berthon-Jones M, Sullivan CE. Studies of oxygenation during sleep in patients with interstitial lung disease. Am Rev Respir Dis 1984; 129:27–32.
64. Perez-Padilla R, West P, Lertzman M, Kryger MH. Breathing during sleep in patients with interstitial lung disease. Am Rev Respir Dis 1985; 132:224–229.
65. Midgren B, Hansson L, Eriksson L, Airikkala P, Elmqvist D. Oxygen desaturation during sleep and exercise in patients with interstitial lung disease. Thorax 1987; 42:353–356.
66. Midgren B. Oxygen desaturation during sleep as a function of the underlying respiratory disease. Am Rev Respir Dis 1990; 141:43–46.
67. Tatsumi K, Kimura H, Kunitomo F, Kuriyama T, Honda Y. Arterial oxygen desaturation during sleep in interstitial pulmonary disease. Correlation with chemical control of breathing during wakefulness. Chest 1989; 95:962–967.
68. George CF, Kryger MH. Sleep in restrictive lung disease. Sleep 1987; 10(5):409–418.
69. Mezon BL, West P, Israels J, Kryger M. Sleep breathing abnormalities in kyphoscoliosis. Am Rev Respir Dis 1980; 122:617–621.
70. Guilleminault C, Kurland G, Winkle R, Miles LE. Severe kyphoscoliosis, breathing, and sleep. The "Quasimodo" syndrome during sleep. Chest 1981; 79(6):626–630.
71. Hill NS, Eveloff SE, Carlisle CC, Goff SG. Efficacy of nocturnal nasal ventilation in patients with restrictive thoracic disease. Am Rev Respir Dis 1992; 145:365–371.
72. Ellis EH, Grunstein RR, Chan S, Bye PTP, Sullivan CE. Noninvasive ventilatory support during sleep improves respiratory failure in kyphoscoliosis. Chest 1988; 94:811–815.
73. Bye PTP, Ellis ER, Issa FG, Donnelly PM, Sullivan CE. Respiratory failure and sleep in neuromuscular disease. Thorax 1990; 45:241–247.
74. Guilleminault C, Cummiskey J, Motta J, Lynne-Davies P. Respiratory and hemodynamic study during wakefulness and sleep in myotonic dystrophy. Sleep 1978; 1(19):19–31.
75. Finnimore AJ, Jackson RV, Morton A, Lynch E. Sleep hypoxia in myotonic dystrophy and its correlation with awake respiratory function. Thorax 1994; 49:66–70.
76. Gilmartin JJ, Cooper BG, Griffiths CJ, et al. Breathing during sleep in patients with myotonic dystrophy and non-myotonic respiratory muscle weakness. Q J Med 1991; 78(285):21–31.
77. Cirignotta F, Mondini S, Zucconi M, et al. Sleep-related breathing impairment in myotonic dystrophy. J Neurol 1987; 235:80–85.
78. Smith PFM, Edwards RHT, Calverley PMA. Ventilation and breathing pattern during sleep in Duchenne muscular dystrophy. Chest 1989; 96:1346–1351.
79. Smith PEM, Calverley PMA, Edwards RHT. Hypoxemia during sleep in Duchenne muscular dystrophy. Am Rev Respir Dis 1988; 137:884–888.
80. Dolmage TE, Avendano MA, Goldstein RS. Respiratory function during wakefulness and sleep among survivors of respiratory and non-respiratory poliomyelitis. Eur Respir J 1992; 5:864–870.

81. Steljes DG, Kryger MH, Kirk BW, Millar TW. Sleep in postpolio syndrome. Chest 1990; 98:133–140.
82. Smith PEM, Edwards RHT, Calverley PMA. Oxygen treatment of sleep hypoxaemia in Duchenne muscular dystrophy. Thorax 1989; 44:997–1001.
83. Bach JR, Penek J. Obstructive sleep apnea complicating negative-pressure ventilatory support in patients with chronic paralytic/restrictive ventilatory dysfunction. Chest 1991; 99:1386–1393.
84. Hill NS, Redline S, Carskadon MA, Curran FJ, Millman RP. Sleep-disordered breathing in patients with Duchenne muscular dystrophy using negative pressure ventilators. Chest 1992; 102:1656–1662.

11

Intimacy and Chronic Lung Disease

SANDRA S. COLE and CAROL J. HOSSLER

University of Michigan Medical Center
Ann Arbor, Michigan

This material was originally developed by the Department of Physical Medicine and Rehabilitation at the University of Michigan Medical Center as a self-help booklet entitled *Intimacy and Chronic Lung Disease*. It was designed to teach patients about relaxation, breath control, postural drainage, percussion, and daily activities that include intimacy. It was intended to demonstrate that application of basic therapeutic techniques to sexual activities would enhance and enrich options for expression of intimacy. The booklet was designed for patients diagnosed with chronic bronchitis, emphysema, chronic obstructive pulmonary disease, and chronic obstructive lung disease.

It is important to include the patient's family when providing information and education, and this material can be particularly relevant for health care professionals as it provides a perspective of how to approach this private and intimate topic with the patient and family.

The single most important task when discussing sexuality with the patient is to desensationalize sexuality and intimacy and provide information as one would with any other activity of daily living. Education and information has proven to be more easily understood and effective when recommendations for accommodating and satisfying positions for intimacy are directly linked to already known instructions regarding energy and stress management with pulmonary disease.

To simplify discussion regarding physical exertion for sexual activity, it should be noted that basic physical therapy instructions have been explained and adapted for specific sexual activities, using familiar physical therapy procedures (i.e., side lying, sitting, head and chest elevation, use of oxygen). A small glossary of physical therapy terms is included. To facilitate discussion of important and natural sexual concerns, a brief description of the sexual response process has been included for both men and women. In addition, positively stated narrative acknowledges, in a respectful way, that the patient is, and is recognized as, a sexual person with legitimate needs for information that will be helpful in maintaining sexual happiness.

Objectives of this patient education material are to stress that:

The patient needs to be able to stay relaxed, to be in control of breathing, and to use effective relaxation and breathing techniques when necessary during intimacy.

The patient needs to be able to independently clear his/her chest of excess mucus and to be trained in postural drainage techniques during times of intimacy.

Most important, the patient and partner desire to be able to continue an active, satisfactory, and intimate life, which includes explicit sexual expression.

It has been our experience that, after having read the booklet and participated in discussion regarding the specific information, the patient (and partner) are better able to:

1. State the need and rationale for relaxation exercises, breath control exercises, postural drainage and percussion, and daily activity suggestions.
2. State potential complications and problems if these techniques are not followed.
3. Demonstrate relaxation exercises and positions, breath control techniques, postural drainage, percussion, suggestions for daily activities.
4. State how the above-mentioned techniques can be safely and positively incorporated.
5. Identify warning signs of physical difficulty and the appropriate action to be taken.

The following patient education information may be worthwhile for distribution by health care professionals to their patients.

I. Introduction*

"What is happening to my lungs? Can it be cured? I'm so short of breath I can't work anymore. I can't do my daily chores. The house is a mess. It's even an effort to bathe and dress some days. I feel so alone. I feel helpless. It's hard for me to depend on other people. I no longer feel close to or interact with my family and friends. I feel badly because my partner and I have stopped being intimate. What can I do?"

You, too, are learning to live with a chronic lung disease (asthma, chronic bronchitis, emphysema) and have probably had many of these thoughts and feelings.

The shortness of breath (whether it be mild or severe) that you may frequently experience during daily activities can be frightening for you and the people around you. The limitations caused by your breathing difficulties may affect all areas of your life, including your intimate times and sexual activity. It can affect how you feel about yourself.

This booklet will explore many topics relating to your daily health and activity. It will offer ideas and suggestions to help you make positive changes and adjustments in your life-style, feel good about yourself, and enjoy a full, meaningful life.

II. Relaxation

When you begin to experience shortness of breath and that familiar feeling of heaviness or tightness in your chest, you may feel anxious. Your entire body may react and become tense. The muscles, especially those in your upper chest, shoulders, and neck (called accessory muscles of breathing), tighten and strain with your efforts to breathe. Panic may set in. Relaxing these muscles, especially in your upper body, can help you maintain control and decrease anxiety feelings and shortness of breath.

Learning to relax is a very important step to breath control and comfort. Try to find a quiet place, away from the noise of the TV, radio, children, grandchildren, the job, etc. Loosen the clothing around your neck, upper chest, and stomach. Sit in a comfortable chair or lie on a couch or bed with your head and shoulders well supported on several pillows.

---

*The rest of this chapter is reprinted, with permission, from Hossler CJ, Cole SS: Intimacy and Chronic Lung Disease, Ann Arbor: University of Michigan, 1983.

A. Exercises

Learn to distinguish between a tense and a relaxed muscle. Make a tight fist. Feel the tenseness in your fingers, hand, and arm. Now loosen the fist and feel the muscles relax. Muscles relax best immediately after they have been tensed. The following exercises are designed to relax those tightened muscles. Repeat each exercise five times.

1. Make large, slow circles with your head, first in one direction, then in the opposite direction.
2. Shrug (or pull) your shoulders all the way up to your ears, then let go and let them drop down.
3. Pull your shoulders back (throw your chest out), then let go and let them fall forward.
4. Make a fist, straighten your arms, and push them down into the bed. Now let go and relax your whole arm.
5. Point your toes, straighten your legs, and push them down into the bed. Now let go and relax your whole leg.
6. Now just lie or sit for a few minutes and let your whole body go. Feel like a rag doll. Imagine you are on a cloud or floating in the water on a comfortable, sunny day.

If you are so relaxed that you feel drowsy and fall asleep, you are doing the relaxation exercises very well.

You should do these exercises several times, especially when you are "feeling well," so that when you do begin to feel tense, short of breath, or panicky you can automatically start relaxing and regain control.

B. Positions

There are a number of positions that you can use to become comfortable and concentrate on relaxing. You may have already discovered some of them on your own. They are nice because they allow you to be up and active and can be used anywhere without calling attention to your breathing difficulties. (See Fig. 1.)

III. Breath Control

Once you start to relax, you can begin to work on breathing skills. Don't rush. These exercises also should be slow, relaxed, and rhythmical.

Let's review the muscles of the chest and neck.

A. Muscles of Breathing

The diaphragm is a dome-shaped muscle that lies right up under your ribs and lungs. It is the main muscle of breathing. It is supposed to do about two-thirds

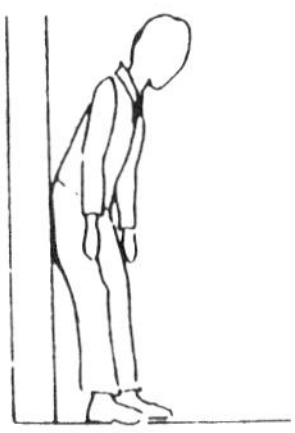

#1) With your feet twelve (12) inches away from the wall, lean against it and slump forward relaxing arms, shoulders, and neck.

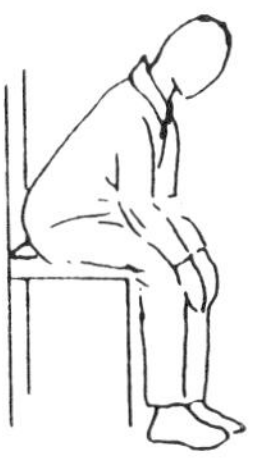

#2) Sitting in a chair, lean forward and place your elbows and forearms on your knees for support.

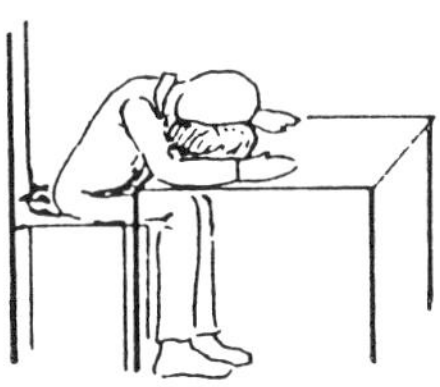

#3) Sitting in a chair, lean forward and place your elbows and forearms on the table, lay your head on your arms. Place a pillow on the table for comfort.

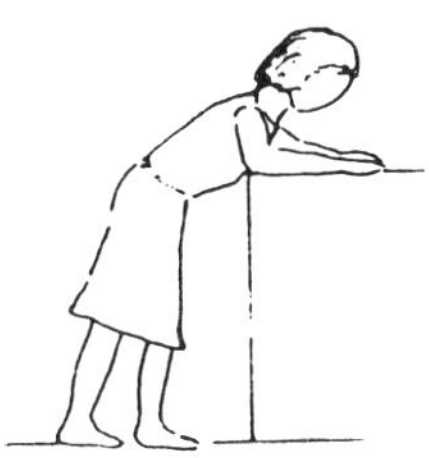

#4) Standing near a counter top, wall, bookcase or anything else of similar height, lean forward leaning on your elbows and forearms for support.

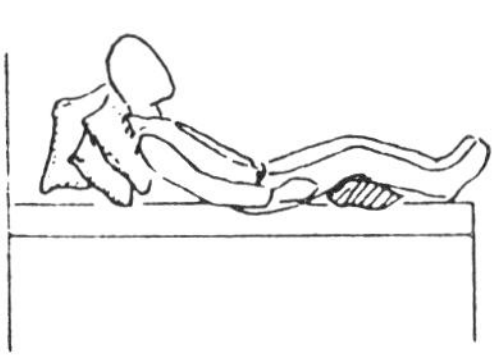

#5) Lie on your back with several pillows or cushions supporting your upper back, shoulders, neck, and head. Place a pillow under your knees for comfort.

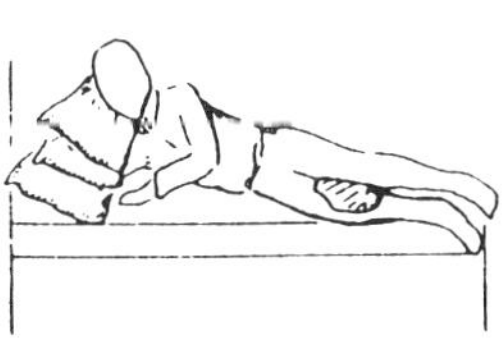

#6) Lie on your side with several pillows or cushions supporting your upper trunk, shoulders, neck and head. Place a pillow between your knees for comfort.

Figure 1 Relaxation positions.

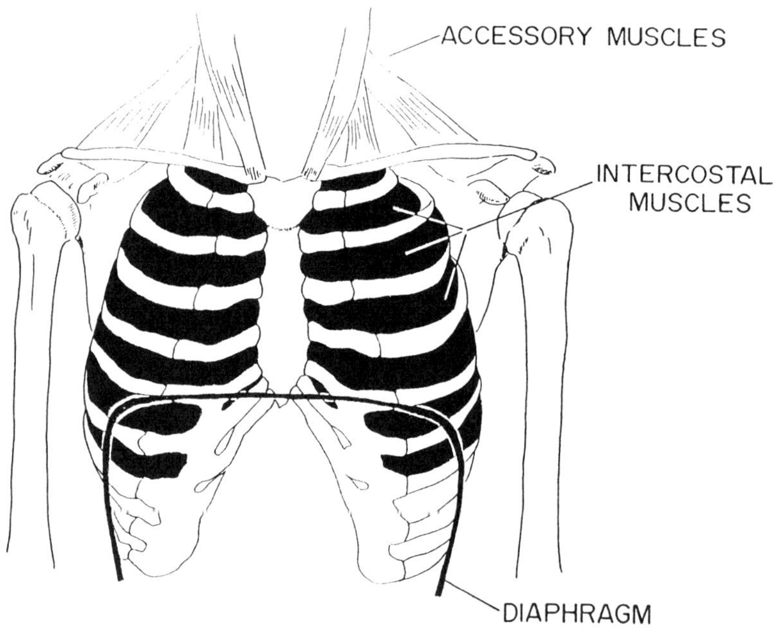

Figure 2 Muscles of respiration.

of the work. The other one-third of the work is done by the muscles (intercostal muscles) that lie between your ribs. Other muscles in the front of your neck and upper shoulders are called accessory muscles, or extra muscles of breathing. These accessory muscles tend to start to work when you become tense and short of breath. Because they are not muscles meant to be used for breathing, they are inefficient and use extra oxygen to work. (See Fig. 2.)

B. Asthma

In asthma, periodically the muscles around your larger airways, or bronchial tubes, go into spasm and clamp down so that it is hard to get air in or out. There may also be extra mucus and swelling on the inside of these airways. (See Fig. 3.)

C. Chronic Bronchitis

In chronic bronchitis the airways are irritated and sometimes infected. This causes extra mucus to be produced, which can obstruct the bronchial tubes.

D. Emphysema

In emphysema the little air sacs, called alveoli, in the lungs actually begin to break apart and the tissue supporting the airways becomes sloppy, like an old sponge. Air has a difficult time moving in or out. (See Fig. 4.)

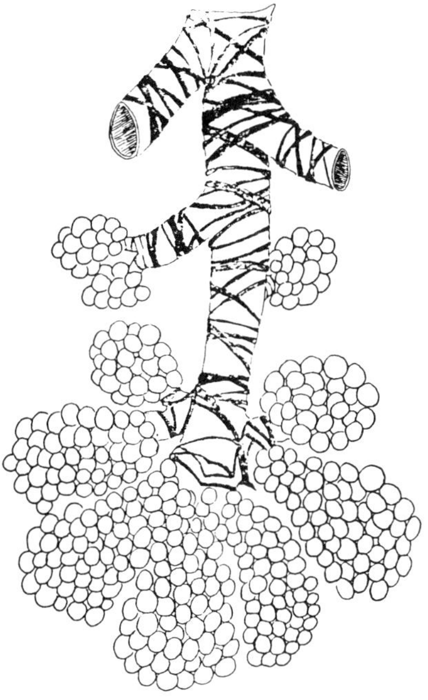

Figure 3 Asthma.

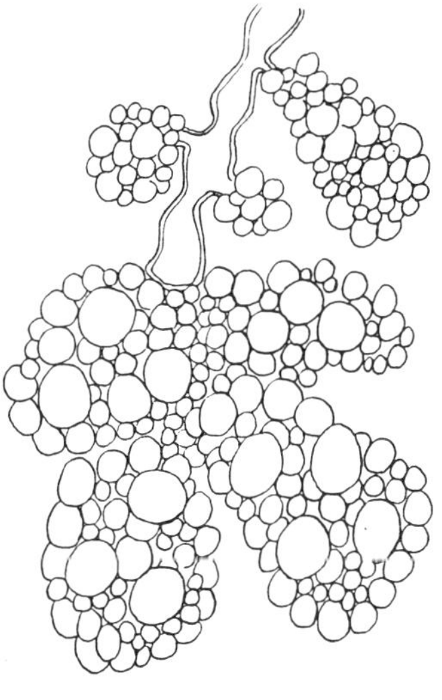

Figure 4 Emphysema.

In these diseases the same thing happens: air becomes trapped inside the lungs. Your body uses up the oxygen. Because you have difficulty getting the stale air out, there is no room to get fresh, oxygen-rich air in. Therefore, you begin to get more and more short of breath. When the lungs become full of stale air, the diaphragm is pushed down into a position where it cannot work properly. The muscles in your neck and upper chest work harder.

E. Diaphragmatic Breathing

To do effective breathing you need to breathe in through your nose and out through your mouth. Breathing in through the nose slows, cleans, warms, and humidifies the air. Your nose is the body's air conditioner. As you breathe in, the diaphragm contracts and moves down, pulling air into the lungs. As the diaphragm moves down, it pushes the stomach out. As you breathe out, the diaphragm relaxes and moves up. Air leaves your lungs through your mouth, and your stomach appears to sink in. (See Fig. 5.)

Try to breathe out for longer than your breathe in. This encourages you to empty the trapped stale air from your lungs.

The best way to find your diaphragm is to put your fingers in the "V" of your ribs and sniff once or twice. The movement you feel is the diaphragm working.

You can practice breathing with your diaphragm when sitting, standing, or lying down. Place one hand on your chest and the other hand on your stomach right below the ribs. Your chest should remain very quiet. When you are breathing in, your stomach will rise. When you breathe out, your stomach will sink in.

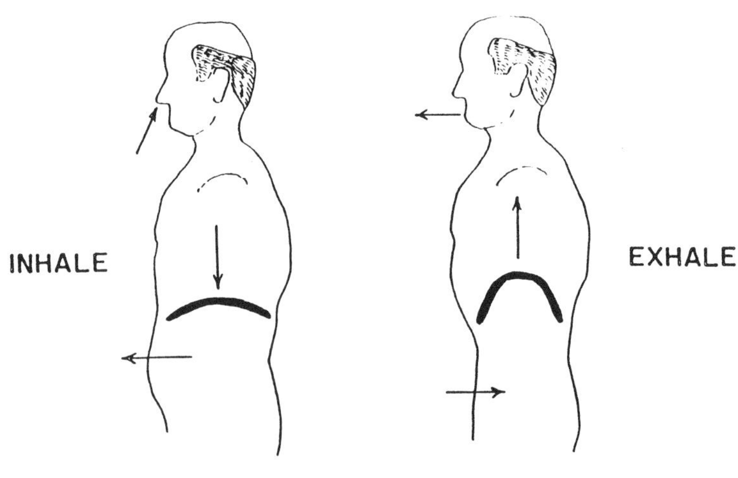

Figure 5 Diaphragmatic breathing.

F. Pursed Lips

Another skill that is helpful while you are doing the diaphragmatic breathing exercises is pursed-lip breathing. You may already be doing this on your own. It is breathing out with your lips puckered up just a little bit, as if you were going to whistle or kiss. It is *not* a hard blowing out, but a very gentle breathing out of the air. This creates just enough backpressure in your airways, helping to keep them open so that the trapped air can be exhaled. It is very important that you not blow out hard.

A good way to practice is to think about having a burning candle in front of you. When you are breathing out, the air is flowing gently from your lips just enough to make the flame of the candle bend over. It is not hard enough to blow out the flame.

Again, it is important that you practice breathing skills several times when you are "feeling well" so that when you do begin to have difficulty breathing you can automatically start to breathe correctly and regain control.

G. Effective Coughing

You may have trouble with extra mucus building up in your chest. One of the things that can help in clearing this is effective coughing. Take in two or three good, deep breaths using your diaphragm, breathing in through your nose and out through pursed lips. On the third breath, hold it for just an instant, then do two or three coughs on the *same* breath. Do not breathe between each cough.

Some people find they need support over their stomachs because these muscles have grown weak. This gives a stronger, more effective cough. You can either hold your stomach with your hands or arms or use a pillow or blanket positioned against your stomach. Do not allow yourself to go into a "fit of coughing." This wastes energy, makes you short of breath, and does not clear the thick, sticky mucus from your lungs.

H. Signs of Infection

Make sure you know the signs of infection so you can call your doctor early, hopefully preventing further illness and possible hospitalization. These signs are: increased shortness of breath and a change in your mucus—increased amount, increased thickness/stickiness, a change in color, or an odor.

IV. Daily Activity

A. Increasing Activity Levels

Now that you have learned to relax and to stay in control of your breathing, you can begin to use these skills in your daily activities. With practice you hopefully will be able to do more with less effort. It is important to pace yourself and not to work into a state of exhaustion during activity. It is also important to exercise *every* day, increasing your effort a little each day. With time and *consistent* practice, your tolerance and endurance will gradually increase. Don't be discouraged if your progress seems slow. Keeping a daily log of your activity will help you to see the progress you really are making.

It is important to recognize that when you start slowly increasing your activity level, you will at first be a little more short of breath. This is normal. The feeling will gradually go away as your body adjusts to working harder.

You can stay in control of your breathing by using a technique called paced activity.

Continue the breathing skills you have just learned. Use your diaphragm. Breathe in through your nose (for a count of two) and out through pursed lips (for a count of four). During activity, the idea is to rest while breathing in, work while breathing out.

B. Walking

Walking is an excellent exercise for your body. It increases your mobility and endurance and strengthens all of your muscles, your heart, and your lungs. It is an activity you can do anywhere, anytime, during your day. The weather (high humidity, high temperatures, rain/snow, pollution, high pollen counts) should not be a reason to skip your daily exercise program. Stores and shopping malls are great places to go. The air is conditioned, there are long areas in which to walk, and there are places to rest and people to watch.

To stay in control of your breathing, follow the "2–4" pattern. Walk two steps while breathing in for a count of two. Walk four steps while breathing out for a count of four. This will seem very mechanical at first. With practice it quickly will become a habit.

Don't expect to cover a great distance on your first walk. Set small goals each day—15 steps today, 20 tomorrow, half a block next week. Or, increase how fast or how long you walk. Over a period of time you'll be able to see the gradual improvement you've made.

C. Stairs

Stairs are a frequently encountered problem. The 2–4 breathing pattern also works well here.

There are two ways to approach this problem:

1. Stop and rest while breathing in for a count of two, slowly walk up four stairs while breathing out for a count of four.
2. Slowly walk up two stairs while breathing in for a count of two,

continue walking up another four stairs while breathing out for a count of four.

Place each foot firmly and flatly on each stair. Remember to use your diaphragm, breathing in through your nose and out through pursed lips.

D. Paced Activity

When doing any activity that is particularly difficult for you, using the 2–4 breathing pattern will help you stay in control and do the job much more easily. It is important not to hold your breath while making an effort to work. Rest and breathe in, work and breathe out.

Such activities could include shaving, bathing, combing your hair, dressing, reaching for things in cupboards/closets/on high shelves, housework, laundry, shopping, yardwork, work on the job, social outings, intimate times, and love making.

E. Energy Conservation

A few more suggestions about your daily activities may be helpful.

Think seriously about all the tasks that need to be accomplished. Do they all *need* to be done? Can someone else help out with a few? Can those tasks you feel need to be done be spaced out over the days of the week, perhaps completing one big task a day?

Plan to do your big chores after a period of rest and/or after you've taken your medication and/or breathing treatments. You will then have a higher energy level and be able to breathe more freely.

Many people with lung disease think, "If I do this quickly I won't get so short of breath." As you've discovered, it doesn't work. Plan to do the activity slowly and deliberately, using your newly learned breathing skills.

V. Helpful Hints

In addition to using relaxation exercises, breathing exercises, and paced activity, you can do a number of other things to help keep yourself as healthy as possible and feeling good.

A. Diet

When you are short of breath, it is sometimes difficult to eat and swallow. You may not eat at all. You may choose foods that are easy to fix and easy to eat, but that do not provide your body with all the nutrients it needs.

Try spacing your eating throughout the day, eating three small meals and two or three snacks. Choose foods from all four food groups—meats, dairy products, fruits and vegetables, grains. Eating several small, well-balanced meals and snacks instead of three large, regular meals keeps your stomach from being distended. Your stomach sits right up under your diaphragm and lungs. It is possible that when the stomach is very full, it pushes up under your diaphragm, making it hard to breathe.

B. Medication

Remember to take your medication in the correct amount, at the correct time. Take breathing treatments if that is a part of your care at home.

C. Fluids

Unless otherwise instructed by your doctor, drink plenty of fluids. This helps to keep the mucus thinned so that you can more easily cough it out.

D. Smoking

Above all, try to stop smoking. Smoking only causes further irritation to lung tissue and makes it hard for your blood to pick up the oxygen your body needs.

VI. Feelings

Your emotional needs, how you feel about yourself, and how other people around you are feeling are as important to adjusting to chronic lung disease as is your physical activity.

There are *many* feelings you may experience as you make adjustments to your lung disease—fear of becoming more and more short of breath as your disease progresses; anger that it happened to you; anger at others around you who don't understand or don't pay enough attention; frustration that you can't do what you used to do; worry over your financial situation; helpless because you've had to become dependent on others; sad and lonely because you feel isolated from your friends; depressed because there is nothing meaningful in your life anymore—and no matter how well you take care of yourself, there are still bad days. What's the use? Even thoughts about death are not easy to deal with.

Your family and friends may also experience many of these feelings—fear because they see you struggling to breathe; helpless because they don't understand and don't know how to help you; anger because they, too, must make changes in their life-style; worry about financial future; sad and depressed because they, too, miss the meaningful interactions and full life you used to have.

Having a close, meaningful relationship is to be able to trust one another and feel comfortable enough to talk honestly and openly.

Try to put into words how you are feeling and, in turn, try hard to listen to how the other person is feeling, too. You could start by simply saying, "I feel ———."

VII. Intimacy

Your physical limitations and your emotional health can greatly affect your sexual feelings. As important as these positive feelings are, this aspect of our lives is frequently ignored during illness. Because it is a very personal, private part of our relationship with another, and because of the way many of us have been raised, it is an area many of us cannot easily talk about.

Satisfying sexual activity adds to feeling good emotionally and physically about ourselves and our bodies.

The need for intimacy is an important part of our emotional makeup. It is important to be close to someone, to care for and be cared for, to share, to give and receive pleasure and fulfillment—particularly if we are in a close relationship with another person. Intimacy is an important part of us whether we are young or old, healthy or ill, alone or involved with another person.

One aspect of intimacy is the ability to physically express ourselves during intimate times. Because your lung disease has affected many of your daily activities, it has probably also affected this personal, yet very important, part of your life.

As you adjust other daily living habits, it may be useful to consider altering some of the familiar ways you and your partner have enjoyed sexual activity.

This section helps you focus on concerns you may be having regarding intimacy and physical limitations. It offers suggestions to help make this important part of your life more fulfilling.

Sexual activity among the "older generation" is frequently a source of jokes, bewilderment, or even disgust among the so-called "young, healthy, beautiful generation." It is often such negative societal attitudes that prevent older persons from being intimate and sexually fulfilled. Frequently, people simply feel guilty about natural sexual feelings.

It will be important for you to carefully consider and evaluate your sexual needs and limitations. Many sexual activities may be important to you or to you and your partner in expressing intimacy: closeness/cuddling, caressing/touching, foreplay, masturbation/manual stimulation of your partner, oral/genital sex, intercourse.

Are you now enjoying any of these activities? How satisfying or enjoyable are they to you and to your partner? How much are you limited in your sexual activities because of your lung disease? What alternate solutions to these limitations have you found enjoyable? How satisfactory are these adjustments? Do any of these adjustments cause concerns? How much distress do you experience when you have an orgasm? Have you quietly stopped activity and closeness altogether? What feelings or concerns does your partner express about your mutual sexual activities? How often do you and your partner discuss your mutual needs and concerns?

It is important to have a good understanding of your own body as well as your partner's body to fully enjoy and make the most of your intimate times.

The following is a brief description of normal male and female anatomy, how the genitals respond to stimulation, and what changes occur as a natural result of aging.

A. Female Anatomy and Sexual Response

In the *female* during stimulation, the labia change in color to darker shades of red and purple. They become moist and swell, slightly exposing the vaginal opening.

The clitoris also swells and becomes more prominent. It is very rich in nerve endings and becomes very sensitive when gently stroked or rubbed.

The walls of the vagina are muscular and wrinkled. With stimulation they quickly produce moisture/lubrication and the vagina becomes larger. (See Fig. 6.)

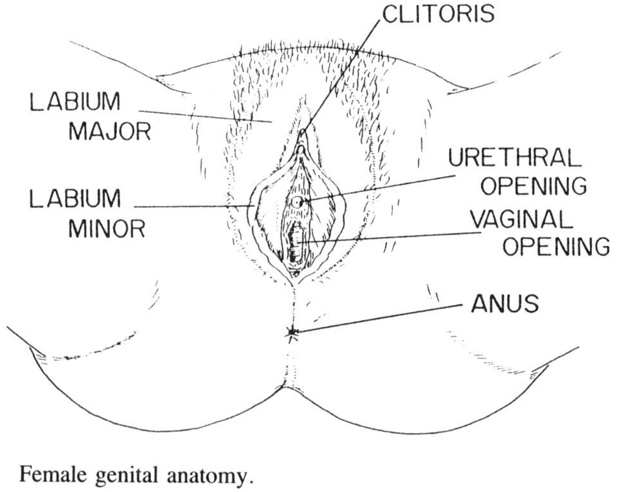

Figure 6 Female genital anatomy.

B. Male Anatomy and Sexual Response

In the *male* during stimulation, the penis quickly becomes firm and erect and the scrotum draws up closer to the body.

The head of the penis, called the glans, is also very rich in nerve endings and becomes very sensitive when stroked. It is especially pleasurable when stroked on the underside.

A clear fluid may be seen seeping from the urethral opening. (See Fig. 7.)

In both men and women, orgasm is characterized by intense, highly pleasurable muscular contractions in the genital area. The overall response of the body is to slightly increase heart rate, respiratory rate, and blood pressure. This increase is about the same as that seen when climbing a flight of stairs. This increase quickly returns to normal levels after sexual tension has been released.

C. Myths

There are many myths surrounding male and female sexuality.

It is a myth that once a woman has had a hysterectomy she is no longer a woman, is not interested in sex, or is not able to have sex any more. Many

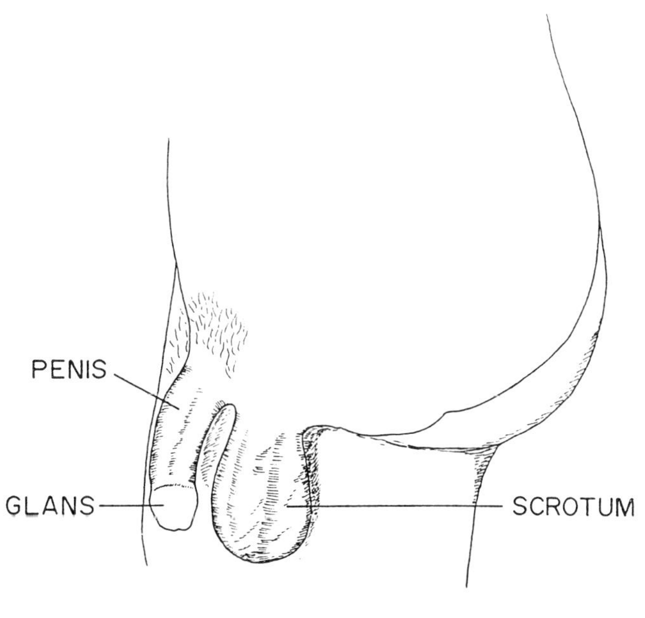

Figure 7 Male genital anatomy.

women who have had a hysterectomy desire, can, and do continue to have pleasurable sexual intercourse. Because the ovaries do secrete the female hormones and may have been removed during the hysterectomy, there may be some drying of the vaginal area. A water soluble lubricant such as K-Y Jelly or hormone creams prescribed by a doctor can be used to make intercourse more comfortable. Vaseline should not be used as a lubrication because it may accumulate bacteria and it does not dissolve.

Another myth is that the size of the woman's vagina determines what size penis can be inserted. In reality, the walls of the vagina stretch, expand, and lubricate with stimulation, thereby accommodating and molding themselves to the size of the penis.

One other myth is that a woman can achieve an orgasm only by stimulation of a penis in her vagina. A woman has many sensitive areas on her body. With adequate stimulation she can achieve orgasm in several different and pleasurable ways, such as stimulating the breast, rubbing the clitoris with fingers, or stimulating with a vibrator.

There are many myths concerning men and the penis: the size of the penis can be judged by the size of a man's hands or feet, the penis must be large to satisfy a woman, he must have an erection to experience orgasm, he must ejaculate to experience orgasm, a man "knows" how to give a woman an orgasm.

D. Aging

It is important to recognize that aging factors in general, the diseases common to bodies growing older, and specifically your lung condition (often found in older people) do not decrease your ability or capacity to enjoy intimate times. These factors may only alter the style, frequency, or intensity of the experience, just as your daily activities in general have been affected.

The normal process of aging does affect your genitals and your sexual response to stimulation.

The ovaries of women who have reached menopause stop producing female hormones. The vaginal walls become thin and are not as elastic. There is less moisture/lubrication. This may cause painful intercourse but can be relieved by using a water-soluble lubrication jelly such as K-Y Jelly. The intensity of orgasm may be less. Some women experience irritability, depression, and/or aggressive behavior; they may or may not have decreased sexual desire.

Men may need more intense and longer stimulation to achieve an erection. The erection will not be as firm and may come and go. There is a decrease in the frequency and intensity of orgasms; the amount of time before another ejaculation is possible is much longer.

For many people, intercourse with orgasm is one of the many ways to enjoy physical sex. A few years ago, in our society, attitudes toward sex suggested that intercourse with orgasm was the only "acceptable" physical activity between partners. Today, societal attitudes toward "acceptable" sexual expression are greatly expanded and include many more options. There is much less emphasis on what is sexually "normal" or "abnormal."

Many options are available to you for expression and fulfilling the need for sexual closeness other than actual intercourse. Some of these might be: cuddling/holding, touching/caressing, foreplay, manual stimulation/masturbation, and oral/genital sex.

A healthy definition of sexual expression between two people could be described as whatever is pleasurable, satisfying, not physically or psychologically harmful or uncomfortable, and mutually desirable.

Exploring new ways to be close can begin during the time you spend practicing your relaxation and breathing exercises. Take advantage of these times to be together. Special things like quiet music, candles, poetry reading, gentle massage, and an unhurried pace can all add to your intimate moods.

Intimate time can mean just being close to each other's body. Lying in one of the previously mentioned relaxation positions that allows for maximum support, relaxation, and breath control will enable you to comfortably hold and touch each other. Talking with your partner about what you are feeling and what you like and dislike is helpful and can reduce anxiety. Many people enjoy becoming aroused and feeling close just as much as they enjoy direct physical union. Arousal in itself can be very pleasurable and satisfying; it need not be just a preliminary to intercourse. Many people don't take enough time to discover the richness of sexual arousal because they are focusing on intercourse and orgasm.

E. Options

Intimacy Without Intercourse

The partner experiencing breathing difficulty can enjoy giving pleasure in love play by lying close to his/her partner, relaxing in a side-lying position, physically quiet, controlling the breathing pattern, while caressing his/her partner's body. The person with lung disease can also receive pleasure and genital caressing in this same position or by lying on his/her back supported on several pillows.

Self-Stimulation or Masturbation

Many people enjoy caressing and stimulating their own genitals as a natural part of their own sexual expression, whether or not they have a sexual partner, or whether or not their partner wants to be sexually close at that particular moment of desire. Men and women have the ability to satisfy their own strong and natural biological/emotional sexual desires by masturbating—touching, rubbing, or stroking one's own genitals in a rhythmical way that is pleasurable. It is also natural to have an orgasm during masturbation if it is desired. Many people enjoy masturbation using their own fingers and hands, as well as using battery-powered or electric vibrator stimulators. These aids are sold in most department stores where massagers are sold.

Throughout history there have been many untrue myths surrounding masturbation—it causes insanity, stunted growth, hair on the palms of the hands, bad complexions. It is medically not true that excessive masturbation will cause physical weakness. Nor is it true that masturbation is limited to any particular age group, sex, or population. Contrary to some beliefs, masturbation is experienced and enjoyed by almost all men and women at some point in their life spans, frequently on a regular basis.

Oral/Genital Stimulation

For many people, caressing a partner's genitals with their mouths by kissing/licking/sucking/gently biting is described as sensuous and enjoyable. It is another form of sexual expression that can be experienced in a relaxed position requiring little physical activity of either partner. However, the partner with breathing difficulty might have more difficulty giving mouth genital pleasure because of the need to maintain breath control, which requires breathing in through the nose and out through pursed lips. In such a situation, the person with the breathing difficulty can caress his/her partner with a hand while experiencing mouth caressing from him/her.

Sexual Intercourse

If you and your partner desire to have intercourse, Figures 8–18 suggest how to use your relaxation positions advantageously to make sexual activity more comfortable for you. You may find some more comfortable or preferable than others. Perhaps you may find new positions and techniques that work better for you. What is important is for you to remain relaxed and in control of your breathing as you continue to enjoy your intimate times. Many couples find it useful to have a special word or signal indicating that activity needs to slow or stop for a moment so that breathing distress can be controlled. This is much better than stopping or totally avoiding activity with no explanation.

It is not essential to have an orgasm with intercourse, even if it has been customary for you. Intercourse is enjoyable by itself, and for some as satisfying without the building pressure of orgasm.

Sharing pleasure and closeness with each other are important in any relationship no matter how severe the disabling disease of one partner may be.

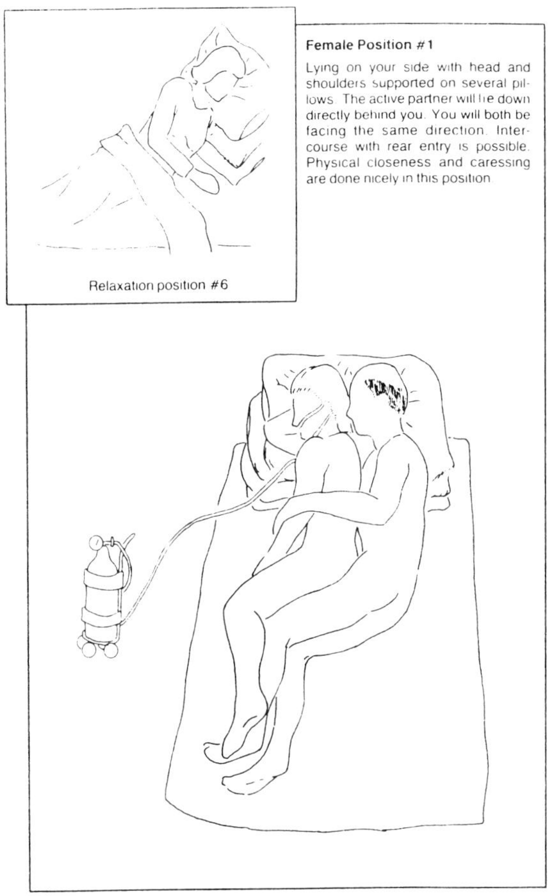

Figure 8 Suggested position for sexual intimacy.

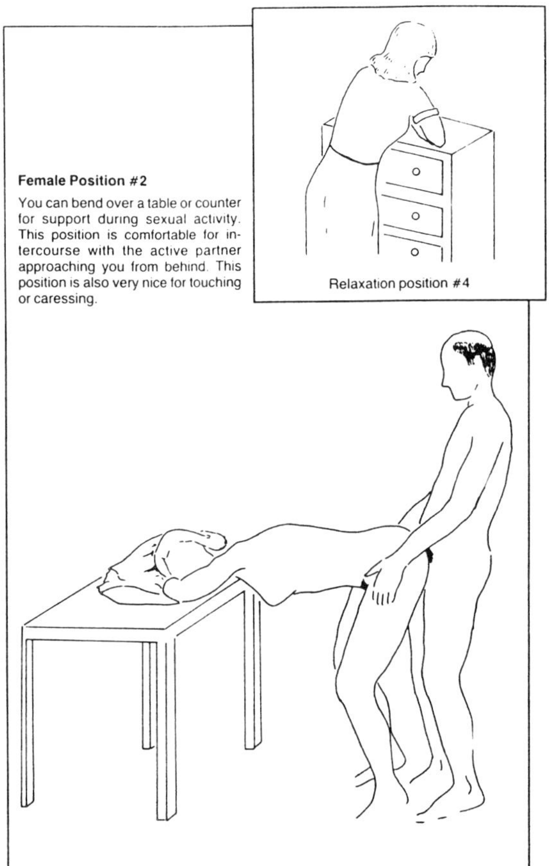

Figure 9 Suggested position for sexual intimacy.

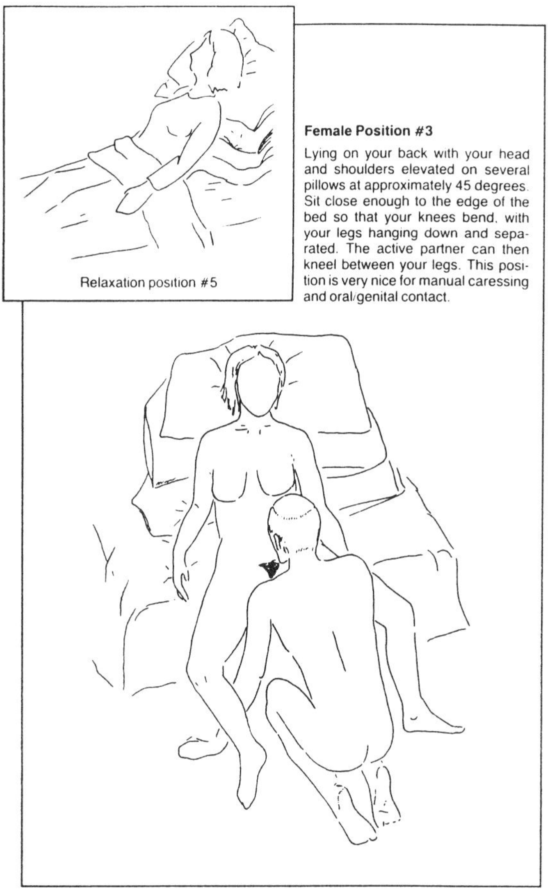

Figure 10 Suggested position for sexual intimacy.

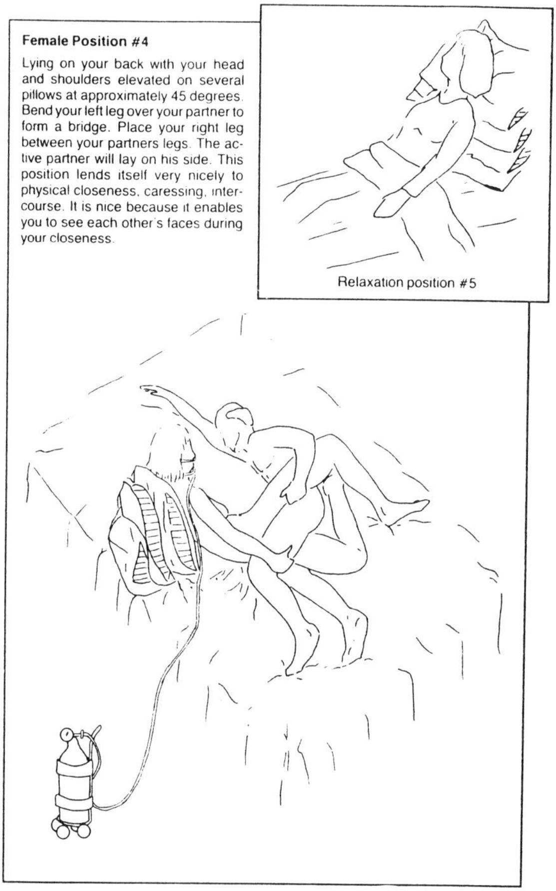

Figure 11 Suggested position for sexual intimacy.

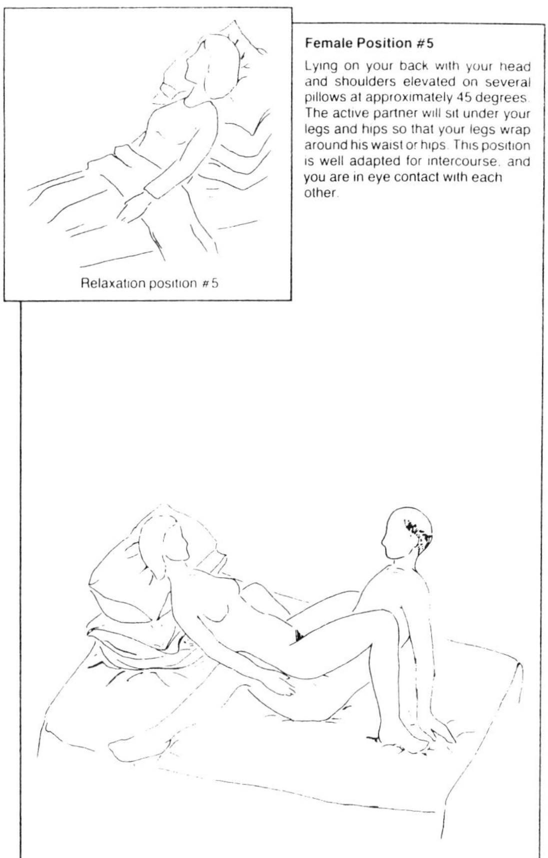

Figure 12 Suggested position for sexual intimacy.

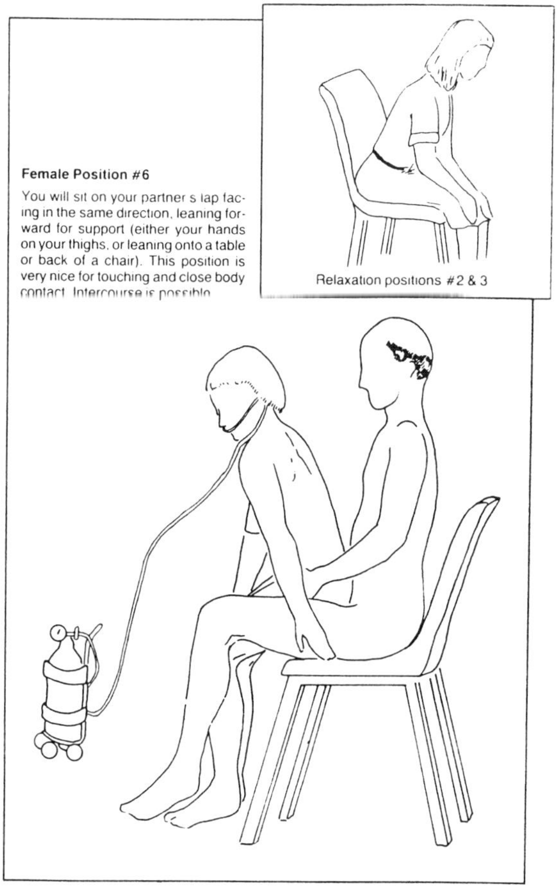

Figure 13 Suggested position for sexual intimacy.

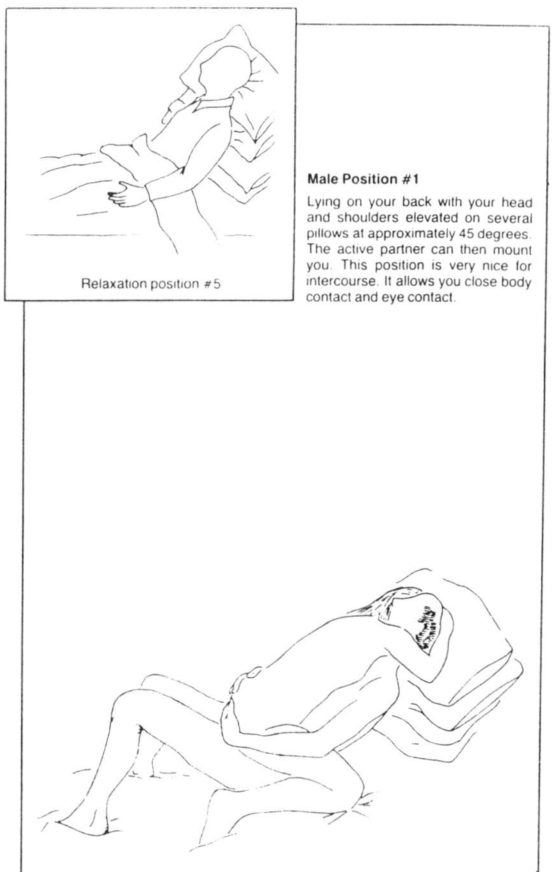

Figure 14 Suggested position for sexual intimacy.

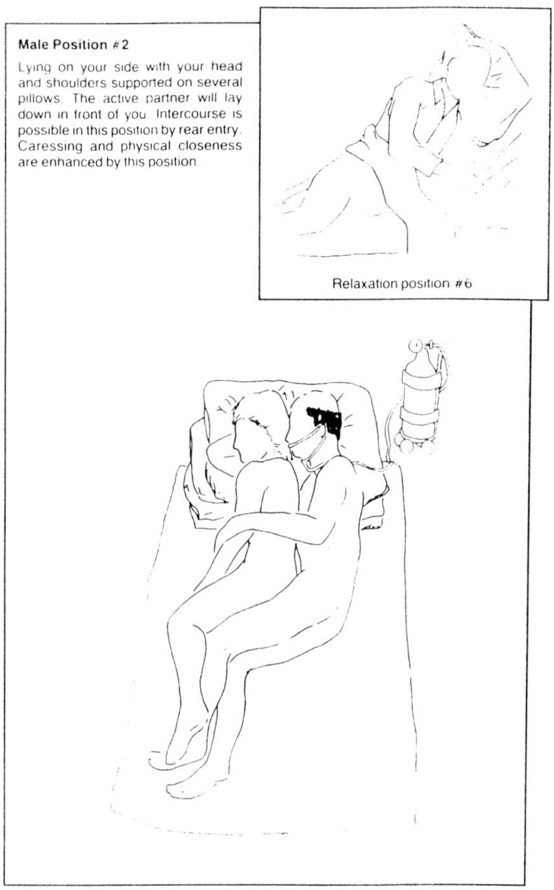

Figure 15 Suggested position for sexual intimacy.

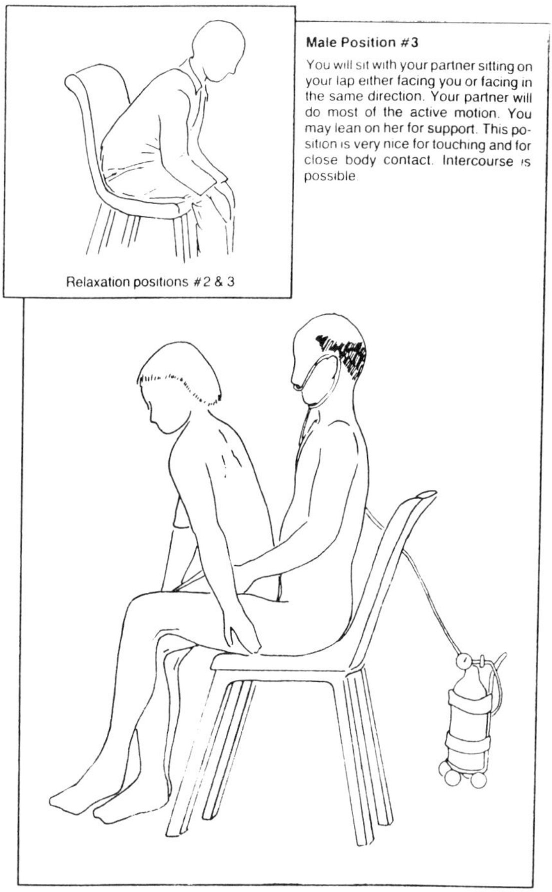

Figure 16 Suggested position for sexual intimacy.

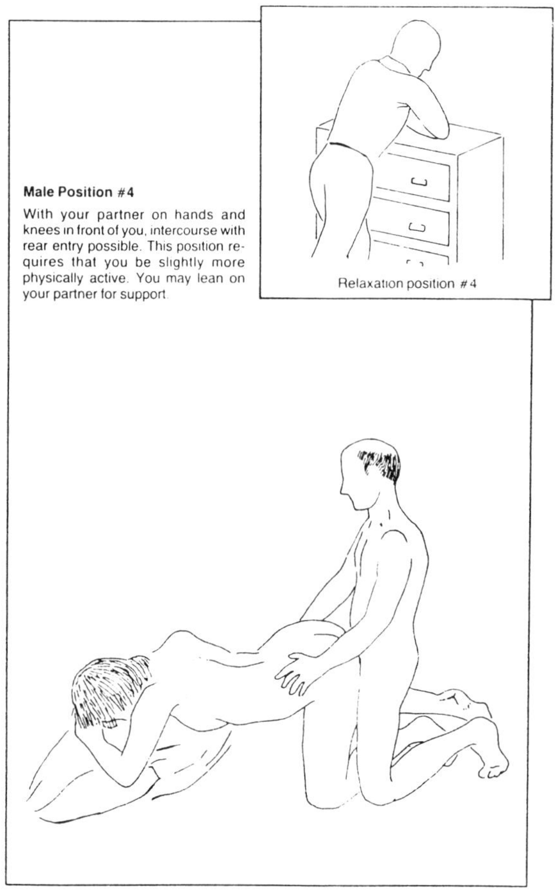

Figure 17 Suggested position for sexual intimacy.

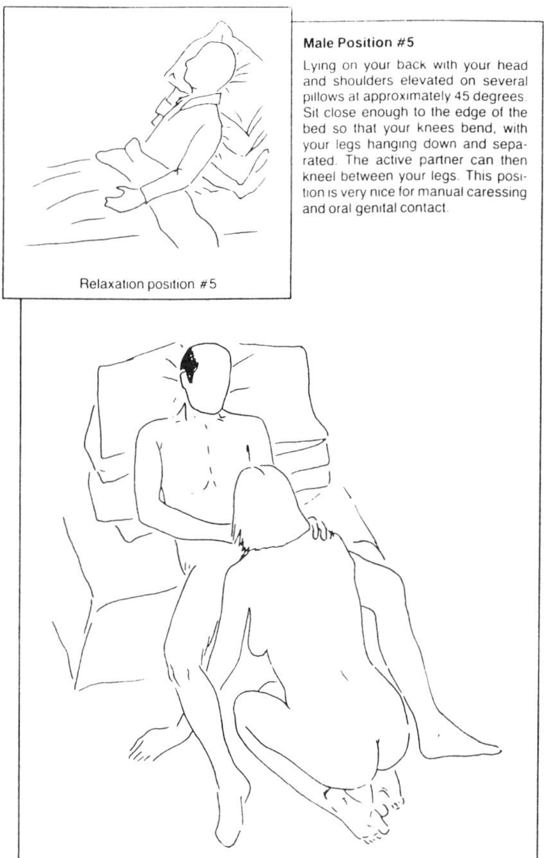

Figure 18 Suggested position for sexual intimacy.

When one partner feels he/she gives more intimacies than are received, it is possible for that partner to feel left out or overlooked. This can easily lead to a loss of interest. This is true of all relationships and is especially important to consider when disease or illness is present and activity may be limited. Lying close to each other, holding each other, and remembering past sexual experiences can make personal times emotionally fulfilling and intimate. Extra patience, care, gentleness, and time are important when you think, explore, and practice old and new ways of being intimate that are most pleasurable and satisfying to you and your partner.

VIII. Summary

As you have read through this booklet, you have been given a lot of material, ideas, and suggestions. If you use all of the things we have presented, you should be able to continue living a relatively active, meaningful, fulfilling life, and do the things that are important to you.

We have reached out to you, sharing what we know to help you understand what is happening to you and showing you ways to be in control of your symptoms. This, in turn, will let you reach out to those people who are important to you. It will help you feel good about yourself and be in control of your disease, instead of the other way around.

To help you pull together all that we have presented, here is a summary list:

Relaxation—exercises and positions
Breath control—muscles of breathing and your disease, diaphragmatic and pursed-lips breathing, effective coughing, and signs of infection
Daily activity—increasing your activity level, walking and stairs, paced activity, and energy conservation
Helpful hints—diet, medication, fluids, smoking
Feelings
Intimacy—anatomy and response, myths, aging, options, intercourse, and suggested positions

Appendix: Postural Drainage

An important factor in your daily regimen may be bronchial or postural drainage. If you are having difficulty removing large amounts of sticky mucus from your lungs, this will be of great help to you.

When mucus becomes thick, it plugs up the smaller airways (bronchial tubes), makes breathing difficult, and makes you susceptible to infections. Postural drainage uses the principles of positioning and gravity to help move mucus out of the respiratory tree. It is a physical means of moving the mucus to a point where coughing can more easily remove it. It is usually most beneficial if done when you get up in the morning (to remove all the secretions that have collected during the night) and at bedtime (so that your sleep will be more comfortable and undisturbed by coughing spells). You can, of course, do it more often during the day if your secretions increase in amount or become harder to get up. You should never do postural drainage directly after a meal, but should wait at least 1 hr.

The positions used for postural drainage are based on the anatomy of the lung. The lungs are not just two big bags of air. They are made up of several small sections (like a cluster of grapes), and each section drains in a different position (see Fig. 19).

You may have had postural drainage if you were in the hospital and you know that it was done with the help of your hospital bed. At home, several pillows, sofa cushions, or a stack of newspapers or magazines 12 in. high, tied securely together, with a pilow on top for comfort, will work just as well.

Try to make this treatment a pleasant part of your day. You should wear loose, cool clothing and make yourself comfortable. You should use the positions suggested by your doctor or therapist in a relaxed, unhurried manner.

For this treatment to be effective, you should stay in each position you use for approximately 10 min; during that time you should work on your breathing exercises. These exercises help to "milk" the airways and get the

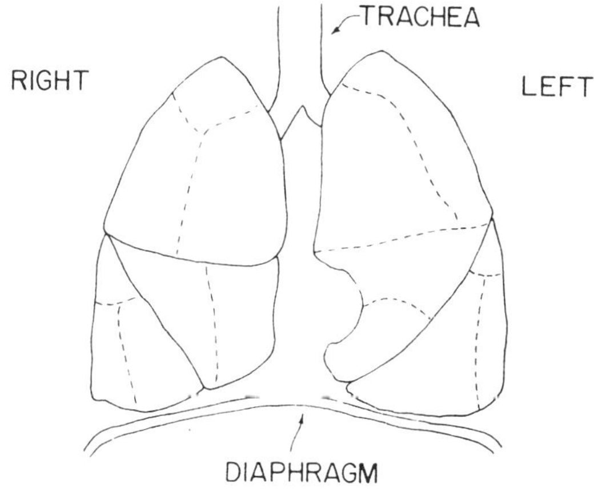

Figure 19 Anatomy of the lung.

mucus moving faster. When finished with your treatment, sit to cough as described earlier in this manual.

If you have *chronic bronchitis* or *emphysema,* the following postural drainage positions have been found helpful in clearing excess mucus from your lungs. You should place your hips on a pile of pillows or papers and: (1) lie on your right side to drain the lower parts of the left lung, (2) lie on your stomach to drain the back parts of both lungs, and (3) lie on your left side to drain the lower parts of the right lung.

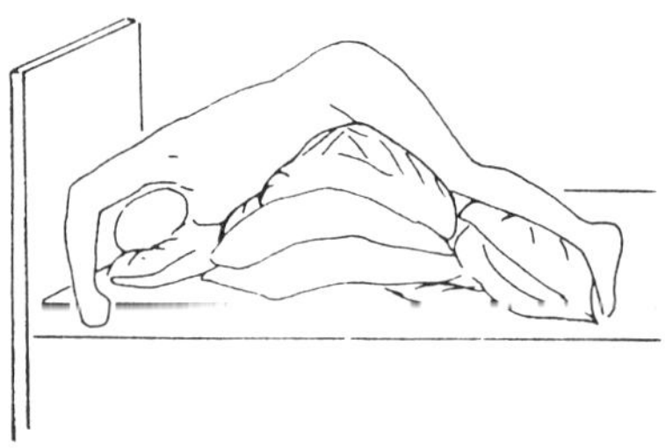

1. lie on your right side to drain the lower parts of the left lung

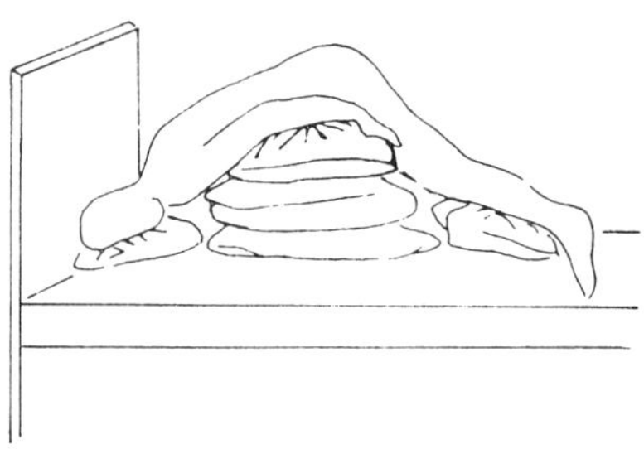

2. lie on your stomach to drain the back parts of both lungs

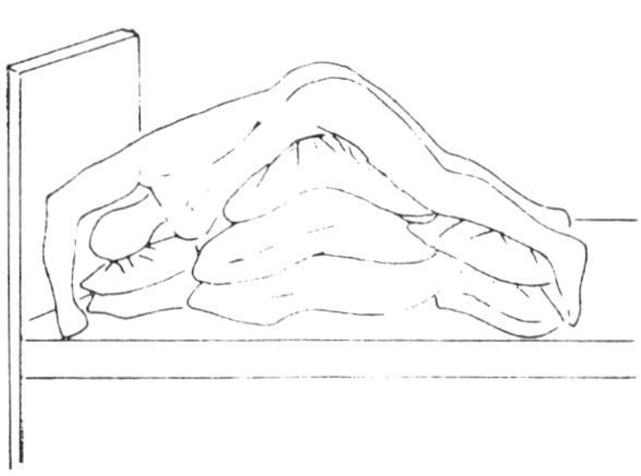

3. lie on your left side to drain the lower parts of the right lung

(a)

Figure 20 (a) Postural drainage positions in emphysema. (b) Postural drainage positions in asthma. (c) Cupped hand for percussion.

1. sit leaning forward about 45 degrees holding a pillow in front of you for comfort, to drain the top backs of your lungs

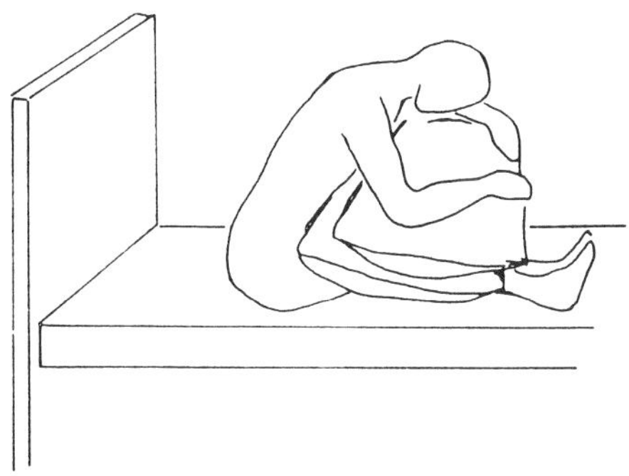

2. sit leaning backward about 45 degrees supported on pillows to drain the top fronts of your lungs

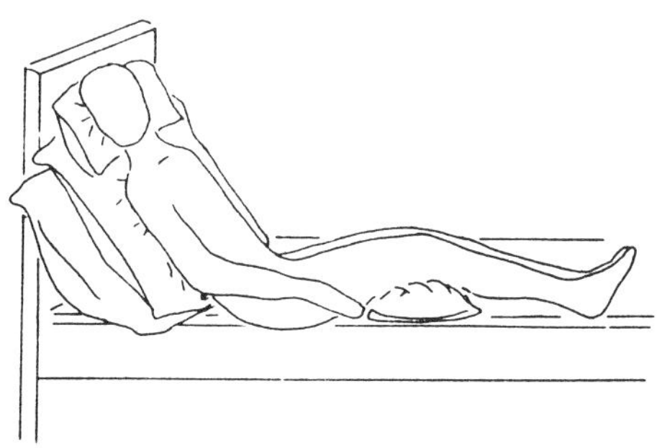

3. lie flat on your back to drain the front parts of your lungs.

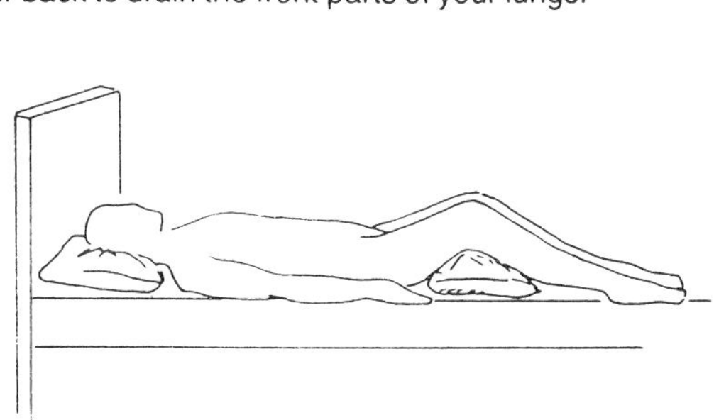

(b)

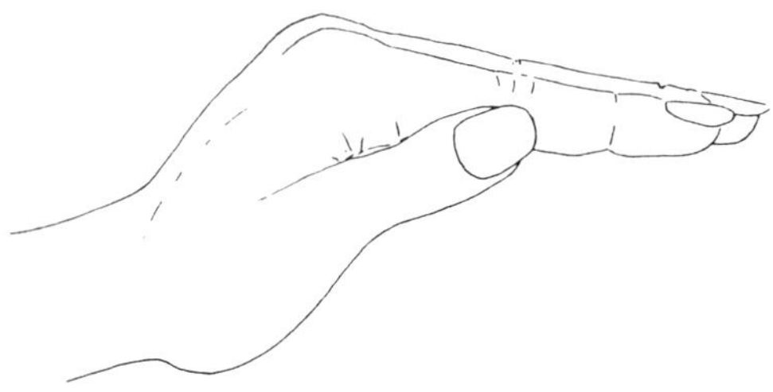

(c)

Figure 20 (Continued)

If you have *asthma,* the following postural drainage positions have been found helpful in clearing excess mucus from your lungs. You should: (1) sit leaning forward about 45 degrees holding a pillow in front of you for comfort, to drain the top backs of your lungs, (2) sit leaning backward about 45 degrees supported on pillows to drain the top fronts of your lungs, and (3) lie flat on your back to drain the front parts of your lungs.

Another method of moving sticky, sluggish mucus is by doing percussion. You may need the help of someone else during this treatment, or in some cases you can do it yourself. To be effective you should percuss for at least 3–5 min in each drainage position that you use, remembering to also do your breathing exercises.

Percussion is clapping on the chest wall with a cupped hand (see Fig. 20c). The hand should not be flat, as if slapping, or fisted, as if for hitting. The cupped hand traps air under it as it moves toward the chest and it is that air cushion, and the clap on the chest wall, that vibrates your airways, dislodges mucus, and helps to move it from the smaller airways in the outer parts of your lungs into the larger airways so that you can cough it out. You should never do percussion on bare skin. The person receiving the treatment should be wearing a shirt, blouse, or pajamas or have a sheet covering the area. Percussion should always be comfortable. It should never be done over delicate areas such as the spine, breastbone, or breasts. The longer you are percussed, the more effective it is. At first the person doing the percussion will tire easily. But with practice, endurance will build up quickly. After each position and at the end of the treatment you should sit and do some effective coughing as discussed earlier in this manual.

Do not be discouraged if your cough is not immediately productive. Although the mucus may have been moved up into the larger airways, it may take up to an hour to arrive at a point where it can be coughed up. Make it a point to always look at your mucus for amount, thickness, and color. If these change, call your doctor.

Glossary

Accessory Muscles of Breathing—extra muscles in the upper chest, shoulders, and neck used for breathing during episodes of shortness of breath.

Airways—bronchial tubes.

Bronchodilator—medication taken by mouth or inhaled that helps to open up airways.

Chronic Lung Disease—conditions of the lung that cannot yet be cured, i.e., asthma, chronic bronchitis, emphysema.

Climax—orgasm, part of sexual response cycle, characterized by highly pleasurable rhythmical contractions of the muscles in and around the genital tissues of both men and women.

Clitoris—highly sensitive tissue of the female external genital anatomy, equivalent to the head of the male penis.

Diaphragm—dome-shaped muscle located between the chest (heart and lungs) and the abdominal cavity, used for 65% of the work of breathing.

Ejaculation—spurting of semen from the penis by rhythmical, muscular contractions.

Erection—firm, hard penis.

Exhale—breathe out.

External Genitals—those sexual organs located outside the body, i.e., breast, clitoris, labia, penis, scrotum.

Foreplay—that sexual closeness occurring by itself, or prior to more active sexual activity, holding, touching, caressing, kissing, etc.

Genitals—sexual organs of male and female.

Hysterectomy—removal of part or all of the female internal genital organs.

Inhale—breathe in.

Intercourse—coitus, act of placing penis into vagina.

Internal Genitals—those genital organs inside the body, i.e., ovaries, uterus, vagina, prostate gland, testes.

Labia Majora—large outer lips of the female external genital anatomy, containing fatty tissue and covered by pubic hair.

Labia Minora—smaller, hairless inner lips of the female external genital anatomy, protected by the labia majora.

Manual Stimulation—the act of touching the genitals in a pleasurable way with the hands.

Masturbation—the act of touching, rubbing, stroking one's own genitals in a pleasurable way with the hands, vibrators, or stimulators.

Oral/Genital Stimulation—the act of placing the mouth on a partner's genitals to kiss/lick/suck/gently bite.

Orgasm—climax, part of the sexual response cycle characterized by pleasurable rhythmical contractions of the muscles in and around the genital tissues of both men and women.

Ovaries—part of the internal female genital anatomy, produce eggs and female hormones.

Ovum—egg, female cell, counterpart of the male sperm.

Penis—part of the male external genital anatomy.

Prostate Gland—part of the male internal genital anatomy, secretes fluid to produce semen.

Pursed-Lips Breathing—the act of puckering the lips as if to kiss or whistle and exhaling through them gently in an effort to keep collapsing airways open.

Respiratory Distress—increased difficulty breathing.

Scrotum—part of the male external genital anatomy, containing the testes.

Semen—the fluid containing sperm that is ejaculated during orgasm in the male.

Sperm—the male tadpole-like cell.

Testes—part of the male internal genital anatomy that produce the sperm.

Urethra—the tube through which urine passes from the bladder to the outside of the body.

Uterus—part of the female internal genital anatomy, small, pear-shaped organ 2½ in. long, the womb.

Vagina—part of the female body that connects the internal and external genital system, the birth canal, entrance for sperm.

Vulva—the whole area of the female external genitals containing the labia majora, labia minora, clitoris, urethra, and the vaginal opening.

Bibliography

Allgeier ER, Allgeier AR. Sexual Interactions, 4th ed. Lexington, MA: DC Heath, 1995.

Boggs J. Living and Loving with Arthritis: Information on Sex and Arthritis. Honolulu: Arthritis Center of Hawaii, 1978.

Brecher EM, and the Editors of Consumer Report Books. Love, Sex, and Aging. Boston: Little, Brown, 1984.

Burnside IM, ed. Sexuality and Aging. Los Angeles: Ethel Percy Andrus Gerontology Center, University of South California, 1975.

Cole TM, Glass DD. Sexuality and physical disabilities. Arch Phys Med Rehabil 1977; 58:585, 586.

Comfort A, ed. The Joy of Sex: A Gourmet Guide to Lovemaking. New York: Simon & Schuster, 1972.

Haas A, Pineda H, Haas F, Axen K. Pulmonary Therapy and Rehabilitation: Principles and Practice. Baltimore: Williams & Wilkins, 1979.

Hodgkin JE, Zorn EG, Connors L, eds. Pulmonary Rehabilitation: Guidelines to Success. Stoneham, MA: Butterworth, 1984.
Kaplan HS. The New Sex Therapy. New York: Brunner/Mazel, 1974.
Kaplan HS. The New Sex Therapy—Disorders of Sexual Desire. Vol. II. New York:Brunner/Mazel, 1979.
Kaplan HS, et al. The Evaluation of Sexual Disorders: Psychological and Medical Aspects. New York: Brunner/Mazel, 1983.
Klein E, Kroll K. Enabling Romance: A Guide to Love, Sex, and Relationships for the Disabled. New York: Harmony Books (a division of Crown Publishers), 1992.
Mooney TO, Cole TM, Chilgren RA. Sexual Options for Paraplegics and Quadriplegics. Boston: Little, Brown, 1975.
Sandowski CL. Sexual Concerns When Illness or Disability Strikes. Springfield, IL: Charles C Thomas, 1989.
Schnarch DM. Constructing the Sexual Crucible: An Integration of Sexual and Marital Therapy. New York: WW Norton, 1991.
Schover LR, Jensen SB. Sexuality and Chronic Illness. New York: Guilford Press, 1988.
Shipes EA, Lehr ST. Sexual Counseling for Ostomates. Springfield, IL: Charles C Thomas, 1980.
Woods NF. Human Sexuality in Health and Illness. C.V. Mosby Co., St. Louis: CV Mosby, 1975, Chapters 1, 3, 7, 8, 11–13.

12

Ethical Considerations in Pulmonary Intensive Care

PAUL N. LANKEN

University of Pennsylvania Medical Center
Philadelphia, Pennsylvania

The intensive care unit (ICU) of a modern hospital serves as two important and contrasting paradigms: the practice of contemporary high-technology medicine with its high potential for depersonalization of patient care, on the one hand, and the close integration of bioethics with its intensely humanistic concerns into clinical practice, on the other hand. The term "bioethics" encompasses the ethics of health care, of health care professionals, and of basic biological and physical scientific research relevant to human health and disease. The aim of the discipline of ethics, in simple terms, is doing the right action for the right reasons.

Although the practice of pulmonary intensive care, in particular, and critical care medicine, in general, involves a broad range of ethical dilemmas, the most distinctive and challenging of these relate to end-of-life decision making. Many share a common theme: that the technological capacity of the ICU can prolong a patient's life markedly and, at times, seemingly indefinitely, but cannot cure the patient to allow him/her to recover and survive outside the ICU. The distinctive ethical dilemmas of ICU medicine often arise from the interface between this capacity of life-prolonging ICU technology and the fundamental question of whether a given patient's life should or should not be prolonged.

Further complexity occurs when different ethical principles addressing this question give different answers.

I. Fundamental Principles of Bioethics

Three fundamental principles of bioethics are particularly relevant to ethical issues in pulmonary intensive care: (1) respect for patient autonomy, (2) beneficence, and (3) justice (Fig. 1). Conflict between two principles often lies at the heart of an ethical dilemma in the ICU as elsewhere. An ethical dilemma is a situation that can only be resolved by violating one or more ethical principles in order to follow another overriding ethical principle. In addition, Figure 1 notes the moral entities that are most closely related to each ethical principle: (1) patients, their families, and other surrogate decision makers relate to the principle of respect for patient autonomy; (2) physicians, nurses, other health care providers, and health care institutions relate to the principle of beneficence, (3) society, communities of recipients and potential recipients of health care services and governmental institutions relate to the principle of justice.

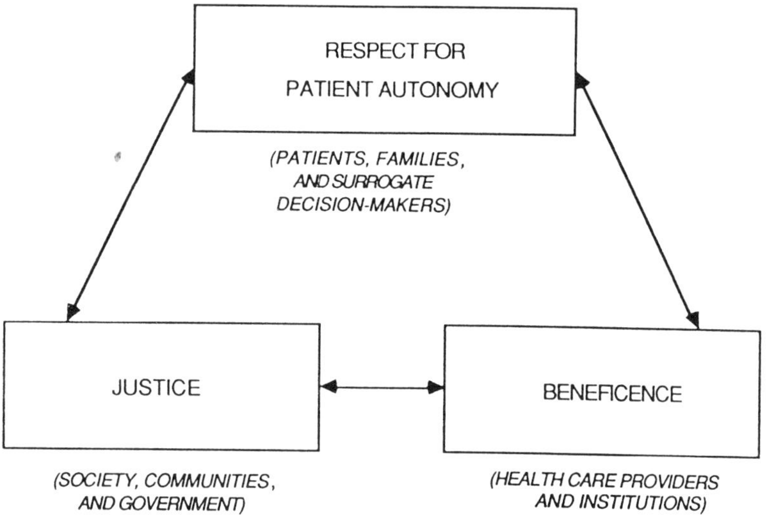

Figure 1 The three basic ethical principles commonly involved in ethical dilemmas in ICU medicine and their associated moral agents. The arrows between the rectangles represent the potential conflicts between principles.

A. Principle of Respect for Autonomy

The principle of *respect for patient autonomy* is grounded in the concept that the patient with a sound mind has an ethical and legal right to determine what happens to his or her body. This principle relates closely to the legal principles of an individual's right to privacy and self-determination. In this context, the patient has the right to decide whether or not to undergo a certain medical intervention. This principle also forms the basis for the legal and ethical concept of informed consent; i.e., under nonemergency circumstances a capable patient must give his/her informed consent prior to undergoing medical care, particularly potentially hazardous interventions; under emergency conditions, consent is assumed. Currently there is a strong consensus in the United States that health care professionals should not only respect, but also support and enhance, their patient's autonomy in the process of medical decision making (1).

B. Principle of Beneficence

The principle of *beneficence* refers to the fundamental purpose of all health care professions, which is to benefit the patient either as an individual or as the aggregate, e.g., public health. Beneficence is closely related to *nonmaleficence*, which is embodied by the Hippocratic maxim of "primun non nocere," i.e., first of all do not harm. The concept of beneficence has evolved from the Hippocratic tradition where the physician determined what was best for the patient to the more contemporary notion that what is best for the patient is determined by the patient albeit with significant input, e.g., information and recommendations, by the physician. When interpreted in this manner, the principle of beneficence is congruent with the principle of respect for autonomy.

C. Principle of Justice

The principle of justice in this context refers to the principle of *distributed justice*. This refers to the fair allocation of limited or expensive health care resources between an individual and the rest of society. The general principle of formal justice is attributed to Aristotle: equals should be treated equally and nonequals unequally (2). However, this statement lacks easy applicability because it lacks specific criteria for judging in what sense two individuals are equal or unequal. There are various applied theories of distributive justice that emphasize different values as the overriding criterion. For example, a utilitarian theory of justice above all values the principle of utility and holds that the right decision should maximize utility as its consequence; the maxim "the greatest good for the greatest number" reflects utilitarianism. On the other hand, there are deontological or rule-based theories of justice. One example is an egalitarian theory of justice whose rule holds that equal access to health care should be available to every member of the society.

II. Principle of Paternalism and Use of Therapeutic Privilege

On the opposite extreme from respect for patient autonomy is the principle of *paternalism*, which has been a guiding principle for medical practice since Hippocrates and continues to be influential in countries other than the United States. Paternalism is defined as interference with the patient's autonomy by the physician for the patient's own sake. Paternalism is closely related to the Hippocratic tradition of beneficence as discussed above.

One aspect of paternalism in medicine has involved the use of therapeutic privilege. This refers to the customary practice of *not* giving the patient complete and truthful information about his/her disease or prognosis to avoid harming the patient, e.g., by the patient suffering loss of hope or other mental anguish. The change in the interpretation of what is best for the patient, i.e., from the physician knowing best (Hippocratic beneficence) to the patient knowing best (respect for patient autonomy), exemplifies the continually evolving nature of bioethics and, specifically, medical (physician) ethics.

This change also illustrates the complex relationship between ethics and the law, e.g., what is ethical versus what is legal. For example, the traditional view of the legal aspect of health care providers was as a type of minimal morality; e.g., one *must* be a licensed practitioner to give medical or nursing care. This view contrasted with that of the professional ethics of health care providers, which were in keeping with the ideals of professional behavior; e.g., one *should* always follow the principle of beneficence in providing health care. For many bioethical issues, the relationship between legal and ethical viewpoints has grown even more complex.

III. Evolving Health Care Law and Ethics

Figure 2 illustrates what has happened with regard to the practice of therapeutic privilege, discussed above, in the United States. In the 1950s it was both legal and ethical to withhold health care information from capable patients. One survey of physicians published in 1961 indicated that 90% of physicians would prefer not to inform patients of a diagnosis of cancer, which was then almost invariably fatal (3). In contrast, 16 years later a survey published in 1977 found that 97% of physicians replied that they routinely told their patients of cancer diagnoses (4). By the 1980s judicial decisions and state statutes firmly established the practice of informed consent (5), and a consensus among those in-

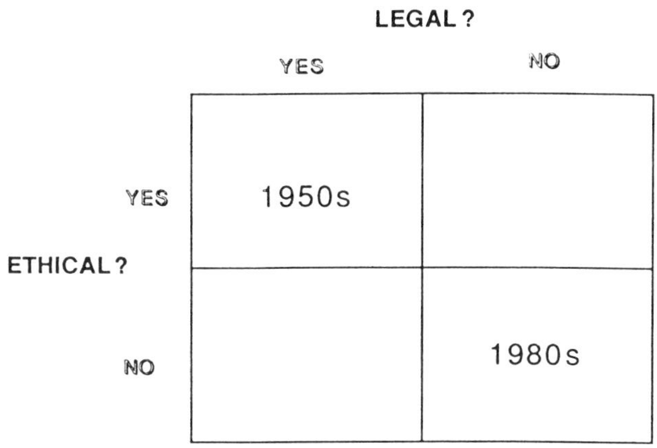

Figure 2 The changing ethical and legal status of use of therapeutic privilege, i.e., intentionally withholding "bad" information from the patient to prevent the patient being harmed by the information. In the 1950s, use of therapeutic privilege was widely practiced and endorsed by the medical profession, i.e., ethical, and since there were no laws against it, legal. The ethical and legal consensus had changed from the 1950s to the 1980s (and beyond) in the United States so that use of therapeutic privilege can now be viewed as both unethical and illegal. Note that it is still ethical and legal to withhold information from a capable patient at the patient's request (but not at the request of a capable patient's family).

volved in ethical decision making endorsed medical decision making that is shared between patient and physician (1). In addition, many states had their own regulations that required hospitals to provide patients with a Bill of Rights. One of the patients' rights was the right to be informed of their medical condition in understandable language. From these considerations, therapeutic privilege can be interpreted to have evolved from the "legal and ethical" quadrant to the "illegal and unethical" quadrant in Figure 2.

Depending on where and when medical care is being provided, some actions by health care professionals may change from legal to illegal or vice versa since health care law varies significantly among different jurisdictions and over time. The same may apply to what is considered ethical or unethical. For example, active euthanasia, which currently is considered unethical by the medical profession (as represented by their organized bodies) and illegal in all states of the United States, may evolve in time to be both ethical and legal. Along these lines, active euthanasia in the Netherlands can be viewed as illegal (since there is a statute against it) but also regarded ethical by that society and by their medical profession (as long as it is performed according to a prescribed process). As these circumstances illustrate, health care practitioners should view bioethics not as a static body of knowledge, but rather as a continuously evolving field.

IV. General Principles Regarding End-of-Life Decisions in the ICU

During the 1970s and 1980s, catalyzed by a number of precedent-setting court decisions, such as the Spence decision with regard to informed consent (5), the New Jersey Supreme Court decision regarding Karen Ann Quinlan (6), and the California Supreme Court decision regarding Bartling (7), a strong societal consensus developed regarding the ethical considerations of withholding or withdrawing life-sustaining therapies (8). From this consensus emerged the following general principles to guide health care professionals in this decision-making process.

Informed adults with decision-making capacity have the right to forgo any life-sustaining medical therapy even if it results in their death.

The key words and phrases in this principle are *adult*, *informed*, and *with decision-making capacity*. This right applies only to adults since children are not considered to have the personal autonomy required by legal or ethical standards. Furthermore, an adult patient must have both appropriate information in order to make an informed decision and sufficient mental capacity to be able to evaluate the specific decision under consideration, i.e., not just decision-making capacity in a general sense. Assessment of decision-making capacity is described below.

Forgoing life-sustaining therapy includes both the withholding of such a therapy, such as cardiopulmonary resuscitation, and its withdrawal, such as stopping mechanical ventilation or nutrition and hydration. There is no ethical difference between withholding and withdrawing life-sustaining therapy.

The debate about whether there are significant moral distinctions between acts of omission and acts of commission has essentially ended with the consensus holding that withdrawing is ethically equivalent to withholding (8). Similarly, no legal distinctions can generally be made between withholding and withdrawing. The legal controversy as to whether medically provided food and water is or is not medical care is also basically over. The end came with the judgment by the U.S. Supreme Court in its decision related to Nancy Cruzan (9) in which medically provided food and water were deemed medical care that could be refused by competent adults or by appropriate surrogate decision makers acting in accord with the patient's previously expressed preference.

A surrogate decision maker should make medical decisions on behalf of a patient who loses decision-making capacity, provided the decisions are made on the basis of knowledge of what the patient would have wanted under similar circumstances or, if such knowledge is lacking, on the basis of the patient's best interests.

In general, one or more members of the patient's immediate family usually serves as a surrogate decision maker. However, a number of circumstances may dictate otherwise. First, if the patient has formally designated a health care proxy by means of a durable power of attorney for health care, the designated proxy should be the surrogate decision maker whether or not he or she is a member of the patient's immediate family. Second, if there is no valid durable power of attorney but the patient has informally designated someone as a health care proxy either in writing or verbally, this choice should be respected. In circumstances where the patient has not designated a health care proxy or in states without a formal legal hierarchy that specifies the order of selection of a surrogate, a close family member who knows the patient well should be presumed to be an appropriate surrogate. In these circumstances, the patient's attending physician has the responsibility, as the patient's advocate, to judge the appropriateness of a surrogate decision maker in order to protect the patient.

The following two ethical and legal standards should guide the decisions of the surrogate decision maker: first, the substituted judgment standard, and second, the best-interests standard. A *substituted judgment standard* should accurately reflect what the patient would have preferred under similar circumstances and requires knowledge or prior information about the preferences of the patient, as expressed in a living will or other written or oral advanced directive, or about the values and life goals of the patient from which extrapolation can be made regarding preferences. If such knowledge is lacking, then the *best-interests standard* should be used. By this standard, the *benefits* of the life-sustaining therapy should be weighed against its *burdens*, e.g., life, chance of survival, and residual quality of life versus pain, discomfort, or the financial impact on the patient or on his/her family. The decision should be made based on the outcome of this weighing.

When in doubt regarding the patient's preferences, err on the side of sustaining life.

This rule is ethically fully justified only if the health care provider who elects to sustain a patient's life is willing to withdraw the life-sustaining therapy if it is later discovered that the patient would not have wanted it. When the effectiveness of a certain life-sustaining therapy is uncertain for a patient, this approach has additional merit since, once the therapy has started, the decision to continue it or not can be based on an objective assessment of its effectiveness rather than only on predictions of its effectiveness. For example, whether or not mechanical ventilation for a bout of respiratory failure in a patient with chronic obstructive pulmonary disease (COPD) will succeed in reversing respiratory failure over a short duration often poses a difficult question that, in some cases, can be resolved only by a limited trial of mechanical ventilation; in this instance, it can be agreed that if the patient is not extubated or does not have a reasonable prognosis for extubation by a certain day, the ventilator is withdrawn allowing the patient to die. This therapeutic trial approach is preferable to not trying a potentially efficacious intervention because of uncertainty or because the patient fears that the therapy, such as mechanical ventilation, once started, would not be curative but would be continued indefinitely.

It is ethical to administer medication to relieve pain or other suffering, such as dyspnea, even if doing so might hasten the patient's death, provided it is done with the informed consent of the patient or the patient's surrogate decision maker.

This administration of medication to relieve pain and suffering should be clearly distinguished from active euthanasia or assisted suicide. In the first instance, the intention of the health care provider is to relieve pain and suffering, which follows from the principle of beneficence. In contrast, the intention of active euthanasia and assisted suicide is to cause the patient's death. Although removal of a patient from a mechanical ventilator and allowing him/her to die from the disease is ethically and legally distinct from active euthanasia or assisted suicide, it is sometimes referred to as "passive euthanasia." Because of the potential to confuse this term with active euthanasia, it seems preferable to avoid use of the term in referring to acts of withholding or withdrawing life support.

A physician or health care provider should not be forced to comply with his/her patient's request regarding withholding or withdrawing life-sustaining therapy if it violates the health care provider's personal moral values; under such circumstances, responsibility for care of the patient should be transferred to another provider who can comply with the patient's request.

This principle acknowledges the pluralistic nature of personal and cultural values in the United States and other countries. It respects the health care provider's values when they conflict with the patient's preferences, while continuing to support the patient's autonomy. In practice it may be difficult to implement this principle if the health care provider in conflict with the patient is uncooperative; e.g., if the attending physician refuses to comply with the patient's or family's request to withdraw life support, the family may have to "fire" that physician in order to have the patient transferred to a more supportive physician.

V. The Ethics of Futile Medical Care

Although lacking the strong consensus that the general ethical principles stated above have and still controversial, support is growing to limit life support when it is futile as expressed in the following principles (10,11):

There is no ethical obligation for health care professionals to provide medical care that is futile even if requested by the patient or family. Life-sustaining therapy that is futile can be limited without the consent of the patient or surrogate decision maker.

The term *futile life support* may seem inherently contradictory and warrants explanation. One approach is to distinguish between physiological futility and medical futility. An intervention that is *physiologically futile* fails to achieve the desired physiological function as an end-point. For example, cardiopulmonary resuscitation (CPR) can be considered to be futile when a "code" is "stopped." In the same sense, CPR can also be regarded as futile in a patient who develops cardiac arrest while in refractory septic shock and whose blood pressure is continuing to spiral downward despite maximal pressors; in this type of patient, CPR has virtually no chance of being successful since the cardiac arrest occurred despite ongoing maximal medical therapy. In effect, CPR in these circumstances would only prolong the patient's dying.

With respect to medical futility, an intervention can be judged to be *medically futile* if reasoning and experience indicate that the intervention would have a high likelihood of failing to result in a meaningful survival for the patient; in this sense, meaningful survival signifies a quality and duration of survival that would have value to that particular individual. Admittedly, medically futile is a more debatable entity than physiologically futility. In applying this designation, the key phrases are *high likelihood*, which acknowledges the lack of absolutes in clinical decision making, and *meaningful survival*. Some specialists and organizations devoted to critical care medicine have recommended that for patients with permanent loss of consciousness, such as those in a persisting vegetative state, survival should be regarded as meaningless for that individual (unless the individual had an advanced directive that explicitly stated otherwise); according to this criterion, life-sustaining therapy for such patients is medically futile. Because the use of physiological or medical futility as grounds for not providing life-sustaining therapy can be subject to misinterpretation, and hence to misapplication, it is advisable to incorporate the appropriate definitions and guides to application of these terms into the institution's policies. In addition, the necessary personnel, such as institutional ethics committees or consulting bioethicists, should be readily available to consult with clinicians in this regard (11). In contrast to the situation relating to patient's request to forgo therapy, case law with regard to use of physiological or medical futility is still extremely sparse.

VI. Specific Ethical Issues in Pulmonary Intensive Care

The general principles expressed above can be used to examine a number of ethical issues that are commonly encountered in the practice of pulmonary intensive care. The following questions are among the more common.

How can intubated ICU patients express their preferences?

Although this may be difficult, some ICU patients on mechanical ventilation may be quite lucid while receiving little or no sedation. If the patient is lucid, it is usually not too difficult for health care professionals to communicate by voice while the patient writes his or her responses or questions. In this manner the patient's decision-making capacity can be assessed.

Are ICU patients really capable of valid decision making?

Under ordinary circumstances in medicine, the usual and appropriate presumption is that the patient has decision-making capability. However, in the ICU or in other dire circumstances, clinical experience suggests that the *opposite* presumption should hold: that the patient is *not* capable. Starting from these vantages, the decision-making capacity of an ICU patient needs to be thoroughly investigated and documented before relying on it for decision making. Among the problems that can compromise the decision-making capacity of an ICU patient are the effects of disease, sedatives, narcotics, and other medications that can cause confusion, sleep deprivation, pain, anxiety, and fear.

What if an incapacitated patient's preferences regarding life-sustaining therapy are known but are overridden by his/her family or surrogate decision maker?

In general, the principle of respect for patient autonomy dictates that the patient's preferences, if known, should be respected irrespective of the contrary opinions of the patient's family or surrogate decision maker. However, if the surrogate has a valid durable power of attorney, the surrogate's opinion would have legal authority over the decision. In the event of a conflict, regardless of the legal status of the surrogate, the first step would be to discuss the situation openly with the surrogate and, if needed, to request consultation by the hospital's ethics committee or bioethicist. In this circumstance, the health care professional is still bound by the principle of beneficence and his/her fiduciary relationship with the patient to act as the patient's advocate. In rare instances, the conflict may need to be referred to a court of law for resolution.

What if the patient's preferences, or those of the surrogate decision maker, regarding forgoing life support are in conflict with the ICU team?

In these circumstances, if the preferences are by an informed patient with decision-making capacity, or by a surrogate with a valid, durable power of attorney, the ICU physician or nurse has little choice except to transfer care to another person. The classic example is a patient who is a Jehovah's Witness and refuses blood products on that ground in the face of life-threatening gastrointestinal bleeding. In this case, the patient has the legal and ethical right to refuse the blood even if his/her death results; i.e., respect for patient autonomy overrides beneficence. However, under this same circumstance, if the patient is a child of a Jehovah's Witness and a minor, judicial permission can be obtained to override the parent's wishes to withhold the blood products.

In instances in which the preferences are expressed by a surrogate decision maker who lacks a valid durable power of attorney, the case for the surrogate's preferences is less compelling if the physicians and nurses do not feel that the surrogate is acting in the best interests of the patient. Resolution of the conflict should then be sought along the lines outlined above.

Is a "slow code" or "Hollywood code" ever an ethical course of action?

"Slow code" refers to the performance of resuscitation at less than standard intensity; its intent is to allow the patient to die based on the premise that the attempt at resuscitation should not have been initiated in the first place. A "Hollywood code" has the same meaning but is accompanied by the pretense that the code is in earnest. Both practices entail deception that makes them unacceptable ethically. These practices arise in cases in which clinicians judge that CPR is medically or physiologically futile in hospitals lacking policies addressing futility. To discourage these types of codes, institutions should support their clinicians by providing them with the authority to exercise professional judgment by applying the principles of physiological or medical futility to such cases.

What should be done if CPR or another therapy is judged to be futile? Can health care professionals be forced to provide what they judge to be futile?

Health care professionals should share their judgment about the futility of a specific intervention with the patient or, more realistically for ICU patients, with the patient's surrogate decision maker. The surrogate or family may agree with the physician's judgment that a certain limitation of the life support is futile; some may even thank the physician for making the decision to stop the intervention on this basis. However, if the surrogate demands that CPR or other interventions judged futile be performed, the physician can attempt to transfer the patient to another physician in the same or another institution who agrees to provide the particular intervention in question. If the patient is not able to be transferred to another hospital, which is usually the case for unstable ICU patients, and if the hospital policy allows, the physician should write an order to limit CPR or other life support on the basis of futility and inform the surrogate of that order. If hospital policy does not allow this practice and if the patient *cannot* be transferred, the physician is faced with a number of alternatives: the physician can elect to acquiese and provide the futile care, resign from the case by transferring care to another physician in the same institution, or go to a court of law to limit therapy on the basis of his/her conviction that limiting therapy is the most ethical course to follow.

What is unjust, if anything, about the current system of "first come, first served" for ICU admissions? Who should be discharged from a full ICU to make room for admission of another patient: the patient who depends on the ICU the least or the patient who has only a minimal chance of survival even if he/she remains in the ICU?

Whether an ICU admissions policy is just or unjust can be assessed by examining the admission criteria according to this basic principle of distributive justice, i.e., that equals be treated equally and unequals treated unequally. In this context, if admissions are based on whether a patient is sufficiently ill to meet the threshold criterion for ICU admission and if beds are available, then the patient should be admitted; i.e., this is an example of equals being treated equally where the overriding criterion for equality or inequality is severity of illness. If the ICU precludes admission of certain categories of patients on the basis of gender, race, ethnicity, or age *per se* even though they meet the threshold criterion for severity of illness, then equals would not be treated equally. Similarly, if patients do not meet the threshold criterion for degree of illness, they should not be admitted even if they or their families insist; this is an example of unequals being treated unequally where degree of illness is the determinating factor.

The concept of "first come, first served" is equivalent to queuing up in line and is based on an egalitarian theory of distributive justice, which states that equal opportunity be available to all. If the ICU is full and another patient who meets the threshold of degree of illness for admission presents, what are the alternative responses? First, one could refuse to admit the new patient irrespective of the relative degrees of illness among the new and old patients, i.e., honoring "first come, first served." Second, one could discharge the least sick patient in the ICU to make room for the new patient if the new patient was sicker than the discharged patient. Third, one could discharge the ICU patient who had the worst prognosis if the new patient had a better prognosis than the one discharged. Consideration of this last alternative raises the issue of using predicted outcomes of ICU patients as one of several criteria for admission and discharge. This is a utilitarian concept in which decisions are made to maximize good outcomes. Customarily, except for ICU patients who are designated as "brain dead" or who have do not resuscitate (DNR) orders that limit interventions, the patient traditionally discharged to make room for a new ICU patient is the least sick patient in the ICU. This generalization applies even if the patient who is discharged from the ICU could still benefit from being in the ICU and would be put at higher risk for death or serious morbidity by being transferred out at that time.

One problem inherent in basing admission policy on outcomes rather than on need for ICU resources is that prognostication for individual ICU patients is generally inexact and, for the most part, subjective. Even systems that attempt to provide objective estimates of outcome may not settle this issue. For example, the worst prediction category in the current generation of objective ICU prognostic systems (12–14), which were meant to apply to groups of patients and not to individuals, does not predict more than a 90% chance of death. It is doubtful if many families of ICU patients would interpret a 10% chance for survival for their loved one as futile or would agree that therapy should be stopped on that basis alone.

Is there a point when health care professionals should limit consumption of scarce or expensive resources by a single patient; i.e., is there a "fair share" of resources beyond which there is no obligation to provide?

These are extreme cases that occur uncommonly. For example, the patient with persistent variceal bleeding despite all attempts at control may need an almost continuous infusion of blood to keep up with his/her bleeding. After a certain point, decided by clinical judgment of the ICU clinicians and consultants and communicated to the family (the patient is invariably encephalopathic by this stage), it is ethical to stop transfusions. Indeed, some would think it unethical to do otherwise. However, making the decision and telling the family are the difficult aspects of this decision-making process.

In this scenario, the ICU physicians face another ethical dilemma relating to their professional roles: on the one hand is their role as patient advocate, which is to keep the patient alive in accord with the principles of beneficence and respect for autonomy (assuming that the family wanted transfusions to continue, perhaps hoping for a miracle); on the other hand is their role as stewards of society's limited resources, especially in cases of medical futility. There are only a few guidelines for ICU clinicians to follow in approaching this quandary (15). In this example the limited resource is blood. However, the same argument holds for financial costs since expenses are a legitimate limited resource when the expenditures of ICU resources are part of a larger health care system that is "closed"; "closed" signifies that dollars spent on behalf of one individual lessen the amount of dollars available for other individuals and, conversely that dollars that are not spent for one individual increase the amount of dollars available for others. If, for example, the institution or health care system had an overall budget that included these interactions, then it would be a closed system for the purposes of this argument.

Although ICU physicians in the United States in the past may have emphasized their role more as patient advocates in providing their patients with vast resources rather than as society's guardians of those resources, it is becoming clearer that one of the most important future ethical challenges for ICU professionals will be how to combine their role as good steward of society's limited resources (respecting the principle of justice) with their role as patient advocate (respecting the principle of beneficence). Similarly, one can anticipate that patients and their surrogates will face more conflicts in the future in trying to get what they want from the health care system (patient autonomy) compared to what is available to them under the terms of their contracts with their health care organization or insurer (distributive justice).

VII. "Do Not Resuscitate" Decision Making in the ICU

A. Initiation of Discussion Regarding Withholding or Withdrawing Life-Sustaining Therapy

Ideally, discussion of withholding or withdrawing life support should have been initiated by the health care provider before admission to the ICU and, preferably, while the patient was an outpatient; this discussion could then take place in the context of an overall medical care plan for the patient that is respectful of his/her life goals. Ideally, the patient's primary care physician should encourage the patient to prepare a written advance directive and to identify a health care proxy or surrogate decision maker; these discussions should also include clarification of the patient's preferences for degrees of medical interventions under various scenarios while being mindful of a particular patient's medical disorders and prognosis. For example, if the patient has severe COPD and has been treated with mechanical ventilation for a COPD flare in the past, the physician should encourage the patient to discuss his/her preferences regarding the levels of intervention that can be anticipated: Does the patient want mechanical ventilation again? Under what circumstances? For how long? What if he/she is judged to be unweanable? Prior discussion like these will solve the most vexing problem in ICU medicine: how to communicate effectively about these considerations with an intubated, ventilated patient whose decision-making capacity has become compromised.

Once the patient is in the ICU, discussions may be initiated by the patient, by a family member or other surrogate decision maker, or by a member of the health care team, e.g., house staff, nurse, or attending physician. If the patient made a living will prior to ICU admission, the meaning of that advance directive should have been clarified prior to, and upon, admission to the ICU. If the patient's living will simply stated that life support be withdrawn when it was judged that there was no reasonable hope for a meaningful recovery, it would be helpful for the ICU personnel to know how to interpret "reasonable" and "meaningful recovery" in making their recommendations regarding continuation or discontinuation of life support. However, the ICU patient usually has no written advance directive. Even if there is no written advance directive, the patient may have verbally expressed his/her preferences regarding some forms of life support with which he/she may have been familiar, e.g., not wanting to be kept alive indefinitely by machines. Alternatively, the patient may not have expressed anything, but the family or close friends might be able to reach sufficient agreement as to what the patient's preferences would be, based on the patient's life goals and values, in order to proceed.

If the health care team judges that the patient's prognosis is hopeless, that the therapy is futile, or that the burdens of the therapy clearly outweigh its benefits, the attending physician is obligated to initiate end-of-life discussions, to share these judgments with the patient's family or surrogate decision maker, and to make recommendations regarding withholding or withdrawing life support.

B. Assessment of a Patient's Decision-Making Capacity

Distinction should be made between *competency* and *capacity*. On the one hand, competency is a legal term: an adult is legally competent unless a court has found that individual incompetent (a child or minor automatically lacks competency). On the other hand, decision-making capacity is a functional determination that is made by the patient's attending physician and that may vary over time and with regard to specific medical decisions. In practice, many legally competent patients have decreased or inadequate decision-making capacity, e.g., when they are sedated in the ICU; conversely, a legally incompetent person may still have some degree of decision-making capacity, e.g., opinions of a young teenager about a medical intervention.

Adequate decision-making capacity is present when the patient has the following attributes in relation to a specific decision: (1) comprehension, (2) comparative judgment, and (3) communication. With regard to comprehension, the patient should be able to understand information about his/her medical condition, its prognosis, and the treatment options to be considered, including the option of no treatment at all. With regard to comparative judgment, the patient should be able to evaluate the medical information received compared to his personal values and life goals in order to assess which course of therapy is most consistent with those goals and values. With regard to communication, the patient should be able to communicate decisions in a consistent and meaningful manner, even if he/she lacks the capacity for speech. The need to specify the context of the assessment for decision-making capacity arises from the observation that some patients have seemingly adequate capacity for certain decisions but not for others.

The attending physician should make the assessment about the adequacy of a patient's decision-making capacity through a process that includes reviewing the patient's medical history, performing of mental status examinations, and soliciting observations of other health care professionals and family members. If there is doubt or conflict about the patient's capacity, additional information should be sought, e.g., reviewing prior written advance directives or obtaining a psychiatric consultation.

C. Identification and Role of Surrogate Decision Makers

If an ICU patient lacks decision-making capacity, to whom should the physician turn to as a surrogate decision maker? As noted above, the choice may be mandated by law either in the form of an individual having a valid, durable power of attorney for health care decisions or in the form of a state-designated legal hierarchy, e.g., spouse first, parents next, and so forth.

Alternatively, in the absence of a legal mandate, if the patient has expressed a preference for having someone as his/her surrogate decision maker, that choice should, in general, be respected. In many cases, the surrogate decision maker is usually, but not necessarily, a close family member. There are two important elements for serving as a surrogate: (1) a willingness to serve in that role and be responsible for making decisions on the patient's behalf, and (2) a personal knowledge of the patient's preferences, values, and life goals. It is through the latter information that the surrogate can provide a substituted judgment of what the patient would have wanted under similar circumstances. If no one can be found with a personal knowledge of the patient's values or preferences, the surrogate can be based only on the first element noted above.

In some instances, the frequency of which varies according to the population served by different hospitals, there may be *no* individual who knows the patient or who is willing to serve as a surrogate decision maker. This is an institutional issue that should be addressed through institutional policy. The policies of some institutions provide for a relatively neutral party, i.e., ideally not a hospital employee, to be available to act as a surrogate; for example, the chairperson of the hospital's ethics committee may play this role. In other hospitals, which lack easy access to a neutral party, DNR decisions are required to be reviewed by health care professionals not involved in the case prior to their implementation to ensure that the process of DNR determination was appropriate, i.e., that a best-interests standard was used by the health care team in weighing the benefits against the burdens of various levels of medical intervention.

D. Defining the DNR Order

The order of DNR consists of more than the instruction "do not resuscitate." Instead, it identifies one or more forms of life-sustaining therapy that are to be discontinued. In the ICU setting these include CPR, cardioversion, intubation, mechanical ventilation, hemodialysis, and administration of blood products, vasoactive agents, such as pressors, administered intravenously, and antibiotics. Faced with this array of treatments, how should health professionals, patients, and families decide whether limitation of a certain therapy is appropriate?

One answer that has proven useful in practice in a number of institutions is to define the specific goals of therapy that should apply to the patient's situation. From these goals, one can consider which therapies are compatible, or incompatible, with that goal. For example, at the Hospital of the University of Pennsylvania, clinicians have used a system consisting of three levels of limiting treatment that are defined by DNR orders (Table 1).

Table 1 Levels of Treatment with Associated Goals of Therapy

Level	Definition of therapy	Description and goals of therapy
DNR A	All therapies but CPR	The patient is to be treated as medically indicated, including all efforts to prevent cardiac or respiratory arrest. However, if the patient has a cardiopulmonary arrest, no cardiac resuscitative efforts will be made, nor will the patient be intubated, be mechanically ventilated, or, in general, be admitted to an intensive care unit.
DNR B	Limited therapy, no CPR	Therapy already initiated should be continued as medically indicated by the patient's condition. In general, no additional treatment will be initiated, except for the purpose of comfort. If cardiac or pulmonary arrest occurs, no resuscitative efforts should be made.
DNR C	Comfort measures only	Treatment is to be limited to nursing and medical therapy appropriate for hygiene and comfort. Treatment that is necessary for comfort may be used even if it contributes to cardiac or respiratory depression. Life-sustaining therapies already initiated may be discontinued by written order.

Source: Reprinted with permission from the Policy Manual, Hospital of the University of Pennsylvania, "The Withholding and Withdrawing of Life-Sustaining Therapy," March 17, 1989.

As a general approach, a meeting of all persons involved is held to discuss the situation and reassess the appropriateness of the level of current treatment. The patient is to be included unless he/she lacks decision-making capacity; if the patient lacks capacity, the surrogate decision maker or makers are included; all other interested members of the patient's family are invited to the meeting. The health care team is represented by the ICU attending physician, the patient's primary care physician (if applicable), consultants relevant for discussions of prognosis, members of the house staff caring for the patient, one or more ICU nurses, and respiratory therapists (if the patient is receiving mechanical ventilation). This meeting ensures open communication among parties during and after the decision-making process; it is especially helpful for all parties to feel involved in this process if they are to understand and accept the result of the process. So-called "family meetings" to address DNR status are now a way of life in the ICU practice of medicine since a growing proportion of deaths in the ICU ensue from a deliberate decision to limit life support (16,17).

E. Carrying Out the DNR Order

The next step after defining the limits of therapy is for the attending physician to document the discussion in the patient's medical record and to write the physician's order to implement the limitation of life support that has been agreed upon. Accurate and complete documentation of the discussion should include the parties involved, the reasoning behind limiting life support, whether the patient has capacity or not, the patient's medical prognosis, and the category of limitation of life-sustaining therapy. Details of policies vary from institution to institution; e.g., in New York a state statute requires the signature of a capable patient or, if the patient lacks capacity, of the surrogate decision maker, in order to write a DNR order. Nonetheless, virtually all acute care and rehabilitation hospitals have policies concerning cessation of life-sustaining therapy, especially since it has been a recommendation of the Joint Commission for Accreditation of Hospitals since 1988 (18).

After the order is written, the nursing and respiratory therapy staff generally will modify their therapies appropriately. For example, if a patient is to be extubated and removed from mechanical ventilation, the nurse will begin or increase an intravenous infusion of narcotics titrated to achieve a certain level of sedation; after the desired level has been achieved, the patient will be extubated by the physician, nurse, or respiratory therapist. It is important to determine whether staff members involved in this process are comfortable with removal of life support so as to give them the option of not participating. As the last resort, the attending physician who writes the DNR order must be prepared to perform the extubation, if necessary.

F. Resolution of Conflicts

If the above process is followed, conflicts are uncommon, whereas conflicts often occur if communication is poor among physicians and nurses. Conflicts between the patient's family and the health care team may arise when one group favors forgoing life support and the other does not; on occasion the family may wish to continue full aggressive ICU care in the face of growing pessimism for the patient's prognosis by members of the health care team, or the family may want life support to stop but find that the attending physician does not agree.

Resolution of conflict benefits from full and open communication among parties. In addition, consultation with the hospital's ethics committee may resolve the conflict in a number of ways, e.g., by clarifying hospital policy or legal limits or simply by getting all the people involved to sit around the same table and talk with one another. The majority of hospitals have ethics committees or other resources, e.g., a consulting bioethicist, available (19). In rare instances, legal advice and judicial review has to be sought if an impass is reached. If the situation deteriorates to this degree, transfer of the patient to another hospital or to another attending physician may be prudent.

VIII. Conclusion

Dying in an ICU today occurs predominantly by limiting varying degrees of life-sustaining therapy. The frequency and complexity of this process of limiting life support has created a rich milieu for ethical issues to arise. Most ethical dilemmas occur when those with decision-making responsibility must violate one or more ethical principles in order to respect an overriding ethical principle. This process of weighing ethical principles in cases of specific ICU patients has been grounded by a general ethical, legal, and professional consensus. As a rule, the overriding principle is respect for patient autonomy. This principle is generally embodied in hospital policies and procedures regarding DNR decision making, i.e., withholding and withdrawing life-sustaining therapy. Nonetheless, conflicts still arise, and local resources, such as a hospital's ethics committee or consulting bioethicist, are commonly available to assist in their resolution. Only in extreme cases should the conflict need to be resolved by legal proceedings.

References

1. President's Commission for the Study of Ethical Problems in Medicine and Biomedical and Behavioral Research. Making health care decisions: the ethical and legal implications of informed consent in the patient-practitioner relationship. Vol. 1. Washington, DC: US Government Printing Office, 1982.
2. Beauchamp TL, Childress JF. Principles of Biomedical Ethics. New York: Oxford University Press, 1989.
3. Oken D. What to tell cancer patients: a study of medical attitudes. JAMA 1961; 175:1120.
4. Novak DH. Changes in physicians' attitudes towards telling the cancer patient. JAMA 1979; 241:897.

5. *Canterbury v. Spence, United States Court of Appeals, District of Columbia Circuit*, 464 F 2nd 772, 1972.
6. *In re Quinlan*, 70 N.E. 10, 355 A2d 647, *cert denied* 429 US 922 (NJ 1976).
7. *Bartling v. Superior Court, California Court of Appeal, Second District*, 163 Cal., App.3d 186, 209 Caal.Rptr. 220, 1984
8. President's Commission for the Study of Ethical Problems in Medicine and Biomedical and Behavioral Research. Deciding to forego life-sustaining treatment: ethical, medical and legal issues in treatment decisions. Washington, DC: U.S. Government Printing Office, 1983.
9. *Cruzan v. Director, Missouri Dept. of Health*, 110 S. Ct 284 (1990).
10. Schneiderman LJ, Jecker NS, Jonsen AR. Medical futility: its meaning and ethical implications. Ann Intern Med 1990; 112:949–954.
11. American Thoracic Society. Withholding and withdrawing life-sustaining therapy. Am Rev Respir Dis 1991; 144:726–731.
12. Knaus WA, Wagner DP, Draper EA, et al. The APACHE III prognostic system: risk prediction of hospital mortality for critically ill hospitalized adults. *Chest* 1991; 100:1619–1636.
13. Lemeshow S, Teres D, Avrunin JS, Gehlbach SH, Rapoport J. Mortality Probability Models (MPM II) based on an international cohort of intensive care unit patients. JAMA 1993; 270:2478–2486.
14. Bone RC, LeGall JR, Lemeshow S, Saulnier F. A new simplified acute physiology score (SAPS II) based on a European/North American multicenter study. JAMA 1993; 270:2957–2963.
15. Lanken PN. Critical care medicine at a new crossroads: the intersection of economics and ethics in the intensive care unit. Am J Respir Crit Care Med 1994; 149:3–5.
16. Smedira NG, Evans BH, Grais LS, et al. Withholding and withddrawal of life support from the critically ill. N Engl J Med 1990; 322:309–315.
17. Teres D. Trends from the United States with end of life decisions in the intensive care unit. Intensive Care Med 1993; 19:316–322.
18. Joint Commission for Accreditation of Hospitals. Accreditation Manual for Hospitals. Chicago: JCAH, 1988.
19. Asch DA, Hansen-Flaschen JH, Lanken PN. Decisions to limit or continue life-sustaining treatment by US critical care physicians: conflicts between physicians' practices and patients' wishes. Am J Respir Crit Care Med 1995; 288–292.

Part Two

EVALUATION

13

Effectiveness of Pulmonary Rehabilitation

ARTHUR A. SIEBENS

The Johns Hopkins University
and Milton J. Dance, Jr., Center
Greater Baltimore Medical Center
Baltimore, Maryland

In commenting on whether pulmonary rehabilitation is effective, the first step is to identify a glossary for "rehabilitation," a popular term so general as to complicate analytical commentary.

I. Definitions

The World Health Organization (WHO) has defined terms commonly used in rehabilitation contexts (1).

Impairment is a pathophysiological circumstance, e.g., loss of lung compliance, weakness of the muscles of respiration, presence of a tracheostomy.

Disability is the effect of impairment on daily personal life, e.g., inability to use an upstairs bathroom because of breathlessness in climbing stairs, reduced intelligibility in telephoning because of low tidal volume, difficulty with speaking to one's spouse while driving because the finger of one hand must be used to occlude the tracheostomy cannula during expiration.

Handicap is interference with fulfilling one's expected role in society, e.g., in the instance of a mail carrier whose breathlessness limits his ability to cover his route or a teacher whose voice no longer projects adequately in the classroom.

It is logical to think of rehabilitation effectiveness, then, in terms of impairment, disability, and handicap. Although lessening impairment facilitates lessening disability and handicap, it does not "lock in" such a consequence, for disability and handicap relate to choices, learning, and behaviors of individuals rather than to pathophysiological variables.

II. Prevention of Lung Impairment

Prevention is a core concept of rehabilitation. Disability and handicap can be reduced or eliminated in proportion to the prevention of impairment. Stiffening and contractures of joints, with their adverse consequences for the metabolic cost of walking and dressing, are preventable by stretching exercises. The prevention of ischial decubitus ulcers carries profound implications for wheelchair mobility as well as health. Avoiding tracheostomy, when alternatives to tracheal positive pressure ventilation are available, may prevent the disabling and handicapping consequences of aphonia.

The elimination of cigarette smoke is the preeminent and obvious measure impacting the prevention of respiratory impairment and consequent disability and handicap (2). Irreversible destruction of alveolar walls is the primary impairment of chronic obstructive pulmonary disease (COPD), (3), the secondary impairments including collapsed airways, ventilation-perfusion mismatches, reduced surface area for diffusion, hypertension of the lesser circulation, and dyspnea. All of these, together with their consequent disabilities and handicaps, indisputably follow exposure of the lung to tobacco smoke (4). Patently, the effectiveness of pulmonary rehabilitation is in proportion to the prevention of smoking.

Current smokers 18 years old and over decreased from 42.4% of the population in 1965 to 25.6% in 1991 (5). Of individuals 26 years old and over, the percent of current users fell from 39.1% of the population in 1974 to 28.2% in 1991 (6). The per capita consumption of all tobacco products was 9.7 lb in 1970 as compared to 5.4 in 1991 (7). These data support the belief that the measures used to limit smoking have had a positive effect on society consistent with the prevention of pulmonary impairment.

However, that at least one-quarter (5) of the population has continued to smoke is hardly occasion for congratulations. Moreover, the productivity of the tobacco industry is unrestrained. A total of 583 billion cigarettes were produced in 1970, 714 billion in 1980 (a record within the last 20 years), and 710 billion in 1990 (7). The beguiling tenor of the advertising to which the tobacco industry exposes the public remains in shameless self-interest at variance with societal health. The virile Marlboro rancher and the Virginia Slims liberated woman who has "come a long way" are familiar examples of selling the cigarette and its harm by appeal to human foibles. A full-page spread questioning "where is the land of the free?" (8) contrasts constraints against smoking in the American work environment with three historic milestones in the elimination of human oppression abroad: the fall of the Berlin Wall, Russia's new constitution, and democracy's victory in South Africa. The thinly veiled implication that protecting the public against self-injurious practices is an un-American abrocation of freedom hopefully is born of desperation within the tobacco industry as legislative outcry against smoking mounts.

The argument has been made (9) that health dollars would not be saved by eliminating tobacco and averting premature death from COPD. The price of additional longevity into advanced ages associated with chronic impairments has been calculated to offset the savings incident to eliminating the morbidities of using tobacco. These economics notwithstanding, the fact of a human cost is certain, one that expresses itself ultimately in disability, handicap, and suffering. As in the instance of tuberculosis and of occupational exposures injurious to the lung, because the etiology is known, so also is the prevention. The decrease in use of cigarettes in the United States over the last 20 years predictably will have lessened disability and handicap incident to pulmonary impairment in this country. Less production and fewer sales are necessary, however, if disability and handicap worldwide are to diminish.

III. Compensations for Secondary Impairments

Although the primary impairment of COPD, loss of air space walls, is irreversible, the secondary or consequent impairments do lend themselves to compensatory strategies. The effectiveness of reducing disability and handicap is in proportion to their implementation.

A. Hypoxia

The adverse effects of hypoxia on mentation, mood, fatigability, and sleep were studiously documented during ascensions to real or simulated altitude by Barcroft and by Haldane, pioneers of respiratory physiology. Their vivid imageries were: "Acute anoxia simulates drunkenness, chronic anoxia simulates fatigue" (10) and "Anoxia not only stops the machine, it wrecks the machinery" (11). Not surprisingly, therefore, COPD patients with hypoxia have clinically significant neuropsychologic deficits (12) and score significantly lower than controls in measures of life quality. These include mobility, social interaction, alertness, emotional behavior, home management, recreation and leisure activity, and employment (13). Furthermore, the relief of hypoxemia by administering supplemental oxygen improves psychological functions (14), reduces pulmonary artery hypertension, and increases survival (15). Breakthroughs in the provision of oxygen to the ambulatory individual, therefore, potentially are monumental contributions to reducing disability and handicap. The "packaging" of oxygen is one example of such a contribution. Whereas a full "D" cylinder weighing 8 lb with its regulator can delivery oxygen at 2 L/min for a maximum of 3 hr (approximately 22 min/lb), a liquid oxygen system (Pentox #3) weighing 9–11 lb can last 11 hr (approximately 60 min/lb) and a pulsed system (Devilbiss Pulsair) of equivalent weight as much as 20 hr (120 min/lb). These and additional developments are remarkable advances for reducing disability and handicap by restoring eupoxia. Additional examples are the surprising demonstration that oxygen by nasal prongs is effective whether one breathes by nose or mouth (16), the introduction of the transtracheal route for delivering oxygen directly into the trachea (17), and the conservation of oxygen by pulsing its flow in phase with inspiration (18).

Facilitating exercise and activity are important consequences of avoiding the hypoxemia incident to raising metabolic requirements. That inactivity, including bed rest, leads to physiological and psychological changes that foster its perpetuation is amply documented (19). To the extent that lung impairment causes a breathlessness that is intensified by activity, the stage is set for superimposing the limitations of the deconditioned state (20). Supplementary oxygen may prevent or lessen the hypoxia incident to exercise, thereby warding off compounding the restrictions for activity imposed by the impaired lung with those resulting from deconditioning (21).

B. Flow of Air

An increased resistance to airflow during expiration is another impairment resulting from the loss of air space walls and the consequent reduction of centrifugal traction on airways, diaphragms, and chest wall. The associated increase in functional residual capacity is an involuntary and obligatory biomechanical response. Regrettably, there is no compensatory strategy comparable to using oxygen in the instance of hypoxemia. However, behaviors to avoid compounding airway collapse have a basis in logic. The Bernouilli theorem observes that pressure is least where flow rate is highest. Accordingly, additional "pinching" can be expected in airways where the stream of air is already narrowed by airway collapse. During forced expiration or unmodified cough, the elevation in pleural pressure is transmitted to all the airways (22), causing narrowing and kinking even in those supported in part by cartilage (23). Slowing airflow and lessening pleural pressure conceptually are advantageous under these circumstances. These can be achieved to the extent that respiratory rate is controlled, expiration is slowed, and forced expiration is moderated. Relaxation and posturing exercises, "huff" coughing rather than the closed-glottis or Valsalva coughing, and expiration through pursed lips have a physiological basis in common. How effective these impairment-reducing breathing exercises and instructions are in terms of disability and handicap is difficult to certify inasmuch as they are unlikely to be used in isolation from other measures. Their champion historically, Dr. Alvan Barach, was himself afflicted by COPD; his studies (24) and personal testimonials to their effectiveness bear emphasis even though their value, as determined by tests of pulmonary function, is not proven (25). Whether this reflects on what is measured rather than on the interventions themselves is moot.

C. Motion of Thorax

Preserving the capacity for motion is a core concept of rehabilitation. When applied to the chest, the concept impacts ventilation. The compliance and angles of the costovertebral and costochondral articulations and the capacity of the diaphragms and intercostal muscles to generate tension that results in motion are the critical variables. It is difficult to conceive of circumstances more adverse to motion than those that characterize the chest of patients with COPD. The costal articulations are positioned at one extreme of their range. Their connective tissues are stiffened by lack of stretch from the motions of normal ventilation. The muscles have shortened to a length that is disadvantageous to their developing additional tension. They are driven to contract abnormally frequently and against abnormally high loads (26). The flattening of the diaphragms reduces their effectiveness for expanding the thorax. Given these circumstances, all of which are consequent to the primary pathology of the lung, it is small wonder that measures to increase motion, as reflected objectively in resting lung function measurements, meet with equivocal success (27). However, the complete elimination of impairment, disability, and handicap rarely is a reality-based definition of effective rehabilitation in any context. Small gains toward limited objectives may contribute nevertheless in terms meaningful for self-care and mobility (28) as well as quality of life (29).

IV. Effectiveness in Neuromuscular Impairment

Weakness of the respiratory muscles independently of lung pathology is an impairment that occurs in a variety of settings: upper motor neuron pathology, e.g., damage to the cervical spinal cord from injury or disease; lower motor neuron pathology, e.g., poliomyelitis, Guillain-Barré syndrome, amyotrophic lateral sclerosis; pathology of neuromyal synaptic transmission, e.g., myasthenia gravis, botulism; and the myopathies, e.g., muscular dystrophy. Ventilation of children and adults is jeopardized in these instances because the forces required to produce the motions of breathing are insufficient. Cessation of breathing occurs also when damage to the brain interferes with the generation of discharges from the respiratory center, e.g., in "central" sleep apnea and brainstem stroke, and when the upper airway is obstructed, e.g., during obstructive sleep apnea. These pathologies are life-threatening and commonly not preventable. Compensation requires devices for rhythmical creation of air pressure gradients between alveoli and atmosphere sufficient to overcome the flow resistance of the airways and the compliance forces of the lungs and chest. The catalogue of effective options is remarkable for the biomechanical versatility that it reflects.

The gradients can be created by lowering alveolar pressure below atmospheric ("negative pressure" ventilation) (30) or by raising pressure in the mouth, nose, or trachea above atmospheric ("positive-pressure ventilation"). Examples of the former approach are the tank respirator (Fig. 1), chest shell or cuirass ventilator (Fig. 2), rocking bed (Fig. 3), pneumobelt, pulmowrap (Fig. 4), and paced stimulation of the phrenic nerves (31, 32). Examples of positive-pressure application are squeezing the Ambu bag, numerous electrically powered pumps incorporated into ventilators, and compressed air systems. All of these approaches, properly applied, are effective compensations for the alveolar

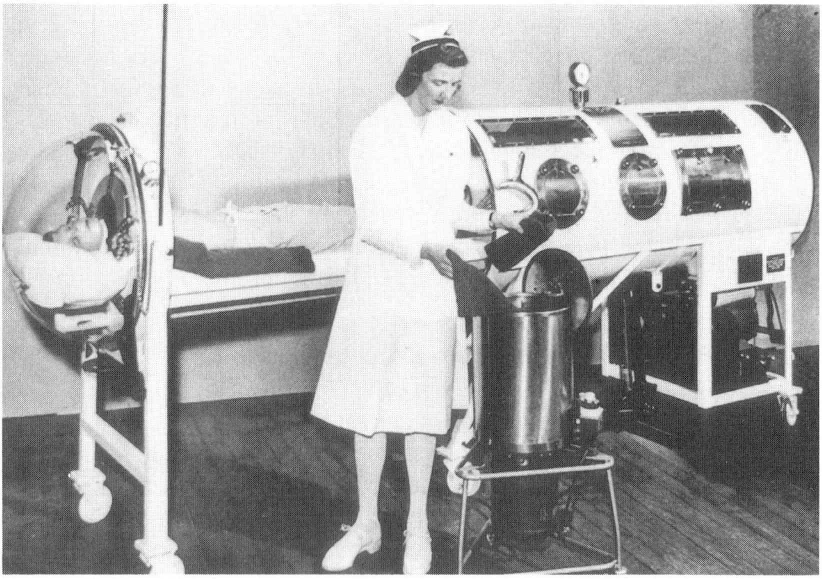

Figure 1 Emerson tank ventilator ("iron lung") opened for nurse to apply hot packs to polio patient circa 1950. Patient is ventilated by intermittent positive pressure in dome within which patient's head is sealed. Tank would be closed for negative-pressure ventilation and dome removed after application of packs.

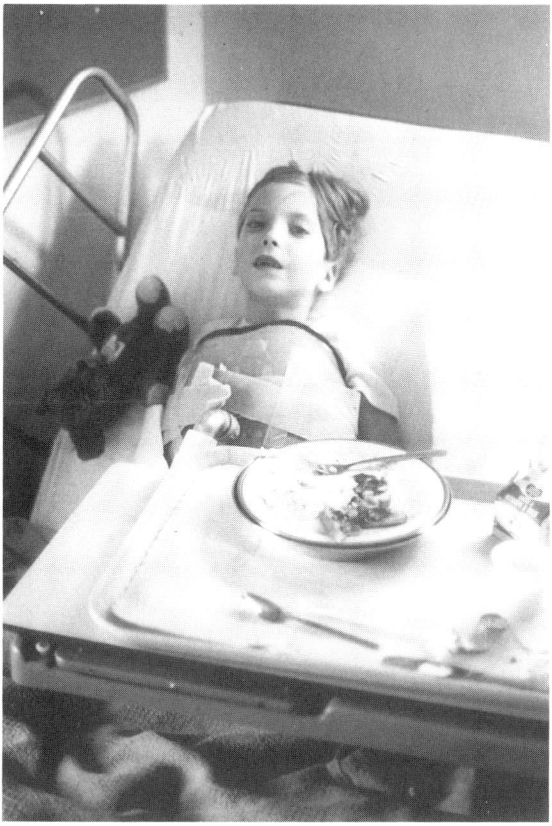

Figure 2 Chest shell or cuirass ventilation in 3-year-old boy with high cervical cord injury. Pump that evacuates space between patient and shell rhythmically is not shown.

hypoventilation consequent to the primary impairment. They vary greatly, however, in their implications for personal care, mobility, and life quality.

The magnitude of the logistical implications is reflected in the dimensions (Fig. 1) and weight (700 lb) of a tank respirator for an adult as compared to a representative positive-pressure ventilator (30 lb). In addition to its compactness, the latter can run on its battery for short periods and is readily adjustable with respect to inspiration and expiration ratio, flow rate, tidal volume, respiratory frequency and the delivery of sighs. It can be mounted on a battery-powered wheelchair, which in turn can use vehicular transportation and reach much of the world at large (Fig. 5). It makes home care of the ventilator-dependent individual a realistic possibility.

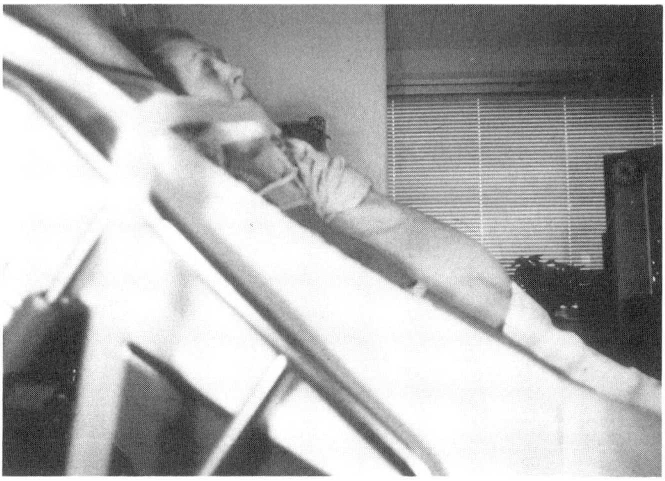

(A)

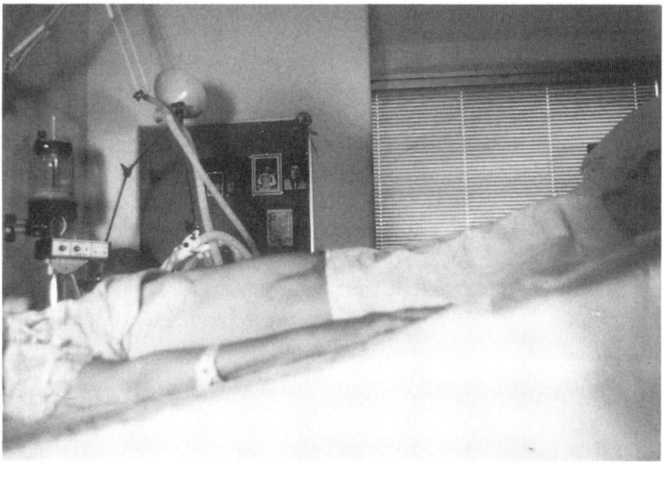

(B)

Figure 3 Ventilation by rocking bed in 65-year-old patient with Guillain-Barré syndrome and paresis of intercostals and diaphragms. Change in configuration of abdomen reflects (A) passive descent and (B) rise of diaphragms.

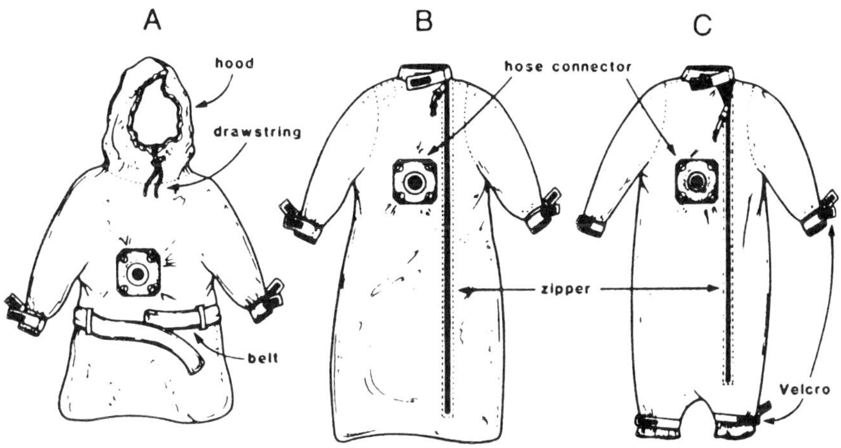

Figure 4 Within each suit, a rigid, perforated frame surrounds patient's chest and abdomen. Rhythmical evacuation of sealed suit expands chest and abdomen into frame during inspiration (From Ref. 30.)

V. Effectiveness with Tracheostomy Present

These technological advances have paralleled accepting tracheostomy as the preferred approach to the airways in many patients who come to rehabilitation as ventilator-dependent individuals (33). The hazards are primarily two: endotracheal damage (Fig. 6) and the consequences of eliminating expiratory airflow through the upper trachea, the larynx, and the pharynx (Fig. 7) (34). Both are the consequence of sealing the cannula within the trachea with an inflatable cuff. The disability resulting from imposing the sacrifice of phonation is difficult to exaggerate.

Cuff inflation is obligatory when precise coupling of the patient to the ventilator is critical for survival, a common intensive care circumstance. Inflation is not necessary, however, for trouble-free respiratory homeostasis of individuals with intact cognition and laryngeal control. These patients quickly learn to vary their glottic resistance so as to apportion tidal output of the ventilator between alveolar ventilation and flow through the larynx (33,34). Both protection from aspiration and oral communication are restored (35–37). During sleep in the supine position, the resistance to outflow through the larynx and pharynx suffices to preserve alveolar ventilation despite the absence of active glottic control or of an inflated cuff. The narrowing of the relaxed pharynx in the supine position doubtless contributes to the explanation (38).

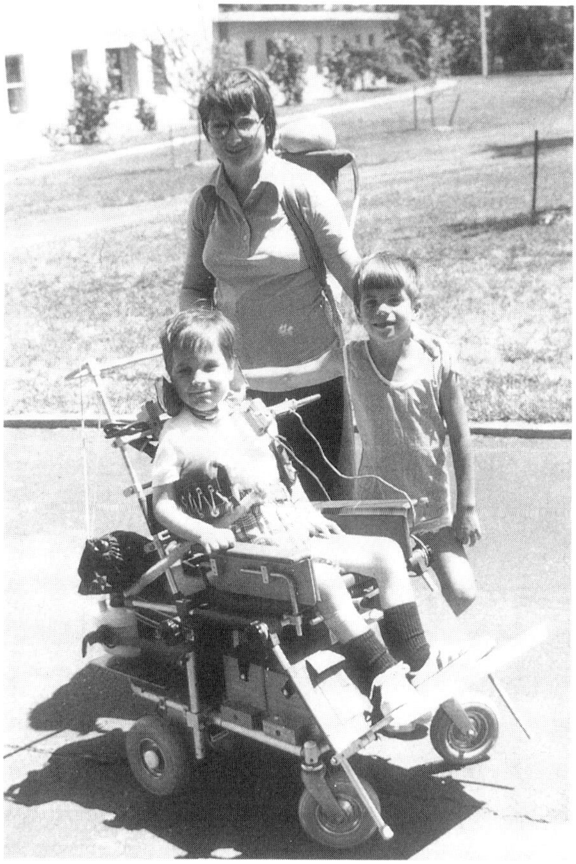

Figure 5 Family picture of 4-year-old boy with high cervical cord trauma and paralysis of intercostals and diaphragms. Ventilation by battery-powered, positive-pressure pump mounted on electric wheelchair. Uncuffed tracheostomy cannula. Chin control allowed independent steering. Patient has graduated from high school.

For the non-ventilator-dependent individual with an open tracheostomy, oral communication may be preserved by valving the tracheostomy cannula to allow only inspiratory flow, forcing expiratory flow through the larynx (Fig. 8) (39–41). This compensation restores not only voice, but the ability to clear the upper airway by airflow during coughing or throat clearing, and frees both hands for bimanual activities rather than requiring finger occlusion of the cannula for speaking.

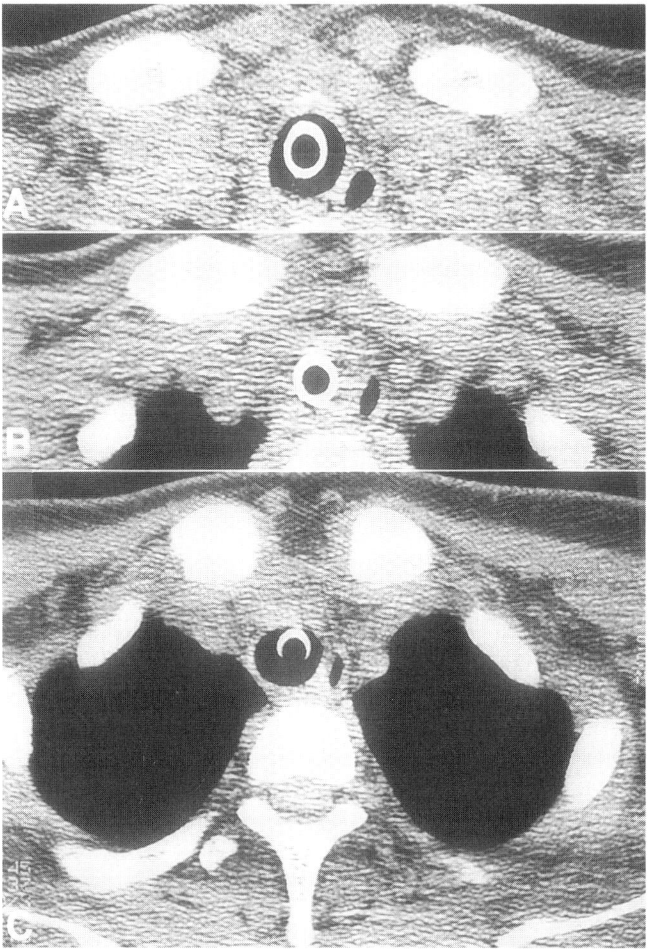

Figure 6 Tracheal stenosis in patient previously on positive-pressure ventilation and cuffed cannula. Magnetic resonance imaging cuts of trachea with #6 Shiley uncuffed cannula. (A) Above stenosis. (B) At stenosis. (C) End of cannula beyond stenosis. Patency of airway (dark shadow) required presence of cannula (open circle).

Accessing the airways through the nose by application of a carefully fitted nasal mask (Fig. 9) that is airtight against the skin at the pressures required for ventilation is a major advance for ventilatory insufficiency and obstructive apnea. When this is added to positive pressure by mouth, electrophrenic respiration (32), and the negative-pressure equipment mentioned previously, the op-

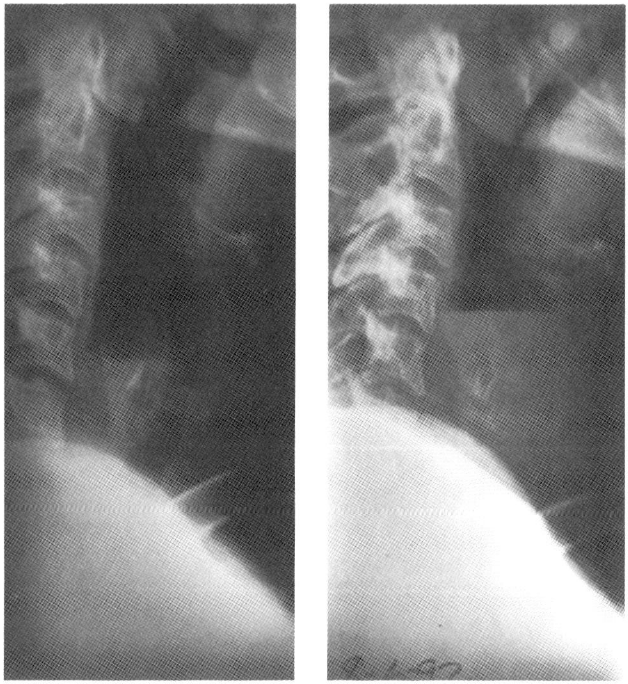

Figure 7 Pharyngeal fluid level before (right) and after (left) deflation of cuff on tracheostomy cannula. Copious secretions were suctioned from trachea after deflation. Patient with brainstem stroke. (From Ref. 37.)

tions for noninvasive alternatives to tracheostomy and positive pressure are several. Their effectiveness in practiced hands justifies the exercise of thoughtful restraint in performing tracheostomy for managing ventilation insufficiency.

VI. Effectiveness with Impaired Cough

Hypoxia and hypercapnia due to alveolar hypoventilation are the secondary impairments consequent to insufficient strength or endurance of the muscles of inspiration. Weakness or paralysis of expiratory muscles usually occurs concurrently but may occur in isolation, as in cervical cord injury. Disabilities arise that are attributable specifically to the inability to raise subglottic pressure beyond relaxation pressure values. These pertain to elimination, parturition, vocal intensity and duration, and cough (42). Because the latter is of particular conse-

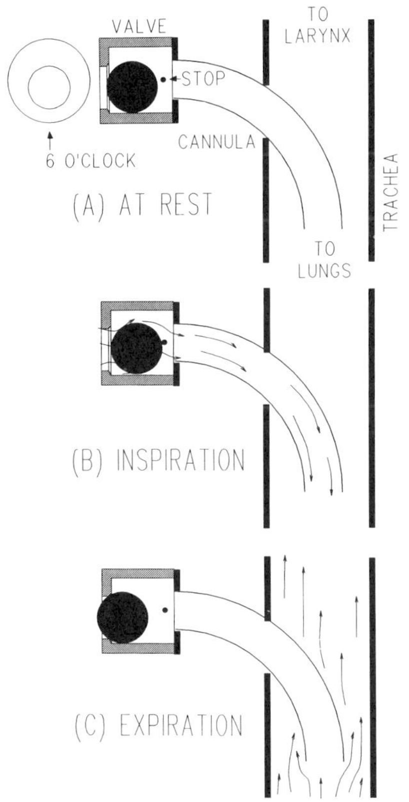

Figure 8 Ball valve for preserving speech in presence of tracheostomy.

quence to bronchopulmonary health, measures to compensate are essential. Figure 10 shows that a normal airflow velocity for coughing can be achieved despite paralysis of abdominal and intercostal muscles simply by combining a deep inspiration under oral positive pressure with a downward and upward thrust on the upper abdomen of the supine patient (43). This "quad cough" variant of the Heimlich maneuver (44) becomes lifesaving when bronchopulmonary secretions are profuse, cough is impaired, and the absence of tracheostomy precludes easy suctioning of the airways. Patients who have learned glossopharyngeal ("frog") breathing can use this technique for inflating their lungs under positive pressure, this being generated by pharyngeal musculature rather than exogenous sources.

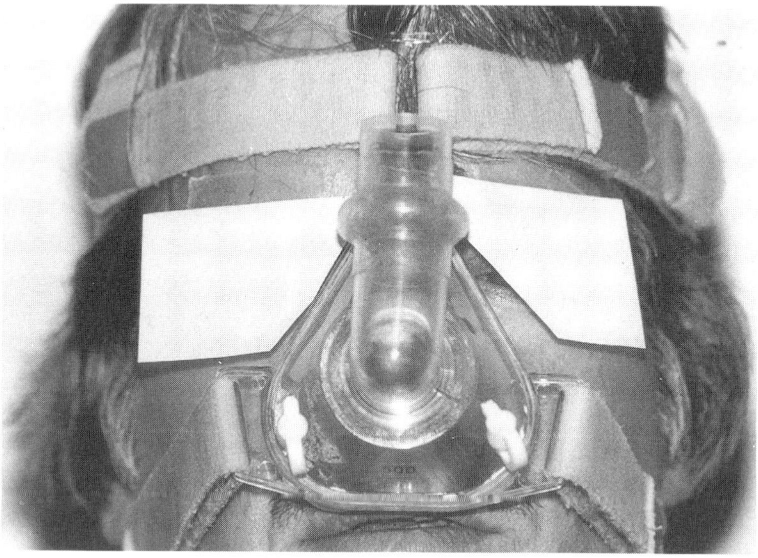

Figure 9 Mask for intermittent positive-pressure ventilation delivered through nose. Hose from pump fits plastic coupler. Leak through open mouth is prevented by seal of velum against tongue. Postpoliomyelitis syndrome. Mask used for sleep.

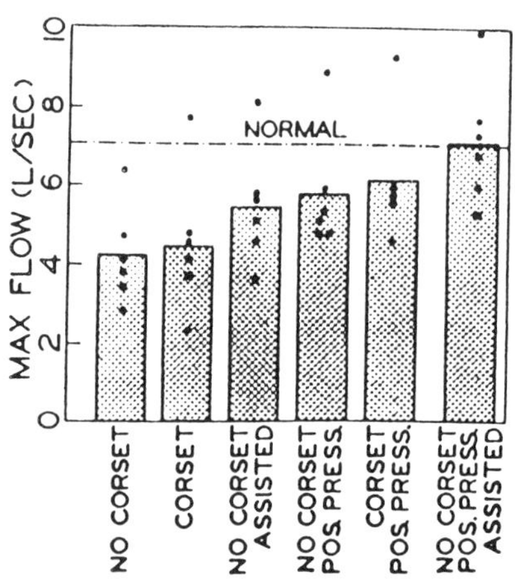

Figure 10 Peak expiratory flow rates (L/sec) during cough in six patients with intercostal and abdominal muscle paralysis but intact diaphragms. Dots are mean of three measurements under circumstances identified. "Assisted" refers to "quad coughing" described in text. (From Ref. 42.)

VII. Teams and Effectiveness

Because rehabilitation is time-intensive and its objectives are broad, effectiveness requires specialization. The strengths of physicians lie primarily in establishing a supportive relationship and applying medical science to the reduction of impairment. Lessening disability and handicap, however, additionally requires assisting cough, managing respiratory equipment, restoring oral communication and safe swallowing, optimizing homemaking, exercising for strength and endurance, and counseling toward personal and family adjustment. These and other objectives require the skills, time, patience, and motivating spirit of nurses, respiratory therapists, speech-language pathologists, occupational therapists, physical therapists, and social workers, respectively. The concept of team function, generic to rehabilitation generally, is indispensable to effective pulmonary rehabilitation.

References

1. International Classification of Impairments, Disabilities and Handicaps. Geneva: World Health Organization, 1980.
2. Bartechi CE, McKenzie TD, Schrier RW. The human costs of tobacco use. N Engl J Med 1994; 330:907:330–975.
3. Snider GL et al. Report of National Heart, Lung and Blood Institute Workshop. Am Rev Respir Dis 1975; 132:182.
4. Holland WW. Chronic obstructive lung disease prevention. Br J Dis Chest 1988; 82:182.
5. Statistical Abstract of the United States, 113th Ed. 1993, Table 210, p. 138.
6. Statistical Abstract of the United States, 113th Ed. 1993, Table 208, p. 136.
7. Statistical Abstract of the United States, 113th Ed. 1993, Table 1271, p. 758.
8. Baltimore Sun, October 25, 1994, p. 14A.
9. Lippiatt BC. Measuring medical cost and life expectancy impacts of changes in cigarette sales. Prev Med 1990; 19:515.
10. Barcroft J. Anoxaemia. Lancet 1920; 2:485.
11. Haldane JS. The symptoms, cause and prevention of anoxaemia. Br Med J 1919; 2:65.
12. Grant I, Heaton AK, McSweeny AJ, et al. Neuropsychologic findings in hypoxemic chronic obstructive pulmonary disease. Arch Intern Med 1982; 142:1470.
13. McSweeny AJ, Grant I, Hecton RK, et al. Life quality of patients with chronic obstructive pulmonary disease. Arch Intern Med 1982; 142:473.
14. Krop HD, Block AJ, Cohen E. Neuropsychologic effects of continuous oxygen therapy in chronic obstructive pulmonary disease. Chest 1973; 64:317.
15. Report of the Medical Research Council Working Party. Long term domiciliary oxygen therapy in chronic hypoxic corpulmonale complicating chronic bronchitis and emphysema. Lancet 1981; 681.

16. Gould, GA, Forsyth IS, Flenly DC. Comparison of two oxygen conserving nasal prong systems and the effects of nose and mouth breathing. Thorax 1986; 41:808.
17. Christopher KL, Spofford BT, Petrum MD, et al. A program for transtracheal oxygen delivery: assessment of safety and efficacy. Ann Intern Med 1987; 107:802.
18. Cooper, CB. Long-term oxygen therapy. In: Casaburi R, Petty TL. Principles and Practice of Pulmonary Rehabilitation. Philadelphia: WB Saunders, 1993:183.
19. Downey RJ, Waissman C. Physiologic changes associated with bed rest and major body injury. In: The Physiological Basis of Rehabilitation Medicine, 2nd ed. Boston: Butterworth-Heinemann, 1994:447.
20. Casaburi R. Exercise training in chronic obstructive lung disease. In: Casaburi R, Petty TL. Principles and Practice of Pulmonary Rehabilitation. Philadelphia: WB Saunders, 1993:204.
21. Bouchard C, Sheppard R. Physical activity, fitness and health: the model and key concepts. In: Bouchard C, Sheppard RJ. Physical Activity, Fitness and Health. Champaign, IL: Human Kinetics, 1994:77.
22. Campbell EJM, Morton HB, Riley RL. Mechanisms of airway obstruction. Bull Johns Hopkins Hosp 1957; 101:329.
23. DiRienzo S. Bronchial dynamism. Radiology 1949; 53:168.
24. Barach AL. Breathing exercises in pulmonary emphysema and allied chronic respiratory disease. Arch Phys Med Rehabil 1955; 36:379.
25. Faling LJ. Controlled breathing techniques and chest physical therapy in chronic obstructive pulmonary disease and allied conditions. In: Casaburi R, Petty TL. Principles and Practice of Pulmonary Rehabilitation. Philadelphia: WB Saunders, 1993:167.
26. DeTroyer A. Respiratory muscle function in chronic obstructive pulmonary disease. In: Casaburi R, Petty TL. Principles and Practice of Pulmonary Rehabilitation. Philadelphia: WB Saunders, 1993:33.
27. Cockcroft A, Saunders M, Berry G. Randomized controlled trial of rehabilitation in chronic respiratory disability. Thorax 1981; 36:200.
28. Foster S, Lopez D, Thomes HM. Pulmonary rehabilitation in COPD patients with elevated Pco_2. Am Rev Respir Dis 1988; 138:1521.
29. Guyatt GH, Berman LB, Townsend M. Long-term outcome after respiratory rehabilitation. Can Med Assoc J 1987; 137:1089.
30. Levine S, Levy S, Henson D. Negative-pressure ventilation. Crit Care Clin 1990; 6:509; Can Med Assoc J 1987; 137:1089.
31. Glenn W, Holeums, McLoughlin A, et al. Total ventilatory support in a quadriplegic patient with radio-frequency electrophrenic respiration. N Engl J Med 1972; 286:513.
32. Esclerin A, Bravo P, Arroyo O, McKenzie J, Garrido H, Alcaraz M. Tracheostomy ventilation versus diaphragmatic pacemaker ventilation in high spinal injury. Paraplegia 1994; 32:687.
33. Bach J, Alba A. Tracheostomy ventilation. Chest 1990; 97:679.
34. Tippett D, Siebens A. Preserving oral communication in individuals with tracheostomy and ventilator dependency. Am J Speech-Lang Pathol (in press).

35. Hoit J, Shea S, Benzett R. Speech production during mechanical ventilation in tracheostomized individuals. J Speech Hearing Res 1994; 37:53.
36. Tippett D, Siebens A. Using ventilators for speaking and swallowing. Dysphagia 1991; 6:94.
37. Siebens A Tippett D, Kirby N, French J. Dysphagia and expiratory airflow. Dysphagia 1993; 8:266.
38. Weller J, Siebens A, Marshall T, Tippett D, Kirby N. The effect of position on cross-sectional area of pharynx. Denver, Colorado, March 12–15, 1995.
39. French J, Siebens A, Kummel J, Kirby N, Eisele J. Preserving communication and airway clearance in tracheotomized children and adults. Arch Phys Med Rehabil 1984; 65:651.
40. Passy V. Passy-Muir tracheostomy speaking valve. Otolaryngol Head Neck Surg 1986; 95:247.
41. Fornataro-Clerici L, Zajac D. Aerodynamic characteristics of tracheostomy speaking valves. J Speech Hearing Res 1993; 529.
42. Siebens A, Kirby N, Poulos D. Cough following transaction of spinal cord at C-6. Arch Phys Med Rehabil 1964; 45:1.
43. Kirby N, Barnerias M, Siebens A. An evaluation of assisted cough in quadriparetic patients. Arch Phys Med Rehabil 1966; 47:705.
44. Heimlich JH. A Life-saving maneuver to prevent food choking. JAMA 1975; 234:398.

14

Assessing Health-Related Quality of Life in Chronic Pulmonary Disease

J. RANDALL CURTIS

University of Washington
Seattle, Washington

Chronic pulmonary diseases, such as chronic obstructive pulmonary disease (COPD), inoperable lung cancer, cystic fibrosis, and severe asthma, are usually incurable and, for many individuals, inexorably progressive. Consequently, health care providers spend much of their efforts trying to minimize these patients' symptoms and improve their ability to function in day-to-day life. While improved survival time is an important goal of therapy, there is growing recognition that improving the *quantity* of an individual's life may not be the only goal; for some, especially those with debilitating and incurable disease, improving the *quality* of life may be far more important. Since reducing symptoms, increasing function, and improving the quality of life are central therapeutic goals for many chronic diseases, it is important for researchers and clinicians to develop a common understanding of what is meant by functional status and quality of life.

Health service researchers have been exploring ways to measure quality of life for many years. In the past 10 years, there has been an increasing body of literature concerning the measurement of quality of life in patients with several chronic pulmonary diseases, and more recently, the efficacy of therapeutic agents has been examined using quality-of-life measures. Studies measuring the quality of life in patients with COPD rose in number in the mid-1980s (1–7).

More recently, these measures have been used in the assessment of theophylline (8), inhaled bronchodilators (9), home respiratory nursing care (10), and pulmonary rehabilitation programs (11). Some work has also been done in assessment of quality of life for individuals with nonoperable lung cancer (12), asthma (13–15), and cystic fibrosis (16). As this trend continues, it is increasingly important for physicians to understand and critically assess these measures to help decide whether a new therapy should be applied to their patients.

This chapter provides an overview of quality-of-life measures as applied to patients with chronic pulmonary diseases, concentrating specifically on COPD, where much of this work has been done. The emphasis is on issues important to the clinician who seeks an understanding of quality-of-life measures as they are used in therapeutic trials. The chapter first deals with general issues concerning the measurement of quality of life and some of the specific instruments that have been developed for COPD. COPD is then used as an example to highlight some of the insights provided by quality-of-life assessment. Finally, the chapter explores potential uses of these instruments in clinical practice.

I. Definition and Relevance of Health-Related Quality of Life

A. Terms and Definitions

The term "quality of life" is widely used in clinical research and clinical care, but rarely defined. In its broadest definition, the quality of an individual's life is a holistic, self-determined evaluation of satisfaction with issues important to the individual and is influenced by many factors that health care does not directly impact. These factors may include financial status, housing, employment, and social support network. Consequently, many researchers favor the more restrictive term "health-related quality of life" (HRQL) to mean the quality of life as it is affected by the individual's health status. The term "functional status" is used to describe an individual's ability to function in such diverse realms as physical, social, and emotional. These two terms, HRQL and functional status, are often used interchangeably. Functional status connotes a stronger basis in ability to perform the tasks of daily life, while HRQL connotes a more subjective experience of the impact of health on the quality of one's life. HRQL is used in this chapter because it has the broadest implications.

In its most general definition, HRQL measures the impact of an individual's health on his or her ability to perform and enjoy the activities of daily life. The operational definition of HRQL depends, in part, on the specific measure being chosen and its purpose. HRQL instruments vary from disease-specific measures assessing the severity of particular symptoms, such as dyspnea or cough (3), to a generic global assessment of many facets of HRQL, which may include emotional functioning (mood changes and other psychiatric symptoms), social role functioning (employment, home management, and social/family relationships), activities of daily living (self-care skills and mobility), and the ability to engage in enjoyable activities (hobbies and recreation) (1).

The operational definition of HRQL also varies somewhat depending on the intended purpose. In general, outcome measures can have at least three purposes: discriminating between subjects at a single point in time, prognosticating, and evaluating changes within a given subject over time. While the intended purpose does not alter development and application of many physiological measures, the design of HRQL measures may vary substantially depending on how it will be used (17). To discriminate among a group of subjects, questionnaire items are selected to represent all important components of HRQL and to be applicable to as many individuals as possible. In contrast, for use in a therapeutic trial, the purpose of a HRQL measure is to detect change over time in an individual. Thus, questionnaire items are chosen only if they reflect features amenable to change. An example from the Sickness Impact Profile was chosen by Deyo in a recent review to illustrate this point (18). A positive response to the statement "I have attempted suicide" would indicate a high level of emotional distress and help discriminate among individuals. However, the response would remain positive at subsequent testing and consequently would not help measure change over time. In contrast, the number of stairs an individual can climb would be an effective gauge of change over time, but it might not be a useful discriminative tool in a group of older adults who have made environmental changes to avoid stairs.

B. Relevance and Usefulness of HRQL

A common criticism of HRQL is that it is highly subjective. This criticism maintains that HRQL is therefore inherently immeasurable or, at best, "soft" data. It is axiomatic that HRQL is subjective, since it is the individual patient's perspective that is the most important measure of HRQL. If we are concerned with the patient's perspective on HRQL, we should measure it directly. Is this subjective quality necessarily immeasurable or "soft"? The crucial attribute of "hardness" is the reproducibility of a measure (19). HRQL measures *are* able to provide adequate and often excellent reproducibility. If physiological measures accurately reflected HRQL, it could be argued that HRQL measures would be unnecessary. However, physiological measures, such as pulmonary function parameters and exercise tolerance, do not correlate strongly with measures of HRQL (1,2,20).

HRQL should not be measured in every therapeutic trial or longitudinal survey. There are circumstances where survival is the paramount outcome measure and HRQL is irrelevant. An example would be a randomized controlled trial of corticosteroids in COPD patients with acute respiratory failure. The goal of this short-term treatment is to improve survival or shorten the course of the acute illness, and HRQL is less important in judging efficacy. In other instances, therapy may be applied to asymptomatic adults to prevent disease, such as a trial of smoking cessation techniques. In this case, HRQL would not be expected to be a sensitive outcome measure and the benefit would be more appropriately demonstrated in terms of smoking cessation.

Finally, HRQL measures can be especially useful in trials designed to assess treatments that differ dramatically in cost, side effects, or degree of invasiveness. For instance, in trials of extensive pulmonary rehabilitation or even lung transplantation, HRQL would be an important component to factor into cost-effectiveness analyses.

II. Measurement Issues

A. Generic Versus Disease-Specific Measures

HRQL instruments may be designed to assess overall quality of life or only those aspects directly related to a single disease. For instance, COPD-specific instruments may assess only a single symptom, such as dyspnea (3). They could also measure a series of symptoms, e.g., dyspnea, cough, and sputum production, plus components of life particularly affected by COPD, e.g., exercise tolerance and mood (4). Generic instruments also represent a spectrum from one question on overall quality of life, to a series of questions about different dimensions of HRQL. The generic HRQL instruments are often divided into sections devoted to different dimensions, such as physical discomfort, role functioning, emotional well-being, and social interactions. In addition, generic HRQL instruments may include a summary score allowing investigators to assign a single number to overall HRQL and use this score for cost-effectiveness analyses.

Disease-specific and generic instruments each have their advantages (21). The optimal choice of the type of instrument depends, in part, on whether it is to be used in an evaluative or a discriminative study and, in part, on the specific question under study. While there may be no single correct approach, an understanding of the issues will help the clinician to assess appropriate use of HRQL instruments. Disease-specific instruments are likely to be more sensitive to small changes in a therapeutic trial (an evaluative study) of an agent targeted at the specific symptoms of COPD. For instance, an instrument to measure dyspnea is more likely to show a benefit of bronchodilators than a generic HRQL instrument. In addition, disease-specific instruments relate closely to the clinical history explored frequently by the pulmonary clinician and, consequently, may be more readily understandable to the clinician.

Generic instruments often have the advantage of being more thoroughly tested in a variety of clinical settings and populations. The breadth of HRQL issues that they cover may reveal important, but unexpected, impacts of the treatment. In addition, they are more likely to appropriately weigh diverse side effects of treatment and establish an overall assessment of the impact of treatment on the patient's life. This may be particularly important in evaluation of chemotherapy for nonoperable lung cancer where diverse nonpulmonary side effects of treatment may have a large impact on HRQL (22,23). Finally, generic instruments are necessary if one wishes to compare the HRQL benefits of interventions for widely disparate conditions; e.g., is lung transplantation as cost-effective as heart transplantation (24,25)?

B. Reproducibility, Validity, and Responsiveness

Three features of a questionnaire are important for clinicians to understand before assessing evidence based on HRQL instruments. The first is the reproducibility (or reliability) of the instrument. The term "reproducibility" is used to indicate whether the instrument is resilient to confounding variation in the environment. There are various components to reproducibility, including test-retest reproducibility (how vulnerable the instrument is to unimportant day-to-day variations in subjects' response), interobserver reproducibility (whether different administrators of the instrument get the same results from the same individual), and internal consistency (whether different parts of the instrument give consistent results). These reproducibility and internal consistency issues are not necessarily reexamined with each study using the instrument, but investigators should be convinced that this work has been done in the past and that the instrument fulfills the basic measurement expectations. It is best to assess these properties in a large study of a diverse population, because reproducibility may vary among clinical populations, depending on education, age, frailty, or other patient characteristics.

Validity is a more difficult issue to assess in HRQL and yet is the primary issue in development of a HRQL instrument. Validity asks the question, is this instrument really measuring the impact of health on an individual's quality of life? In the area of HRQL, there is no reference standard against which to measure an instrument. Consequently, correlations with biological indicators of disease severity, such as FEV_1 and exercise tolerance, and with other HRQL instruments must be used as proxies for a "gold standard." In this situation, very high correlations are not expected, since the goal is not to duplicate these other measures and thereby produce a redundant measure. Nonetheless, the instrument should correlate in the expected direction with important markers of disease severity and with other HRQL instruments. This process, known as "construct validation," is an ongoing process since no single critical observation or "criterion" can definitively establish validity. This is in contrast to "criterion validity," in which a true "gold standard" or criterion exists. Some of these correlations should be provided with each use of an instrument in a clinical trial so the reader can be reassured that the instrument is valid in the population under study.

For clinical trials or other longitudinal evaluations, responsiveness is a key feature of HRQL instruments. In this setting, responsiveness evaluates whether the instrument can distinguish small, but clinically important, changes over time. In other words, how sensitive is the instrument to important changes in HRQL? This is a critical issue for the use of HRQL instruments in clinical trials since the intent is to demonstrate a benefit (or lack of benefit) from a specific therapy. A HRQL instrument should be demonstrated to be responsive prior to its use in a clinical trial. Conversely, a large controlled trial might easily be able to identify statistically significant differences in HRQL that are clinically irrelevant. This is less an issue in biological measures, since clinicians are often more familiar with these measures. For example, a clinician can examine a statistically significant improvement of 10 ml in FEV_1 from a large study and dismiss it as clinically unimportant. However, with HRQL measures, it is usually the responsibility of the researchers to identify the minimal clinically important difference (26).

C. Statistical Issues

In any research, it is important for the investigators to identify the key hypotheses prior to data collection and to honestly report when hypotheses were generated by analysis of associations in the data. This is particularly important in HRQL because these instruments often have multiple components and are conducive to "data torturing" (27). If post hoc analyses are performed, some attempt should be made to adjust the level of statistical significance appropriately for the problem of multiple comparisons (28).

Sample size, or power, calculations are a critical part of designing and evaluating clinical studies. Sample size calculations are problematic in trials using HRQL instruments because the relative inexperience with these measures may make it difficult to estimate the minimal clinically important difference, a central component of these calculations. The difficulty with power calculations is usually considered to be the problem of the researcher, not the clinician. However, in a trial showing no benefit of therapy, the power of the trial to find a benefit becomes of foremost interest to the clinician trying to decide whether to abandon this therapy. If power calculations are unreliable, it becomes difficult to judge the value of the trial.

III. Selected HRQL Instruments

A. Generic HRQL Instruments

Four generic HRQL instruments have been used extensively in patients with chronic pulmonary diseases. Table 1 shows some important features of each of these instruments.

The generic HRQL instrument that has been used most extensively in patients with COPD is the Sickness Impact Profile (SIP). This comprehensive, 136-item, self-administered questionnaire was developed to measure HRQL in a wide variety of chronic diseases. The instrument assesses a broad range of areas, including ambulation, body care, mobility, emotional behavior, social behavior, work, sleep, eating, home management, and recreational activities. It is one of the longest instruments, requiring 20–30 min to complete. It has undergone extensive testing to establish its reproducibility and validity (29), although its responsiveness has not been studied in patients with chronic pulmonary diseases. The SIP has been used to describe the HRQL in patients with COPD (1,2,30,31). It has also been used in patients with asthma (14,15) and patients with inoperable lung cancer (32,33). In addition, the SIP has been used in patients with COPD to assess the value of continuous oxygen therapy (5), antidepressant therapy (34), home respiratory nursing care (10), and intermittent positive-pressure breathing (6).

Another generic instrument was developed from the Medical Outcomes Study (MOS), a physicians' office-based, cross-sectional study of 9385 adults (35). This is a 20-item, self-administered instrument developed from a large number of questions and divided into two components. The first component examines physical functioning, role functioning, and social functioning. The second component examines mental health, health perceptions, and bodily pain. This instrument requires approximately 5 min to complete and was shown to be reproducible and valid (35). COPD was one of the diseases examined in this survey (36). A related instrument has been shown to be valid in assessing HRQL in cystic fibrosis (37). The MOS instruments have the advantage of brevity, but, like the SIP, responsiveness in patients with chronic lung diseases has not been thoroughly examined. More recently, the authors of the MOS instruments have prepared a 36-item "short form," known as the MOS SF-36 (38). This generic health status instrument is being widely disseminated for outcomes research and has been adopted by a number of researchers and health care organizations. Its validity has been well described (39), but studies among COPD populations are limited (40).

The Quality of Well Being (QWB) is a 50-item, interviewer-administered questionnaire developed as a subcomponent of a larger health outcomes measure, the Health Status Index (41). The QWB is divided into three scales: mo-

Table 1 Selected HRQL Instruments Used in Patients with COPD

Instrument	Domains and dimensions examined	Length	Administration	Reproducible, valid, and responsive
Generic				
Sickness Impact Profile (SIP)	Physical: ambulation, mobility, body care Social: general well-being, work/social role performance, social support and participation, global social function, personal relationships, and global emotional functioning	136 items (30 min)	Self-administered	Reproducibility, validity, and responsiveness well demonstrated
Medical Outcomes Study (MOS)	Functioning: physical, role, and social Well-being: mental health, health perceptions, and bodily pain	20 items (3 min)	Self-administered	Reproducibility and validity well demonstrated; responsiveness in COPD not well studied
Quality of Well Being (QWB)	Mobility: access to modes of transportation Physical: limits to activity Social: limits to activity Symptoms: review of systems	50 items (12 min)	Trained interviewer administered	Reproducible and valid; responsiveness in COPD not well demonstrated
Nottingham Health Profile (NHP)	Health: energy, pain, emotional reactions, sleep, social isolation, physical mobility Life functioning: employment, relationships, personal life, sex, hobbies, vacations, housework	45 items (10 min)	Self-administered	Reproducible and valid; responsiveness in COPD not well demonstrated

COPD-specific				
Chronic Respiratory Disease Questionnaire (CRDQ)	Dyspnea, fatigue, mastery over disease, emotional dysfunction	20 items (20 min)	Trained interviewer administered	Reproducibility, validity, and responsiveness well demonstrated
St. George's Respiratory Questionnaire (SGRQ)	Symptoms: cough, sputum, wheeze, breathlessness Activity: physical functioning, housework, hobbies Impact on daily life: social and emotional impact	76 items (? min)	Self-administered	Reproducibility, validity, and responsiveness well demonstrated
Oxygen Cost Diagram (OCD)	Single vertical line to be marked in location to indicate degree of disability caused by dyspnea	1 item (<5 min)	Self-administered	Intermediate reproducibility and validity; not as responsive as SGRQ
Baseline Dyspnea Index (BDI)	Functional impairment, magnitude of task evoking dyspnea, magnitude of effort evoking dyspnea	3 indices with four grades (<5 min)	Trained interviewer administered	Reproducibility, validity, and responsiveness well demonstrated

bility, physical activity, and social activity. The QWB score is expressed as the value that subjects associate with a particular combination of function and symptoms. Consequently, the QWB can be used for quantitative assessment and cost-effectiveness analysis. It has been shown to be reproducible and valid (42,43) and has been used to describe HRQL in patients with COPD (44) and cystic fibrosis (16). In addition, the QWB has been used to assess home respiratory nursing care (10) and pulmonary rehabilitation programs (11) in COPD, and lung transplantation (24) and antibiotic therapy (45) in cystic fibrosis. Although the QWB does not assess as many domains as the SIP or the MOS, it has the unique advantage of being applicable to cost-effectiveness analysis.

Finally, the Nottingham Health Profile (NHP) is a 45-item, self-administered questionnaire composed of two parts. The first part contains 38 items assessing energy, pain, emotional reactions, sleep, social isolation, and physical mobility. The second part contains seven items covering the areas of life functioning most often affected by health problems. This self-administered instrument takes 10 min to complete. It is reproducible and valid in the assessment of chronic diseases (46) and has been used to describe HRQL in patients with COPD (47). The NHP has recently been used to assess inhaled bronchodilators in patients with COPD (48) and is also being used to assess HRQL in heart-lung transplantation for cystic fibrosis (49).

Several other instruments that measure mood, depression, anxiety, and other psychiatric symptoms have been used to assess patients with chronic lung disease. These include the Minnesota Multiphasic Personality Inventory (MMPI), the Profile of Mood States (POMS), and the Beck Depression Inventory (1,2,34,50). While these instruments have provided insights into the HRQL of persons with COPD and may provide important information in the assessment of therapy, they are not strictly measures of HRQL and will not be discussed in detail in this chapter.

B. Disease-Specific HRQL Instruments: Chronic Obstructive Pulmonary Disease

The Chronic Respiratory Disease Questionnaire (CRDQ) was developed by Guyatt and colleagues through in-depth, unstructured interviews with 100 COPD patients. The result of these interviews was a 20-item questionnaire dealing with dimensions of dyspnea, fatigue, patients' sense of control over the disease (mastery), and emotional dysfunction. This interviewer-administered questionnaire takes 20 min to complete and has been shown to be reproducible, valid, and responsive (51,52). In a head-to-head comparison, the CRDQ was shown to be more valid and more responsive than two other measures of dyspnea, the Oxygen Cost Diagram and the Medical Research Council Dyspnea Questionnaire (52). The CRDQ has been used to assess inhaled bronchodilators (9), theophylline (9,53,54), and nocturnal nasal intermittent positive pressure (55).

The St. George's Respiratory Questionnaire (SGRQ) is a 76-item instrument divided into three components: symptoms, activity, and impact on daily life. This self-administered questionnaire has been shown to be reproducible, valid, and responsive (20). In a comparison with SIP, SGRQ was shown to be twice as responsive as the generic instrument. Jones and colleagues excluded questions explicitly designed to assess anxiety and depression, since other questionnaires are available for this purpose (20).

The Oxygen Cost Diagram (OCD) represents a single vertical line with common activities listed beside it ascending in order of increasing exertional requirements. The activities range from sleeping, at the bottom, to brisk walking uphill, at the top. Patients are asked to indicate the point above which they think their dyspnea would limit their activity. The instrument is moderately reproducible and, as mentioned, less responsive than the CRDQ (51).

The Baseline Dyspnea Index (BDI) was designed by Mahler and colleagues to measure degree of dyspnea as well as the impact of dyspnea on an individual's life. The instrument obtains an interviewer-based rating on three scales: functional impairment, magnitude of task needed to evoke dyspnea, and magnitude of effort needed to evoke dyspnea. These are combined into a baseline score. In addition, Mahler and colleagues developed a transition dyspnea index specifically to measure changes from the baseline condition (3). These indexes have been shown to be reproducible and valid in patients with COPD (3,36,50,56), and are more responsive than the oxygen cost diagram (56). While this instrument concentrates on a single symptom, it is an important symptom in chronic pulmonary diseases and often the target of therapeutic agents. The BDI has been used to assess the value of theophylline for individuals with COPD (8).

C. Disease-Specific HRQL Instruments: Other Pulmonary Diseases

A number of disease-specific instruments have been developed and validated for individuals with asthma. A recent review summarized some of these instruments (13). Those instruments that have been most extensively validated are the Living with Asthma Questionnaire (57,58) and two instruments that have both been titled the Asthma Quality of Life Questionnaire (14,15,59,60). So far, research demonstrating these instruments to be responsive to change in clinical trials is limited.

A number of clinical trials have used cancer-specific HRQL instruments for individuals with inoperable lung cancer. Such instruments include the Functional Living Index-Cancer Scale (61–63) and the European Organization for

Research and Treatment of Cancer Questionnaire (64–66). Several questionnaires have been developed specifically for individuals with lung cancer (67–69). Finally, some studies have used daily diary cards (66,70) or visual analog scales (71,72) to assess HRQL in patients with lung cancer.

IV. Features of the HRQL of Patients with COPD

A. Description of HRQL in Patients with COPD

COPD is the chronic pulmonary disease for which the most extensive HRQL research has been performed, and this research offers an example of the insights HRQL measures can provide. There have been a number of studies describing the HRQL of patients with COPD. These studies vary in their inclusion criteria and consequently examine the HRQL of patients with varying severity of disease. The severity of disease examined has ranged from patients eligible for continuous oxygen therapy having a mean FEV_1 of 0.75 L/sec (30% of predicted) (1) to patients seen in a family practice with a mean FEV_1 of 1.86 (70% predicted) (73). Despite this heterogeneity of disease severity, a clear picture emerges demonstrating that patients with COPD have marked decrements in their HRQL. Stewart and colleagues, using the MOS instrument called the SF-20, showed that patients with COPD had decreased HRQL in all six domains of this instrument: physical functioning, role functioning, social functioning, mental health, health perceptions, and bodily pain (35). Furthermore, COPD patients consistently scored worse on all domains than patients with hypertension, arthritis, and diabetes, and worse than those with chronic back pain on all domains except bodily pain. Similarly, McSweeny and colleagues showed that patients with severe COPD had diminished HRQL in all domains of the SIP except employment (1). Employment is not a sensitive marker of HRQL in COPD because a large proportion of COPD patients are retired. In McSweeny's study, patients with COPD showed the largest decrements of HRQL in the domains of emotional disturbances (primarily depression), recreational activities, home management, and sleep and rest. Likewise, Prigatano and colleagues found diverse decrements of HRQL in a group of COPD patients with moderate disease having a mean FEV_1 of 1.02 L/sec (2). It is interesting to compare the HRQL of patients from these two large studies. The patients studied by Prigatano and colleagues had a mean FEV_1 that was 0.25 L/sec higher and a mean Pao_2 at rest that was 20 mmHg higher than those in the study by McSweeny and colleagues. Although the patients with less severe disease had markedly less impairment on the physical domains of the SIP, they had very similar impairment in psychosocial domains. This suggests that while degree of physical limitation is associated with severity of disease, the degree of psychosocial limitation may not be as strongly influenced by severity of disease once some threshold degree of COPD is present. Another interesting feature of HRQL in patients with COPD is that regardless of the instrument used or the severity of disease studied, sleep and rest are markedly disturbed (1,2,4,47,73).

A final feature of HRQL in COPD worth mention is the association between continued smoking and HRQL. Prigatano and colleagues found that those who continued to smoke had a markedly lower HRQL than those who had quit despite the fact that the smokers were younger and had a higher mean FEV_1 (2). While this does not prove a causal relationship between continued smoking and HRQL, it is intriguing and worthy of further study.

B. Depression, Emotional Dysfunction, and HRQL

One of the most striking findings of the studies describing the HRQL in patients with COPD, is the prominent role that depression and emotional dysfunction play in this disease. In the study of Stewart and colleagues using the SF-20, patients with COPD scored lower on the mental health domain than patients with hypertension, diabetes, congestive heart failure, myocardial infarction, angina, arthritis, and chronic back pain. Only patients with chronic gastrointestinal disorders scored lower in mental health than those with COPD (35).

The influence of depression on the overall HRQL of a group of patients with COPD depends on the prevalence of depression in these patients and the effect of depression on HRQL. McSweeny and colleagues, using the MMPI, found that 42% of patients fit the category of reactive depression compared to 9% of age-matched controls (1). Light and colleagues used a questionnaire designed to detect depression, the Beck Depression Inventory, and found the same prevalence of depression in a group of patients with less severe COPD (50). Prigatano and colleagues used POMS to quantify depression and anxiety and found that both depression and anxiety strongly correlated with the HRQL as measured by the SIP (2). In fact, both depression and anxiety predicted the overall SIP score substantially better than the physiological parameters FEV_1, PaO_2, and exercise tolerance.

C. Physiological Measurements and HRQL

Intuitively, we would expect HRQL to correlate with physiological measures of the severity of COPD. In other words, as the severity of COPD progresses, the HRQL would presumably decrease. Most studies that have compared physiological measures with HRQL measures have shown some weak correlation between these measures. Correlations have been demonstrated for the generic HRQL instruments including the SIP (1,2,20), the QWB (44), and disease-specific instruments such as the BDI (3) and the SGRQ (20). However, not all studies demonstrate such correlations (1,31) and these correlations, when present, are weak.

The most widely used measure of the severity of COPD is the FEV_1. The FEV_1 has been shown to be an accurate predictor of prognosis and survival (74). While most studies have shown that FEV_1 is statistically correlated with various measures of HRQL (2,3,20,44,73), a few have shown no significant correlation (1,47). Even studies demonstrating a correlation have found that FEV_1 is less well correlated with HRQL than are emotional dysfunction (2,20) and dyspnea (20,36). Similarly, measures of oxygenation, such as Pao_2 and Sao_2, are either weakly correlated with HRQL (44) or not significantly correlated (1,2,47).

Exercise tolerance is a physiological measure that is not well predicted by ventilatory capacity or pulmonary function parameters (75,76). Exercise tolerance correlates with HRQL better than either FEV_1 or oxygenation correlates with HRQL (1,2,20,44,47). Exercise tolerance also correlates with many dyspnea measures better than do pulmonary function parameters (3,77,78). In a study by Jones and colleagues, all the correlation between pulmonary function and HRQL could be accounted for entirely by exercise tolerance (20). However, correlations between exercise tolerance and HRQL are not strong.

Since dyspnea is often used as a marker of disease-specific HRQL, one would expect dyspnea and HRQL instruments to correlate fairly well. Dyspnea, as measured by the Medical Research Council dyspnea scale, the BDI, and a visual analog scale, does correlate well with HRQL and is a better predictor of HRQL than either pulmonary function or oxygenation (20,36,47,73).

In general, summary statistics of correlation from different studies should be compared with caution, since studies have different entry criteria, use different outcome measures, and use different statistical techniques. Nonetheless, the

---

Figure 1 Squared correlation coefficients (R^2) between health-related quality of life (HRQL), dyspnea scale, pulmonary physiological parameters, demographic characteristics, and psychological states. The numbers represent the median of the R^2 values found in the studies cited below with the ranges in parentheses. R^2 can be viewed as an estimate of the proportion of the variability in HRQL or dyspnea that is explained by the given parameter. The arrows do not imply demonstrated causality, but represent the direction of the relation of interest in understanding the role of HRQL measures. (a) Correlation of HRQL and dyspnea with each other and with measures of pulmonary function, oxygenation, and exercise tolerance. (b) Correlation of HRQL with psychological states and demographic variables, and socioeconomic status (SES) (1–3,14,20,29,31,33,35,42,43). Demonstrated is the moderate correlation between HRQL, dyspnea, anxiety, and depression, as well as the weaker correlation between HRQL and the physiological measures such as FEV_1 and Pao_2.

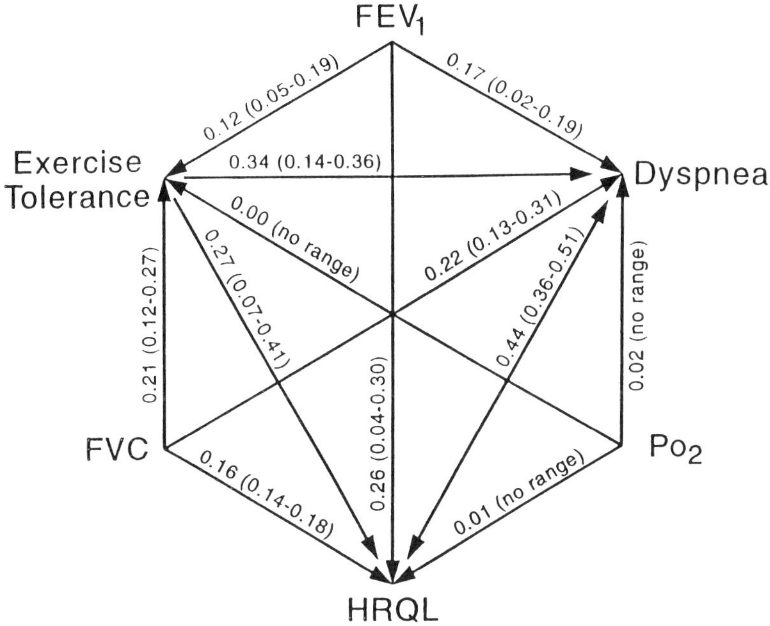
FEV1
Exercise Tolerance
Dyspnea
FVC
Po2
HRQL
0.12 (0.05-0.19)
0.17 (0.02-0.19)
0.34 (0.14-0.36)
0.00 (no range)
0.22 (0.13-0.31)
0.21 (0.12-0.27)
0.27 (0.07-0.41)
0.26 (0.04-0.30)
0.44 (0.36-0.51)
0.02 (no range)
0.16 (0.14-0.18)
0.01 (no range)

(a)

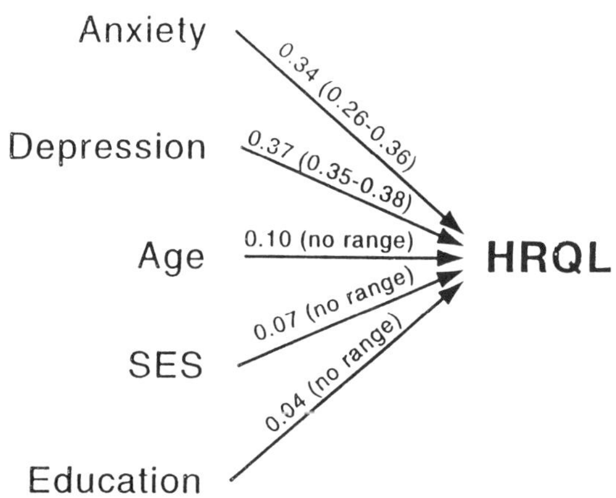
Anxiety
Depression
Age
SES
Education
HRQL
0.34 (0.26-0.36)
0.37 (0.35-0.38)
0.10 (no range)
0.07 (no range)
0.04 (no range)

(b)

squared correlation coefficients (R^2) between different variables in studies of patients with COPD have shown some homogeneity across studies. Figure 1 shows the squared correlation coefficient between HRQL and dyspnea and several physiological, psychological, and descriptive variables. HRQL and the dyspnea scale correlate better with each other than the physiological parameters and descriptive variables correlate with either of them. Depression and anxiety have an intermediate correlation with HRQL and the dyspnea scale.

In summary, several studies have shown than HRQL does correlate with physiological measures of COPD severity and they correlate in the expected direction. That the correlation is not strong or universal to all studies suggests that the physiological parameters do not predict HRQL well and that HRQL instruments provide additional information in the assessment of patients with COPD.

D. Impact of Therapy on HRQL in Patients with COPD

Although descriptive data on the HRQL of patients with COPD are useful, the main concern of clinicians caring for patients with COPD is whether therapeutic interventions will improve HRQL. The instruments described in this review have been used to evaluate a number of specific therapies, and these studies provide insight into both the specific therapies and the role of HRQL instruments in clinical practice.

HRQL has been used to assess pulmonary rehabilitation and home respiratory nursing care. Toshima and colleagues used QWB to evaluate a comprehensive pulmonary rehabilitation program compared to an education-only control program (11). They demonstrated improvements in exercise tolerance with the rehabilitation program, but showed no difference in HRQL. Wijkstra and colleagues, however, demonstrated improved HRQL (using the CRDQ) and exercise tolerance in a randomized-controlled trial of home pulmonary rehabilitation (79). In a controlled trial, Bergner and colleagues showed no benefit in HRQL (using SIP and QWB) from specialized respiratory home care and concluded that current limited coverage of home care services by third-party payers was appropriate (10).

Guyatt and colleagues used the CRDQ to assess inhaled salbutamol and oral theophylline. In 19 patients they showed that both agents individually improved HRQL, FEV_1, exercise tolerance, and peak flow. Although some patients had additional benefit from the two agents used together, this was not statistically significant for the group (9). Mahler and colleagues used the BDI in a cross-over, double-blind trial of theophylline. In this study, the dyspnea scale demonstrated a benefit of theophylline, while spirometry, arterial blood gases, and exercise tolerance did not significantly change (8). More recently, McKay and colleagues have shown improved HRQL, as assessed by CRDQ, with the addition of theophylline to maximal inhaled bronchodilator therapy (53), and Kirsten and colleagues used CRDQ to demonstrate decline in HRQL after short-term withdrawal of theophylline (54).

van Schayck and colleagues examined the impact of routine versus symptomatic inhaled salbutamol and ipratropium therapy on HRQL (using the NHP) and on spirometry (48). Although they found no difference between salbutamol and ipratropium in either HRQL or spirometry, there was a significantly greater decline in FEV_1 in the group receiving continuous therapy compared to those receiving symptomatic therapy. The more rapid decline in FEV_1 was not associated with a decline in HRQL. Since changes in FEV_1 and HRQL did not move in the same direction, this trial emphasizes the importance of measuring HRQL rather than assuming HRQL will change with a physiological parameter such as FEV_1.

Borson and colleagues examined the impact of antidepressant therapy on depression, HRQL (using SIP), spirometry, and exercise tolerance in 36 patients with COPD and depression (34). They found that therapy improved not only anxiety and depression, but also HRQL. There was no significant change in FEV_1, arterial blood gases, or exercise tolerance.

The Nocturnal Oxygen Therapy Trial (NOTT) Group examined the impact of nocturnal versus continuous oxygen therapy in patients with COPD and hypoxemia (5). There was a decreased mortality with continuous oxygen in conjunction with a significant benefit in HRQL as assessed by the SIP. HRQL has been used to assess intermittent positive-pressure ventilation in two separate trials. In the Intermittent Positive Pressure Breathing (IPPB) Trial, 985 patients used either IPPB or a routine compressor nebulizer to receive inhaled bronchodilators and completed the SIP to assess HRQL (6). The authors demonstrated no benefit of IPPB over the nebulizer in HRQL, survival, duration of hospitalization, or lung function. In the second trial, Elliott and colleagues used the CDRQ to assess nocturnal nasal intermittent positive pressure in 12 patients, using each patient as his or her own historical control (55). They found improved sleep time and sleep efficiency, but no change in HRQL.

These controlled trials show a range of possible outcomes from trials using HRQL instruments. The HRQL instrument may agree with other outcome measures and thereby provide additional evidence either for or against the use of a specific therapy. The HRQL instrument may show no benefit when other outcomes show clear benefit, as was the case with routine versus symptomatic salbutamol (48). In this case, it is important that clinicians and patients be aware of this discrepancy and consider this discrepancy in the decision to use the therapy. If the benefit of the therapy is considered to outweigh the lack of improvement in HRQL, the patient's awareness of this lack of benefit in HRQL may minimize disappointment with the therapy and consequent noncompliance. Finally, HRQL instruments may demonstrate a benefit when traditional outcomes do not. In this circumstance, these instruments may allow patients to receive important and effective therapy that would otherwise be assessed as ineffective.

V. Applicability of HRQL Measures to Clinicians

A. Use of HRQL Instruments in Clinical Practice

In general, the practicing clinician assesses the HRQL of a patient with chronic pulmonary disease by taking a careful history. The major component of this history is eliciting the patient's symptoms and assessing how these symptoms impact on the patient's functional capacity and ability to perform the recreational and social activities the patient enjoys. The clinician generally does not need a HRQL instrument to perform this task of HRQL assessment. However, there may be circumstances in which these instruments may be directly useful to the practicing clinician. First, a clinician may decide to use a self-administered generic or disease specific HRQL instrument as a screening instrument for patients to complete in the waiting room. This practice may identify specific areas of concern or changes over time that might not be obvious during the routine office visits. For this purpose, the HRQL instrument would need to be not only reproducible, valid, and responsive, but also easily administered and interpreted in the clinical setting. Candidate instruments for patients with COPD include the MOS SF-36 and the SGRQ. However, to date, these instruments have not been modified for easy use and interpretation in clinical practice.

In addition, a HRQL instrument could be useful in the N-of-1 trial. The N-of-1 trial is a clinical trial using a single patient in which a clinician uses two sequential therapeutic agents, or a therapeutic agent and a placebo, and compares the patient's response in each phase of the trial. Guyatt and colleagues have described the utility and practice of N-of-1 randomized controlled trials in detail (80). This technique can be useful to assess an individual's response to different therapeutic approaches. In the N-of-1 trial, HRQL is an ideal outcome measure since the point of these trials is often to determine the therapy that provides individual patients with the best HRQL (26,80).

B. Lessons for the Clinician Regarding HRQL in COPD

Previous research on HRQL has pointed out several important, but not widely known, features of the HRQL of patients with COPD. First, maximal improvement in physiological measures of disease severity, such as FEV_1 or oxygenation, may not be sufficient to maximally improve HRQL. If we are interested in improving HRQL, we must assess it directly. As a corollary of this point, it is possible to improve patients' HRQL without changing any physiological measures of disease severity. The use of antidepressants in individuals with COPD and depression improved HRQL without changing FEV_1 or exercise tolerance (34).

A second important lesson to the clinician provided by the studies of HRQL in COPD patients is that COPD has a major impact on specific facets of HRQL that might not be obvious. These facets include depression, anxiety, sleep, and rest. It is not clear from the literature whether depression and anxiety cause a decrease in HRQL or whether diminished HRQL causes depression and anxiety. It seems likely that there is a complex interdependence of these factors. Regardless, it is clear that treating depression and anxiety can improve HRQL (34).

A final generic lesson of HRQL studies is that individuals vary as to what they consider to be the most important aspects of HRQL and these aspects are not well correlated with disease severity, exercise tolerance, or other terms familiar to clinicians. In the assessment of an individual patient's HRQL, it is important to directly ask what each person values about his or her life. This should include the patient's religious beliefs, value system, and priorities. This is especially important in chronic pulmonary diseases in part because these diseases predispose patients to acute respiratory failure. In the event of acute respiratory failure, it may be appropriate to consider withholding or withdrawing life support measures such as mechanical ventilation. The decision to withhold or withdraw life support measures in the event of acute respiratory failure depends on the likelihood of a reversible component to the acute or chronic disease and the patient's acceptance or rejection of the therapy based on risks and benefits that the therapy offers. A patient's assessment of the risks and benefits of life support therapy will depend in large part on the patient's HRQL prior to the acute event. Discussion of HRQL and goals of treatment should occur prior to an episode of acute respiratory failure. Often patients will be unable to make a decision about life support based on a hypothetical scenario, but this discussion will give clinicians and family members a better understanding of the patient's views should the patient not be able to participate in the discussion after acute respiratory failure. Without these discussions, many physicians and families do not have a good understanding of the patient's wishes. This was documented by Uhlmann and colleagues, who asked patients whether they wished to receive cardiopulmonary resuscitation and mechanical ventilation if they had COPD and became critically ill. The same situation was presented to both the patient's physician and spouse. In approximately 40% of these instances, both the patient's spouse and the physician differed from the patient in what they thought the patient would have wanted (81). This emphasizes the importance of discussion, not only of issues of resuscitation, but also of patients' current HRQL and their concerns about future HRQL.

VI. Summary

Assessment of HRQL is an important feature of the care of patients with chronic disease. HRQL instruments will be used increasingly to assess the quality of life of patients with specific diseases and to help assess the impact of various therapies on patients' lives. In addition, as outcome assessment becomes an increasing part of the assessment of health care technology, HRQL will become an increasingly useful outcome measure. To assess the importance or applicability of a HRQL measure, clinicians must have a basic understanding of the field of HRQL assessment. Clinicians should expect evidence that the instrument used is reproducible, valid, and responsive in patients with the disease under study. Studies describing new HRQL instruments should be expected to demonstrate the need for a new instrument as opposed to one already developed and tested.

HRQL instruments have provided important insights into the lives of persons with moderate to severe chronic pulmonary diseases. In addition, these instruments have been important in the demonstration that some therapies improve the lives of persons with chronic pulmonary diseases while other therapies do not. We can expect that the HRQL instruments will continue to play this role in future research.

References

1. McSweeny AJ, Grant I, Heaton RK, Adams KM, Timms RM. Life quality of patients with chronic obstructive pulmonary disease. Arch Intern Med 1982; 142:473–478.
2. Prigatano GP, Wright EC, Levin D. Quality of life and its predictors in patients with mild hypoxemia and chronic obstructive pulmonary disease. Arch Intern Med 1984; 144:1613–1619.
3. Mahler D, Weinber D, Wells C, Feinstein A. The measurement of dyspnea: contents, interobserver agreement, and physiologic correlates of two new clinical indexes. Chest 1984; 85:751–758.
4. Guyatt G, Townsend M, Berman L, Pugsley S. Quality of life in patients with chronic airflow limitation. Br J Dis Chest 1987; 81:45–54.
5. Nocturnal Oxygen Therapy Trial Group. Continuous or nocturnal oxygen therapy in hypoxemic chronic obstructive lung disease. Ann Intern Med 1980; 93:391–398.
6. Intermittent Positive Pressure Breathing Trial Group. Intermittent positive pressure breathing therapy of chronic obstructive pulmonary disease. Ann Intern Med 1983; 99:612–620.
7. Curtis JR, Deyo RA, Hudson LD. Health-related quality of life among patients with chronic obstructive pulmonary disease. Thorax 1994; 49:162–170.
8. Mahler DA, Matthay RA, Snyder PE, Wells CK, Loke J. Sustained-release the-

ophylline reduces dyspnea in non-reversible obstructive airway disease. Am Rev Respir Dis 1985; 131:22–25.
9. Guyatt GH, Townsend M, Pugsley SO, et al. Bronchodilators in chronic air-flow limitation: effects on airway function, exercise capacity, and quality of life. Am Rev Respir Dis 1987; 135:1069–1074.
10. Bergner M, Hudson LD, Conrad DA, et al. The cost and efficacy of home care for patients with chronic lung disease. Med Care 1988; 26:566–579.
11. Toshima MT, Kaplan RM, Ries AL. Experimental evaluation of rehabilitation in chronic obstructive pulmonary disease: short-term effects on exercise endurance and health status. Health Psychol 1990; 9:237–252.
12. Fergusson RJ, Cull A. Quality of life measurement for patients undergoing treatment for lung cancer. Thorax 1991; 46:671–675.
13. Richards JM, Hemstreet MP. Measures of life quality, role performance, and functional status in asthma research. Am J Respir Crit Care Med 1994; 149:S31–S39.
14. Rowe BH, Oxman AD. Performance of an asthma quality of life questionnaire in an outpatient setting. Am Rev Respir Dis 1993; 148:675–681.
15. Marks GB, Dunn SM, Woolcock AJ. An evaluation of asthma quality of life questionnaire as a measure of change in adults with asthma. J Clin Epidemiol 1993; 46:1103–1111.
16. Orenstein DM, Nixon PA, Ross EA, Kaplan RM. The quality of well-being in cystic fibrosis. Chest 1989; 95:344–347.
17. Kirshner B, Guyatt G. A methodological framework for assessing health indices. J Chronic Dis 1985; 38:27–36.
18. Deyo R. Measuring the functional status of patients with low back pain. Arch Phys Med Rehabil 1988; 69:1044–1053.
19. Feinstein AR. Clinical biostatistics: hard science, soft data, and the challenges of choosing clinical variables in research. Clin Pharmacol Ther 1977; 22:485–498.
20. Jones P, Quirk FH, Baveystock CM, Littlejohns P. A self-complete measure of health status for chronic airflow limitation. The St. George's Respiratory Questionnaire. Am Rev Respir Dis 1992; 145:1321–1327.
21. Guyatt G, Feeny D, Patrick D. Issues in quality of life measurement in clinical trials. Controlled Clin Trials 1991; 12:81S–90S.
22. Kassa S, Mastekaasa A, Naess S. Quality of life of lung cancer patients in a randomized clinical trial evaluated by a psychosocial well-being questionnaire. Acta Oncol 1988; 27:335–342.
23. Kaasa S, Mastekaasa A. Psychosocial well-being of patients with inoperable non-small cell lung cancer. Acta Oncol 1988; 27:829–835.
24. Busschbach JJV, Horikx PE, van den Bosch JJM, de la Riviere AB, de Charro FT. Measuring the quality of life before and after bilateral lung transplantation in patients with cystic fibrosis. Chest 1994; 105:911–917.
25. Orenstein DM, Kaplan RM. Measuring the quality of well-being in cystic fibrosis and lung transplantation: the importance of the area under the curve. Chest 1991; 100:1016–1018.
26. Jaeschke R, Guyatt GH, Keller J, Singer J. Interpreting changes in quality of life score in N of 1 randomized trials. Controlled Clin Trials 1991; 12:226S–233S.

27. Mills JL. Data torturing. N Engl J Med 1993; 329:1196–1199.
28. Pocock SJ. A perspective on the role of quality of life assessment in clinical trials. Controlled Clin Trials 1991; 12:257S–265S.
29. Bergner M, Bobbitt RA, Carter WB, Gilson BS. The sickness impact profile: development and final revision of a health status measure. Med Care 1981; 19:787–805.
30. McSweeny AJ, Heaton RK, Grant I, Cugell D, Solliday N, Timms R. Chronic obstructive pulmonary disease; socioemotional adjustment and life quality. Chest 1980; 77:309–311.
31. Jones P, Baveystock CM, Littlejohns P. Relationships between general health measured with the sickness impact profile and respiratory symptoms, physiological measures, and mood in patients with chronic airflow limitation. Am Rev Respir Dis 1989; 140:1538–1543.
32. Bergman B, Sullivan M, Sorenson S. Quality of life during chemotherapy for small cell lung cancer. I. An evaluation with generic health measures. Acta Oncol 1991; 30:947–957.
33. Bergman B, Sullivan M, Sorenson S. Quality of life during chemotherapy for small cell lung cancer. II. A longitudinal study of the EORTC Core quality of life questionnaire and comparison with the Sickness Impact Profile. Acta Oncol 1992; 31:19–28.
34. Borson S, McDonald GJ, Gayle T, Deffebach M, Lakshminarayan S, Van Tuinen C. Improvement in mood, physical symptoms, and function with nortriptyline for depression in patients with chronic obstructive pulmonary disease. Psychosomatics 1992; 33:190–201.
35. Stewart AL, Greenfield S, Hays RD, et al. Functional status and well-being of patients with chronic conditions: results from the Medical Outcomes Study. JAMA 1989; 262:907–913.
36. Mahler DA, Faryniarz K, Tomlinson D, et al. Impact of dyspnea and physiologic function on general health status in patients with chronic obstructive pulmonary disease. Chest 1992; 102:395–401.
37. Shepherd SL, Hovell MF, Slymen DJ, et al. Functional status as an overall measure of health in adults with cystic fibrosis: further validation of a generic health measure. Clin Epidemiol 1992; 45:117–125.
38. Ware JE, Sherbourne CD. The MOS 36-item short form health survey (SF-36). Med Care 1992; 30:473–483.
39. McHorney CA, Ware JE, Rogers W, Raczek AE, Lu J. The validity and relative precision of MOS short- and long-form health status scales and Dartmouth COOP charts. Med Care 1992; 30:MS253–MS265.
40. Viramontes JL, O'Brien B. Relationship between symptoms and health-related quality of life in chronic lung disease. J Gen Intern Med 1994; 9:46–48.
41. Fanshel S, Bush JW. A Health-Status Index and its application to health-services outcomes. Oper Res 1970; 18:1021–1066.
42. Kaplan RM, Bush JW, Berry CC. Category rating versus magnitude estimation for measuring levels of well-being. Med Care 1979; 17:501–521.
43. Anderson JP, Kaplan RM, Berry CC, Bush JW, Rumbaut RG. Interday reliability of function assessment for a health status measure: the Quality of Well-Being Scale. Med Care 1989; 27:1076–1083.

44. Kaplan RM, Atkins CJ, Timms R. Validity of a Quality of Well-Being Scale as an outcome measure in chronic obstructive pulmonary disease. J Chronic Dis 1984; 37:85–95.
45. Orenstein DM, Pattishal EN, Nixon PA, Ross EA, Kaplan RM. Quality of well-being before and after antibiotic treatment of pulmonary exacerbation in patients with cystic fibrosis. Chest 1990; 98:1081–1084.
46. Hunt SM, McKenna SP, McEwen J, Backett EM, Williams J, Papp E. A quantitative approach to perceived health status: a validation study. J Epidemiol Commun Health 1980; 34:281–286.
47. Alonso J, Anto JM, Gonzalez M, Fiz JA, Izquierdo J, Morera J. Measurement of general health status of non-oxygen-dependent chronic obstructive pulmonary disease patients. Med Care 1992; 30:MS125–MS135.
48. van Schayck CP, Rutten-van Molken MPMH, van Doorslaer EKA, Folgering H, van Weel C. Two-year bronchodilator treatment in patients with mild airflow obstruction: contradictory effects on lung function and quality of life. Chest 1992; 102:1384–1391.
49. Caine N, Sharples LD, Smyth R, et al. Survival and quality of life of cystic fibrosis patients before and after heart-lung transplantation. Transplant Proc 1991; 23:1203–1204.
50. Light RW, Merrill EJ, Despars JA, Gordon GH, Mutalipassi LR. Prevalence of depression and anxiety in patients with COPD: relationship to functional capacity. Chest 1985; 87:35–38.
51. Guyatt G, Berman L, Townsend M, Pugsley S, Chambers L. A measure of quality of life for clinical trials in chronic lung disease. Thorax 1978B; 42:773–778.
52. Guyatt G, Townsend M, Keller J, Singer J, Nogradi S. Measuring functional status in chronic lung disease: conclusions from a randomized control trial. J Respir Med 1989; 83:293–297.
53. McKay SE, Howie CA, Thomson AH, Whiting B, Addis GJ. Value of theophylline treatment in patients handicapped by chronic obstructive lung disease. Thorax 1993; 48:227–232.
54. Kirsten DK, Wegner RE, Jorres RA, Magnussen H. Effects of theophylline withdrawal in severe chronic obstructive pulmonary disease. Chest 1993; 104:1101–1107.
55. Elliott MW, Simonds AK, Carroll MP, Wedzicha JA, Branthwaite MA. Domiciliary nocturnal nasal intermittent positive pressure ventilation in hypercapnic respiratory failure due to chronic obstructive lung disease: effects on sleep and quality of life. Thorax 1992; 47:342–348.
56. Mahler D, Rosiello R, Harvver A, Lentine T, McGovern J, Daubenspeck J. Comparison of clinical dyspnea ratings and psychophysical measurements of respiratory sensation in obstructive airway disease. Am Rev Respir Dis 1987; 135:1229–1233.
57. Hyland ME, Finnis S, Irvine SH. A scale for assessing quality of life in adult asthma sufferers. J Psychosom Res 1991; 35:99–110.
58. Hyland ME. The Living with Asthma Questionnaire. Respir Med 1991; 85(Suppl B):13–16.
59. Marks G, Dunn S, Woolcock A. A scale for the measurement of quality of life in adults with asthma. J Clin Epidemiol 1992; 45:461–472.

60. Juniper EF, Guyatt GG, Epstein RS, Ferrie PJ, Jaeschke R, Hiller TK. Evaluation of impairment of health-related quality of life in asthma: development of a questionnaire for use in clinical trials. Thorax 1992; 47:76–83.
61. Ganz PA, Haskell CM, Figlin RA, La Soto N, Siau J. Estimating the quality of life in a clinical trial of patients with metastatic lung cancer using the Karnofsky performance status and the Functional Living Index—Cancer. Cancer 1988; 61:849–856.
62. Finkelstein DM, Cassileth BR, Bonomi PD, Ruckdeschel JC, Ezdinli EZ, Wolter JM. A pilot study of the Functional Living Index—Cancer Scale for the assessment of quality of life for metastatic lung cancer patients. Am J Oncol 1988; 11:630–633.
63. Buccheri GF, Ferrigno D, Curcio A, Vola F, Rosso A. Continuation of chemotherapy versus supportive care alone in patients with inoperable non-small cell lung cancer and stable disease after two or three cycles of MACC. Cancer 1989; 63:428–432.
64. Regan J, Yarnold J, Jones PW, Cooke NT. Palliation and life quality in lung cancer; how good are clinicians at judging treatment outcome? Br J Cancer 1991; 64:396–400.
65. Hurny C, Bernhard J, Joss R, et al. Feasibility of quality of life assessment in a randomized phase III trial of small cell lung cancer. Ann Oncol 1992; 3:825–831.
66. Geddes DM, Dones L, Hill E, et al. Quality of life during chemotherapy for small cell lung cancer: assessment and use of a daily diary card in a randomized trial. Eur J Cancer 1990; 26:484–492.
67. Spitzer WD. Measuring the quality of life of lung cancer patients. J Chronic Dis 1981; 35:585–597.
68. Kaasa S. Mastedaasa, Stokke I, Naess S. Validation of a quality of life questionnaire for use in clinical trials for treatment of patients with inoperable lung cancer. Eur J Cancer Clin Oncol 1988; 24:691–701.
69. Hollen PJ, Gralla RJ, Kris MG, et al. Measurement of quality of life in patients with lung cancer in multicenter trials of new therapies: psychometric assessment of the Lung Cancer Symptom Scale. Cancer 1994; 73:2087–2098.
70. Fayers PM, Bleehen NM, Girling DJ, Stephens RJ. Assessment of quality of life in small-cell lung cancer using a daily diary card developed by the Medical Research Council Lung Cancer Working Party. Br J Cancer 1991; 64:299–306.
71. Fernandez C, Rosell R, Abad-Esteve A, et al. Quality of life during chemotherapy in non-small cell lung cancer patients. Acta Oncol 1989; 28:29–33.
72. Maasilta PK, Rautonen JE, Mattson MT, Mattson KV. Quality of life assessment during chemotherapy for non-small cell lung cancer. Eur J Cancer 1990; 26:706–708.
73. Schrier A, Dekker FW, Kaptein AA, Dijkman JH. Quality of life in elderly patients with chronic nonspecific lung disease seen in family practice. Chest 1990; 98:894–899.
74. Hudson LD. Survival data in patients with acute and chronic lung disease. Am Rev Respir Dis 1990; 140:519–524.
75. Killian KJ, LeBlanc P, Martin DH, Summers E, Jones NL, Campbell EJM. Exercise capacity and ventilatory, circulatory, and symptom limitation in patients with chronic airflow limitation. Am Rev Respir Dis 1992; 146:935–940.

76. Morgan AD, Peck DF, Buchanan DR, McHardy GJR. Effect of attitudes and beliefs on exercise tolerance in chronic bronchitis. Br Med J 1983; 286:171–173.
77. McGavin C, Artvinli M, Naoe H, McHardly G. Dyspnea, disability, distance walked: comparison of estimates of exercise performance in respiratory disease. Br Med J 1978; 2:241–243.
78. Guyatt G, Thompson P, Berman L, et al. How should we measure function in patients with chronic heart and lung disease? J Chronic Dis 1985; 38:517–524.
79. Wijkstra PJ, Van Altena RV, Kraan J, Otten V, Postma DS, Koeter GH. Quality of life in patients with chronic obstructive pulmonary disease after rehabilitation at home. Eur Respir J 1994; 7:269–273.
80. Guyatt GH, Keller JL, Jaeschke R, Rosenbloom D, Adachi JD, Newhouse MT. The N-of-1 randomized controlled trial: clinical usefulness. Ann Intern Med 1990; 112:293–299.
81. Uhlmann RF, Pearlman RA, Cain K. Physicians' and spouses' predictions of elderly patients' resuscitation preferences. J Geronto 1988; 43:M115–M121.

15

Assessing Outcomes in Pulmonary Rehabilitation

LEWIS E. KAZIS

Edith Nourse Rogers Memorial Veterans Hospital
Bedford, Massachusetts
and Boston University School of Public Health
Boston, Massachusetts

ALFREDO J. SELIM

Edith Nourse Rogers Memorial Veterans Hospital
Bedford, Massachusetts

Interventions in pulmonary rehabilitation have evolved from approaches that focus on physiological outcomes to those that focus on improvement in functional status and well-being (1–3). Instead of single intervention modalities based on a traditional biomedical model, rehabilitation medicine has moved to broader types of interventions designed to impact on health-related quality of life (HRQL) defined as the functional status and well-being of the individual (4). To achieve these goals, the traditional physiological measures of outcome have proved inadequate for purposes of evaluation.

The expanded goals of rehabilitation call for methodologies for assessing outcomes that are reliable, valid, and sufficiently precise for evaluative applications. This chapter provides a historical overview and conceptualization of approaches for evaluating pulmonary rehabilitation programs. It emphasizes methods for assessing which measures of outcome are appropriate for use in rehabilitation settings and application of these measures to patient management, program evaluation, and clinical research.

I. Historical Overview and Conceptualization of Health

Historically, broadening of the concept of health is not new. The World Health Organization definition of health includes the physical, psychological, and social functioning of the individual, not merely the absence of disease (5). According to this definition, health is a multidimensional concept that involves the individual's ability to perform physically, psychologically, and socially in the community. Each of these concepts also includes a range of functional states from the vigorous and vital to the disabling.

In recent years, the technology of outcomes assessment has provided new methods for evaluation and for their application in research, management, and practice. Early classifications of the severity of disease were relatively insensitive and focused on the more severely disabled and impaired. Some examples of these measures included the New York Heart Association Functional Classification for patients with cardiac disease, the Katz Index of ADL (activities of daily living), and the American College of Rheumatology Functional Classification for patients with arthritis (6–8). For the most part, these measures focused on the most basic functional status, including bathing, dressing, toileting, and continence. They were administered by the providers appropriate for the more severely disabled and involved in rehabilitation programs. These early measures focused on a narrow range of health status, targeted at the most basic physical functioning. They were coarse and tended to lump broad functional categories into a few grades or classes. For example, the cardiovascular and arthritis classifications had only four functional groupings that ranged from bedbound to the ability to perform normal activities. Because the scales were crude, these approaches were fairly insensitive for monitoring patient outcomes. However, these early efforts laid a framework for developing a future technology of multidimensional assessments of patient health.

Previous attempts to apply assessment of functional status to the field of rehabilitation have been problematic. In addition to narrow therapeutic goals for treating patients, the measures of HRQL were too circumscribed and the scales for measuring functional disability were relatively crude and not standardized. The technical quality of the measurement was beset with inherent problems of reliability, validity, and responsiveness to change.

In more recent years, both the conceptualization and operationalization of measures for use in rehabilitation have made considerable progress. Jette and Deniston (9) developed assessments based in "pathology" that manifests itself in physical disability and/or symptoms. Functional assessment in this context has been evaluated through the impact of disease on physical, mental, emotional, and social performance. Schipper et al. (10) define functional status more broadly to include physical ability, psychological status and well-being, and social activities. Their approach involves a comprehensive set of assessments that target the interaction between the individual and his/her environment.

Building on the work of Nagi (11), Wood (12), and Granger (2), a conceptual model was developed that incorporates impairment, disability, and handicap into measures of HRQL (Fig. 1). *Impairment* is the biological/physiological problem arising from dysfunction of an organ or body system. *Disability* refers to a reduction in physical or psychological functioning and energy levels often, but not always, accompanied by symptoms because of underlying disease. *Handicap* is the social disadvantage resulting from the impairment and/or the disability and is manifested by social and role functioning and/or the perceptions of the patients of their general health or well-being. The severity of the impairment, disability, and handicap is often related to specific levels of biological dysfunction, symptoms (when present), functional status, and HRQL.

More recently, multidimensional concepts of HRQL that include physiological status, functional status, and well-being have been linked to the more traditional relationships among impairment, disability, and handicap. For the purposes of outcomes research, impairment has usually been linked to biological and physiological status. With the emerging comprehensive goals of medical rehabilitation, the earlier focus on impairment is now inadequate to address the full complement of outcomes related to rehabilitation therapy. Proximate to physiological functioning are "symptoms." Assessment of symptoms is often a clinical summary of a patient's subjective statement about a feeling related to his/her body. These subjective reports may be physical, emotional, or cognitively driven. While a symptom is often directly tied to an impairment that is physiologically based, that relationship may not always be straightforward. Some physiological parameters may be quite abnormal without a corresponding relationship to symptoms or functional status. For example, measures of established disease, such as joint erosion in osteoarthritis of the knee measured by anterior-posterior radiographs during weight bearing, bear little or no relationship with pain (13).

In another study of a group of diabetic patients, Weinberger et al. (14) found a very limited relationship between the baseline glycohemoglobin (GHB) concentrations and general perceptions of health. Similarly, no significant correlations were found between GHB concentrations and changes in functional status as defined by physical, social, role functioning, energy/fatigue, and general perceptions of health. Patients with GHB levels and fasting blood glucose levels outside of normal ranges also showed little or no correlation with patient-reported HRQL as defined by the SF-36 (short-form health survey).

Previous radiological studies have also shown little or no correlation with radiological abnormalities and chronic low back pain, either by radiographs or

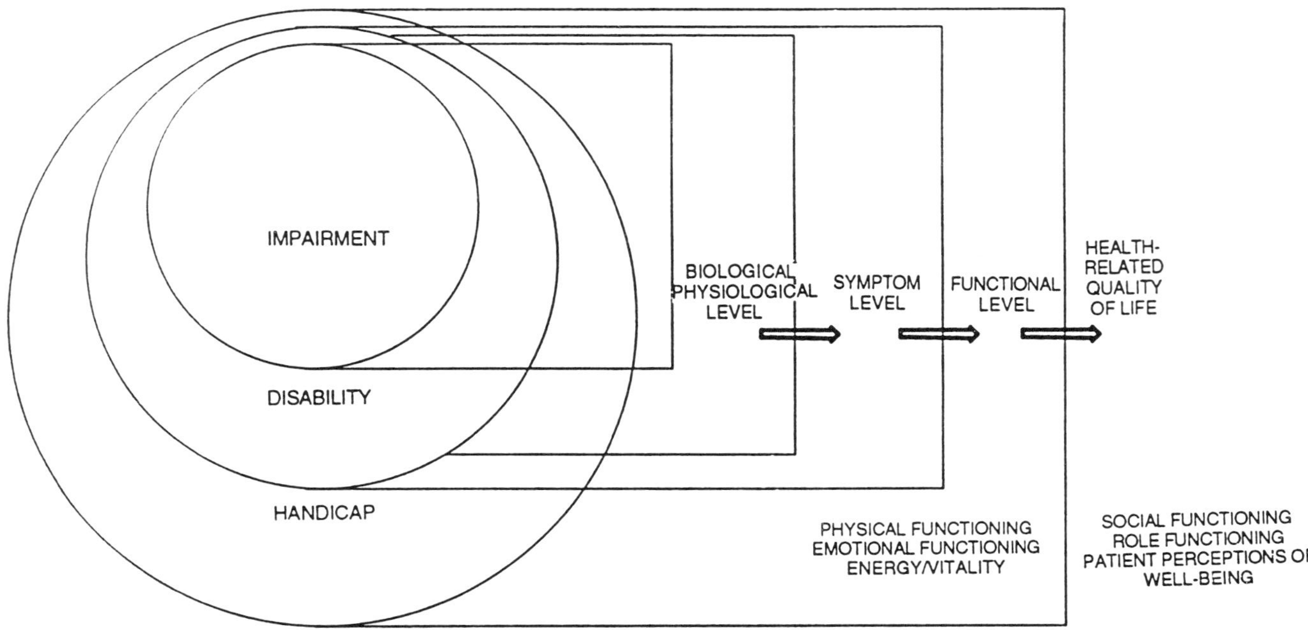

Figure 1 A framework for patient assessment of outcomes in pulmonary rehabilitation.

by magnetic resonance imaging (15). Several studies have shown that there are small, nonsignificant correlations between FEV_1 (forced expiratory volume) and changes in dyspnea as well as measures of functional status.

In contrast, Mahler et al. (16) reported that in a population of patients with chronic obstructive pulmonary disease (COPD), the FEV_1 was a significant predictor of physical and social functioning. Prigatano et al. (23), in an earlier study of patients with COPD, had found a highly significant relationship between physical function using the Sickness Impact Profile and PO_2, (R^2 = 0.42). Anthonisen et al. (17), in a study of patients with COPD, found a significant correlation ($p < 0.05$) between the psychosocial functioning index, measured by the Sickness Impact Profile, and future change in FEV_1. Finally, Jones et al. (18) found a highly significant relationship between the total score for the Sickness Impact Profile and FVC ($R^2 = 0.60$).

The above studies illustrate the complexity of the relationship between impairment and symptoms. Symptoms are important because they are often the reason why patients seek medical care and sometimes they are tied to their functional status and considerations of HRQL. The following discussion describes the functional impacts of disability and handicap in terms of physical functioning, emotional and energy/fatigue status, social and role functioning, and patients' perceptions of their general well-being.

A. Physical Functioning, Psychological Status, and Energy/Fatigue

Physical Functioning

Disabilities often refer to physical functioning, psychological status, and vitality (energy/fatigue). *Physical functioning* refers to limitations in performing the activities of daily life; these activities range from self-care, at the more disabling end of the spectrum, to vigorous day-to-day activities, at the enabling end of the spectrum. In contrast to physiological impairments, which are not always related to utilization of health care, functional limitations are more directly tied to the need for such services (19).

Mahler et al. (20), Bergner et al. (21), and Ware et al. (22) have provided scales for measuring functional status which emphasize physical functioning. Questionnaires (see below) focus on physical functioning ranging from the most limiting, e.g., difficulties in bathing, dressing, and eating, to limitations in less essential functions, e.g., running and strenuous sports.

Psychological Status

The patient's psychological status or mental health is defined in terms of the patient's psychological well-being, affect (negative subjective feelings of anxiety and depression, as well as positive feelings of pleasure, happiness, and satisfaction with life), and cognitive functioning. Cognitive functioning involves orientation to time, place, and person; it also refers to memory, attention span, ability to perform mental tasks, and alertness. The emotional status of the patient is measured by the frequency and intensity of patient-perceived feelings of psychological distress and well-being. Structured questions that are as simple as "how often do you feel tense?" are included as part of several questions that derive standard ratings assessing the patient's overall mental health.

Energy/Fatigue

Energy and vitality refer to patient-perceived feelings about "pep" and "energy" at one end of the continuum to "tired" and "fatigued" at the opposite end. This dimension provides a broad definition of subjective well-being. In patients with COPD, measures of energy/fatigue have correlated well with the severity of the disease (23).

B. Social and Role Functioning

Handicap refers to the social disadvantages and role limitations that are associated with impairment and/or disability. Handicap in rehabilitation can be divided into two components: limitations in the social functioning of the individual and limitations in role activities.

Social functioning is tied to the social contacts with relatives and/or friends as well as the strength of these associations. This concept considers the frequency of visits with friends and/or relatives as well as the satisfaction derived from such contacts. Measures of social functioning have been developed by Donald and Ware (24) and Brownell and Shumaker (25).

Role functioning relates to the quality of the patient's work at home, on the job, or at school. The impact of illness on role functioning calls for separate assessment. For example, patients with COPD may not be able to perform their job as well as might be required. They may also have role limitations at home because they are unable to complete their routine household tasks as completely and carefully as is necessary. Ware et al. make the distinction between role limitations due to emotional problems and role limitations due to physical problems (26). This dichotomy suggests that role problems can be attributed to a specific dimension of physical or emotional functional limitations or disabilities (29). Recreational activities are also influenced by the inability to participate in these activities as often and completely as desired.

Social, role, and recreational activities are components of the HRQL. Although handicap refers to the negative disabling end of the continuum, the concepts of social and role functioning outlined above apply to the full range, i.e., from the most limiting and disadvantaged to the most active.

C. General Health Perceptions or Perceptions of General Well-Being

General health perceptions refers to the patient's subjective ratings of his or her own overall health. Many assessments of general well-being have been developed. For the most part, many of these typologies represent a synthesis of the salient feelings and experiences that patients report about their health. This kind of assessment is very valuable, since it can capture aspects of health that are not included in earlier definitions of health status.

Measures of overall health extend assessments into the positive range of health status. This is especially useful with respect to clinical outcome studies in which the therapeutic goals may be to improve the status of the patient's health so that they can function in the positive range of health. Traditional concepts and measures of health may not detect these changes since their focus has been on the negative aspects of health and its associated limitations. Positive perceptions of health, as defined by measures of general well-being, have been shown to be important determinants of the outcomes of health care. Self-reported perceptions about health in patients with COPD have correlated well with respiratory symptoms, physiological measures, and emotional status (27).

Global evaluations of health also relate to use of health services and morbidity and mortality. An example of a simple structured question about health perceptions is "In general, is your health excellent, very good, good, fair, or poor?" This specific self-rating about health is an important consideration in defining HRQL and has been associated with feelings of well-being and of energy level and vitality.

II. Standards for Assessing Outcomes in Pulmonary Rehabilitation

Measures of HRQL are assessments of patient outcomes that require standardization before they can be used in outcomes studies and in clinical care. Standardization of questions entails examination of measures for reliability, validity, responsiveness to change, and generalizability.

A. Reliability

Reliability is defined in terms of the stability and reproducibility of the item or scale. Approaches used to assess reliability include internal consistency (Cronbach's Alpha) and test-retest reliability. Tests of reliability are often used in publications about quality of life to assess the consistency or stability of a measure. These approaches are useful in determining the degree of error in the scales used to assess a population of patients involved in a rehabilitation program. Minimizing error has important tradeoffs in terms of requirements for proper sample size and in the precision with which differences between study groups can be ascertained. Although reliability is a critical standard, it does not necessarily mean that the measure is also valid. A measure that is reliable need not be valid.

B. Validity

Validity is another essential standard for assessments of outcomes. Validity is the extent to which a scale or concept measures what it purports to measure. Several types of validity are useful to consider with respect to outcomes studies. First, *content validity* refers to the adequacy with which a specific domain of content is sampled, e.g., bathing, toileting, dressing, walking, and running. Frequently, content validity is assessed by clinical experts and information is gathered by focusing on a targeted area of content.

Other measures of validity include criterion validity, convergent validity, and divergent validity. *Criterion validity* tests a concept against a gold standard: the gold standard and the new measure are administered concurrently and the results are statistically compared using a measure of the degree of association, e.g., Pearson or Spearman correlation coefficient. For example, a measure of physical functioning obtained by several standard questions correlates strongly with certain clinical parameters, such as forced vital capacity (FVC) and forced expiratory volume (FEV_1). However, in practice, for most functional assessment scales it is difficult to determine a proper gold standard. Evidence for criterion validity is often gathered by using more than one standard.

Divergent and convergent validity test the expected magnitude and direction of the association of a scale or measure against another instrument or clinical test. *Divergent validity* of a test refers to a correlation that is expected to be weak when compared with another valid instrument that measures an unrelated concept. *Convergent validity* refers to a test that correlates strongly with a related measure. An example of convergent validity might be a measure of dexterity by self-administered questionnaire that is expected to be highly correlated with a clinical measure such as strength of grip. On the other hand, if the clinical standard was walking time, this might be an illustration of divergent validity in which correlation is expected to be low. To summarize, the validation test is used to determine whether a reliable measure is measuring what it intends to measure. Validation approaches should be multifaceted and usually involve more than one approach.

C. Responsiveness to Change

Responsiveness is another important criterion for selecting outcomes in rehabilitation studies. Responsiveness refers to the ability of a measure or scale to detect clinically meaningful changes in terms of either their improvement or worsening. The ability of a measure to distinguish between different severities of disease may be important in determining whether an intervention alters the prognosis, e.g., mortality and morbidity, or HRQL outcomes, e.g., functional status and subjective measures of well-being. For example, Anthonisen (28) noted that the initial value of FEV_1, a measure of severity of disease in patients with COPD, was one of the most accurate predictors of prognosis. The initial measure of severity was related to subsequent physical disability and morbidity as well as mortality over 3 years of follow-up.

D. Generalizability

Generalizability refers to the ability of a measure to maintain the properties of reliability, validity, and responsiveness to change for different diseases, different levels of severity of disease, and different socioeconomic groups. For example, in patients with severe lung disease, spirometry may be highly associated with a patient-reported measure of functional status whereas it may be poorly associated in those with mild disease. In this case, the validity of the patient-reported assessment cannot be generalized to cover the full range of severity of disease.

Finally, the assessments must be practical in the rehabilitation setting. Practical considerations include a matching of the assessment with the goals of the evaluation or of the research. A psychometrically sound instrument must also be relevant to the needs of the user in terms of the content of the scales applied. The assessment should be acceptable to the patients who are the target of the administration, e.g., the length of the questionnaire. Ware and Sherbourne (29) have noted that a general population should be able to complete three to four standardized items per minute on a categorical or ordinal scale, e.g., ranging from severely limited to unlimited. However, in a patient population with severe pulmonary dysfunction, this may take longer, e.g., an average of two items per minute.

In recent years, questionnaires have been developed that are short and psychometrically sound for use in specific clinic populations. Since the burden of illness in the rehabilitation setting may be considerable, a short questionnaire that places minimal burden on the respondent may have considerable utility. Examples of such assessments include the SF-36 (short-form 36-item health survey) (29) and the Nottingham Health Profile (30). Both are relatively short and require less than 10–15 min to complete.

E. Additional Standards for Assessing Functional Status

Mode and Location of Administration

The mode and the location of the administration are other important practical considerations in the use of HRQL assessments. For example, attention has focused recently on questioning by telephone versus questionnaires self-administered by mail. The SF-36 scores were found to be lower (worse health status) for the mailed questionnaires than for the surveys by telephone; more reports of chronic conditions were found in the group that answered by mail (33). Interestingly, the mailed survey reports resulted in higher response rates and cost less. The mode of administration may have influenced the reported levels of health since the mail survey may have allowed more candor because of the greater anonymity.

In a separate study, Miller et al. (31) found that the setting in which the structured questionnaire is administered may have an effect on the levels of the scores for the HRQL. Using the SF-36 questionnaire, self administered questions were completed by patients at home and in a clinic; less than a week separated the two administrations. The scores from questionnaires completed in the clinic were significantly higher ($p < 0.05$) (better health status). Both the mode of administration and the location should be given careful consideration in designing studies that entail assessment of the HRQL.

Scale Development

Standards used to develop scales for functional assessment are often applied to instruments that are questionnaire-based. These consist of a set of structured questions, usually on ordinal scales ranging from three to five points, e.g., excellent to poor, extremely to not at all, all of the time to none of the time, definitely true to definitely false. Individual items or questions are aggregated or grouped with other questions related to the same concept and a single score is computed. This aggregation is often determined empirically through principal-component or factor analysis and testing for internal consistency reliability. Based on sound psychometric properties, the principles for defining a specific item within a concept or construct are validated.

An example is the Mental Health Inventory questionnaire (32). This set of five questions includes items related to feelings of anxiety, depression, positive affect, and behavioral-emotional control. Prior work has demonstrated that these items are internally consistent (Chronbach's Alpha = 0.90) and a principal-component analysis yields a single factor that is separate and distinct from physical functioning and other health status concepts. These items are aggregated using a single arithmetic sum. Total scores are calculated with a range of 0–100, where 100 indicates perfect mental health. The Mental Health Inventory has a long history of testing and use and is a good example of a measure that has become a universal assessment for mental health functioning.

Practical Considerations

Another standard concerns the practical considerations involved in the administration of instruments in clinical settings. These points include ease of administration, scoring of the measures, and costs. McHorney et al. (33) have noted that the cost difference between mail and telephone surveys is considerable and that savings can accrue when mailed surveys are implemented in lieu of questioning by telephone. Other studies have indicated that a self-administered questionnaire implemented in a clinic setting is clearly more cost-efficient than a questionnaire administered by an interviewer (34). The interviewer also adds another source of variability to the assessment and may reduce the reliability or precision of the measures. Consequently, self-administered questionnaires are well suited for patient settings, for research applications, for policy studies, or for integration into routine clinical practice for evaluations.

F. Summary of Standards

Standards for outcome assessments using health status questionnaires have a history of rigorous scientific development and use (35). Standard clinical parameters and laboratory tests often have not been evaluated with equal scientific rigor. For example, in the rheumatology literature, measures of strength of grip, range of motion, and walk time have demonstrated poor interobserver reliability and test-retest reliability (36). Further, some radiology studies have noted that radiologists may differ as much as 30% of the time in reading radiographs (37).

Compared to standard clinical parameters, functional status assessments have demonstrated exceptionally good properties of measurement when judged by the standards outlined above. Patient self-administered questionnaires have been increasingly applied to rehabilitation outcome programs. These questionnaires have been tested in a range of socioeconomic groups and different chronic diseases involving a range of illness severities.

The discussion that follows describes some of the more prominent measures that are used to assess the HRQL of patients undergoing rehabilitation.

III. General and Disease-Specific Assessments of Functional Rehabilitation Status

Both general and disease-specific assessments of function with strong psychometric properties, have been developed for rehabilitation populations. *General measures* are assessments that have broad applications across different socioeconomic groups and chronic disease populations. These measures are often used for comparisons between different subgroups of a heterogeneous population and are relevant to health policy. *Disease-specific measures* have been tested on a population with a chronic illness or a particular clinical problem, e.g., arthritis, COPD, congestive heart failure, hip arthroplasty. Disease-specific measures that focus on the specific disabilities and handicaps of an illness may be more sensitive to clinical changes or interventions than are the general measures of function. While these assessments have generally been developed independently, it is often useful to include both a general and disease-specific set of assessments in clinical trials. However, application of these measures frequently depends on the objectives and goals of the user. The following section describes several prominent instruments that are general and disease-specific for rehabilitation populations (Table 1).

A. General Assessments

Sickness Impact Profile

The Sickness Impact Profile (SIP) is one of the most widely used assessments of general health status (38). This questionnaire has been used for more than two decades. The SIP profiles scale scores for 12 dimensions of functional status and subjective measures of health. The dimensions include physical function as it relates to ambulation, mobility, and body care; a psychosocial dimension that includes social interaction, communication, alertness, and emotional behavior; and other dimensions including sleep/rest, eating, work, home management, and recreational pastimes.

Although this questionnaire is general, it has demonstrated strong discriminatory power in capturing the impact of COPD on the quality of life. McSweeny et al. (39) noted substantial impairment in functioning; employment was not affected probably because the population consisted primarily of elderly patients. The percentage of impairment in functioning ranged from 10% for eating to 45% for recreation and pastime. The areas of functional status most influenced were management of the home and sleep/rest.

The SIP is a valid and reliable assessment in patients with pulmonary disease in the rehabilitation setting. In patients with COPD, the overall test-retest reliability has been as high as 0.92 while internal consistency reliability has been 0.94. The instrument is designed to provide measures of patient outcomes of care for evaluation of program planning and clinical trials of therapeutic interventions. However, the SIP includes 136 items and is often administered by the interviewer. Self-administration is often difficult in populations that are severely ill. The interviewer administration takes from 45 min to 1 hr. The questionnaire may be less practical in routine clinical settings.

Table 1 Selected General and Disease-Specific Measures for Rehabilitation

General measures
Sickness Impact Profile
SF-36 Short-Form 36-Item Health Survey
Duke–University of North Carolina Health Profile
McMaster Health Index
Nottingham Health Profile
Quality of Well-Being Index
Coop Charts
Disease-specific measures
Katz Index of ADL
Barthel Index
Functional Status Index
Arthritis Impact Measurement Scales (AIMS I and II)
Health Assessment Questionnaire
Dyspnea Index
Chronic Respiratory Disease Questionnaire
The Veterans Health Study—Disease Severity Index for Chronic Lung Disease
Functional Assessment Inventory
Rehabilitation Indicator
Rapid Disability Rating Scale
Social Adjustment Scale

SF-36 (Short-Form 36-Item Health Survey)

The Health Insurance Experiment and the Medical Outcomes Study have developed many questionnaire batteries that include physical functioning, role functioning, mental health, social contacts, and health perceptions (40,41). These batteries have had more than two decades of use. More recently, the items developed through these two major health policy studies have been condensed for economy and utility. The SF-36 reflects the best and most powerful item scales that have evolved from many years of testing and work (42). This questionnaire includes 36 items that tap eight scales or dimensions of health status, including physical functioning, role limitations due to emotional problems, role limitations due to physical problems, social functioning, mental health, energy or vitality/fatigue, pain, and general health perceptions. Each of these domains or concepts is made up of two (social functioning) to 10 (physical function inventory) items and scored on scales ranging from 0 to 100, with 100 indicating the best health. This questionnaire is quickly becoming a standard in the health service research industry. Based on a Medical Outcomes Study of ambulatory patients, those with COPD had substantially lower scores for HRQL (between 50 and 80% of a standard deviation worse for eight health concepts) than did those with hypertension. The strong psychometric properties of this questionnaire (internal consistency reliability in patients with pulmonary disease ranges from 0.80 to 0.92) and the practical aspects of its short form make it a strong candidate for administration in pulmonary rehabilitation populations. The instrument takes between 10 and 15 min to administer in patients with COPD.

Duke-UNC Health Profile

The Duke-University of North Carolina Profile is a 63-item questionnaire developed for use in clinical practice (43). This questionnaire is self-administered and has a long history of use in populations of patients undergoing ambulatory care. This assessment has been used in patients with pulmonary disease and reliability coefficients range from 0.85 to 0.95. However, the questionnaire is somewhat lengthy and does impose some respondent burden in patients with severe disease.

McMaster Health Index, Nottingham Health Profile, and Quality of Well-Being Index

The McMaster Health Index, the Nottingham Health Profile, and the Quality of Well-Being Index are other general instruments developed for measuring the functional status of patient populations (44). These questionnaires have all been administered to populations of patients with pulmonary disease and to patients undergoing rehabilitation. The questionnaires are all patient self-administered and have for the most part a decade of use in clinical practice. The McMaster Health Index and the Nottingham Health Profile each include measures of physical, psychological, and social functioning dimensions. The Quality of Well-being Index includes assessments of mobility, physical activity, and social activity. These questionnaires have been used in general ambulatory and rehabilitation populations.

Coop Charts

The final example of general measures of HRQL is the Coop Charts (45). This approach uses a cartoon layout depicting various characters of health. This layout provides a set of figures for each of the ordinal choices related to a dimension of health status. The areas include global ratings of physical, mental, role, social, pain, and overall health. The questionnaire is simple to administer in clinical settings and takes less than 1 min to be completed. The charts have undergone considerable psychometric testing and have been shown to be reliable and valid when compared with the SF-36 as a standard. This instrument has also been applied to pulmonary rehabilitation populations and, in cross-sectional studies, has been shown to be capable of discriminating between clinically relevant groups.

B. Disease-Specific Measures for Rehabilitation Populations

Disease-specific measures for rehabilitation populations include assessments developed for chronic lung disease, for arthritis, and, specifically, for rehabilitation. For the most part, these instruments have been used to evaluate therapeutic programs for various chronic diseases and in clinical trials to assess the outcomes of specific interventions. A number of them have been used to describe the impact of illness on the health status of patients.

The Katz Index of ADL and the Convery Index are early measures of functional assessment that focused on physical disabilities related to activities of daily living (7,46). Interestingly, although widely used, until recently these measures had not undergone rigorous psychometric testing. The Functional Status Index, the Arthritis Impact Measurement Scales versions 1 and 2, and the Health Assessment Questionnaire are several assessments developed in rheumatology; because pain is an important dimension in arthritis, each of these instruments includes a comprehensive pain battery for its assessment (47–49). The measures also capture physical functioning, psychological status, and social functioning that are specific to musculoskeletal problems. These assessments have been applied to rehabilitation populations and to populations of patients with chronic lung disease. They have been shown to discriminate between clinical groups, and in patients with chronic pulmonary disease, the measures have also been shown to detect clinically important differences in the effects of interventions.

The Chronic Respiratory Disease Questionnaire developed by Guyatt et al. was specifically developed for those with COPD (50). This assessment includes the following dimensions: dyspnea, fatigue, mastery over disease, and emotional dysfunction. The questionnaire is administered by a trained interviewer. The results indicate that this assessment is reproducible, valid, and responsive to clinical changes. The assessment also includes both the positive and negative aspects of health status. By direct comparison, this assessment was shown to be more valid and more responsive than two other measures of dyspnea, i.e., the Oxygen Cost Diagram and the Medical Research Council Dyspnea index.

The Veterans Health Study, a large-scale observational study of the processes and outcomes of ambulatory care of veterans, had, as one of its foci, the development of an index of disease severity for chronic lung disease (CLD) (51,52). Case identification was performed on the basis of reports by patients of the diagnosis, made by physicians, of chronic bronchitis, emphysema, and asthma and of the use of either inhaled medications or a productive cough for most days of 3 months. Identification was confirmed by chart review (93% agreement, kappa = 0.81). Clinic visits included a questionnaire administered by an interviewer relating to CLD. For a measure of the severity of the CLD, an expert panel selected a parsimonious set of questions about symptoms. Items in the severity measure included the frequency of dyspnea, wheezing, cough, and sputum production (grade 1–4, with 4 most severe). Factor analysis confirmed that the four clinical symptoms grouped together into a single dimension. Validity was evaluated by correlation analysis with the SF-36. Statistically significant correlations were found with physical functioning, role functioning due to physical limitations, general health perceptions, energy/vitality, and social functioning (correlations ranged from 0.26 to 0.38). Interestingly, peak flow did not correlate significantly with any of the SF-36 scales. This index has been shown to be both reliable and valid using clinical symptoms that are self-reported by patients. It provides a useful approach to severity of illness as a basis for assessment of outcomes in patients with CLD.

Specific assessments for rehabilitation include the Functional Assessment Inventory (FAI), the Rehabilitation Indicator (RI), the Rapid Disability Rating Scale (RDRS), and the Social Adjustment Scale (SAS) (53–56). These assessments have been extensively used in rehabilitation settings for evaluating outcomes of care. The FAI and the RI provide assessments of the illness burden related to functional limitations including physical, mental, emotional, and social.

The FAI is reasonably short and takes about 5–10 min to complete. This assessment is completed by a rehabilitation counselor by abstracting records, patient interviews, and other observations. A summary score as well as seven subscale scores are produced for ordinal ratings. The instrument has been validated and shown to be internally consistent using factor analytical approaches.

The RI is somewhat more broadly based and includes assessments of 51 descriptors in six areas of functioning, including vocation, income, education, self-care, transportation, and family role. A separate set of activity pattern indicators describe the individual's profile of daily activity, i.e., the types of activity, location, assistance required, and strengths of social contact through direct observation. Finally, skill indicators relate to several hundred skills representing behaviors necessary for functioning in vocational, educational, recreational, family, role, self-care, and other settings. These three components produce numerical scores that give a comprehensive behavioral profile of the functioning of the patients. The assessments are obtained by interviews, observations, and medical records. The comprehensive assessment requires more than 2 hr to administer. Both the FAI and RI can be applied to evaluating both rehabilitation programs and clinical outcome studies.

The RDRS was developed as a measure of the physical capacity of elderly long-term-care and community-based patients. This functional assessment consist of 18 items on four-point rating scales completed by a provider knowledgeable about the patient. The assessment consists of activities of daily living, degree of disability in terms of communication, diet, and incontinence, and questions about confusion, uncooperativeness, and depression. Items are then summed to provide an overall score. Although the assessment is short and useful, it has not undergone extensive testing for reliability and validity. Finally, the SAS provides an assessment of emotional and social functioning and has been applied to both long-term-care and community-wide populations. The assessment can be administered as an interview or self-report. It consists of 42 items. Areas covered include functional status at work, social-leisure activities, relationship with extended family, and role functioning at home. Subscales and overall scores can be computed for this set of assessments. This instrument has been used as a measure of outcome for purposes of evaluation and can be applied to clinical studies.

To summarize, both general and specific assessments have been developed for application to rehabilitation settings. General assessments tend to be comprehensive and include measures of functional status and well-being. Specific measures target particular chronic illnesses and the disabilities as well as symptoms associated with them. Specific assessments for rehabilitation often include measures of disability related to physical, emotional, and social functioning. The following section describes the application of these assessments to rehabilitation-based populations.

IV. Applications of Health Outcome Assessments to Rehabilitation Settings

Assessment of health outcome assessments have served a variety of purposes in rehabilitation settings. Measures of health status outcome have frequently been applied to evaluate treatments in the rehabilitation setting (57). Interventions that focus on medical therapy, adaptive equipment to reduce physical and mental barriers, and integration of multidisciplinary services to provide a network of support have been evaluated using methods for outcomes. These approaches have also been applied to patient management through the direct feedback of information to clinicians and other providers about the patient's functional status. Assessments have also been used in clinical trials to compare the efficacy of a specific therapeutic intervention with alternative approaches.

A. Program Evaluation

The use of outcome assessments for program evaluation involves identifying and specifying a target population, describing the changes resulting from health care services delivered, and examining the outcomes in terms of cost-benefit.

In recent years, considerable attention has been given to the outcomes obtained from certain services and their associated cost.

B. Clinical Practice

The second major application of outcome assessments is in routine clinical practice in rehabilitation settings. Quantifiable assessments of health status have been shown to be at least as reliable and valid as standard clinical parameters. Structured questionnaires are fairly simple to administer and score in the rehabilitation setting. Questionnaires can be administered and scored in the clinicians office. Functional status results can be fed back as a quantitative score and compared with reference populations. These assessments can be used to pinpoint or flag specific problems at a given visit based on repeated assessments over time.

These assessments also provide important screening information so that the provider can obtain more detailed assessments. A good example of this is the Mental Health Inventory described previously. This assessment can be used as a basis for administering more detailed mental health batteries in accordance with responses to five items. This approach might also be cost-saving. In a similar vein, information on functional assessment can provide baseline data relating to an initial diagnosis.

Some studies have confirmed the clinical utility of functional assessment measures in clinical practice. Kazis et al. (58) indicated that health status summary reports could be interpreted by clinicians in a reproducible fashion. Rubenstein et al. (59) indicated that the feeding back of functional status assessments to clinicians in routine practice, using summary reports of the individual patient's data base, resulted in significant improvement in the patient's physiological status and social functioning.

C. Research

The application of these measures to clinical studies has been widespread. This approach has broadened traditional assessments. Measures of functional status provide important descriptive information about the natural history of illness. Guyatt et al. (60) describe specific profiles related to patients with pulmonary illness. Functional status assessments in addition to standard mortality and morbidity outcomes provide a broad set of assessments that overlaps with the multidimensional goals frequently involved in rehabilitation interventions.

V. Controversies

The development and expanded use of assessments of functional status have resulted in controversies. One debate is about the use of general versus disease-specific assessments. Use of these measures frequently depends on the purpose of the user and the setting in which the measures are applied. Frequently in rehabilitation settings where the purpose is individual client feedback, a hybrid of general and disease-specific measures is used. Lengthier assessments are often used that may assure greater reliability or precision in the measures. Research applications may involve disease-specific measures when the objective is to describe the underlying epidemiological course of the disease. Users interested in clinically based approaches that address specific therapeutic outcomes are likely to select the disease-specific ones. Another approach is to use general measures with disease-specific supplements. This approach is meant to capture both specific and general concepts of health-related quality of life. Continued experience with alternative approaches will shed light on this debate.

Another debate involves the recent emergence of both long- and short-form assessments for measuring health status. Long forms for use in rehabilitation settings provide important advantages over short-form approaches since they provide a wide net of concepts and scales for detecting health status that may be more reliable and responsive over time. However, these instruments tend to be burdensome in clinical settings and may be logistically less satisfactory. On the other hand, short forms have recently appeared on the scene with excellent properties for measurement. These batteries meet standards of reliability, validity, ease of administration, and scoring. The instruments are practical for use in routine clinical settings. Further implementation of these short-form assessments in rehabilitation settings will help to resolve this debate.

A third controversy involves determining the appropriate application of health status assessments for different purposes. Assessments can be used to evaluate programs to provide routine feedback of information to providers and patients and for clinical research. The purpose behind the use of health status assessment may dictate the type of assessment that is to be used. For example, short forms may be more appropriate for research purposes and less appropriate for routine client assessments. Disease-specific measures may be more appropriate for routine feedback of information to clients, whereas both general and disease-specific assessments might be used for program evaluation. As this field continues to grow, and familiarity with the use of instruments develops, the specific application of these assessments will be better understood.

VI. Future Directions

Assessment of health-related quality of life in rehabilitation is closely related to the multidimensional goals that are the outcomes of patient care. As this field has evolved from acute management of physical impairment to chronic management of disability and handicap, measurement of functional status using a more comprehensive set of dimensions, emotional, social, and role functioning has emerged. Standards for assuring the reliability, validity, and responsiveness to clinically important change have been applied to these assessments. These measures are conceptually relevant, practical, and useful in rehabilitation settings.

In recent years, computer technologies, such as personal computers and optical scanner technologies for processing and feeding back summary health status information, have been developed. These technologies have increased the ability to summarize information in a timely fashion to providers and to practice managers in their respective organizations. This information can be summarized at the time of a clinic visit and fed back to the client and provider. Further study is needed to determine the most appropriate approaches to summarizing health status information so that it can be integrated into the patient treatment plan. Ultimately, administrators, providers, and researchers will have this technology, instrumentation, and analysis training for the interpretation and use of this information on a routine basis. These future systems will provide important data bases for programmatic evaluation, client feedback of clinical information, and research.

Acknowledgment

This work was supported by the VA Health Services Research and Development Service (Health Related Quality of Life in Veterans Study—SDR 91006-S).

References

1. Nagi SZ. Disability and Rehabilitation. Columbus, OH: Ohio State University Press, 1969.
2. Granger CV. A conceptual model for functual assessment. In: Granger CV, Gresham GE, eds. Functional Assessment in Rehabilitation Medicine. Baltimore: Williams & Wilkins, 1984.
3. Keith RA. Functional assessment measures in medical rehabilitation: current status. Arch Phys Med Rehabil 1984; 65:74–78.
4. Frey WD. Functional assessment in the '80s: A conceptual enigma, a technical challenge. In: Halpern AS, Fuhrer MJ, eds. Functional Assessment in Rehabilitation. Baltimore: Paul H. Brookes, 1984.
5. World Health Organization. The First Ten Years of the World Health Organization. Geneva, World Health Organization, 1948.
6. Criteria Committee of the New York Heart Association. Diseases of the Heart and Blood Vessels: Nomenclature and Criteria for Diagnosis, 6th ed. Boston: Little, Brown, 1964.
7. Katz S, Ford AB, Moskowitz RW, et al. Studies of illness in the aged: the Index

of ADL, a standardized measure of biological and psychosocial function. JAMA 1963; 185:914.
8. Steinbroker O, Traeger CH, Batterman RC. Therapeutic criteria in rheumatoid arthritis. JAMA 1949; 140:659–662.
9. Jette AM, Deniston DL. Inter-observer reliability of a functional status assessment instrument. J Chronic Dis 1978; 31:573.
10. Schipper H, Clinch J, McMurray A, et al. Measuring the quality of life of cancer patients: the functional living index—cancer: development and validation. J Clin Oncol 1984; 2:472.
11. Nagi SZ. Some conceptual issues in disability and rehabilitation. In: Sussmann MB, ed. Sociology and Rehabilitation. Columbus, OH: Ohio State University Press, 1965.
12. Wood PHN. Classification of impairment and handicap. Document WHO/ICDP/REV-CONF/75.15. Geneva: World Health Organization, 1975.
13. Felson DT. Epidemiology of hip and knee osteoathritis. Epidemiology reviews. 1988; 10:1–28.
14. Weinberger M, Kirkman MS, Sansa GP, Cowper PA. The relationship between glycemic control and health-related quality of life in patients with non-insulin dependent diabetes mellitus. Med Care 1994; 32:1173–1181.
15. Deyo RA. Back pain revisited: newer thinking on diagnosis and therapy consultant. 1993; 88–98.
16. Mahler OA, Farynialz K, Tomlinson D, Colice GL, et al. Impact of dyspnea and physiologic function on general health study in patients with chronic obstructive pulmonary disease. Chest 1992; 102:395–400.
17. Anthonisen NR, Wright EC, Hodgkin JE, et al. Prognosis in chronic obstructive pulmonary disease. Am Rev Respir Dis 1986; 133:14–19.
18. Jones PW, Baveystock CM, Littlejohns P. Relationship between general health measured with the sickness impact profile and respiratory symptoms physiological measures and mood in patients with chronic airflow limitation. Am Rev Respir Dis 1989; 140:1538–1543.
19. Ware JE. Analysis of Relationships Among Health Status Measures. Santa Monica, CA: RAND Corp., 1979.
20. Mahler DA, Weinberg DH, Wells CK, Feinstein AR. The measurement of dyspnea: contents, interobservor agreement and physiologic correlations of two new clinical indexes. Chest 1984; 85:751–758.
21. Bergner M, Bobbitt RA, Pollard WE, et al. The Sickness Impact Profile: validation of a health status measure. Med Care 1976; 14:57.
22. Ware JE, Brook RH, Davies-Avery A, et al. Conceptualization and Measurement of Health for Adults in the Health Insurance Study. Vol 1: Model of Health and Methodology. R-1987/1-HEW. Santa Monica, CA: RAND Corp., 1980.
23. Prigatano GP, Wright EC, Levin D. Quality of life and its predictors in patients with mild hypoxemia and chronic obstructive pulmonary disease. Arch Intern Med 1984; 144:1613–1619.
24. Donald CA, Ware JE. The quantification of social contacts and resources. Santa Monica CA: RAND Corp., 1982.

25. Brownell A, Shumaker SA. Social support on introduction to complex phenomena. J Soc Issues 1984; 4:1–11.
26. McHorney CA, Ware JE, Raczek A. The MOS 36-Item Short Form Health Survey (SF-36). II. Psychometeric and clinical tests of validity in measuring physical and mental health constructs. Med Care 1993; 31:247.
27. Jones PW. Measuring the quality of life of patients with respiratory diseases. In: Walker SR, Rosser RN, eds. Quality of Life Assessment and Applications. London: MTP, 1987:235–251.
28. Anthonisen NR. Prognosis in chronic obstructive pulmonary disease: results from multicenter trials. RN Respir Dis 1989; 140:595–599.
29. Ware JE, Sherbourne CD. The MOS 36-Item Short-Form Health Survey. I. Conceptual framework and item selection. Med Care 1992; 30:473.
30. Jenkinson C, Fitzpatrick R, Argyle M. The Nottingham Health Profile: an analysis of its sensitivity in differentiating illness groups. Soc Sci Med 1988; 27:1411–1414.
31. Miller DR, Skinner K, Desai M, Kazis LE. Quality of life assessments; the white coat effect. National Health Services Research and Development Meeting, 1993 (abstract).
32. Veit CT, Ware JE Jr. The structure of psychological distress and well-being in general populations. J Consult Clin Psychol 1983; 51:730.
33. McHorney CA, Kusinski M, Ware JE. Comparisons of the costs and quality of norms for the SF-36 health survey collected by mail verses telephone interview: results from a national survey. Med Care 1994; 32:551–567.
34. Brambilla DJ, McKinlay SM. A comparison of responses to mailed questionnaires and telephone interviews in a mixed mode health survey. Am J Epidemiol 1987; 126:962.
35. Nelson EC, Berwick DM. The measurement of health status in clinical practice. Med Care 1989; 27:S77.
36. Meenan RF, Gertman PM, Mason JR. Measuring health status in arthritis: the Arthritis Impact Measurement Scales. Arthritis Rheum 1980; 23:146–152.
37. Fries JF, Spitz P, Kraines RG, Holman HR. Measurement of patient outcome in arthritis. Arthritis Rheum 1980; 23:143–152.
38. Bergner M, Bobbitt RA, Carter WB, et al. The Sickness Impact Profile: development and final revision of a health status measure. Med Care 1981; 19:787.
39. McSweeny AJ, Grant I, Heaton RK, et al. Life quality of patients with chronic obstructive pulmonary disease. Arch Intern Med 1982; 142:473–478.
40. Brook RH, Ware JE, Rogers WH, et al. Does free care improve adults' health? Results from a randomized controlled trial. N Engl J Med 1983; 309:1426.
41. Tarlov AR, Ware JE, Greenfield S, et al. The Medical Outcomes Study—an application of methods for monitoring the results of medical care. JAMA 1989; 262:925.
42. Ware JE, Snow KK, Kosinski M, et al. SF-36 Health Survey Manual and Interpretation Guide. Boston, MA: The Health Institute, New England Medical Center Hospitals, 1993.
43. Parkerson GR, Gehlbach SH, Wagner EH, et al. The Duke-UNC health profile: an adult health status instrument for primary care. Med Care 1981; 19:806.

44. Patrick DL, Erickson P. Health Status and Health Policy. New York: Oxford University Press, 1993.
45. Nelson E, Wasson J, Kirk J, et al. Assessment of function in routine clinical practice: description of the COOP chart method and preliminary findings. J Chronic Dis 1987; 40(Suppl 1):55S.
46. Convery FR, Minteer MA, Amiel D, et al. Polyarticular disability: a functional assessment. Arch Phys Med Rehabil 1977; 58:494.
47. Meenan RF, Gertman PM, Mason JR, Dunaif R. The arthritis impact measurement scales: further investigations of a health status measure. Arthritis Rheum 1982; 25:1048–1055.
48. Meenan RF, Pincus T. The status of patient status measures. J Rheumatol 1987; 14:411–414.
49. Pincus T, Summey JA, Soraci SA, Wallston KA, Hummon NP. Assessment of patient satisfaction in activities of daily living using a modified Stanford Health Assessment Questionnaire. Arthritis Rheum 1983; 26:1346–1353.
50. Guyatt GH, Berman LB, Townsend M, et al. A measure of quality of life for clinical trials in chronic lung disease. Thorax 1987; 42:773–778.
51. Kazis LE, Miller D, Clark J, et al. Quality of life in veterans: preminary results from the Veterans Health Study. Presented at National Meeting of Association for Health Services Research, 1993 (abstract).
52. Selim AJ, Fincke G, Clark J, et al. A short measure of illness severity for chronic lung disease from the Veterans Health Study. Society of General Internal Medicine, 1995 (abstract).
53. Crewe NM, Athelstan GT. Functional assessment in vocational rehabilitation: a systematic approach to diagnosis and goal setting. Arch Phys Rehabil 1981; 62:299–305.
54. Brown M, Diller L, Fordyce W, Jacobs D, Gordon W. Rehabilitation indicators: their nature and uses for assessment. In: Bolton B, Cook D, eds. Rehabilitation Client Assessment. Baltimore: University Park Press, 1980.
55. Linn MW, Linn DS. The Rapid Disability Rating Scale-2. J Am Geriatr Soc 1982; 30:378–382.
56. Weissman MM, Gothwell S. Assessment of social adjustment by patient self-report. Arch Gen Psychiatry 1976; 33:1111–1115.
57. Halpern AS, Fuhrer MJ. Functional Assessment in Rehabilitation. Baltimore: Paul H. Brookes, 1984.
58. Kazis LE, Anderson JJ, Meenan RF. Health status information in clinical practice—the development and testing of patient profile reports. J Rheum 1988; 15:338.
59. Rubenstein LV, McCoy JM, Cope DW, et al. Improving patient functional status—a randomized trial of computer-generated resource and management suggestions. Clin Res 1989; 37:801A.
60. Guyatt GH, Townsend M, Berman LB, et al. Quality of life in patients with chronic airflow limitation. Br J Dis Chest 1987; 81:45–54.

16

Cost-Effectiveness of Pulmonary Rehabilitation

ROBERT M. KAPLAN and ANDREW L. RIES

University of California, San Diego
San Diego, California

Pulmonary rehabilitation has become an accepted modality of care for patients with chronic obstructive pulmonary disease (COPD) and other chronic lung diseases (1–3). However, rehabilitation typically involves multidisciplinary care and it is not always reimbursed by third-party payers. The American Lung Association (ALA) and the American Thoracic Society (ATS) formed a Health Policy Task Force that offered a position statement on the reform of the U.S. health care system. The statement was general, but it did specifically advocate pulmonary rehabilitation. In particular, the ALA and ATS noted, "The ALA/ATS also is concerned that some rehabilitation services, such as pulmonary rehabilitation may not be covered. Their [Clinton administration] criteria for continuation of such services indicates that 'improvement' must be documented. Many types of rehabilitation, including pulmonary rehabilitation, ensure non-deterioration in a condition—not necessarily improvement" (4).

Should rehabilitation services be included in basic benefit packages? How should these services be treated in health care reform? In this chapter we introduce several topics that may be useful in evaluating these issues. The chapter will review general issues in health care reform, the need for outcomes research, and the application of cost-effectiveness models. Then, we will consider the evidence that rehabilitation programs are valuable in relation to other alternative uses of health care resources. The relative cost-effectiveness of rehabilitation programs will also be addressed.

I. Why Is the Issue Important?

American health care is in a state of turmoil. Physicians' autonomy is being challenged as never before. They must submit their judgment to second opinions, have the hospital stays of their patients preauthorized, and undergo time-consuming and frustrating encounters with utilization review. What went wrong? Is this really necessary?

A. Is There a Crisis?

Some people argue that there is no health care crisis and that we need only minor changes in our current system. However, the problems in contemporary health care are hard to ignore. Three important problems in American health care are affordability, access, and accountability (5). The affordability problem results from the inability to pay for all health services that are desired. Health care costs in the United States have grown exponentially since 1940 and the rate of increase has continued to accelerate through the 1990s. Health care in the United States now consumes 14.5% of the gross domestic product, while no other country in the world spends more than 10% (6). The problem is not only that health care is expensive, but that the rate of increase in health care costs exceeds that of other sectors in the economy. For example, over the last few decades, health care costs have risen at a rate of about 11.5% per year. Since the rate of growth of health care costs exceeds that of other sectors of the economy, health care is steadily gaining larger proportions of the gross domestic product (GDP) at a rate of about 1% per year. As a result of devoting a higher portion of the GDP for health care, we have less to devote to other sectors. For example, in 1965, health care accounted for less than 5% of federal spending. By 1990 that figure had risen to 15% and it is projected to be 30% by the year 2000 (7). There are consequences of devoting an increasingly larger portion of the federal budget to health care. Unless we raise taxes or other revenues, we will have less to spend for other activities, such as defense, education, and criminal justice.

Access is the second major challenge. Even with our high expenditures on health care, 58 million Americans have no health insurance for part of each year and 38 million are uninsured throughout the entire year (8). Programs designed to serve the poor, such as Medicaid, have evolved peculiar rules of eligibility. The costs of Medicaid programs have grown dramatically and all states must now consider cost-cutting strategies (9). The accountability problem is perhaps the most challenging. Despite the fact that we spend more on health care than any other country in the world, we have a great deal of difficulty demonstrating that our high expenditures result in health benefits (10).

The three problems (affordability, access, and accountability) are connected. Access has become limited because health care is unaffordable, and care may be too expensive because there is poor accountability. Better accountability may preserve resources that could be used to provide greater access to care.

II. Opportunity Cost Problem

One of the problems in reforming health care is that advocacy groups often fail to consider the total picture. Successful lobbying to obtain reimbursement for a specific service may necessarily mean that another service is excluded. This is called the opportunity cost problem. Opportunity costs are the foregone opportunities that are surrendered as a result of using resources to support a particular decision. If we spend a lot of money in one sector of health care, we necessarily spend less money elsewhere. Part of the problem in the U.S. health care system is that we have tended to follow a "rule of rescue." The rule of rescue, in the words of philosophers, is a moral obligation to provide rescue services whenever saving a life is a possibility (1). However, the decision to invest in rescue may necessarily mean two decisions have been made. For instance, with limited resources, a decision to perform an expensive transplantation surgery for one person often means giving up the opportunity to perform less expensive rehabilitation services for large numbers of people. In some cases a transplant may have limited potential for producing a health benefit, while the rehabilitation services that are neglected have substantial potential to help other people. Indeed, the U.S. health care system is rich with applications of the rule of rescue. Large investments in dramatic and often futile care have resulted in the unfunding or underfunding of important opportunities in primary care, prevention, and rehabilitation (11).

When confronted with the choice between two good programs, it is always tempting to do both. The difficulty is that it is expensive to offer multiple programs. The cost of programs is represented in the fees for health insurance or the cost of health care to taxpayers. A society can choose to offer as many health programs as it wants. However, programs require funding. Employees do not want the fees for their health insurance to rise and taxpayers do not want tax increases. The goal of formal decision models is to get higher-quality health care at a lower cost (11). This chapter focuses on the cost-effectiveness of rehabilitation services for patients with COPD. However, we must recognize the larger context. Pulmonary rehabilitation programs compete for limited resources with many other and different health care services. Thus, consideration of funding programs for the rehabilitation of patients with COPD must be taken in the context of all programs. This requires the application of generic methods for assessing cost-effectiveness and cost-utility.

A. Cost-Utility Versus Cost-Benefit

The terms "cost-utility," "cost-effectiveness," and "cost-benefit" are used inconsistently in the medical literature (12). The key concepts are summarized in Table 1. Some economists have favored the assessment of cost-benefit. These approaches measure both program costs and treatment outcomes in dollar units. For example, treatment outcomes are evaluated in relation to changes in use of medical services or the economic productivity of patients. Treatments are cost-beneficial if the economic return exceeds treatment costs. Patients with COPD who are aggressively treated with antibiotics, for example, may need fewer emergency medical services. The savings associated with decreased services might exceed treatment costs. Russell argued that the requirement that health care treatments reduce costs may be unrealistic (13). Patients are willing to pay for improvements in health status just as they are willing to pay for other desirable goods and services. We do not treat chronic lung disease in order to save money. Allowing patients to die would certainly be less expensive. Treatments are given to achieve better health outcomes.

Cost-effectiveness is an alternative approach in which the unit of outcome is a reflection of treatment effect. In recent years, cost-effectiveness has gained considerable attention. Some approaches emphasize simple, treatment-specific outcomes. For example, Nichol and colleagues estimated the cost per hospitalization prevented by vaccinating the elderly against influenza (14). The major difficulty with cost-effectiveness methodologies is that they do not allow for comparison across very different treatment interventions. For example, health care administrators often need to choose between investments in very different alternatives. They may need to decide between supporting transplantation for a few patients versus prenatal counseling for a large number of patients. For the same cost, they may achieve a large effect for a few people or a small effect for a large number of people. The treatment-specific outcomes used in cost-effectiveness studies do not permit these comparisons.

Table 1 Comparison of Cost-Effectiveness, Cost-Utility, and Cost-Benefit Analysis

Type of analysis	Compares	To
Cost-effectiveness	$ value of resources used	Clinical effects
Cost-utility	$ value of resources used	Quality of life produced
Cost-benefit	$ value of resources used	$ value of resources saved or created

Cost-utility approaches use the expressed preference or utility of a treatment effect as the unit of outcome. As noted in World Health Organization documents, the goals of health care are to add years to life and to add life to years (15). In other words, health care is designed both to make people live longer (increase the life expectancy) and to allow them to have a higher quality of life in the years prior to death. Cost-utility studies use outcome measures that combine mortality outcomes with quality-of-life measurements. The utilities are the expressed preferences for observable states of function on a continuum bounded by 0 for death to 1.0.0 for optimum function (16–24). In recent years, cost-utility approaches have gained increasing acceptance as methods for comparing many diverse options in health care (13,25). Recently, Kassirer and Angell urged the consistent use of these terms for all reports on cost-effectiveness analyses submitted to the *New England Journal of Medicine* (5).

III. Estimating the Effects of Rehabilitation Programs

COPD has a profound effect on functioning and everyday life. Current estimates suggest that COPD affects nearly 11% of the adult population and the incidence is increasing. Newer trends indicate that the rate of COPD among women is increasing to reflect the increase in tobacco use among women in the latter part of this century (26). Reviews of the medical management of COPD justify the use of symptomatic measures including bronchodilators, corticosteroids, and antibiotic therapy. In addition, long-term oxygen therapy has been shown to be beneficial in patients with severe hypoxemia (27). However, it is widely recognized that these measures cannot cure COPD and that much of the effort in the management of this condition must be directed toward preventive treatment strategies, improving symptoms, patient functioning, and quality of life.

There have been few controlled studies evaluating pulmonary rehabilitation programs or their components. Reports from these trials as well as nonrandomized studies typically suggest that the objectives can be achieved (2,28). In one of our recent studies, 119 COPD patients, were randomly assigned to either comprehensive pulmonary rehabilitation or an education control group. Pulmonary rehabilitation consisted of 12 4-hr sessions over an 8-week period. The content of the sessions was education, physical and respiratory care, psychosocial support, and supervised exercise. The education control group attended four 2-hr sessions that were scheduled twice per month, but did not include any individual instruction or exercise training. Topics included medical aspects of COPD, pharmacy use, breathing techniques, and a variety of interviews about smoking, life events, and social support. Lectures covered pulmonary medicine, pharmacology, respiratory therapy, and nutrition. Outcome measures included lung function, maximum and endurance exercise tolerance, symptoms, perceived breathlessness, perceived fatigue, self-efficacy for walking, CES-D depression, and the Quality of Well-Being Scale. In comparison to the educational control group, rehabilitation patients demonstrated a significant increase in exercise endurance (82% versus 11%), maximal exercise workload (32% versus 14%), and peak Vo_2 (8% versus 2%). These changes in exercise performance were associated with significant improvement in symptoms of perceived breathlessness and muscle fatigue during exercise (29,30).

Several studies have documented the benefits of exercise programs for patients with COPD. In a recent review, Casaburi summarized 37 reports of exercise training in the literature up to 1991 (31). These studies included 933 patients with COPD with an average $FEV_{1.0}$ of 1.1 L. A wide improvement in exercise performance was noted, with maximal level or duration being reported in 31 of the 32 studies in which exercise tolerance was evaluated. A few of these studies were controlled trials.

Cockcroft et al. randomly assigned 39 patients to a 6-week exercise training program or to a no-treatment control group (32). In comparison to the control group, patients in the exercise group experienced subjective benefits and increased the amount of distance they could walk in 12 min. However, the length of follow-up was only 2 months. McGavin and co-workers randomly allocated 24 patients with COPD to a 3-month unsupervised stair-climbing home exercise program or to a nonexercise control group. The 12 patients in the exercise group noted subjective improvements and an increased sense of well-being and decreased breathlessness. They also reported an objective increase in the 12-min walk distance and maximal level of exercise on a cycle ergometer. These changes did not occur in the control group. However, the length of follow-up was limited to 3 months (33). Ambrosino and co-workers randomly assigned 23 patients to a 1-month medical and rehabilitative therapy group and 28 patients to medical therapy alone (without exercise training). The experimental group improved in exercise tolerance and ventilatory pattern (as evidenced by decrease in respiratory rate and increase in tidal volume). Again, these changes were not present in the control group (34).

Developing exercise programs for patients with COPD is difficult for several reasons. First, principles of training that have been well studied for normals or for cardiac patients do not necessarily apply to patients with COPD (35,36). Adherence is often a major problem for the patient with COPD. Some studies suggest that the degree of benefit is associated with compliance to the exercise regimen (37). Although patients can benefit from exercise, the routine is typically not comfortable for them. Many participants in rehabilitation programs have become physically deconditioned over a long period of time. Exertion may be uncomfortable and commonly leads to the frightening symptom of breathlessness (dyspnea). Because of these problems, discontinuation of the exercise regimen is common.

In summary, some evidence suggests that rehabilitation is effective. Establishment of these benefits is a crucial step in estimating the cost-effectiveness of programs. However, there are limitations in the current evidence for the effectiveness of these programs. In particular, few studies have been systematic clinical trials and most studies have had limited follow-up.

IV. Economic Evaluations in COPD

Despite the interest and the cost-effectiveness of pulmonary rehabilitation, there have been relatively few investigations of this topic. Molken and Associates, in The Netherlands, systematically reviewed economic appraisals of asthma and COPD care for the years 1980–1991 (38). They found only 20 economic appraisals of treatments. Among these, only one used cost-utility methods. Two of the 20 studies focused on pulmonary rehabilitation, while the majority of the studies emphasized health education for asthma. Nine of the 20 studies focused on patients with COPD, while the others considered patients with other lung diseases. Their review suggested that use of control groups characterized less than half of the studies (eight of 20 studies), and most of these trials evaluated education for children with asthma. We extended the review through 1994, but found only one additional reference. The new study was a review rather than an original research contribution (39).

V. Cost-Benefit Studies

The literature on the cost-benefit of pulmonary rehabilitation programs was recently reviewed (40). Although the title of this review was "Cost-Effectiveness of Pulmonary Rehabilitation Programs," the majority of the studies that were reviewed emphasized cost-benefit. In other words, these were studies that considered the financial savings associated with investments in pulmonary rehabilitation programs. The various studies are summarized in Table 2. The studies are consistent in their methodology and in the obtained results. Dunham and colleagues considered the number of hospital days used by patients before and after a pulmonary rehabilitation program conducted by Loma Linda University. Initially, 80 patients participated in the study, but only 53 survived 1 year. The mean $FEV_{1.0}$ at entry to the study was 1.33 L. The study demonstrated that the average number of hospital days dropped from 17.41 for the year prior to the study to 7.78 the year following the study. The same effect was observed when patients who died were eliminated from the analysis (41).

A similar result was reported by Hudson and associates. They began their study in 1966 at the University of Colorado School of Medicine and studied 44 patients (mean $FEV_{1.0} = 1.07$ L). Hospitalizations prior to a rehabilitation pro-

Table 2 Summary of Cost-Benefit Studies on Rehabilitation of Patients with COPD

Study	Design	Finding	Comment
Durham et al., 1984	Pretest-posttest using hospital records	Hospital days dropped from 17.41 to 7.78	One-third of the patients died, but the result holds with adjustments for mortality
Hudson et al., 1976	Pretest-posttest evaluation of 44 patients followed over 5 years	Hospital days dropped from an average of 12 the year prior to the program to 3 the year after; average hospital days remained at about 5 or 3 additional years	Results were similar with inclusion of 20 additional patients who died prior to the end of the study
Johnson et al., 1980	Pretest-posttest follow-up of 74 survivors from among 96 registrants in a program	Hospital days dropped from 38 preprogram to 12 postprogram	Results were similar when all 96 patients were included in the analysis
Wright et al., 1983	Pretest-posttest evaluation of 57 completers of a 10-week program	Hospital days dropped from 8.72 pretreatment to 0.60 after treatment	All preprogram hospital days were among 16 patients
Bria et al., 1987	Nonequivalent control group comparison of individual ($n=25$) versus group ($n=30$) treatment	Hospital days dropped by 5.43 days for the individual treatment and 4.52 days for the group treatment	Phone calls to program increased
Ries et al., 1994	Randomized comparison of rehabilitation versus education control in 119 patients	Hospital days were reduced by 2.9 in the rehabilitation group and increased by 1.6 days in the control group	Although not statistically significant, the results were in the expected direction
Sneider et al., 1988	Nonrandomized self-selection of 150 patients into three groups: interview only, education, and comprehensive rehabilitation; hospital days compared 5 years pre- and postprogram	Hospital days increased in the interview-only and education-only groups; days decreased by 1.53 days in the comprehensive rehabilitation group	Self-selection into groups rather than treatment may account for the results

gram and after the rehabilitation program were determined from hospital records. Hospital days dropped from 12 the year prior to the program to about 5 for each of 4 follow-up years. The results were more dramatic when the subset of patients who had been hospitalized prior to the program were separated. Among these 14 patients, the number of hospitalizations dropped from 38 to 10 in the first year and remained less than 17 throughout the rest of the 4-year follow-up. Among the 44 patients, approximately one-third of all preprogram hospitalizations were accounted for by a single patient who was hospitalized for 178 days. After rehabilitation, this patient was hospitalized for only 1 day over the next 4 years. Elimination of this one patient reduced the magnitude of the pre-post programs difference from about 7 days to about 4 days (42).

Another group, at Barlow Hospital, evaluated 96 patients and obtained follow-up data on 74 patients 1 year after completing pulmonary rehabilitation. The mean $FEV_{1.0}$ value was 0.87 L. There was an average of 38 hospital days prior to the program, which was reduced to 12 days after completion of the program (10).

Wright and associates, at St. Joseph's Hospital in Stockton, California, evaluated a 10-week outpatient education and exercise program among 74 COPD patients (mean $FEV_{1.0}$ not reported). Hospitalizations were obtained from patients' self-reports on a questionnaire. On average, the patients had been hospitalized for 8.7 days the year prior to the program and only 0.60 days the year following the program (43). A similar result was reported in an abstract of a program at the Basystate Medical Center in Springfield, Massachusetts. In this study 55 COPD patients (mean $FEV_{1.0}=1.17$ L) were randomly assigned to pulmonary rehabilitation in the form of individual sessions ($n=30$) or group sessions ($n=25$). The pretreatment hospital days were not reported. However, there was a significant decrease in the number of hospital days for those in the individual treatment (mean = 5.43) and for those in the group treatment (mean = 4.52). The abstract suggests that many patients replaced hospital visits with phone calls to their providers (44).

One of the most detailed studies was reported by Sneider et al. from the Eisenhower Medical Center in Rancho Mirage, California. These investigators evaluated 150 patients who self-selected themselves into a pulmonary rehabilitation program. Using hospital records, Sneider et al. compared hospitalizations for the 5 years prior to the program with those for the 5 years after the program among three different groups of patients. One group was interviewed for the program but did not participate. A second group received the education component but did not complete the exercise portion. The third group completed all phases of pulmonary rehabilitation. There was a significant decrease in hospital days only for those who had completed the program. In the other two groups, there was a significant increase in the number of days of hospitalization (45).

More recently, in our randomized clinical trial at the University of California, San Diego, patients were assigned to either a comprehensive pulmonary rehabilitation program or an education control group. The mean $FEV_{1.0}$ for the 119 participants was 1.23 L. In comparison to baseline, rehabilitation patients decreased days of lung disease–related hospitalizations by an average of 2.4 days while the education control group increased hospital days by 1.3 days. Although they were in the expected direction, these differences were not statistically significant (29,46).

To summarize, cost-benefit studies compare monetary investments in pulmonary rehabilitation against monetary savings attributable to the programs. To date, studies consistently suggest that the costs of pulmonary rehabilitation programs may be offset by reductions in health care costs. However, the interpretation of almost all of these studies can be challenged on various accounts. We reviewed seven different investigations. Four of the seven studies did not use a control group. Among the three studies using a control group, only one randomly assigned patients to the treatment or control conditions. The studies consistently show that pulmonary rehabilitation reduces hospital utilization and costs. However, a recent randomized experimental trial failed to show that this benefit was statistically significant.

Other methodological issues must also be considered. For example, patients with high rates of hospitalization are likely to be referred preferentially. In fact, many patients are referred at the point of a hospitalization. The selection process may also screen out patients who are unlikely to get better. Another problem is the changing health care scene with its emphasis on decreased length of stay and increased use of outpatient facilities. All in all, despite strong evidence that pulmonary rehabilitation reduces hospitalizations, randomized controlled clinical trials are needed to substantiate the cost-benefit of pulmonary rehabilitation.

One of the important problems in cost-benefit studies is that cost reduction may not necessarily translate into patient benefit. For example, recent policies of utilization review have greatly reduced hospital use. However, it has not been clearly established that reduced hospital use benefits patient. Further, these studies do not clearly evaluate the relationship between reduced hospitalization and reduced disability.

VI. Cost-Utility Studies

Despite the attractiveness of cost-benefit studies, there are also some disadvantages. Limiting the evaluation to only economic criteria may neglect the primary mission of health care. For example, the development of guidelines for appropriate care might exclude expensive services that save lives and produce changes in function. If cost is the only criterion, the cheapest alternative might always be selected. To choose between alternatives, it is necessary to value the health benefits of patient outcomes as well as the cost (47). Clinical measures of benefit are often poorly understood with respect to their implications for the patient. For example, improvement in arterial blood gas values may not mean much to a patient or to a public policy maker. On the other hand, restoration or preservation of the ability to perform activities of daily living, the goal of many therapies, is meaningful to all concerned. These outcomes are measurable, and a paradigm shift in medicine is beginning to embrace patient-centered reports.

Despite the improvements in measuring patient outcomes, determining the value of health services has been particularly difficult. In economics, the value of a product is related to the willingness of consumers to pay for it. For example, the value of a Mercedes Benz automobile is set by the price consumers are willing to pay to obtain the car. If the price is set too high, few cars will be sold. Health services are difficult to value because consumers rarely pay for them directly. Instead, the charges are paid by third parties. Third-party payment has left consumers out of the loop and made it difficult to establish whether the services are valuable to patients. Cost-utility analysis considers both costs and patient outcomes in determining the value of treatment. In contrast to cost-benefit analysis, which focuses on the dollar returns for investing in particular programs, cost-utility analysis considers the health benefit of a program, weighted by patient preferences for outcomes, in relation to the financial costs of the program.

There are several methods for evaluating patient outcome. One approach combines morbidity and mortality into a single index. Survival analysis is a common method for considering mortality outcomes. In survival analysis each patient is coded as 1.0 if he/she is alive and 0.0 if dead. Thus, a patient is given 1 year of credit for each year that he/she survives and no credit if he/she is dead. A patient who survives to 83 years would be given 83 points while someone in the same birth cohort who survives to age 50 would be given 50 credits. The appeal of survival analysis is that it is general and can be used to describe any patient cohort or disease classification. The disadvantage is that survival analysis does not recognize levels of wellness between death and optimum function.

We prefer methods of adjusted survival analysis that consider the continuum of wellness between death and optimum function. The outcomes are assessed using a general measure known as the Quality of Well-being Scale (QWB) (19–22). If a patient with COPD was limited by the illness in some, but not all, activities, his score on this scale might be 0.60 on the 0.0–1.0 continuum. Instead of being given a year credit for survival, he might be given 0.60 years for surviving the year in the disabled state. In other words, survival time is "quality adjusted." The outcome is defined as a quality-adjusted life year (QALY). A treatment that boosted the patient from 0.6 to 0.7 would produce the equivalent of one-tenth of a year of life. Aggregated across 10 patients, the treatment would produce the equivalent of 1 year. Determining the quality weights is a complex task that is described in several other papers (16–24). The goal of cost-utility analysis is to divide the cost of a program by the equivalents of life years that the program produces. Since the goal of all interventions in health care is to increase quality-adjusted life expectancy, programs and treatments with different specific objectives can be directly compared to one another.

Only a few attempts have been made to evaluate the cost-utility of rehabilitation programs for patients with COPD. In one experimental trial, patients with COPD underwent exercise testing and were given an exercise prescription. They were then randomly assigned to one of five experimental or control groups. The experimental groups were based on the principles of behavior modification or a variant of behavior modification known as "cognitive behavior modification." These methods involve setting goals, analyzing the reinforcers for walking, and using behavioral contracts. The experimental programs included six weekly sessions in the patient's home. One control group received attention but did not have the behaviorally based sessions, while the other control group received no treatment. After 3 months, the three experimental groups showed greater compliance with the exercise program than did the two control groups. These changes were reflected in changes in exercise tolerance measured 1 month after the treatment. However, there were no significant changes in spirometric parameters (48).

Several additional analyses were performed using the QWB measure (49). Over the course of 18 months, the experimental and control groups showed significant differences on a quality-of-life index (Fig. 1). These analyses pooled together the three experimental groups and the two control groups. These same patients were studied again 3 years after the beginning of the program. At this time, observed differences between the experimental and control groups remained for the quality-of-well-being measure (50). However, substantial increases in variability precluded statistically significant effects. The differences were used to calculate QALY and perform cost-utility studies. There is considerable debate about the economic value of behavioral and rehabilitation programs. The cost-utility analyses suggested that behavioral programs designed to increase adherence for patients with COPD produce a QALY for approximately $23,000. The cost per QALY has been analyzed for a wide range of medical, surgical, and public health interventions. The cost per QALY for the behavioral intervention is comparable to that of other widely advocated health care programs (51). Figure 2 shows the cost-utility of this program in relation to other widely advocated treatments or programs. The behavioral programs were significantly more cost-effective than coronary artery bypass sur-

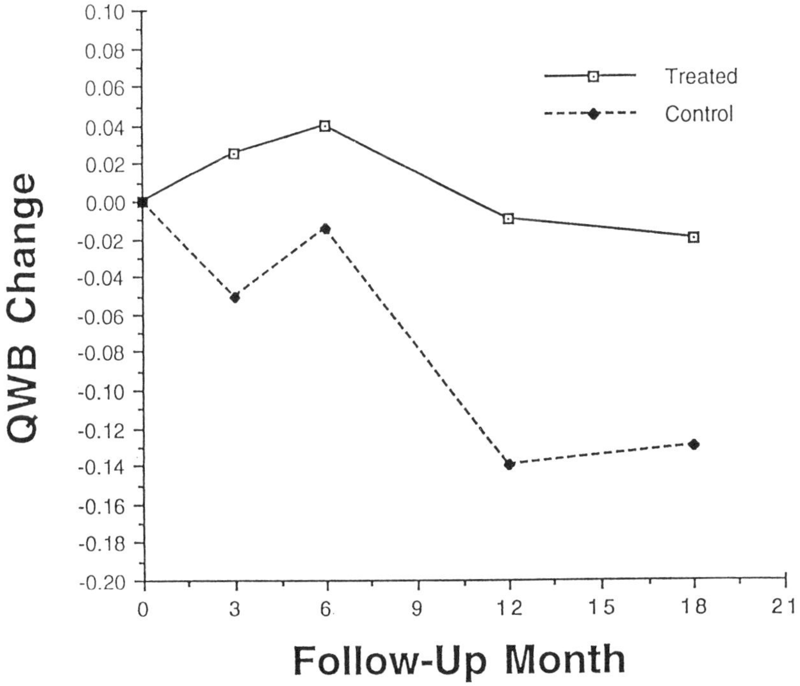

Figure 1 Quality of well-being differences between patients who had completed a behavioral rehabilitation program and controls during an 18-month follow-up. Scores did not change significantly for the treatment groups and showed significant decline for those in the control groups. (Adapted from Ref. 51.)

gery for one-vessel coronary heart disease ($670,000/QALY) or mammography screening programs ($175,000/QALY), but less cost-effective than pnemonococcal vaccine for the elderly ($1000/QALY) or laws requiring children to be in infant restraints and adults to wear seatbelts while in motor vehicles (<$100/QALY). Figure 2 also shows a hypothetical pay line where a policy maker might separate those programs to be supported from those not recommended for funding.

VII. Other Results

Not all studies have supported the cost-utility of pulmonary rehabilitation. For example, our clinical trial that compared comprehensive pulmonary rehabilitation versus an educational control group demonstrated highly significant improvement in exercise performance and relief of symptoms. In the comprehen-

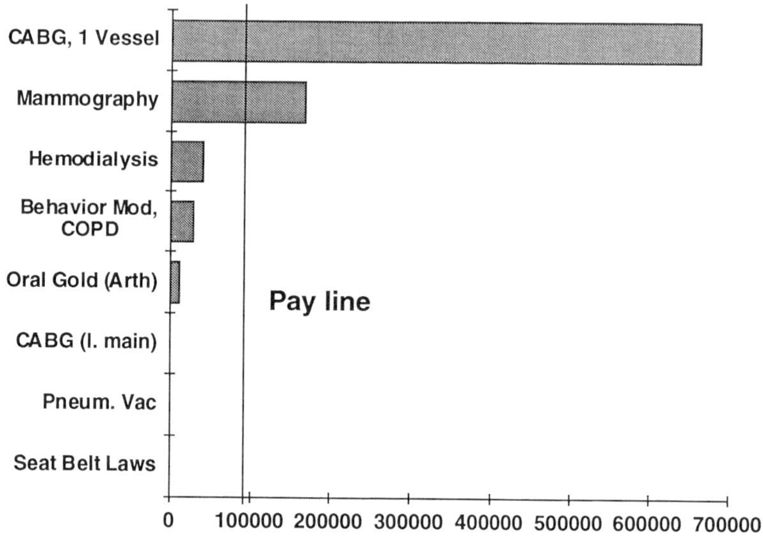

Figure 2 Relative cost/quality-adjusted life year for various programs. CABG, coronary artery bypass graft; 1 vessel, single-vessel disease; Mammography, screening all women older than age 40; Oral Gold, Auranofin for rheumatoid arthritis; CABG (l. main) is surgery for patients with left main artery disease; Pneum. Vac, pnemonococcal vaccine for adults older than 65 years; seat belt laws refers to policies requiring children to be in carseats and adults to use seatbelts. Behavioral modification for patients with COPD produces a QALY for about $23,000. This is significantly more cost-effective than CABG for one-vessel disease ($670,000/QALY) or mammography screening programs ($175,000/QALY), but less cost-effective than pnemonococcal vaccine ($1000/QALY) or seatbelt laws (<$100/QALY). The hypothetical pay line shows where a policy maker may draw the line between those programs to be supported and those not funded.

sive rehabilitation group, however, there were no significant differences between groups for measures of lung function, depression, or general quality of life. Both groups experienced reductions in quality of life over long-term follow-up, partly due to the mortality that is incorporated in the quality-of-well-being measure. For the exercise and symptom variables, the benefits in the comprehensive pulmonary rehabilitation group tended to relapse toward baseline after 18 months of follow-up (29).

The failure of pulmonary function to improve was not unanticipated. Nearly all previous studies have also failed to show significant changes in lung function (52–54). The failure to demonstrate benefits of pulmonary rehabilitation for measures of quality of life, e.g., well-being, and depression were somewhat unexpected. Long-term benefits beyond 12 months were observed only for measures of exercise endurance and perceived breathlessness.

There are several potential explanations for the absence of long-term benefits in this controlled trial of comprehensive pulmonary rehabilitation. One explanation is that short-term behavioral interventions, such as rehabilitation, are inadequate to produce long-term change. Long-term maintenance of behavior change has also been difficult to demonstrate in research on smoking cessation (55), weight loss (56), and exercise adherence (57). The finding that patients experience behavior change during treatment that is not maintained after treatment is consistent across a variety of different behavioral interventions (58). It is also important to recognize that few controlled studies have followed patients longer than 6 months. Thus, conclusions about long-term effectiveness may be premature.

The failure to obtain significant differences on quality-of-life outcomes is a problem because these measures are the denominator in the cost-utility ratio. With a small denominator, the ratio tends to be large, discouraging support for the program. In this study, the small effect on the quality of well-being may be explained by the insensitivity of these measures to small changes in general health status from interventions of this type. However, this measure has been used in a variety of outcomes studies and has shown significant associations with clinical measures for patients with lung diseases (20,59,60). It is possible that questionnaires that are more specific to lung diseases may offer a more sensitive assessment. For example, one recent trial did show that patients improved on measures of quality of life relevant to lung disease following a rehabilitation program (15).

VIII. Summary of Cost-Utility Studies

Most observational studies support the cost-benefit of pulmonary rehabilitation. Although these studies rarely use control groups, they often have long-term follow up. The outcome measures have emphasized the financial savings that may be attributable to participation in pulmonary rehabilitation. In contrast to cost-benefit studies, cost-utility analysis emphasizes patient-reported outcomes and measures of quality of life. One experimental trial estimated the QALYs contributed by participation in a behavioral rehabilitation program. The cost per QALY was comparable to that of many widely advocated medical and surgical treatments. However, another randomized clinical trial showed positive effects for exercise performance and relief of symptoms, but not for pulmonary function, quality of life, or depression.

Future research is necessary to evaluate these issues further. We have five specific suggestions. First, more controlled clinical trials are needed in which COPD patients are randomly assigned to comprehensive pulmonary rehabilitation or to control conditions. The outcome measures should include pulmonary function, quality of life, and cost. Follow-up should be at least 2 years. Second, if comprehensive programs are shown to produce positive outcomes in terms of functioning and quality of life, research will be necessary to demonstrate which components of the comprehensive program are essential to the package. Third, better research is necessary to determine whether standardized measures of functioning and quality of life, commonly applied in cost-utility studies, are sensitive and reliable measures of outcome in pulmonary rehabilitation. A fourth need for future research is an estimate of the duration of benefit for rehabilitation treatments. Evidence suggests that the treatment effect may attenuate over the course of time. Methods for making the benefit long-lasting should be developed and evaluated. Finally, we encourage more studies that consider the cost-utility of pulmonary rehabilitation in relation to other investments of health care resources. For example, managed-care organizations may limit their services to those deemed basic or essential. Other services might be added to the basic benefits package if they produce health benefit at a reasonable cost. Studies documenting the cost-utility of pulmonary rehabilitation, in comparison to other programs, are needed to justify inclusion in the basic services package.

IX. Conclusions

Rehabilitation programs for patients with COPD are widely advocated. Studies on the cost-benefit of these programs consistently demonstrate that following pulmonary rehabilitation, patients are hospitalized less often than they were prior to the program. Since the cost of a rehabilitation program approximates just 1 hospital day, reductions in hospital days are meaningful. However, few of the evaluations have used systematic experimental designs, and it is usually not possible to rule out other explanations for reductions in hospital days.

Only two studies have evaluated the cost-utility of pulmonary rehabilitation programs. One of these showed that rehabilitation produces one QALY, or the equivalent of one well-year of life, for about $23,000. This compares favorably with many widely advocated health care programs. For example, commonly accepted mammography screening programs cost about $175,000 to produce one QALY. However, the other cost-utility study of pulmonary rehabilitation failed to demonstrate that pulmonary rehabilitation produced significant benefits when measured in QALY units.

Cost-effectiveness analysis and outcomes research present important research challenges. Currently, there are too few studies that systematically evaluate the effectiveness of various treatments. For example, only one clinical trial has evaluated the health benefits of pulmonary rehabilitation. The new outcomes research paradigm emphasizes the documentation of benefits using outcome measures that capture the patient's perspective. Another challenge is in showing the relative cost-utility of rehabilitation interventions. Many cost-effectiveness analyses measure benefits using measures specific to lung diseases. These studies cannot be used for general policy analysis. For example, changes in exercise tolerance for pulmonary patients cannot be compared directly with changes in blood glucose for patients with diabetes mellitus. However, programs for these two patient groups compete for the same resources. New methods in outcomes research use general metrics, such as the QALY, to facilitate cross-illness comparisons. In the future, it will become increasingly important to document that expenditures on pulmonary rehabilitation are a good investment of resources in relation to alternative uses of the same funds. To accomplish this, we encourage continuing studies that apply cost-utility methodologies.

References

1. Hadorn DC. Setting health care priorities in Oregon: cost-effectiveness meets the rule of rescue. JAMA 1991; 265:2218–2225.
2. Ries AL. Position paper of the American Association of Cardiovascular and Pulmonary Rehabilitation: scientific basis of pulmonary rehabilitation. J Cardiopulm Rehabil 1990; 10:418–441.
3. Ries AL. The importance of exercise in pulmonary rehabilitation. Clin Chest Med 1994; 15(2):327–337.
4. American Lung Association/American Thoracic Society. Position Statement of the ALA/ATS Health Care Policy Task Force. Reform of the US Health Care System. New York: American Lung Association, 1994.
5. Kassirer JP, Angell M. The *Journal*'s policy on cost-effectiveness analyses. N Engl J Med 1994; 331(10):669–670.
6. Health Care Financing Administration. Office of the Actuary Report. Washington DC: US Government Printing Office, 1994.
7. Burner ST, Waldo DR, McKusick DR. National health expenditures projections through 2030. Health Care Financ Rev 1992; 14(1):1–29.
8. Levit KR, Olin GL, Letsch SW. American's health insurance coverage, 1980–91. Health Care Financ Rev 1992; 14:31–57.
9. Merritt RE, Demkovich L. Exhausting alternatives. There are disadvantages to relying on the states, but many feel forced to take aggressive steps to cover the uninsured. Health Manage Q 1991; 13:11–15.
10. Johnson NR, Tanzi F, Balchum OJ, Gunderson MA, DeFlorio G, Hoyt A. Inpatient comprehensive pulmonary rehabilitation in severe CODP: Barlow Hospital study. Respir Ther 1980; May/June:17.
11. Eddy, DM. Rationing resources while improving quality. How to get more for less. JAMA 1994; 272:817–824.

12. Doubelet P, Weinstein MC, McNeil BJ. Use and misuse of the term "cost effectiveness" in medicine. N Engl J Med 1986; 314:253–256.
13. Russell L. Is Prevention Better than Cure? Washington, DC: The Brookings Institution, 1986.
14. Nichol KL, Margolis KL, Wuorenma J, Von Sternberg T. The efficacy and cost effectiveness of vaccination against influenza among elderly persons living in the community. N Engl J Med 1994; 331(12):778–784.
15. World Health Organization. Health Promotion: A Discussion Document on the Concept and Principles. Copenhagen: WHO Regional Office for Europe, 1984.
16. Kaplan RM, Anderson JP. The general health policy model: an integrated approach. In: Spilker B, ed. Quality of Life Assessment in Clinical Trials. New York: Raven Press, 1990:131.
17. Kaplan RM, Anderson JP, Erickson P. Estimating well-years of life for a new public health indicator. Proceedings of the 1989 Public Health Conference on Records and Statistics. HDDS, National Center for Health Statistics. DHHS Publication Number (PHS), 1989; 90–1214, pp 298–303.
18. Kaplan RM, Anderson JP, Ganiats TG. The quality of well-being scale: rationale for a single quality of life index. In: Walker SR, Rosser RM, eds. Quality of Life Assessment: Key Issues in the 1990s. London: Kluwer, 1993:65–94.
19. Kaplan RM, Anderson JP, Wu AW, Mathews WC, Kozin, F, Orenstein D. The quality of well-being scale: applications in AIDS, cystic fibrosis, and arthritis. Med Care 1989; 27(Suppl 3):S27–S43.
20. Kaplan RM, Atkins CJ, Timms R. Validity of a quality of well-being scale as an outcome measure in chronic obstructive pulmonary disease. J Chronic Dis 1984; 37:85–95.
21. Kaplan RM, Bush JW. Health related quality of life measurement for evaluation research and policy analysis. Health Psychol, 1982; 1:61–80.
22. Kaplan RM, Bush JW, Berry CC. Health status: types of validity for an index of well-being. Health Serv Res 1976; 11:478–507.
23. Kaplan RM, Bush JW, Berry CC. The reliability, stability and generalizability of a health status index. Am Statist Assoc Proc Soc Statist Sect 1978; 26:415–418.
24. Kaplan RM, Hartwell SL, Wilson DK, Wallace JP. Effects of diet and exercise interventions on control and quality of life in non-insulin-dependent diabetes mellitus. J Gen Intern Med 1987; 2:220–228.
25. Weinstein MC, Stason, WB. Foundations of cost-effectiveness analysis for health and medical practice. N Engl J Med 1977; 296:716–721.
26. Spiezer RE. Overview and summary: the rise in chronic obstructive pulmonary disease mortality. Am Rev Respir Dis 1989; 140:5106–5107.
27. Edelman, NH, Kaplan, RM, Buist, S, et al. Chronic obstructive pulmonary disease. Chest 1992; 102:234S–256S.
28. Casaburi R, Petty TL, eds. Principles and Practice of Pulmonary Rehabilitation. Philadelphia: WB Saunders, 1993.
29. Ries AL, Kaplan RM, Limberg TM, Prewitt LM. Effects of pulmonary rehabilitation on physiologic and phychosocial outcomes in patients with obstructive pulmonary disease. Ann Intern Med 1995; 122:823–832.

30. Toshima MT, Kaplan RM, Ries AL. Experimental evaluation of rehabilitation in chronic obstructive pulmonary disease: short-term effects on exercise endurance and health status. Health Psychol 1990; 9:2337–2352.
31. Casaburi R. Exercise training in chronic obstructive lung disease. In: Casaburi R, Petty TL, eds. Principles and Practice of Pulmonary Rehabilitation. Philadelphia: WB Saunders, 1993:204–224.
32. Cockcroft AE, Saunders MT, Berry G. Randomized controlled trial of rehabilitation in chronic respiratory disability. Thorax 1981; 36:200.
33. McGavin CR, Gupta SP, Lloyd EL, McHardy JR. Physical rehabilitation of chronic bronchitis: results of a controlled trial of exercises in the home. Thorax 1977; 32:307.
34. Ambrosino N, Paggiaro PL, Macchi M, et al. A study of short-term effect of rehabilitative therapy in chronic obstructive pulmonary disease. Respiration 1981; 41:40.
35. Belman MJ, Wasserman K. Exercise training and testing in patients with chronic obstructive pulmonary disease. Basics RD, 1981; 10:1.
36. Shephard RJ. On the design and effectiveness of training regimens in chronic obstructive lung disease. Bull Eur Physiopathol Respir 1977; 13:457–469.
37. Mertens DJ, Shephard RJ, Kavanagh T. Long-term exercise therapy for chronic obstructive lung disease. Respiration 1978; 35:96.
38. Molken MP, Van Doorslaer EK, Rutten FF. Economic appraisal of asthma and COPD care: a literature review 1980–1991. Soc Sci Med 1992; 35(2):161–175.
39. Folgering H, Rooyakkers J, Herwaarden C. Education and cost-benefit ratios in pulmonary patients. Monaldi Arch Chest Dis 1994; 49(2):166–168.
40. Radovich J, Hodgkin JE, Burton GG, Yee AR. Cost-Effectiveness of pulmonary rehabilitation programs. In: Hodgkin JE, Connors GL, Bell CW, eds. Pulmonary Rehabilitation: Guidelines to Success, 2d ed. Philadelphia: JB Lippincott, 1993:548–561.
41. Dunham JL, Hodgkin JE, Nicol J, Burton GG. Cost effectiveness of pulmonary rehabilitation programs. In: Hodgkin JE, Zorn EG, Connors GL, eds. Pulmonary Rehabilitation: Guidelines to Success. Boston: Butterworth, 1984:389.
42. Hudson LD, Tyler ML, Petty TL. Hospitalization needs during an outpatient rehabilitation program for severe CAO. Chest 1976; 70:606.
43. Wright RW, Larsen DF, Monie RG, Aldred RA. Benefits of a community-hospital pulmonary rehabilitation program. Respir Care 1983; 28:1474.
44. Bria W, Stillerman R, Lemoine M, Niles D, Soldega A. Effect of pulmonary rehabilitation on health care utilization. Chest 1987; 92:153s.
45. Sneider R, O'Malley JA, Kahn M. Trends in pulmonary rehabilitation at Eisenhower Medical Center: an 11-year's experience (1976–1987). J Cardiopulm Rehabil 1988; 11:453.
46. Toshima MT, Blumberg E, Kaplan RM, Ries AL. Social support and health care utilization in patients with chronic obstructive pulmonary disease. Proc Soc Behav Med 1990; 11:171 (abstract).
47. Sturm R, Wells KB. How can care for depression become more cost-effective? JAMA 1995; 2731:51–58.

48. Atkins CJ, Kaplan RM, Timms RM, Reinsch S, Lofback K. Behavioral programs for exercise compliance in COPD. J Consult Clin Psychol 1984; 52:591.
49. Kaplan RM. Hippocratic Predicament: Affordability, Access, and Accountability in Health Care. San Diego: Academic Press, 1993.
50. Atkins CJ, Hayes J, Kaplan RM. Four year follow-up of behavioral programs in COPD. University of California Health Psychology Conference. Lake Arrowhead, CA, June 1984.
51. Toevs CD, Kaplan RM, Atkins CJ. The costs and effects of behavioral programs in chronic obstructive pulmonary disease. Med Care 1984; 22(12):1088–1100.
52. Moser KM, Bokinsky GE, Savage RT, Archibald CJ, Hansen PR. Results of a comprehensive rehabilitation program: physiologic and functional effects on patients with chronic obstructive pulmonary disease. Arch Intern Med 1980; 140:1596.
53. Bass H, Whitcomb JF, Forman R. Exercise training: therapy for patients with chronic obstructive pulmonary disease. Chest 1970; 57:116.
54. Fishmen DB, Petty TL. Physical, symptomatic and psychological improvement in patients receiving comprehensive care for chronic airway obstruction. J Chronic Dis 1971; 24:775.
55. Lichtenstein E, Brown RA. Current trends in the modification of cigarette dependence. In: Bellack AS, Hersen M, Kazdin AE, eds. International Handbook of Behavior Modification and Therapy. New York: Plenum Press, 1983.
56. Wadden TA, Brownell KD. The development and modification of dietary practices in individuals, groups, and large populations. In: Matarazzo JD, Weiss SM, Herd JA, Miller NE, Weiss SM, eds. Behavioral Health: A Handbook of Health Enhancement and Disease Prevention. New York: Wiley, 1984:608–631.
57. Martin JE, Dubbert PM. Exercise applications and promotion in behavioral medicine: current status and future directions. J Consult Clin Psychol 1982; 30:1004–1017.
58. Marlatt GA. Relapse prevention: a self-control program for the treatment of addictive behavors. In: Stuart RB, ed. Adherence, Compliance and Generalization in Behavioral Medicine. New York: Brunner/Mazel, 1982.
59. Orenstein, DM, Nixon, PA, Ross, EA, Kaplan, RM. The quality of well-being in cystic fibrosis. Chest 1989; 5:344–347.
60. Orenstein DM, Pattishall EN, Ross EA, Kaplan RM. Quality of well-being before and after antibiotic treatment of pulmonary exacerbation in cystic fibrosis. Chest 1990; 98:1081–1084.
61. Hodgkin JE, Connors GL, Bell CW, eds. Pulmonary Rehabilitation: Guidelines to Success, 2d ed. Philadelphia: JB Lippincott, 1993.

Part Three

THERAPEUTIC INTERVENTIONS

17

Smoking Cessation and Pulmonary Rehabilitation

DAVID B. COULTAS

University of New Mexico Health Sciences Center
Albuquerque, New Mexico

JONATHAN M. SAMET

School of Public Health and Hygiene
The Johns Hopkins University
Baltimore, Maryland

While a multidisciplinary approach to pulmonary rehabilitation can benefit patients with chronic obstructive pulmonary disease (COPD), most cases of this crippling, chronic disease can be prevented by smoking prevention and cessation. In 1986, over 80% of cases were attributable to cigarette smoking (1). Mortality from COPD has steadily increased in this century as the full impact of the widespread smoking of cigarettes that began early in the century took effect (2). Present mortality rates from COPD place the disease among the leading causes of death in the United States (3). Prevalence estimates for clinically diagnosed COPD and related conditions range from a few percent up to about 10%, depending on the criteria for establishing the presence of the conditions (3,4). Unfortunately, the disease is long-lasting and inexorably progressive.

The increasing frequency of the disease and its poor prognosis provide a strong imperative for prevention. Fortunately, the gradual decline of lung function that leads to COPD in most cases provides a lengthy window for intervention with a program of smoking cessation. Clinicians need to understand the natural history of COPD and the associated opportunity for intervention at a time before smoking-caused decline of lung function has resulted in overt disease. Health care professionals can also favorably impact on tobacco control through engagement in public health and regulatory initiatives; as acknowledged community experts on health issues, they can offer both expertise and leadership.

This chapter considers the epidemiological data on smoking and COPD and the clinical implications of the evidence for prevention of COPD through identification of the high-risk smoker. It also addresses the physician's responsibility for identifying cigarette smoking as a clinically relevant problem and the approaches that the individual physician can apply to achieve smoking cessation.

I. The Benefits of Smoking Cessation

A. Natural History of Chronic Airflow Obstruction

The occurrence of clinically manifest COPD reflects the development of underlying chronic airflow obstruction in sufficient severity to produce symptomatic impairment. In normals, beginning in the fourth decade of life, ventilatory function begins to decline after reaching a maximum level by approximately the end of the second decade. Longitudinal studies of ventilatory function, indexed in most studies by the forced expiratory volume in 1 sec (FEV_1), show that smokers have higher rates of decline than nonsmokers (Fig. 1) (1,4,5). On average, current smoking approximately doubles the rate of decline, from approximately 25 ml/year to 50 ml/year. However, the rates of decline vary widely among smokers, and the FEV_1 may decrease at even higher rates in those who are more susceptible (1,6). As the number of cigarettes smoked daily increases, the rate of decrease in FEV_1 becomes steeper. In those who continue to smoke cigarettes, the increased rate of decline eventually reduces the FEV_1 to a level associated with dyspnea and limitation of activities; at this level, the clinical diagnosis of COPD can be made.

Studies of mortality from COPD provide complementary evidence. Mortality rates from COPD are approximately 10-fold greater in current smokers than in never smokers (1,7,8). Dose-response relationships between number of cigarettes smoked and mortality rates have been consistently demonstrated (4,8). Former smokers tend to have mortality rates from COPD that are comparable to, or only somewhat lower than, the rates for current smokers. After 40 years of follow-up of 34,439 British male doctors, Doll and co-workers (8) determined annual mortality rates for COPD and compared mortality rates of current and former smokers to never smokers. They found mortality ratios of 12.7 and 5.7 deaths per year, respectively. Curiously, mortality rates from COPD have been reported to be higher in recent quitters than in current smokers (1). One possible explanation for this result may be that these individuals quit smoking after developing irreversible and progressive disease.

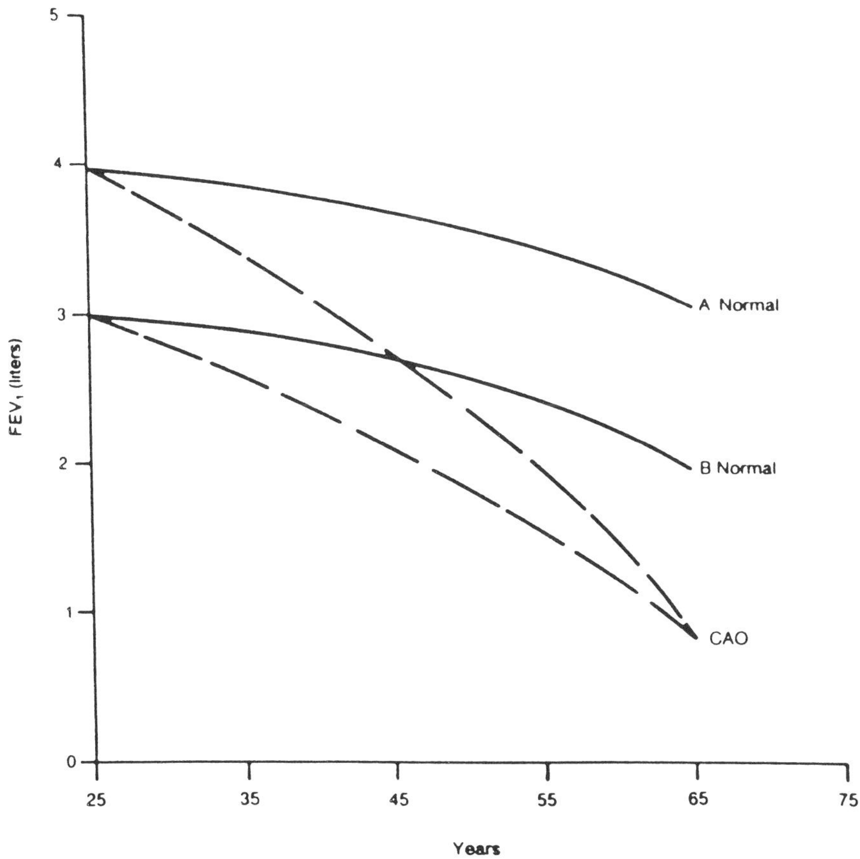

Figure 1 Decline of FEV_1 at a normal rate (solid line) and at an accelerated rate (dashed line). Line A indicates a person who has attained "normal" maximal FEV_1 during lung growth and development. Line B indicates a person whose maximal FEV_1 has been reduced by childhood respiratory infection or exposure to environmental tobacco smoke. The accelerated decline of FEV_1 (dashed line) results in chronic airways obstruction (CAO). (From Ref. 4.)

With few exceptions, little is known about the factors that determine the rate of decline of ventilatory function in individual smokers (1,5). One exception is the group with homozygous α_1-antitrypsin deficiency or other genotypes that lead to deficiency in the important antiprotease (5). However, other genetic determinants of rate of decline have not been identified. Additional factors that are suspected of being relevant are respiratory illnesses in childhood and airways hyperresponsiveness (9). Also, decrease in lung function from occupational exposures may add to the decrease in function caused by smoking, thereby accelerating the development of COPD (10).

Fortunately, in smokers who have not developed manifest COPD, smoking cessation is followed by a return of the rate of decline to that in never smokers (1,6). Thus, cessation of smoking before the onset of COPD may either prevent or delay the occurrence of disease, depending on the level to which ventilatory function has decreased. As a rule, little improvement in lung function occurs immediately after cessation. However, after a few months of abstinence, lung function improves about 5%.

In 1986, the Lung Health Study, a multicenter clinical trial, undertook to determine the effects of smoking cessation and/or ipratropium bronchodilator therapy on the rate of decrease in FEV_1 in middle-aged smokers with mild impairment of lung function (11). Between 1986 and 1994, 5887 smokers, 35–60 years of age, with a FEV_1/FVC ratio of 70% or less and FEV_1 between 50% and 90% of predicted, were enrolled. They were randomized to three groups: (1) usual care; (2) smoking cessation plus placebo inhaler; (3) smoking cessation plus ipratropium metered-dose inhaler. Among the smokers who underwent intense smoking intervention and placebo inhaler (group 2), smoking cessation was clearly of benefit: at the first annual visit, FEV_1 increased on average by 57 ml in those who had quit smoking and decreased by 38 ml in those who had not quit. Subsequently, in the interval between the first and fifth annual visits, the FEV_1 decreased at a rate of 34 ml/year in those who continued to abstain compared to 63 ml/year in those subjects who continued to smoke.

B. Opportunities for Prevention of COPD

Strategies for the prevention and cessation of smoking can avoid the development of COPD in most individuals. The natural history of COPD suggests that screening for FEV_1 can be helpful in programs designed to prevent clinically overt COPD; a reduced FEV_1 indicates an abnormally accelerated rate of decline, the "horse-racing" effect (6), which is predictive of a future rapid rate of decline. Thus, one strategy for preventing COPD is to apply principles of secondary prevention and to screen for adult smokers who have lung function that is less than predicted. In order to obtain reliable results in screening, the testing equipment should meet American Thoracic Society standards and standardization of test procedures (12–14).

Other indices of lung function, in addition to the FEV_1, may be helpful in pinpointing the smoker at risk for accelerated decrease in FEV_1 (15–17). These include low FEV_1/FVC ratio (15,16), low diffusing capacity (16), low weight (16), and respiratory symptoms (17). Cauberghs and co-workers (16), in a study lasting 6 years, compared anthropometric features and pulmonary function tests in 24 male smokers who experienced the normal rate of decrease in FEV_1 with the same number of male smokers in whom the rate of decline was more rapid. In a discriminant analysis, they found that a negative score based on the following formula:

$$Z = 0.076\ DL_{CO}\ (\%\ \text{predicted}) + 0.044\ W\ (\text{kg}) + 0.067\ FEV_1/VC - 15.788$$

had a 75% sensitivity for categorizing smokers with a rapid decline in FEV_1 and 85% specificity for categorizing smokers with normal decline.

The benefit of screening for lung function impairment as part of a comprehensive smoking intervention strategy is likely to be greatest among smokers who are less than 40 years of age (18,19). In a cross-sectional analysis of lung function and cigarette smoking among 5201 men and women 65 years of age and older, Higgins and co-workers (18) examined the relationship between the level of FEV_1 and the age at which smokers quit. Never smokers and those who quit before 40 years of age had similar levels of FEV_1; also, the FEV_1 levels were 7% lower in smokers who quit at age 40–60 years and 14% lower in smokers who quit at 60 years of age and older. In a longitudinal study that included 1705 adults from Tucson, Arizona, Camilli and co-workers (19) found that most of the excess decline in FEV_1 occurs between 50 and 70 years of age, and that quitting smoking before 35 years of age was associated with an increase in FEV_1.

Although smoking cessation offers the greatest potential for slowing the rate of decline in lung function, the possibility has been examined that pharmacological interventions might play a role in the prevention of COPD. In the Lung Health Study, those who received the ipratropium inhaler increased their FEV_1 on average by 40 ml during the first year, but inhaler treatment did not improve the annual rate of decline in those who were given the placebo inhaler (11). Dompeling and co-workers (20) determined the rate of decline in FEV_1 over 4 years in 22 subjects with COPD and in 26 with asthma; these subjects were randomized to bronchodilator therapy alone or to bronchodilator therapy combined with inhaled beclomethasone dipropionate. In the subjects with COPD, 61% continued to smoke during the beclomethasone treatment; their annual change in prebronchodilator FEV_1 was −146 ml/year before beclomethasone and −104 ml/year after beclomethasone. The rate of decline in the postbronchodilator FEV_1 was greater during beclomethasone treatment (−120 ml/year) than in the period before beclomethasone treatment (−79 ml/year). The limited information available on pharmacological interventions and the rate of lung function decline suggests that bronchodilator therapy alone is not effective, and that inhaled corticosteroids may produce a small benefit. Additional studies are needed on larger numbers of subjects.

Once COPD has developed to the stage of clinical diagnosis, smoking cessation is of limited benefit (1). A few studies have shown a decrease in the rate of decline of lung function in former smokers with COPD than in those who continue to smoke (21,22). Evidence on smoking cessation and subsequent mortality is limited and inconsistent (1).

II. Process of Smoking and Smoking Cessation

Both continuation and cessation of cigarette smoking are complex phenomena that entail psychological, social, and physiological factors that interact to make quitting extremely difficult (23). An understanding of these complex factors equips the physician to assist smokers who are trying to quit.

Smoking begins in childhood and adolescence, and by 18 years of age, approximately 90% of adult smokers have started to smoke (24). The major determinants of the initiation of smoking are social factors, including peer pressure and familial influences, i.e., parental smoking and family dynamics that may be reinforced by cigarette advertising (24). Children who begin to smoke at least at monthly intervals early in life are likely to continue to smoke into adulthood (25).

The act of cigarette smoking and the pharmacological effects of nicotine are frequently "paired" with environmental stimuli, i.e., extrinsic cues, which may act together to trigger the desire to smoke, i.e., intrinsic or psychological cues, to make cigarette smoking a highly conditioned response (23,26). Common cues that may trigger the desire to smoke include smoking by others, finishing a meal, drinking coffee and/or alcohol, and feeling stressed. Because of the strong influence of extrinsic and intrinsic cues on the desire to smoke, simple nicotine replacement with a patch or gum may not eliminate the desire to smoke when the smoker is confronted with environmental and psychological cues (27).

Physiological effects of nicotine and conditioned responses to extrinsic and intrinsic factors are known to be linked to the development of tobacco dependence (23). Along this line, the 1988 report of the U.S. Surgeon General (28) offered the following conclusions: (1) cigarettes and other forms of tobacco are addicting; (2) nicotine is the drug in tobacco that causes addiction; and (3) the pharmacological and behavioral processes that determine tobacco dependence are similar to those that determine addiction to drugs such as heroin and cocaine.

Nicotine has a wide range of pharmacological effects on neural, endocrine, cardiovascular, and skeletal muscle functions, with particularly powerful psychoactive effects on the central nervous system (29). In the tobacco-dependent person, nicotine has a euphoriant effect and may reduce stress and anxiety, facilitate learning and memory, and help control appetite and weight. The physiological effects of nicotine on the central nervous system may reinforce the conditioned response to environmental and psychological cues and/or be the primary mechanism resulting in nicotine addiction. Within 24 hr of discontinuing smoking, withdrawal symptoms may result (Table 1), thereby contributing to relapse.

Smoking cessation has been conceptualized as a dynamic process with consecutive stages (30) defined by motivation to quit and intention to quit (Table 2, Fig. 2). Successful cessation usually requires multiple cycles through these stages, which may extend over several years. Since the original description by Prochaska and DiClemente (30), a variety of definitions have been used to classify the stages of smoking cessation. Despite this variability, categorization does afford a clinically useful method for targeting advice and assistance and for predicting the success of smoking cessation efforts (30,31). In an investigation of smokers referred to the Nicotine Dependence Center at the Mayo Medical Center, Rohren and co-workers (31) found that smokers in the "action" stage were twice as likely to be abstinent at 6 months (41.5%) than were the "contemplators" (20.3%).

III. Effectiveness of Smoking Cessation Methods

Although many methods for smoking cessation have been used (32), the effectiveness of these methods varies widely and their public health impact needs to be addressed with respect to the smokers' intentions to quit and the methods they choose to accomplish this goal. In a recent survey in the United States, of 4700 current smokers and 4614 former smokers 17 years of age and older, Fiore and co-workers (33) found that 66% of current smokers had made a serious attempt to quit; i.e., 34% had not. Among those who had attempted to quit, individual methods of cessation were used by 80–90%, and program assistance was used by the remaining 10–20%. The methods involving assistance did not include advice or assistance by a physician. Furthermore, among smokers who attempted to quit in the 10 years prior to the survey, 48% of those

Table 1 Common Symptoms/Signs that May Result from Nicotine Withdrawal

Craving for nicotine
Irritability, frustration, or anger
Anxiety
Difficulty concentrating
Restlessness
Decreased heart rate
Increased appetite or weight gain

Source: From Ref. 28.

Table 2 Definitions Used to Categorize Smokers' Stage of Change at the Nicotine Dependence Center of the Mayo Medical Center (31)

Precontemplation	A patient who is currently smoking or using tobacco and not motivated to make changes
Contemplation	A patient who is currently using tobacco and is motivated to stop but either has not set a stop date or has set one that is more than 1 month from the time of consultation
Action	A patient has a stop plan and date that were (or will be) implemented within 1 month of the consultation
Maintenance	A patient has discontinued the use of tobacco for a minimum of 1 month and has not used tobacco on a regular daily basis during this time

who quit on their own were successful compared with only 24% of those using a smoking cessation program.

The limited usefulness of referring patients to smoking cessation programs was further emphasized by the findings of a study conducted by Lichtenstein and Hollis (34). They randomized 1387 smokers attending primary care clinics at a large health maintenance organization either to receive brief advice to quit from their physician with subsequent reinforcement by a nurse or to receive the same advice and a referral and encouragement to attend a free nine-session smoking cessation program. Although a higher proportion of subjects given the referral attended the program (11%) compared to those only given advice to quit (0.6%), the overall proportion attending the program was low despite specific measures designed to facilitate attendance. Predictors of not attending the program included not contemplating quitting compared to contemplating quitting [odds ratio (OR) = 0.17; 95% confidence interval (CI), 0.07–0.44], age less than 40 years (OR = 0.44; 95% CI, 0.25–0.76), and smoking 19 cigarettes per day or less (OR = 0.56; 95% CI, 0.56–0.98).

Based on the information about the intentions of smokers to quit and the methods used by smokers to quit, it is clear that for the majority of smokers, physicians need to direct their efforts toward motivating smokers who have never made a serious attempt to quit and toward improving the efforts of those attempting to quit on their own. The next sections focus on the effectiveness of physicians in helping smokers to quit and on the specific methods that physicians can use to promote smoking cessation.

A. Effectiveness of Physician Interventions

The effectiveness of physician counseling about smoking cessation must be evaluated in terms of the financial costs to patient and physician as well as

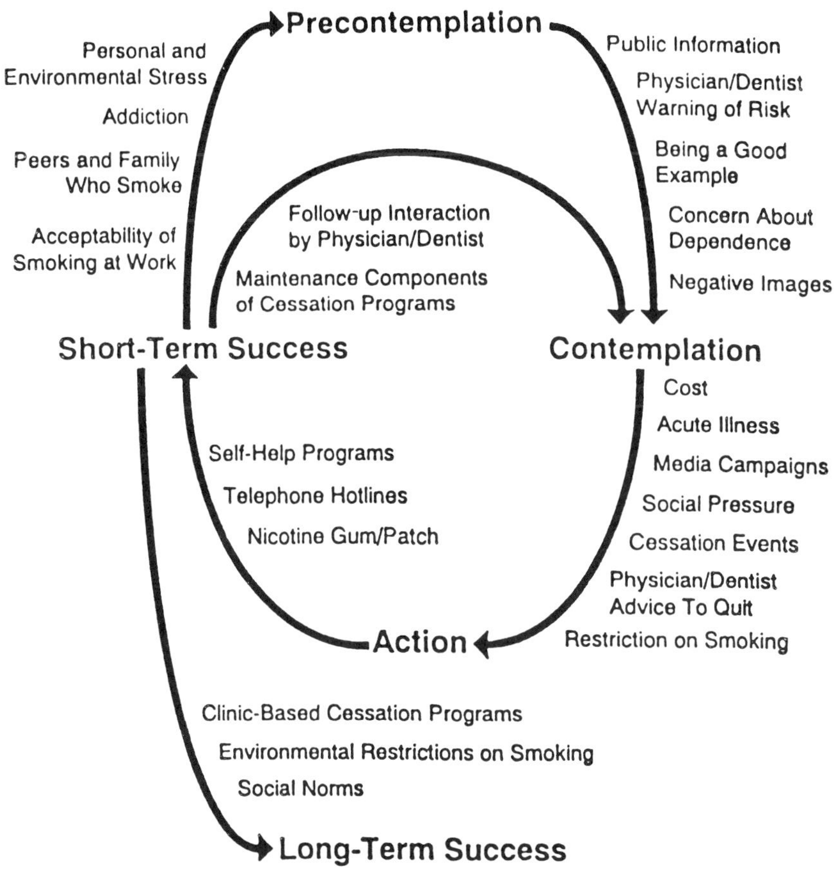

Figure 2 Stages of change in the process of smoking cessation and factors that may influence a smoker in his or her movements between the different stages. (From Ref. 51.)

whether the counseling is effective in getting smokers to quit. Physician advice to quit, even though resulting in only a few percent of additional smokers quitting, is a highly cost-effective preventive intervention, e.g., compared with treatment interventions for such chronic conditions as hypertension or hypercholesterolemia (35).

The effectiveness of physician intervention in smoking cessation has been examined primarily in randomized trials of smokers attending general practices (32,36). Although the intensities of the interventions used in the investigations of physicians and smoking cessation have varied, the overall results are favorable. Simple physician advice, compared to no advice, may result in an additional 5% of smokers quitting in 1 year (32). In general, the physician's role in these trials has simply been to advise patients to stop smoking. Cessation rates may be increased by additional interventions, including self-help pamphlets, feedback on exhaled carbon monoxide concentrations, counseling by a trained nurse, nicotine replacement, and follow-up to provide ongoing assistance. In a review of 10 trials that involved physician counseling and other interventions, Schwartz (32) found that the proportion of smokers who quit at 1 year ranged from 13 to 38%, with a median of 23%.

B. Pharmacological Interventions

Withdrawal symptoms, which are most intense during the first several weeks of quitting, may present a substantial barrier for some smokers during attempts at quitting. Consequently, pharmacological interventions to lessen these symptoms should be considered as potentially useful adjuncts for selected smokers during the smoking cessation process. However, these interventions may have limited usefulness for alleviating the desire to smoke that is cued primarily by extrinsic factors. Of the four categories of pharmacological interventions potentially available, i.e., nicotine replacement, nicotine blockade, nonspecific pharmacotherapy, and deterrent therapies, only the categories of nicotine replacement and nonspecific pharmacotherapies are considered here because of their ready availability for clinical practice (27).

Nicotine replacement therapy with nicotine polacrilex gum or transdermal nicotine has been found to be effective in assisting the smoker to quit (37,38). Nicotine polacrilex gum in doses of 2 and 4 mg, offered in conjunction with physician advice, facilitates smoking cessation (28,38) and is cost-effective (39). Silagy and co-workers (38) recently reported a meta-analysis of nicotine replacement therapies based on 39 trials that enrolled smokers from a variety of settings, i.e., community volunteers, smoking clinics, primary care, and hospitals. Subjects treated with nicotine polacrilex had an overall quit rate of 18.2% after at least 6 months of follow-up compared to 10.6% among controls. The benefit of replacement was less in the 15 trials that enrolled patients from primary care settings, i.e., 10.9% in treated smokers versus 6.8% in controls. Despite the potential benefit of the gum for smoking cessation, it is infrequently prescribed by physicians or used by smokers (7,40), and patients often are improperly instructed or not instructed in its use (40).

Although no direct comparisons have been made of the effectiveness of nicotine polacrilex gum and of nicotine patches, the patch offers a simpler method for the administration of nicotine replacement and may partly contribute to its efficacy. Indirect evidence from the meta-analysis of nicotine replacement therapies conducted by Silagy and co-workers (38) suggests that nicotine patches may be slightly more efficacious than nicotine polacrilex: the OR was 2.1 (95% CI, 1.6–2.6) for quitting by use of the patches (nine trials) as compared to an OR of 1.6 (95% CI, 1.5–1.8) for quitting with the use of nicotine polacrilex (39 trials). Based on these comparative figures for effectiveness, they estimated that up to 60% fewer smokers would have to be treated with nicotine patch to reach the same number of smokers who would quit by using nicotine polacrilex.

Fiore and co-workers (37) conducted a meta-analysis of 17 randomized clinical trials of nicotine patches conducted through September 1993. They found that overall abstinence at 6 months was 22% for subjects treated with an active patch compared to 9% for subjects treated with a placebo patch. Efficacy was not substantially improved by extending treatment beyond 8 weeks or by weaning the nicotine dose. While intensive counseling, i.e., at least weekly sessions during the first 4 weeks, seven or more sessions in the first 12 weeks, and sessions lasting for greater than 40 min with the nicotine patch, contributed to higher abstinence, lower levels of counseling still provided substantial benefits at 6 months.

Although the nicotine patch is a useful adjunct for smoking cessation, its effectiveness can be limited by inadequate patient education. Orleans and co-workers (41) assessed the use of the nicotine patch among 1070 elderly smokers from Pennsylvania who had been prescribed a nicotine patch in 1992. Overall, only 54% received any advice or materials with the prescription for the patch, and 47% continued to smoke while using the patch. Smokers abstinent for 7 or more days during the 6 months after receiving the patch were more likely to have received advice from a physician or pharmacist.

Nonspecific pharmacological interventions that do not directly affect nicotine levels include a wide range of agents, such as clonidine, anxiolytics, and antidepressants (27). Clonidine, an α-adrenergic agonist, may help lessen withdrawal symptoms and increase success in smoking cessation acutely (42). Covey and Glassman (42) conducted a meta-analysis of the use of clonidine for smoking cessation that included nine placebo-controlled trials; this analysis showed that at the end of treatment, overall 39% of subjects treated with clonidine quit smoking compared to 21% of control subjects. However, only limited and conflicting data are available on the long-term effectiveness of clonidine.

Although few data are available on the use of antiantibody agents or antidepressants for smoking cessation, anxiety and depression are common problems among smokers (23) and among patients with COPD (43). Because these psychological problems may interfere with quitting, judicious use of antianxiety and antidepressant agents may be beneficial.

C. Interventions in COPD

Few randomized, controlled clinical trials have been conducted to specifically examine the efficacy of smoking cessation interventions as part of pulmonary rehabilitation programs for COPD (4). In a review of six trials that involved physician intervention among pulmonary patients, Schwartz (32) found that the proportion of smokers who quit at 1 year ranged from 25 to 75%, with a median of 32%. Information on control groups was not provided.

Recent evidence suggests that the presence of pulmonary risk factors, symptoms, or disease is not sufficient to predict successful smoking cessation (44,45). Two randomized trials were conducted by the British Thoracic Society and involved 2854 smokers (87.5% COPD, 8.0% heart disease, 4.5% other smoking-related conditions). The smokers were seen as outpatients by chest physicians or general physicians who had an interest in chest medicine (46). The cessation rates at 12 months in those receiving advice from chest physicians were similar to those achieved by those seeing general physicians. With simple advice to quit, 5% of smokers (whose report of not smoking was verified by carboxyhemoglobin or thiocyanate) did quit. One or more follow-up visits that included simple advice within 6 months increased the proportion who quit to 9%. Simple advice that was followed by an encouraging letter, but no follow-up visits, resulted in a 9% quitting rate, and 13% quit if one or more follow-up visits were added. Overall, among patients with lung disease, the proportion who quit was lower than that of patients with heart disease, i.e., 7.5% and 14.4%, respectively. Other investigators have also reported a lower smoking cessation rate in patients with COPD than in patients with heart disease (32,47).

In the Lung Health Study (11), 5887 smokers with mild airflow obstruction were randomized into three groups: usual care, smoking cessation intervention plus placebo inhaler, smoking cessation intervention plus active bronchodilator inhaler. After 5 years of follow-up, 22% of subjects remained continuously abstinent after an intensive smoking cessation intervention whereas in only 5% of subjects in the usual care group was abstinence sustained.

Cox and co-workers (48) examined the effectiveness of pulmonary rehabilitation among consecutive patients with asthma ($n = 27$) and COPD ($n = 17$) referred for rehabilitation and compared their outcomes to those of 43 patients with the same diagnoses recruited from outpatient clinics. The comprehensive rehabilitation program consisted of 38 hr/week for 3 months. Except for being provided with information about the hazards of smoking, patients in the rehabilitation group did not receive any other smoking cessation interventions. Patients in the two groups were followed for 2 years: 40% of smokers ($n = 10$) in the rehabilitation group quit smoking whereas none of the 12 smokers in the control group did so.

Pederson and co-workers (49) conducted a randomized trial of the effectiveness of counseling in smoking cessation among 74 patients hospitalized with COPD. All patients were advised to quit smoking by their physician and the intervention group received a self-help manual and three to eight counseling

tion. In 1991, an estimated 70% of the 51 million smokers in the United States had at least one outpatient visit with a physician or other health professional during the previous year (52).

The desire of many cigarette smokers to stop smoking coupled with a perception of physician advice that is generally positive should motivate physicians to promote smoking cessation among patients. Surveys of smokers indicate that 60–70% of current smokers want to stop, and 70–90% consider that a physician's advice would be important in their decision to stop smoking (36). However, in the general population, only about 50% of current smokers report ever being advised by a physician to quit smoking (51).

Numerous factors contribute to the low rate of advice by physicians. In 1984, the National Cancer Institute began funding 12 clinical trials in an effort to develop effective smoking cessation methods for use by physicians and other health professionals. These have added greatly to our understanding of how to increase physicians' interventions directed at smoking cessation (51). Although all of these trials are as yet incomplete, preliminary results suggest that simply training physicians is insufficient. In addition, office systems and procedures will have to be implemented to enable systematic identification of all smokers and to remind both the physician and the office staff to address the patient's smoking. Furthermore, the office staff needs to be trained in how to implement interventions aimed at smoking cessation.

C. Tertiary Prevention

By decreasing respiratory symptoms and slowing the rate of decline in lung function, smoking cessation can benefit patients with clinically evident COPD (1). However, only 15–20% of all smokers develop COPD, and smoking cessation interventions targeting only these patients will produce limited public health benefit. Furthermore, continued smoking by patients with COPD or other smoking-related diseases indicates that these individuals may be highly dependent on tobacco and, therefore, have great difficulty in quitting. Accordingly, comprehensive efforts at tobacco control by health professionals begins with primary and secondary prevention.

D. How to Help

Because cigarette smoking and smoking cessation are complex processes that involve social (e.g., peer pressure to smoke), psychological (e.g., environmental cues), and physiological influences (e.g., nicotine addiction), an intervention to help smokers quit that addresses only one of these areas (e.g., nicotine addiction) is not likely to be successful (53). Therefore, a comprehensive and structured approach is needed to maximize effectiveness and efficiency when helping smokers to quit. The intervention described here is adapted from available programs designed to improve physicians' skills in counseling about smoking cessation (51,54,55). A manual prepared by the National Cancer Institute entitled *How to Help Your Patients Stop Smoking* (54) includes four components described as the four A's: (1) ask about their smoking status at each visit; (2) advise them in a clear, direct manner to quit smoking; (3) assist the interested smoker to quit by setting a quit date, provide self-help materials, and consider prescribing nicotine replacement therapy; and (4) arrange follow-up visits.

Although an initial determination of a patient's smoking status is essential in helping smokers to quit, additional information for the current cigarette smoker is necessary to provide appropriate advice and assistance in the smoking cessation process (Table 2, Fig. 2). The appropriate intervention will vary with the stage of change of each smoker; the possible interventions for the various stages have been reviewed extensively elsewhere (31,53,56,57). The physician should assess and provide feedback on factors that may influence the smoker's stage of change, including his or her perceptions about the effects of smoking, past experience with quitting, current concerns about quitting, resources available to assist in quitting, and specific plans for quitting (55). Careful questioning and discussion of these topics provides the physician and the patient with necessary information for formulating realistic goals and plans for smoking cessation.

Goldberg and co-workers (57) found that physicians who provide brief, stage-specific interventions for smoking cessation are effective in moving smokers through the stages of change. Six months after training internal medicine residents in how to provide brief, stage-specific interventions, smokers seen by trained residents were less likely to be precontemplators (25%) compared to smokers seen by untrained residents (36%). However, no difference was found between the proportion of smokers who quit smoking when the results of trained residents and untrained residents were compared (14.7% versus 16.2%).

For smokers in the precontemplation or contemplation stage, physician advice will largely be directed toward motivating them to think about quitting or to begin making specific plans for quitting, respectively. Because no single message will motivate all smokers, the first approach is to identify specific, personal reasons to quit. Although "scare" tactics should be avoided, current, personal health reasons, i.e., symptoms, physical findings, test findings, provide an immediate opportunity for the physician to provide simple and direct advice about quitting. Rohren and co-workers (31) found that a patient's report of a current disease, but no past history of disease worsened by smoking, was predictive of successfully quitting. For asymptomatic smokers, determination of levels of carbon monoxide in expired air and "lung age" from spirometric testing offer other objective measures that may motivate smokers to quit (58,59).

For smokers in the contemplation and action stages appropriate advice and assistance should focus on specific techniques for quitting. These techniques may concern methods to overcome obstacles to quitting (e.g., nicotine replacement, weight control, environmental cues) or resources for quitting (e.g., self-help pamphlets, group programs, family members).

High nicotine dependence decreases the likelihood of success in quitting. Identification of highly nicotine-dependent smokers and the use of nicotine replacement offer a specific and effective method for assisting smokers to quit (37). Smokers with high dependence can be recognized by certain characteristics: withdrawal symptoms in previous attempts at quitting, the smoking of more than 20 cigarettes per day, difficulty refraining from smoking where it is forbidden, smoking of the first cigarette soon after awakening, smoking while bedridden with illness, or a great depth of inhalation (60).

Because of the cardiovascular effects of nicotine, therapies designed at nicotine replacement may be contraindicated or relatively contraindicated in certain patients with cardiovascular diseases (27). Patients unwilling to stop smoking while using nicotine replacement may develop nicotine poisoning; in these individuals, replacement is contraindicated. Although the levels of nicotine are lower with nicotine replacement therapies than with active smoking, nicotine replacement is relatively contraindicated for patients immediately after myocardial infarction and for those with unstable angina or life-threatening arrhythmias.

Many self-help materials for smoking cessation are available to provide guidance for smokers (36). Investigations of the effectiveness of self-help materials with or without physician advice, although limited, suggest that these materials may benefit smokers in their efforts to quit. Furthermore, self-help materials are cost-effective compared to smoking cessation classes. Because of their potential effectiveness, the physician should provide self-help materials to all smokers.

As with any medical intervention, ongoing monitoring of the patient's status is critical for success. The patient's smoking status and stage of change should be reviewed at each follow-up visit. Furthermore, because relapse is most common during the first several weeks to months after smoking cessation, follow-up by mail, telephone, or in person is warranted. For those patients for whom nicotine replacement has been prescribed, follow-up contact 2 weeks after quitting increases effectiveness (61).

V. Conclusions

The physician's role in smoking cessation by individual patients may involve different levels of intervention, from brief advice to quit to assessment of the stage of change and assistance with specific behavioral changes and nicotine replacement. The intensity of intervention by the physician will be determined by training, available time, and interest. Many programs are available to provide physicians with training and materials for implementing smoking cessation counseling in their practices (36). To identify the essential attributes for successful smoking cessation interventions in medical practice, Kottke and coworkers (62) reviewed 39 controlled trials, in which the most effective characteristics were the use of more than one modality for motivating behavioral change, individualized face-to-face contact between patient and the health professional providing the counseling, and messages encouraging motivation and reinforcement provided on many occasions over the longest possible time.

References

1. Department of Health and Human Services. The Health Benefits of Smoking Cessation. A Report of the Surgeon General. DHHS Publication No. (CDC) 90-8416. Rockville, MD: Centers for Disease Control, 1990.
2. Speizer FE. The rise in chronic obstructive pulmonary disease mortality. Overview and summary. Am Rev Respir Dis 1989; 140 (Suppl):S106–S107.
3. Redline S. The epidemiology of COPD. In: Cherniack NS, ed. Chronic Obstructive Pulmonary Disease. Philadelphia: WB Saunders, 1991:225–234.
4. U.S. Department of Health and Human Services. The Health Consequences of Smoking: Chronic Obstructive Pulmonary Disease. A report of the Surgeon General. DHHS Publication No. 84-50205. Washington, DC: U.S. Government Printing Office, 1984.
5. Samet JM. The relationship of smoking to COPD. In: Cherniack NS, ed. Chronic Obstructive Pulmonary Disease. Philadelphia: WB Saunders, 1991:249–258.
6. Fletcher C, Peto R, Tinker C, et al. The Natural History of Chronic Bronchitis and Emphysema: An Eight-Year Study of Early Chronic Obstructive Lung Disease in Working Men in London. New York: Oxford University Press, 1976.
7. U.S. Department of Health and Human Services. Reducing the Health Consequences of Smoking: 25 Years of Progress. A report of the Surgeon General. DHHS Publication No. (CDC) 89-8411. Washington, DC: U.S. Government Printing Office, 1989.
8. Doll R, Peto R, Wheatley K, et al. Mortality in relation to smoking: 40 years' observations on male British doctors. Br Med J 1994; 309:901–911.
9. Parker DR, O'Connor GT, Sparrow D, et al. The relationship of nonspecific airway responsiveness and atopy to the rate of decline of lung function. Am Rev Respir Dis 1990; 141:589–594.
10. Becklake MR. Occupational exposures: evidence for a causal association with chronic obstructive pulmonary disease. Am Rev Respir Dis 1989; 140 (Suppl):S85–S91.
11. Anthonisen NR, Connett JE, Kiley JP, et al. Effects of smoking intervention and the use of an inhaled anticholinergic bronchodilator on the rate of decline of FEV_1. JAMA 1994; 272:1497–1505.

12. Becklake MR, Permutt S. Evaluation of tests of lung function for "screening" for early detection of chronic obstructive lung disease. In: Macklem PT, Permutt S, eds. The Lung in the Transition Between Health and Disease. New York: Marcel Dekker, 1980:345–387.
13. Becklake MR, White N. Sources of variation in spirometric measurements: identifying the signal and dealing with noise. In: Eisen EA, ed. Occupational Medicine: Spirometry. Philadelphia: Hanley & Belfus, 1993:241–264.
14. American Thoracic Society. Standardization of spirometry—1987 update. Am Rev Respir Dis 1987; 136:1285–1298.
15. Burrows B, Knudson RJ, Camilli AE, et al. The "horse-racing effect" and predicting decline in forced expiratory volume in one second from screening spirometry. Am Rev Respir Dis 1987; 135:788–793.
16. Cauberghs M, Clement J, Van de Woestijne KP. Functional alterations accompanying a rapid decline in ventilatory function. Am Rev Respir Dis 1993; 147:379–384.
17. Sherrill DL, Lebowitz MD, Knudson RJ, et al. Smoking and symptom effects on the curves of lung function growth and decline. Am Rev Respir Dis 1991; 144:17–22.
18. Higgins MW, Enright PL, Kronmal RA, et al. Smoking and lung function in elderly men and women: The Cardiovascular Health Study. JAMA 1993; 269:2741–2748.
19. Camilli AE, Burrows B, Knudson RJ, et al. Longitudinal changes in forced expiratory volume in one second in adults. Am Rev Respir Dis 1987; 135:794–799.
20. Dompeling E, van Schayck CP, van Grunsven PM, et al. Slowing the deterioration of asthma and chronic obstructive pulmonary disease observed during bronchodilator therapy by adding inhaled corticosteroids. Ann Intern Med 1993; 118:770–778.
21. Hughes JA, Hutchison DCS, Bellamy D, et al. The influence of cigarette smoking and its withdrawal on the annual change of lung function in pulmonary emphysema. Q J Med 1982; 51:33–45.
22. Postma DS, De Vries K, Koeter GH, et al. Independent influence of reversibility of air-flow obstruction and nonspecific hyperreactivity on the long-term course of lung function in chronic air-flow obstruction. Am Rev Respir Dis 1986; 134:276–280.
23. Fisher EB, Lichtenstein E, Haire-Joshu D. Multiple determinants of tobacco use and cessation. In: Orleans CT, Slade J, eds. Nicotine Addiction: Principles and Management. New York: Oxford University Press, 1993:59–88.
24. Lynch BS, Bonnie RJ, eds. Growing Up Tobacco Free: Preventing Nicotine Addiction in Children and Youths. Washington, DC: National Academy Press, 1994.
25. Chassin L, Presson CC, Sherman SJ, et al. The natural history of cigarette smoking: predicting young-adult smoking outcomes from adolescent smoking patterns. Health Psychol 1990;9:701–716.
26. Henningfield JE, Nemeth-Coslett R. Nicotine dependence: interface between tobacco and tobacco-related disease. Chest 1988; 93:37S–55S.
27. Jarvik ME, Henningfield JE. Pharmacological adjuncts for the treatment of to-

bacco dependence. In: Orleans CT, Slade J, eds. Nicotine Addiction: Principles and Management. New York: Oxford University Press, 1993:245–261.

28. U.S. Department of Health and Human Services. The Health Consequences of Smoking: Nicotine Addiction. A report of the Surgeon General. DHHS (CDC) Publication No. 88-8406. Washington, D.C.: U.S. Government Printing Office, 1988.
29. Henningfield JE, Cohen C, Pickworth WB. Psychopharmacology of nicotine. In: Orleans CT, Slade J, eds. Nicotine Addiction: Principles and Management. New York: Oxford University Press, 1993:24–45.
30. Prochaska JO, DiClemente CC. Stages and processes of self-change of smoking: toward an integrative model of change. J Consult Clin Psychol 1983; 51:390–395.
31. Rohren CL, Croghan IT, Hurt RD, et al. Predicting smoking cessation outcome in a medical center from stage of readiness: contemplation versus action. Prev Med 1994; 23:335–344.
32. Schwartz JL. Methods for smoking cessation. Clin Chest Med 1991; 12:737–753.
33. Fiore MC, Novotny TE, Pierce JP. Methods used to quit smoking in the United States: do cessation programs help? JAMA 1990; 263:2760–2765.
34. Lichtenstein E, Hollis J. Patient referral to a smoking cessation program: who follows through? J Fam Pract 1992; 34:739–744.
35. Tsevat J. Impact and cost-effectiveness of smoking interventions. Am J Med 1992; 93(Suppl):43S–47S.
36. Coultas DB. The physician's role in smoking cessation. Clin Chest Med 1991; 12:755–768.
37. Fiore MC, Smith SS, Jorenby DE, et al. The effectiveness of the nicotine patch for smoking cessation. JAMA 1994; 271(24):1940–1947.
38. Silagy C, Mant D, Fowler G, et al. Meta-analysis on efficacy of nicotine replacement therapies in smoking cessation. Lancet 1994; 343:139–142.
39. Oster G, Huse DM, Delea TE. Cost-effectiveness of nicotine gum as an adjunct to physician's advice against cigarette smoking. JAMA 1986; 256:1315–1318.
40. Cummings SR, Hansen B, Richard RJ. Internists and nicotine gum. JAMA 1988; 260:1565–1569.
41. Orleans CT, Resch N, Noll E, et al. Use of transdermal nicotine in a state-level prescription plan for the elderly: a first look at "real-world" patch users. JAMA 1994; 271:601–607.
42. Covey LS, Glassman AH. A meta-analysis of double-blind placebo-controlled trials of clonidine for smoking cessation. Br J Addict 1991; 86:991–998.
43. Kellner R, Samet J, Pathak D. Dyspnea, anxiety, and depression in chronic respiratory impairment. Gen Hosp Psychiatry 1992; 14:20–28.
44. Fisher EB, Haire-Joshu D, Morgan GD. Smoking and smoking cessation. Am Rev Respir Dis 1990; 142:702–720.
45. Pederson LL, Wanklin JM, Baskerville JC. The role of health beliefs in compliance with physician advice to quit smoking. Soc Sci Med 1984; 19:573–580.
46. Research Committee of the British Thoracic Society. Smoking cessation in patients: two further studies by the British Thoracic Society. Thorax 1990; 45:835–840.

47. Gritz ER, Kristeller JL, Burns DM. Treating nicotine addiction in high-risk groups and patients with medical co-morbidity. In: Orleans CT, Slade J, eds. Nicotine Addiction: Principles and Management. New York: Oxford University Press, 1993:279–309.
48. Cox NJM, Hendricks JC, Binkhorst RA, et al. A pulmonary rehabilitation program for patients with asthma and mild chronic obstructive pulmonary diseases (COPD). Lung 1993; 171:235–244.
49. Pederson LL, Wanklin JM, Lefcoe NM. The effects of counseling on smoking cessation among patients hospitalized with chronic obstructive pulmonary disease: a randomized clinical trial. Int J Addict 1991; 26:107–119.
50. Gruman J, Lynn W. Worksite and community intervention for tobacco control. In: Orleans TC, Slade J, eds. Nicotine Addiction: Principles and Management. New York: Oxford University Press, 1993:396–411.
51. National Institutes of Health. Tobacco and the Clinician: Interventions for Medical and Dental Practice. NIH Publication No. 94-3693. Washington, DC: U.S. Government Printing Office, 1994.
52. Centers for Disease Control. Physician and other health care professional counseling of smokers to quit—United States, 1991. MMWR 1993; 42:854–857.
53. Abrams DB. Treatment issues: towards a stepped-care model. Tobacco Control 1993; 2:517–529.
54. Glynn TJ, Manley MW. How to Help Your Patients Stop Smoking—a National Cancer Institute Manual for Physicians. NIH publication 909-3064. Washington, DC: U.S. Dept. of Health and Human Services, Public Health Service, National Institutes of Health, 1990.
55. Ockene JK, Kristeller J, Goldberg R, et al. Increasing the efficacy of physician-delivered smoking interventions. J Gen Intern Med 1991; 6:1–8.
56. Orleans CT. Treating nicotine dependence in medical settings: a stepped-care model. In: Orleans CT, Slade J, eds. Nicotine Addiction: Principles and Management. New York: Oxford University Press, 1993:145–180.
57. Goldberg DN, Hoffman AM, Farinha MF, et al. Physician delivery of smoking-cessation advice based on the stages-of-change model. Am J Prev Med 1994; 10:267–274.
58. Morris JF, Temple W. Spirometric "lung age" estimation for motivating smoking cessation. Prev Med 1985; 14:655–662.
59. Risser NL, Belcher DW. Adding spirometry, carbon monoxide, and pulmonary symptom results to smoking cessation counseling: a randomized trial. J Gen Intern Med 1990; 5:16–22.
60. Heatherton TF, Kozlowski LT, Frecker RC, et al. The Fagerstrom Test for nicotine dependence: a revision of the Fagerstrom Tolerance Questionnaire. Br J Addict 1991; 86:1119–1127.
61. Kenford SL, Fiore MC, Jorenby DE, et al. Predicting smoking cessation: who will quit with and without the nicotine patch? JAMA 1994; 271:589–594.
62. Kottke TE, Battista RN, DeFriese GH. Attributes of successful smoking cessation interventions in medical practice: a meta-analysis of 39 controlled trials. JAMA 1988; 259:2882–2889.

18

Pharmacological Approaches in Pulmonary Rehabilitative Medicine

RICHARD K. MURRAY and REYNOLD A. PANETTIERI, JR.

University of Pennsylvania Medical Center
Philadelphia, Pennsylvania

A number of pharmacological agents are useful in supporting the goals of pulmonary rehabilitation (1,2). Drug therapy, as part of pulmonary rehabilitation, is based on the assumption that there are specific pathophysiological components of the patient's disability that are either reversible, e.g., airway narrowing, pulmonary hypertension, or at least limited by inadequate supply of a substance that can be provided exogenously, e.g., oxygen. In some cases, pharmacological agents that have been used in pulmonary rehabilitation may operate at multiple sites, e.g., theophylline effects on airway narrowing versus effects on diaphragmatic contractility.

This chapter reviews the scientific basis for drug therapy in rehabilitation medicine as well as the current status of specific pharmacological agents used in this area. It is important to point out that most, if not all, pharmacotherapy used in rehabilitation is supportive. *As such, it is intended to optimize the functional status of the individual given certain physiological disabilities.* At the same time, this optimization of functional status may be crucial in facilitating a more rapid recovery after an illness or slowing the tempo of a progressive one. These therapeutic effects may lead simply to improved functional status by minimizing the effects of anxiety or depression, while in others they may facilitate more definitive forms of therapy such as organ transplantation.

A number of pathophysiological events occur in chronic pulmonary diseases which may provide targets for relatively specific pharmacological intervention. In some cases, these targets may be the root cause of the patient's disability, e.g., chronic obstructive lung disease, while in others they may be superimposed, but reversible contributing factors to the patient's total disability, e.g., reactive airways disease in a severe acute respiratory distress syndrome (ARDS) survivor. Table 1 lists the current targets of pharmacological therapy used in rehabilitation medicine and examples of agents used in therapy.

Pulmonary disability may also be exacerbated by the effects of other, more indirect, disease processes that alter either pulmonary mechanics, gas exchange, or the function of the respiratory pump (chest wall and diaphragm and associated accessory muscles of respiration). Examples of such diseases include congestive heart failure (worsened pulmonary mechanics, worsened gas exchange), pulmonary emboli (impaired $\mathring{V}/\mathring{Q}$ matching), progressive pulmonary restriction [interstitial lung disease (ILD), kyphoscoliosis], and muscular weakness (myopathy, neuropathy, malnutrition). While all of these causes of pulmonary disability have therapeutic approaches, e.g., diuretics, angiotensin-converting enzyme inhibitors, heparin, anti-inflammatory agents, a complete discussion of such approaches is beyond the scope of this chapter. Instead, this chapter focuses on common causes of reversible pulmonary disability, with an emphasis on the scientific basis for treatment as well as a discussion of the clinical utility of the appropriate therapeutic agents.

In this chapter, we first review the clinical syndromes of obstructive airways disease focusing on their common features and the broad aspects of their treatment. We also summarize current pharmacotherapy for obstructive airways disease as well as other treatable aspects of respiratory impairment in the context of pulmonary rehabilitation.

I. Obstructive Lung Disease

A great deal of pulmonary disability is the result of obstructive lung disease, particularly chronic obstructive pulmonary disease (COPD) (1–3). In addition, many patients undergoing pulmonary rehabilitation for other disease processes also have concurrent obstructive airways disease. Operationally, these may be classified as those with a large reversible component (asthma) and those with insufficient reversibility to ever restore the patient to normal (COPD).

Other disorders that may be associated with substantial pulmonary disability share certain features of obstructive lung disease. These include cystic fibrosis, bronchiectasis, congenital bullous disease, survivors of severe ARDS, and bronchiolitis obliterans; the latter is distinguished from bronchiolitis obliter-

Table 1 Targets of Pharmacological Agents Used in Pulmonary Rehabilitation

Pathophysiological target	Specific disease	Drug
Airway resistance	COPD	Bronchodilators
Airway inflammation	COPD	Anti-inflammatory agents
Sputum production	COPD	Mucolytics/expectorants
Diaphragmatic dysfunction	COPD	Theophylline
Pulmonary HTN	Various	Vasodilators
Low oxygen saturation	COPD/ILD	Continuous oxygen
Desaturation with exercise	ILD	Intermittent oxygen
Anxiety/depression	Various	Anxiolytics/antidepressants

COPD, chronic obstructive lung disease; HTN, hypertension; ILD, interstitial lung disease.

ans organizing pneumonia (BOOP), a restrictive disease. In addition, the pathophysiological changes characteristic of obstructive lung disease may be part of other more complex disorders, including sarcoidosis, the vasculitides involving the lung, e.g., Wegener's disease, and lymphangiomyomatosis (LAM). It is important to remember that asthma, because of its prevalence, may coexist with other diseases or may be exacerbated by other causes of bronchial inflammation (3,4). For example, a significant subset of patients with cystic fibrosis also suffer from asthma. The guiding principle of management in all of these diseases is to search for a reversible component and to treat aggressively in order to optimize the patient's functional status. Since asthma and emphysema account for the majority of obstructive lung disease, their clinical features will be briefly reviewed.

A. Clinical Features of Asthma

Asthma is a chronic disease characterized by reversible obstruction to airflow within the lungs (5–7). It affects about one person in 15. In contrast to emphysema or chronic bronchitis, patients with asthma may have essentially normal lung function between episodes. Although the etiology of asthma remains unknown, airway hyperreactivity in response to inhalational challenge using methacholine or aerosolized allergen is a hallmark of this disease. In some patients, narrowing of the airways may be part of an allergic reaction triggering the release of biologically active mediators. In other patients, specific stimuli trigger episodes and suggest an etiological relationship (exercise, airway cooling, or stress). In the majority of patients, the cause of the airway hyperreactivity is unknown. Specific causes that have been proposed include imbalances within the nervous system, deficiency of β-receptors, excess contraction of airway smooth muscle, imbalances in mediator production, and immune regulatory defects (8). It is important to try to understand which triggers are involved in exacerbating the patient's asthma, particularly if such symptoms are interfering with progress through a rehabilitation program.

The pathology of asthma includes narrowing of the airway lumen and thickening of the walls of the airways (9,10). Mucus and sloughed epithelial cells are seen within the airway lumen, and an infiltrate of inflammatory cells, especially eosinophils, is seen within the airway wall. Edema within the airway wall is also a prominent finding. Recent studies of biopsies in asthmatics have shown increased numbers of T lymphocytes, mast cells, macrophages, and eosinophils compared to normals (11,12).

Increased resistance to airflow is the sine qua non of the asthmatic attack. In large part, the increase in airway resistance is due to contraction of airway smooth muscle cells. Other mechanisms—notably thickening of the airways by edema and cellular infiltration as well as intraluminal collections of mucus secretions, and cellular debris—also contribute to the obstruction to airflow. Small changes in airway diameter have dramatic effects on airway resistance, due to r^4 relationship between radius and resistance.

An increase in resistance to airflow causes a series of physiological alterations, including abnormalities of lung mechanics and gas exchange (13,14). Spirometry reveals an obstructive pattern manifested by a decrease in FVC and FEV_1 and a decrease in the FEV_1/FVC ratio. The functional residual capacity (FRC) is increased and the lungs appear hyperinflated on the chest radiograph. The work of breathing is increased and the efficiency of the respiratory pump is decreased because of altered compliance and a pressure-volume relationship that places the respiratory muscles at a suboptimal length-tension relationship. Thus, as airflow is restricted, the work of breathing is increased.

Regional inhomogeneity in the distribution of inspired air leads to ventilation-perfusion ($\mathring{V}/\mathring{Q}$) mismatch and impaired gas exchange (6). Areas of low $\mathring{V}/\mathring{Q}$ contribute to the development of hypoxemia. Dead space ventilation is increased, but adequate elimination of CO_2 is maintained in mild to moderate asthma by a compensatory increase in minute ventilation. In severe asthma, the combined effects of augmented CO_2 production, impaired CO_2 elimination, and respiratory muscle fatigue lead to the development of hypercapnia and respiratory acidosis, eventuating in respiratory failure if therapy is unsuccessful (13,14).

Although asthma is generally thought of as a disease with a favorable prognosis, recent studies suggest that chronic severe asthma can be disabling (15). In addition, the chronic use of systemic steroids to treat airway inflammation may induce a number of severe complications, such as myopathy, which may further increase the extent of disability. Pulmonary rehabilitative medicine may play an important role in improving the quality of life in many of these patients (1,2).

B. Clinical Features of COPD

Although the term "chronic obstructive pulmonary disease" is used to describe a variety of pulmonary disorders, including asthma, chronic bronchitis, emphysema, cystic fibrosis, and bronchiectasis, COPD usually refers to chronic bronchitis and emphysema. Unlike asthma, COPD implies, in part, irreversible airways obstruction. There also exists considerable overlap in the clinical manifestations of these diseases such that many of the features of asthma, emphysema, and/or chronic bronchitis may coexist in an individual with airways obstruction. *Chronic bronchitis* may be defined as a clinical disorder characterized by excessive mucus secretion in the bronchial tree and manifested by a chronic or a recurrent productive cough. These symptoms should be present on most days for a minimum of 3 months in the year and for not less than 2 consecutive years. By contrast, *emphysema* refers to an anatomical alteration of the lung characterized by an abnormal enlargement of air spaces distal to the terminal, nonrespiratory bronchiole, accompanied by destructive changes of the alveolar walls.

Although defined as a clinical disorder, chronic bronchitis is manifested by chronic excessive secretion of mucus that is associated with airway obstruction and mucus plugging. Pathologically, there exists enlargement of bronchial mucus glands with an increase in the number of mucus-secreting cells (hyperplasia).

Emphysema is characterized by a permanent, abnormal increase in the size of air spaces distal to the terminal bronchiole (acinus). Emphysema is also classified according to the site where the terminal bronchiole is affected. Centrilobular emphysema, which occurs most commonly as a result of, or in association with, cigarette smoking, affects the proximal segment of the respiratory bronchiole. Panacinar emphysema, which occurs in the elderly and in patients with α_1-antiprotease deficiency, uniformly affects the entire respiratory bronchiole. Such classifications are not unique to specific disorders since panacinar and centrilobular emphysema may coexist in the same lung. *It is the degree of functional impairment from emphysema, not the type, that determines the clinical significance of the disease.*

In the United States, the majority of patients with emphysema and chronic bronchitis smoke cigarettes or were former smokers (16–19). Only a minority of smokers (approximately 15%) develop COPD. The benefits of smoking cessation are well established. Studies have demonstrated that smoking cessation has been associated with dramatic reductions in respiratory symptoms within a month of cessation. At 1 year after cessation, former smokers reduce their risk of ischemic heart disease by 50%, and after 15 years of abstinence, risk from all smoking-related mortality approaches that of individuals who never smoked. Many centers have taken a renewed interest in a variety of approaches to help patients discontinue the use of tobacco, and no effort should be spared in this important therapeutic goal. Smoking cessation is an important aspect in any pulmonary rehabilitation program.

Chronic airflow limitation is the hallmark of emphysema and of chronic bronchitis; it occurs through several mechanisms, including partial occlusion of the airway lumen by excessive and tenacious secretions as described in patients with chronic bronchitis, airway narrowing as a consequence of smooth muscle contraction, and/or bronchial wall edema and inflammation as is also seen in asthma. In addition, in COPD, destruction of lung parenchyma, as described in patients with emphysema, may alter the tethering forces exerted on the airway lumen, allowing the moderate-sized airways, which are those not surrounded by cartilage, to become "floppy" and limit airflow especially during forced expiratory maneuvers. Importantly, all three mechanisms may occur concomitantly; therefore, therapeutic efforts should be directed at reversing airway smooth muscle contraction, decreasing airway inflammation, and augmenting sputum expectoration. Unfortunately, the loss of radial traction of the airways and decrease in the elastic recoil of the lung, as seen in emphysema, are irreversible.

Despite a variety of mechanisms that can induce airway obstruction, chronic airway obstruction alters pulmonary mechanics in a predictable manner. Expiratory flow rates and volumes are diminished throughout the expiratory cycle. Since airflow limitation prolongs expiration time and prevents complete emptying of affected alveoli, lung volumes also increase. These increases in lung volume alter the length-tension relationship of the diaphragm, which then places respiratory muscles at a mechanical disadvantage.

In patients with COPD, ventilation-perfusion mismatch occurs commonly and induces hypoxemia with or without CO_2 retention. The alveolar-arterial difference for Po_2 is usually increased with a large proportion of ventilation preferentially directed to areas of the lung with high ventilation-perfusion ratios (increased dead space ventilation). Although patients with severe airflow limitation (less than 0.8 L) are more likely to retain CO_2, there exists considerable individual variation. Some patients with COPD, particularly those with severe chronic bronchitis, develop CO_2 retention while others with comparable airflow limitation do not.

Patients with COPD may experience an increased work of breathing due, in part, to increased airway resistance and altered respiratory muscle mechanics. In addition, these patients may have a blunted ventilatory response to inhaled CO_2 as compared with normal subjects. Despite the concept that patients with COPD may retain CO_2 to compensate for an increased work of breathing, the exact mechanism that induces CO_2 retention in these patients is likely to be multifactorial and remains unknown. In addition, because exercise is limited by the patient's ventilatory capacity, traditional training exercises are often not successful in improving functional status (20,21).

The prognosis in COPD correlates, in part, with measurements of the FEV_1. In young smokers (<35 years old) who have mild obstructive airways disease (80% predicted > FEV_1 > 60% predicted), the FEV_1 will return to normal after smoking cessation. In older patients, smoking cessation will slow, but not eliminate, further decrements in the FEV_1. The advent of cor pulmonale and hypercapnia in COPD indicates a poor prognosis. The FEV_1 can also be useful in prognosis: in patients presenting with values of FEV_1 less than 0.75 L, the mortality rate at 1 year is 30%, and at 10 years is 95% (16,17,19,22).

Respiratory failure is the most common cause of death in these patients. Recent studies suggest that some patients with severe airway obstruction may survive significantly longer than current median survival rates. In these studies, aggressive management of acute exacerbations of COPD appeared to improve overall survival rates (23–25).

II. General Features of Therapy of Obstructive Lung Disease

Because the approach to treatment of the two major classes of obstructive lung disease is somewhat different, they will be discussed separately here.

A. Treatment of Asthma

Successful treatment of the patient with asthma requires the appropriate choice of medication as well as an emphasis on patient education (6,7). The goals of patient education include avoidance strategies for specific trigger events as well as treatment strategies for exacerbations. Frequent contact between the physician and asthmatic can play a major role in decreasing the severity of episodes (3,6,7,26).

The pharmacotherapy of asthma is focused mainly on bronchodilation and on reducing inflammation within the airways (6–8). Bronchodilators, acting primarily on smooth muscle to effect relaxation, include β-adrenergic agents, anticholinergic agents, and theophylline.

Anti-inflammatory agents include inhaled steroids and systemic steroids. Other agents such as cromolyn sodium are more difficult to classify (4,7).

While the use of inhaled β-agonists may cause a prompt increase in airway caliber and thus make the patient feel better, they do not treat the airway inflammation and hyperresponsiveness that characterize the late phase of asthma. For these reasons, as well as recent studies demonstrating inordinate mortality in patients treated with long-acting or regularly scheduled β-agonists, combination therapy with β-agonists and anti-inflammatory drugs, e.g., inhaled steroids, is the most appropriate approach for most patients (7).

An approach to the chronic management of patients with asthma is shown in Figure 1. Inhaled bronchodilators and corticosteroids are essential therapies in the treatment of asthma. Other drugs, such as methylxanthines, long-acting β-agonists, and cromolyn sodium, may be useful in some, but not all, patients (7). In chronic severe asthma, a major therapeutic goal is prevention of side effects induced by systemic corticosteroid use. The role and use of each of these drugs in the treatment of asthma and COPD will be discussed in greater detail below.

B. Treatment of COPD

Many patients with COPD have some component of reversible airways disease that can be treated, in a manner analogous to asthma. The modalities that have been shown to be useful therapeutically in patients with COPD include bronchodilators and anti-inflammatory drugs (27–29). Bronchodilators act to relax airway smooth muscle and thus decrease overall airway resistance. Bronchodilators may be either specific receptor antagonists or functional antagonists of airway smooth muscle contraction. The muscarinic antagonist, ipratropium bromide (Atrovent), is the only available specific receptor blocker shown to be clinically useful in COPD. It is more effective in patients with COPD than it is in asthmatics (30,31). β-Adrenergic agonists and theophylline compounds, which act as functional antagonists of a variety of smooth muscle contractile agonists, act primarily through augmentation of cAMP levels within smooth muscle cells leading to a decrease in airway resistance. Theophylline may also have therapeutic effects at other sites such as the diaphragm (see below).

An approach to the chronic management of COPD patients is shown in Figure 2. Although some similarities do exist with therapies designed to treat patients with asthma, the management of COPD is clearly different from that of asthma. Smoking cessation is by far the most important initial step in improving pulmonary function in patients with COPD (19). The role of each of these drugs in the treatment of COPD will be discussed in greater detail below.

III. Basic Mechanisms of Bronchodilators

Most inflammatory mediators, which induce bronchoconstriction, depend on their ability to interact with specific surface receptors on target cells. The common mechanism by which these signals are translated into biological effects is shared by many different cell types as well as types of receptors. For example, in airway smooth muscle, a large variety of contractile agonists that have been implicated in asthma, e.g., acetylcholine, histamine, leukotriene D_4 (LTD_4),

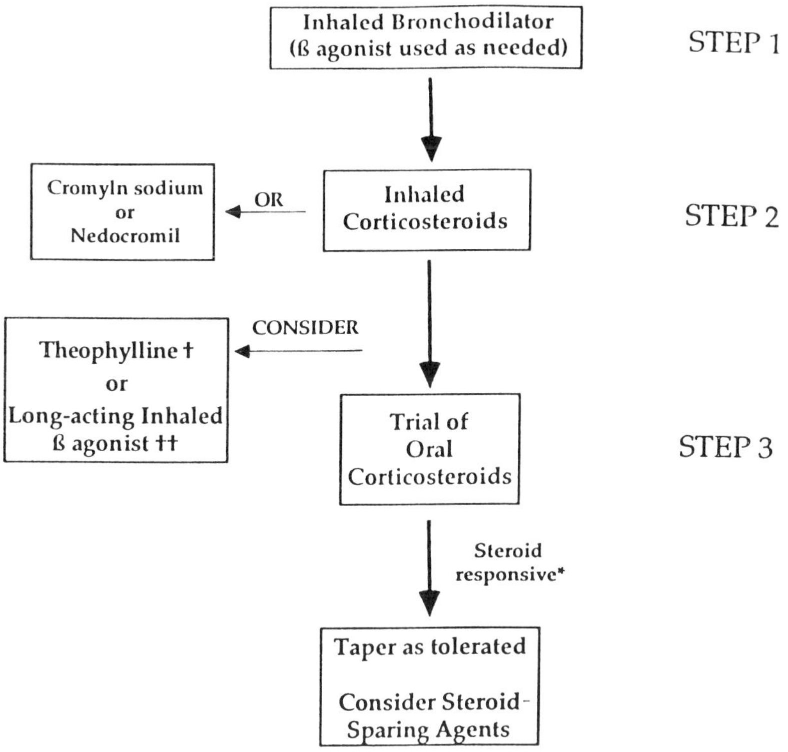

Figure 1 Stepwise approach to the management of patients with asthma. *Step 1*: Inhaled bronchodilators, used on an as-needed basis, is the initial step in the management of asthma. Metered-dose-inhaler technique should be evaluated frequently to confirm adequate use. *Step 2*: Inhaled corticosteroids are a mainstay in reversing airflow obstruction due to airway inflammation and edema. In some patients, especially children and/or those with exercise-induced asthma, cromoyln sodium or nedocromil may be substituted for inhaled steroids. Methylxanthines (†) and/or long-acting inhaled β-agonists (††) are beneficial in those asthmatics who have difficulty using metered-dose inhalers or who have nocturnal symptoms. *Step 3*: Some patients with asthma may only respond to oral corticosteroids with improvement in pulmonary function. Therefore, a trial of oral prednisone (0.5 mg/kg daily) should be considered. If the forced expiratory volume in 1 sec (FEV_1) increases by at least 20% after 2 weeks of oral prednisone therapy, the patient is considered to be steroid-responsive (*). Attempts can then be made to taper the dosage of oral corticosteroids to the lowest maintenance dose that preserves pulmonary function. If the patient remains on more than 10 mg prednisone daily for more than 3 months, steroid-sparing agents should be considered (methotrexate, cyclosporine, or gold).

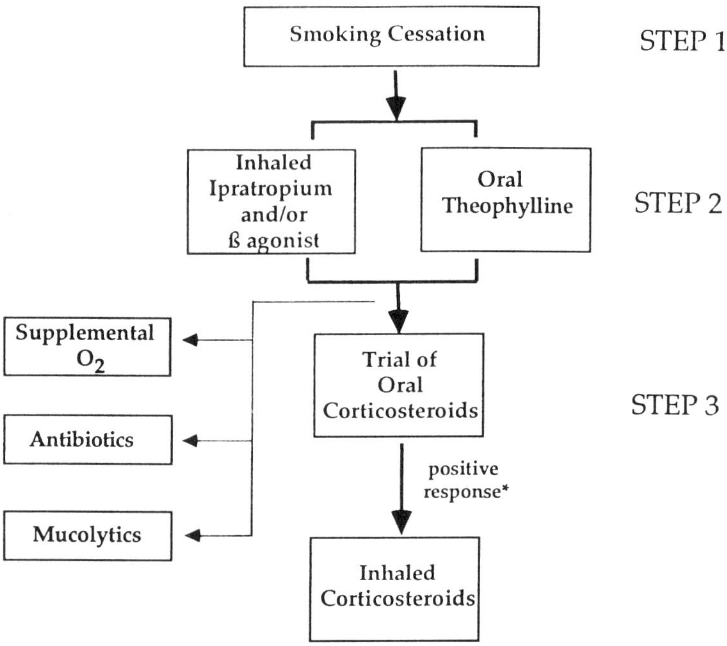

Figure 2 Stepwise approach to the management of patient with chronic obstructive lung disease. *Step 1*: Smoking cessation is critically important as the initial step in slowing further deterioration in lung function as well as decreasing the frequency of acute exacerbations of COPD. *Step 2*: Inhaled bronchodilators are a mainstay in reversing airflow obstruction due to airway smooth muscle contraction. Methylxanthines, such as oral theophylline, are not only used as adjunct bronchodilators but also serve to improve diaphragmatic function and decrease pulmonary hypertension. *Step 3*: Since some patients with COPD may respond to corticosteroids with improved pulmonary function, a trial of oral prednisone (0.5 mg/kg daily) should be considered. If there is at least a 20% improvement in the forced expiratory volume in 1 sec (FEV_1) after 2 weeks of oral prednisone therapy, then this is considered a positive response (*). Attempts can then be made to taper the oral corticosteroids and start inhaled steroids. Adjunct therapy for COPD includes antibiotics, supplemental O_2, and mucolytics as described in the text.

platelet-activating factor (PAF), substance P, and bradykinin, appear to act by augmenting the concentration of intracellular calcium and the production of force arising from the interaction of actin and myosin. A major requirement for effective drugs in obstructive lung disease is to oppose the effects of these contractile agonists, either at the level of the surface receptor or at postreceptor mechanisms to effect relaxation of airway smooth muscle.

Of all the agents capable of relaxing airway smooth muscle, the best example is the β-agonist. β-Agonists increase the concentration of intracellular cyclic adenosine monophosphate (cAMP), thereby affecting a number of intracellular processes via the enzyme cAMP-dependent protein kinase A (32–34). The relaxant effects of protein kinase A appear to include alterations in the ability of contractile agonists to augment cytosolic calcium as well as alterations in the sensitivity of the contractile proteins to calcium (32,34). In addition, β-agonists cause specific G-protein subunits to activate membrane potassium channels, leading to a stabilization of membrane potential (33). This additional mechanism provides yet another way in which β-agonists lead to relaxation of smooth muscle and underscores the point that drugs may have multiple mechanisms of action.

Attempts designed to relax airway smooth muscle or to prevent cell activation by *multiple* mediators contrast with approaches using the *individual* antagonists to cell surface receptors (e.g., anticholinergics, LTD_4, PAF). The search for individual antagonists presupposes that a particular molecule is of key importance in the pathogenesis of the disease. Unfortunately, no single mediator has been shown to be primarily responsible for asthma, although in COPD, cholinergic stimulation is clearly important, as evidenced by the efficacy of its blockade in this disease.

IV. Specific Agents and Their Use in Rehabilitation Medicine

A. β-Adrenergic Agents

These agents act to increase cAMP within airway smooth muscle and cause a decrease in force production leading to a widening of the airway. They are available as both oral and inhalational agents (and i.v. in a few cases). β-Adrenergic agents that are inhaled have a wider therapeutic index than do adrenergic agents taken orally. Table 2 summarizes the currently recommended use of inhaled bronchodilators in asthma. Long-acting β-agonists, such as salmeterol, are now available in the United States and may be useful in patients with nocturnal awakenings due to asthma and in patients with exercise-induced asthma. The utility of these agents is marginal and their advantages over conventional therapy are unknown (35,36). Long-acting agents may be most useful for active individuals who need extended periods of drug effect (37–39). They are not indicated for the acute relief of symptoms, and under no circumstances do they entirely replace short-acting β-agonists.

B. Theophylline

Despite the use of methylxanthines in the treatment of COPD for over 100 years, the mechanism by which this agent improves dyspnea or decreases air-

Table 2 Aerosolized β-Adrenergic Agents

Drug	β_2-specific	Onset of action (min)	Peak effect (min)	Duration (hr)	Aerosol dose by nebulizer[a]	Aerosol dose by metered-dose inhaler
Isoproterenol	No	5	15	1	2.5–5 μg	250 μg/2 puffs
Isoetharine	Yes	10	30	2–3	5 μg	680 μg/2 puffs
Metaproterenol	Yes	10	45	3–6	15 μg	1300 μg/2 puffs
Albuterol	Yes	10	60	4–6	2.5–5 μg	180 μg/2 puffs
Terbutaline	Yes	10	60	4–6		400 μg/2 puffs
Pirbuterol	Yes	10	60	4–6		400 μg/2 puffs
Bitolterol	Yes	10	60	3–8		1050 μg/3 puffs
Fenoterol[b]	Yes	10	6	4–8		400 μg/2 puffs
Salmeterol[c]	Yes	10	60	8–10		50 μg/puff
Formoterol[b]	Yes	10	60	8–10		12 μg/puff

[a] Aerosol dose by nebulizer diluted in 3 ml saline.
[b] Not available in the United States.
[c] Not indicated for the acute relief of symptoms.

way obstruction remains unknown (40,41). Theophylline is a weak bronchodilator in comparison to β-agonists or ipratropium. Given the narrow therapeutic window, the use of theophylline should be tailored to the individual patient and "optimal" bronchodilator effects may occur in the low therapeutic range (5–15 mg/L) (Table 3). Theophylline clearance may be affected by a variety of other medications, and dosing regimens should be individualized and serum levels checked regularly (Table 4).

In COPD patients, the therapeutic benefit of theophylline may be a consequence of its nonbronchodilator actions (42–44). Apart from increasing cAMP levels by inhibiting phosphodiesterase activity, methylxanthines have been reported to increase the contractility of "fatigued" diaphragms and increase mucociliary action in normal airways (42,43). Moreover, methylxanthines also increase hypoxic drive to ventilation in hypercapnic COPD patients and increase right and left ventricular ejection fractions through vasodilation and through direct myocardial stimulation (44).

Theophylline preparations have been prescribed frequently for asthma for many years, though their role in therapy is declining. The dosing of theophylline is confounded by erratic absorption, unpredictable excretion kinetics, and a narrow therapeutic range. Despite serum levels in the therapeutic range, many patients experience anxiety, tremor, palpitations, and gastrointestinal symptoms. In addition, aminophylline effects only slightly improve indices of airflow beyond that achieved by inhaled β-agonists. For asthmatics, theophylline

Table 3 Dosing of Aminophylline Administered Intravenously in Adults with Acute Bronchospasm[a,b]

Loading Dose	
History of theophylline use	
None	6 mg/kg over 20 min
Oral theophylline use	0–3 mg/kg over 20 min
Maintenance Dose	
Patient category	
Nonsmoker	0.5 mg/kg/hr
Smoker	0.3 mg/kg/hr
Critically ill	0.5 mg/kg/hr
Congestive heart failure	0.2 mg/kg/hr
Severe pneumonia	0.2 mg/kg/hr

[a] Dosing expressed in aminophylline equivalents (theophylline dose = 0.8 × aminophylline dose). If possible, serum theophylline levels should be obtained prior to administration. Initial target serum concentration for theophylline is 10 μg/ml.

[b] Theophylline levels should be measured 12–24 hr after loading and more frequently if symptoms or signs of theophylline toxicity are evident.

preparations are generally reserved for those patients who cannot be adequately treated with β-agonists (7). For those patients receiving theophylline, the target concentration in the blood is 6–12 mg/ml. A variety of drugs affect theophylline metabolism through interaction with the hepatic P450 enzyme system; concurrent use of these drugs necessitates that the dose of theophylline be adjusted according to measured blood levels.

C. Anticholinergics

Although inhaled atropine has been used as a form of anticholinergic therapy for obstructive lung disease, ipratropium bromide is currently the only indicated anticholinergic for use in asthma or COPD. In COPD patients, inhaled ipratropium bromide as a single agent is at least equal to and, in many studies, is better than methylxanthines or inhaled β-agonists (24,30,31,45). Ipratropium bromide, which blocks muscarinic receptors on airway smooth muscle, decreases vagal tone, inhibits smooth muscle contraction, and decreases mucus secretion. In a few studies, the addition of anticholinergics to β-agonist therapy appeared to have an additive effect (30). For many patients with COPD, inhaled quaternary anticholinergic agents (ipratropium) represent first-line therapy; they offer greater bronchodilator effect and fewer side effects than do

Table 4 Physiological Factors and Drug Interactions that Alter Theophylline Metabolism

Increases serum levels	Decreases serum levels
Advanced age	Carbamazepine
Obesity	Dilantin
Erythromycin	Rifampin
Cimetidine	Cigarette smoking
Oral contraceptives	Phenobarbital
Propranolol	
Allopurinol	
Hepatic disease/congestion	
Congestive heart disease	
Quinolones (ciprofloxacin, etc.)	

other available bronchodilating agents. In addition, the bronchodilator potency of the anticholinergic agents is not attenuated by continued administration whereas patients treated with β-agonists for prolonged periods may experience blunted bronchodilator responses to β-agonists. Further, β-agonists may also induce pulmonary vasodilation, which worsens ventilation-perfusion matching and occasionally results in a decrease in the arterial Po_2. Ipratropium is delivered by metered dose inhaler (18 μg/puff), two puffs four times daily to a maximum of four puffs four times daily. Although inhaled anticholinergic therapy is as effective as β-agonist therapy in patients with COPD, the same is not true in asthma. Thus, the role of ipratropium in asthma remains as a second-line therapy to β-agonists in asthmatics.

D. Leukotriene Antagonists

Several pharmaceutical companies have LTD_4 antagonists or inhibitors of leukotriene synthesis in various phases of clinical trials (46–50). Exercise-induced asthma is often used as an experimental model to investigate the bronchodilator efficacy of these compounds, and several have been shown to be useful in exercise-induced asthma. When released, these compounds may play a role in controlling airway obstruction in patients undergoing pulmonary rehabilitation.

E. Corticosteroids

Corticosteroids, unlike bronchodilators, act to treat the consequences of airway inflammation that include cellular infiltration, edema, and mediator release. Corticosteroids have no acute effects on airway caliber and exert their effects only after a delay of 3–6 hr (51). The most significant recent advance in the use of steroids in asthma has been the introduction of inhaled corticosteroids that achieve an anti-inflammatory effect localized to the airways without significant systemic side effects (4,6,7). Interestingly, studies have shown that inhaled corticosteroids may also be of value in patients with COPD (29). The three agents currently available in the United States are beclomethasone diproprionate, triamcinolone acetonide, and flunisolide. Inhaled steroids are given via a metered-dose inhaler (MDI), and as with β-agonists, the patient must learn the effective use of an inhaler to assure delivery of the drug to the airways. Although inhaled steroids at currently approved doses are free from systemic side effect, delivery of a significant amount of the steroid to the oropharynx may result in symptomatic *Candida* infections. Such infections may be prevented by proper MDI technique, by the use of a spacer, or by gargling after each dose of the inhaled steroid.

Systemic steroids play an important role in the management of acute and chronic asthma as they represent the most effective anti-inflammatory therapy available (51). In acute exacerbations of asthma, short courses of prednisone or methylprednisolone (i.v. or p.o.) may be necessary in patients already taking inhaled steroids or too sick to use them (52). There is little evidence that doses higher than 40–60 mg of prednisone four times a day result in further improvement of airway obstruction. Despite the well-known complications of chronic steroid use, short courses of even high-dose corticosteroids are generally well tolerated. Hyperkalemia, hyperglycemia, muscle weakness, and alterations in mental status can occur but usually resolve promptly. The optimum method to taper steroids is unclear. Patients are usually switched from parenteral methylprednisolone to either p.o. prednisone or methylprednisolone once symptoms and airflow are clearly improving. Dosing frequency is cut to either q.d. or b.i.d. and the patient is tapered to a target of 20 mg/day over 10–14 days. In many patients, inhaled steroids can fully replace this dose of prednisone and the oral steroids can be discontinued.

Although the benefit of steroids in the management of asthma is well established, the efficacy of steroids in the management of COPD is less well established (27,28). Therapy with corticosteroids has been reported to provide both subjective and objective benefits in some patients with COPD (28,29). Unfortunately, there are few clinical predictors that identify which patients will respond. The popular notion is that patients with COPD in whom the airways disease is reversible may respond to steroids. Less familiar is the fact that some patients with COPD who are not bronchodilator-responsive also improve with steroid therapy. Thus, a therapeutic trial of corticosteroids seems justified in any patient with COPD. After pretreatment pulmonary function testing, the patient undergoes a 2-week course of methylprednisolone or prednisone at a dose of 20–40 mg/day. Repeat pulmonary function testing is then performed, and if objective improvement occurs, the dose of steroids is slowly tapered to maintenance level; if there is no improvement by objective criteria, steroid therapy is discontinued. Patients with COPD do not seem to benefit from inhaled or alternate-day steroid therapy.

F. Cromolyn

Cromolyn, which inhibits mast cell degranulation, can inhibit both the early and late phases of allergen-induced bronchoconstriction (6,7). It is most effective when used as prophylaxis in patients with exercise-induced asthma. Cromolyn is not a bronchodilator, and it is ineffective in treating acute asthma and adults with chronic severe asthma. In addition, it has no role in the treatment of COPD.

G. Mucolytics

Adjunctive use of mucolytics-expectorants appears to improve the quality of life, decreases cough, and decreases the duration of acute exacerbations of dyspnea in some COPD patients with excessive mucus production (53,54). Although 1–8 weeks of iodinated glycerol therapy at a dose of 60 mg four times daily has been reported to reduce symptoms in these patients, other mucolytic agents such as acetylcysteine (inhaled or oral), glycerol guaiacolate (guanifesin), and ambuxol have not been shown to be consistently effective. If conventional therapy fails to improve symptoms of cough or chest tightness, then an 8-week trial of oral iodinated glycerol may determine whether a patient will respond to mucolytic therapy.

H. Antibiotics and Vaccines

Antibiotics (trimethaprim-sulfamethoxizole, amoxacillin, or doxycycline) used in patients with acute exacerbations of COPD decrease the duration of the COPD exacerbation and result in more rapid improvement of peak expiratory flow rates when compared with controls (55–57). There is, however, no evidence to support the prophylactic use of antibiotics in COPD patients. Current data support the use of antibiotics for 7–10 days in the management of acute exacerbations of COPD.

Although *Pneumococcus* is one of the two most commonly cultured pathogens in the sputum of patients with COPD exacerbations, most exacerbations are not due to bacterial infections. There is no evidence that pneumococcal bacteremia or sepsis is more common or more severe in COPD patients. Although the cost-benefit ratio of pneumococcal vaccine is low, this therapy should be regarded as potentially useful but not yet of proven efficacy (58).

I. Supplemental Oxygen

When administered for a minimum of at least 12 hr/day, supplemental O_2 is the ONLY DRUG that has reduced mortality in the management of COPD (59–61). The current indications for home O_2 therapy include: (1) resting Pao_2 <55 mmHg or an arterial oxygen saturation $<90\%$; (2) Pao_2 55–59 mmHg with evidence of cor pulmonale or polycythemia; or (3) significant exercise- or sleep-induced hypoxemia/arterial oxygen desaturation that reverses with supplemental O_2 therapy. Supplemental O_2 should be titrated to maintain the Pao_2 between 65 and 80 mmHg. The benefit of supplemental O_2 in patients with severe restrictive lung disease has been clearly established. When the DL_{CO} drops below 50% of predicted, patients with restrictive lung disease usually become hypoxemic during exercise. Such patients will improve their capacity to exercise if given sufficient supplemental oxygen to block the oxyhemoglobin desaturation.

J. Antielastase Therapy

Since emphysema may be induced by an imbalance between neutrophil elastases and serum antiproteases, therapy directed toward increasing serum antiproteases or decreasing neutrophil elastases may prove beneficial in the management of patients with emphysema. In patients with α_1-antitrypsin (α1-AT) deficiency, plasma α1-AT may be given intravenously once weekly (60 mg/kg) or once monthly (250 mg/ml) to maintain serum α1-AT levels above 11 μM (62). These doses increase lung α1-AT levels and restore lung antineutrophil elastase defense mechanisms into the normal range. Although α1-AT replacement therapy is efficacious in restoring serum levels of antiprotease activity, clinical efficacy remains unproven in regard to reducing the decline in lung function or improving survival in patients with α1-AT deficiency.

K. Experimental Agents

A number of therapeutic agents useful in some patients with asthma are under various stages of investigation. Investigational bronchodilators include leukotriene receptor antagonists, calcium channel blockers, potassium channel agonists, intravenous magnesium, and inhaled diuretics.

The immune modulatory effects of low-dose methotrexate and cyclosporine are currently under investigation as steroid-sparing agents in patients requiring chronic high-dose systemic steroids. Although both agents appear to be able to decrease the required daily dose of steroids, their use is limited by substantial toxicity. Some agents, such as the macrolide antibiotics troleandomycin and erythromycin, also appear to be "steroid-sparing" in some patients.

V. Summary

In conclusion, many patients with severe pulmonary disability have some component of their impairment that is reversible. This "dynamic" component represents the opportunity for the physician to impact on the well-being of the patient. Aggressive approaches toward optimization of any reversible component will be rewarded by an improvement in functional status and quality of life for the patient. Nevertheless, the pathophysiological mechanisms of the pharmacological agents, as well as their propensities for adverse effects or drug interactions, must be kept clearly in mind. In addition, the most aggressive management plan will fail if patient compliance with medication is a problem. Time spent with patients in educating them with respect to the basic mechanisms of their impairment and the rationale for the continued use of their medications, will pay off with many patients.

REFERENCES

1. Make BJ. Introduction to pulmonary rehabilitation. Clin Chest Med 1986; 7:519–540.
2. Petty TL. Pulmonary rehabilitation for COPD. In: Petty TL, ed. Intensive and Rehabilitative Respiratory Care, 3d ed. Philadelphia: Lea & Febiger, 1982:385–413.
3. Irwin RS, Curley FJ, French CL. Difficult-to-control asthma. Contributing factors and outcome of a systematic management protocol. Chest 1993; 103:1662–1669.
4. Kay AB. Asthma and inflammation. J Allergy Clin Immunol 1991; 87:893–910.
5. Goldstein RA, ed. The rising problems of asthma: mechanisms and management. Chest 1992; 101:355S.
6. Murray RK, Panettieri RA. Management of asthma: the changing approach. In: Fishman AP, ed. Update: Pulmonary Diseases and Disorders. New York: McGraw-Hill, 1992:67–82.
7. NHLBI, National Asthma Education Program, Executive Panel Report: Executive Summary: Guidelines for the Diagnosis and Management of Asthma. US DHHS/PHS Publication No. 91-3042A, June 1991.
8. Barnes PJ. Control of airway caliber. In: Fishman AP, ed. Update: Pulmonary Diseases and Disorders. New York: McGraw-Hill, 1992:53–66.
9. Busse WW, Calhoun WF, Sedgwick JD. Mechanism of airway inflammation in asthma. Am Rev Respir Dis 1993; 147:S20–S24.
10. Jeffery PT. Morphology of the airway wall in asthma and COPD. Am Rev Respir Dis 1991; 143:1152–1158.
11. Robinson DS, Hamid Q, Ying S, et al. Predominant TH2 like bronchoalveolar T lymphocyte population in atopic asthma. N Engl J Med 1992; 326:298–304.
12. Corrigan CJ, Haczku A, Gemou-Engesaeth V, et al. CD4 T-lymphocyte activation

in asthma is accompanied by increased serum concentrations of interleukin-5. Effect of glucocorticoid therapy. Am Rev Respir Dis 1993; 147:540–547.
13. Ferrer A, Roca J, Wagner PD, et al. Airway obstruction and ventilation-perfusion relationships in acute severe asthma. Am Rev Respir Dis 1993; 147:579–584.
14. Coates AL, Desmond KJ, Demizio D, Allen PD. Sources of variation in FEV_1. Am J Respir Crit Care Med 1994; 149:439–443.
15. Juniper EF, Guyatt GH, Ferrie PJ, et al. Measuring quality of life in asthma. Am Rev Respir Dis 1993; 147:832–838.
16. Camilli AE, Burrows B, Knudson RJ, Lyle SK, Lebowitz MD. Longitudinal changes in FEV_1 in adults. Effects of smoking and smoking cessation. Am Rev Respir Dis 1987; 135:794–799.
17. Smoking-Attributable Mortality and Years of Potential Life Lost—United States, 1988. Atlanta, GA: Centers for Disease Control, HHS Publication No. (CDC) 91-8017, 1991.
18. Postma DS, de Vries K, Koeter GH, Sluiter HJ. Independent influence of reversibility of airflow obstruction and non-specific hyperreactivity on the long-term course of lung function in chronic airflow obstruction. Am Rev Respir Dis 1986; 134:276–280.
19. U.S. Department of Health and Human Services. The Health Benefits of Smoking Cessation. A Report of the Surgeon General. DHHS Publication No. CDC 90-8416, 1990.
20. Sonne L, Davis J. Increased exercise performance in patients with severe COPD following inspiratory resistive training. Chest 1982; 81:436–439.
21. Harver A, Mahler DA, Daubenspeck JA. Targeted inspiratory muscle training improves respiratory muscle function and reduces dyspnea in patients with chronic obstructive pulmonary disease. Ann Intern Med 1989; 111:117–124.
22. Panettieri RA, Murray RK. Chronic obstructive pulmonary disease. In: Fishman AP, ed. Pulmonary Diseases and Disorders, 2nd ed. Companion Handbook. New York: McGraw-Hill, 1994:170–181.
23. Anthonisen NR, Wright EC, and the IPPB Trial Group. Response to inhaled bronchodilators in COPD. Chest 1987; 91:36S–39S.
24. Guyatt GH, Townsend M, Pugsley SO, et al. Bronchodilators in chronic airflow limitation. Effects on airway function, exercise capacity, and quality of life. Am Rev Respir Dis 1987; 135:1069–1074.
25. Vollmer VM, Johnson LR, Buist AS. Relationship of response to a bronchodilator and decline in forced expiratory volume in one second in population studies. Am Rev Respir Dis 1985; 132:1186–1193.
26. Busse WW, Maisiak R, Young KR Jr. Treatment regimen and side effects of treatment measures. Am J Respir Crit Care Med 1994; 149(2, Pt 2):S44–50, discussion S51–53.
27. Mendella LA, Manfreda J, Warren CPW, Anthonisen NR. Steroid response in stable chronic obstructive pulmonary disease. Ann Intern Med 1982; 96:17–21.
28. American Thoracic Society. Standards for the diagnosis and care of patients with chronic obstructive pulmonary disease (COPD) and asthma. Am Rev Respir Dis 1987; 136:225–244.

29. Shim CS, Williams MH. Aerosol beclomethasone in patients with steroid dependent chronic obstructive pulmonary disease. Am J Med 1985; 78:655–658.
30. Easton PA, Jadue C, Dhingra S, Anthonisen NR. Comparison of the bronchodilating effects of a beta adrenergic agent (albuterol) and an anticholinergic agent (ipratropium bromide) given by aerosol alone or in sequence. N Engl J Med 1986; 315:735–739.
31. Gross NJ, Skorodin MS. Anticholinergic, antimuscarinic bronchodilators. Am Rev Respir Dis 1984; 129:856–870.
32. Kotlikoff MI. Ion channels in airway smooth muscle. In: Coburn RF, ed. Airway Smooth Muscle in Health and Disease. New York: Plenum Press, 1989:169–182.
33. Kume H, Hall IP, Washabau RJ, Takegi K, Kotlikoff MI. Beta adrenergic agonists regulate K_{Ca} channels in airway smooth muscle by cAMP dependent and independent mechanisms. J Clin Invest 1994; 93:371–379.
34. Raeburn D, Giembycz MA. Relaxation of airway smooth muscle. In Farmer SG, Hay DWP, eds. The Airway Epithelium. New York: Marcel Dekker, 1991:401–436.
35. Sears MR, Taylor DR, Print CG, et al. Regular inhaled beta agonist treatment in bronchial asthma. Lancet 1990; 336:1391–1396.
36. O'Connor BJ, Aikman SL, Barnes PJ. Tolerance to the nonbronchodilator effects of inhaled β_2-agonists in asthma. N Engl J Med 1992; 327:1204–1208.
37. D'Alonzo GE, Nathan RA, Henochowicz S, Morris RJ, Ratner P, Rennard SI. Salmeterol xinafoate as maintenance therapy compared with albuterol in patients with asthma. JAMA 1994; 271:1412–1416.
38. Chapman KR, Kesten S, Szalai JP. Regular vs as needed inhaled salbutamol in asthma control. Lancet 1994; 343(8910):1379–1382.
39. Pearlman DS, Chervinsky P, LaForce C, et al. A comparison of salmeterol with albuterol in the treatment of mild-to-moderate asthma. N Engl J Med 1992; 327:1420–1425.
40. Banner AS. Theophylline: should we discard an old friend? Lancet 1994; 343(8898):618.
41. Epstein PE. Hemlock or healer? The mercurial reputation of theophylline. Ann Intern Med 1993; 119:1216–1217.
42. Rice KL, Leatherman JW, Duane PG, et al. Aminophylline for acute exacerbations of chronic obstructive pulmonary disease. A controlled trial. Ann Intern Med 1987; 107:305–309.
43. Aubier M, DeTroyer A, Sampson M, Macklem PT, Roussos C. Aminophylline improved diaphragmatic contraction. N Engl J Med 1981; 305:249–252.
44. Belman MJ, Sieck G, Mazar A. Aminophylline and its influence on ventilating endurance in humans. Am Rev Respir Dis 1985; 131:226–229.
45. Gross NJ, Bankwala Z. Effects of an anticholinergic bronchodilator on arterial blood gases of hypoxemic patients with chronic obstructive pulmonary disease. Am Rev Respir Dis 1987; 136:1091–1094.
46. Hui KP, Barnes NC. Lung function improvement in asthma with a cysteinyl-leukotriene receptor antagonist. Lancet 1991; 33:1062–1063.
47. Taylor IK, O'Shaughnessy KM, Fuller RW, et al. Effect of cysteinyl-leukotriene

receptor antagonist ICI 204.219 on allergen-induced bronchoconstriction and airway hyperreactivity in atopic subjects. Lancet 1991; 337:690–694.
48. Makker HK, Lau LC, Thomson HW, et al. The protective effect of inhaled leukotriene D_4 receptor antagonist ICI 204,219 against exercise-induced asthma. Am Rev Respir Dis 1993; 147:1413–1418.
49. Impens N, Reiss TF, Teahan JA, et al. Acute bronchodilation with an intravenously administered leukotriene D_4 antagonist, MK 679. Am Rev Respir Dis 1993; 147:1442–1446.
50. Israel E, Rubin P, Kemp JP, et al. The effect of inhibition of 5-lipoxygenase by zileuton in mild-to-moderate asthma. Ann Intern Med 1993; 119:1059–1066.
51. Engel T, Heinig JH. Glucocorticosteroid therapy in acute severe asthma—a critical review. Eur Respir J 1991; 4:881–889.
52. McFadden ER Jr. Dosages of corticosteroids in asthma. Am Rev Respir Dis 1993; 147:1306–1310.
53. Petty TL. The national mucolytic study: results of a randomized, double-blind, placebo controlled study of iodinated glycerol in chronic obstructive bronchitis. Chest 1990; 97:75–83.
54. Wanner A. The current status of mucolytic drugs. Contemp Intern Med 1991; 3:29–37.
55. Anthonisen NR, Manfreda J, Warren CPW, Hershfield ES, Harding GKM, Nelson NA. Antibiotic therapy in exacerbations of chronic obstructive pulmonary disease. Ann Intern Med 1987; 106:196–204.
56. Williams JH, Moser KM. Pneumococcal vaccine and patients with chronic lung disease. Ann Intern Med 1986; 104:106–109.
57. Simberkoff MS, Cross AP, Al-Ibrahim M, et al. Efficacy of pneumococcal vaccine in high-risk patients. Results of a Veterans Administration cooperative study. N Engl J Med 1986; 315:1318–1327.
58. Davis AL, Aranda CP, Schiffman G, Christianson LC. Pneumococcal infection and immunologic response to pneumococcal vaccine in chronic obstructive pulmonary disease. A pilot study. Chest 1987; 92:204–212.
59. Medical Research Council Working Party. Long-term domiciliary oxygen therapy in chronic hypoxic cor pulmonale complicating chronic bronchitis and emphysema. Lancet 1981; 1:681–686.
60. Nocturnal Oxygen Therapy Trial Group. Continuous or nocturnal oxygen therapy in hypoxemic chronic obstructive lung disease: a clinical trial. Ann Intern Med 1980; 93:391–398.
61. Anthonisen NR. Long-term oxygen therapy. Ann Intern Med 1983; 99:519–527.
62. Guidelines for the approaches to the patient with severe hereditary α_1-antitrypsin deficiency. Am Rev Respir Dis 1989; 140:1494–1497.

19

Psychosocial Factors in the Rehabilitation of Patients with Chronic Respiratory Disease

A. JOHN McSWEENY

Medical College of Ohio
Toledo, Ohio

SUSAN M. CZAJKOWSKI

Behavioral Medicine Branch
National Heart, Lung, and Blood Institute
National Institutes of Health
Bethesda, Maryland

KAREN T. LABUHN

Wayne State University
Detroit, Michigan

The integration of behavioral science in medical practice and research is now widely appreciated. Recent reviews on topics related to health psychology and behavioral medicine have noted the role of psychosocial factors in the etiology, development, maintenance, treatment, and management of medical disorders (1).

A major conceptual impetus to the scientific application of psychosocial concepts in health care was provided by George Engel's papers on the biopsychosocial model of medicine (2,3). Using a systems theory framework, Engel argued that the inclusion of psychosocial information in the formulation of medical concepts, research, and patient care serves to make medicine a more scientific enterprise compared to more narrow biomedical models or to nonscientific "holistic" models.

However, much of the development of the fields of behavioral medicine and health psychology has resulted from practical needs. Thus, discussions of behavioral factors in the development and treatment of coronary artery disease are now commonplace in family practice journals, and the use of psychological approaches to the assessment and treatment of chronic pain has become standard practice in many major medical centers. Although the use of behavioral outcomes in medical research and treatment is a relatively recent phenomenon, the use of measures of quality of life (QL) or, more narrowly, health-related quality of life (HRQL) to measure the efficacy of medical treatment has enjoyed a rapid growth in the last 20 years (1,4,5).

I. Psychosocial Factors in Rehabilitation

The appreciation of psychosocial factors in evaluation and treatment of patients has perhaps been greater in rehabilitation than in any other field. Psychological services are routinely included in most rehabilitation programs and are required for accreditation by the Committee on Accreditation of Rehabilitation Facilities (CARF) (6). In addition, the National Heart, Lung, and Blood Institute is widely recognized for its support of behavioral research in relation to lung disease (7).

The goals of this chapter are to review some of the psychosocial difficulties associated with pulmonary disease, to discuss some of the factors that moderate psychosocial status, and to describe psychosocial interventions.

A. Psychosocial Difficulties Associated with Chronic Respiratory Disease

Neurocognitive Effects

Although cognitive difficulties associated with hypoxemia secondary to chronic obstructive pulmonary disease (COPD) were described as early as 1954 by Westlake and Kaye (8), systematic neuropsychological investigations of hypoxemic COPD have appeared relatively recently. However, in the past 25 years, several studies have clearly established that patients with moderate to severe COPD suffer deficits in brain function as reflected in standardized neuropsychological measures (9). These studies have employed batteries of psychological tests known to be sensitive to brain function; the one most commonly used is the Halstead-Reitan Neuropsychological Test Battery (HRB) (10). Neuropsychological evaluations provide a "comprehensive sampling of general, as well as specific, indicators of cerebral functioning" (9). Neuropsychological batteries have the advantage of being noninvasive and measure the results of brain activity that are likely to have relevance to everyday life functioning (9).

The first systematic neuropsychological study by Krop et al. (11) involved 10 patients evaluated before and after oxygen therapy. These patients were compared to a second sample of 12 patients who were similar in terms of airway obstruction and demographic characteristics, but less hypoxemic than the first sample. The authors found significant differences between the samples on tests of simple motor speed (finger tapping) and perceptual-motor skills, but not on tests of general intellectual functioning or memory. Assuming that the essential difference between the samples was the level of hypoxemia, the results indicated that hypoxemia does have an impact on certain aspects of neuropsychological function.

The Krop et al. study involved a relatively small sample and a limited neuropsychological battery. These issues were addressed by Grant et al. (12) and Prigatano et al. (13). These two studies used essentially identical neuropsychological test batteries—an expanded version of the HRB that permitted the assessment of a wide variety of neuropsychological functions. Because the two studies used identical neuropsychological testing procedures, the data from them could be combined, resulting in a total sample size of 302 patients with mild to severe hypoxemic COPD and 99 health control subjects (14). Univariate statistical tests showed generalized neuropsychological deficits in the patients.

To enhance the meaningfulness of the findings, subjects were divided on the basis of blood gas studies into normal (control subjects; $n=99$), mildly hypoxemic ($Pao_2 \geq 60$ mmHg; $n=86$), moderately hypoxemic ($Pao_2=50$–59 mmHg; $n=155$), and severely hypoxemic ($Pao_2<50$ mmHg; $n=61$) groups. The results are shown in Figure 1. Despite some similarities, it is clear that differences exist both in the level and in the patterns of results between the

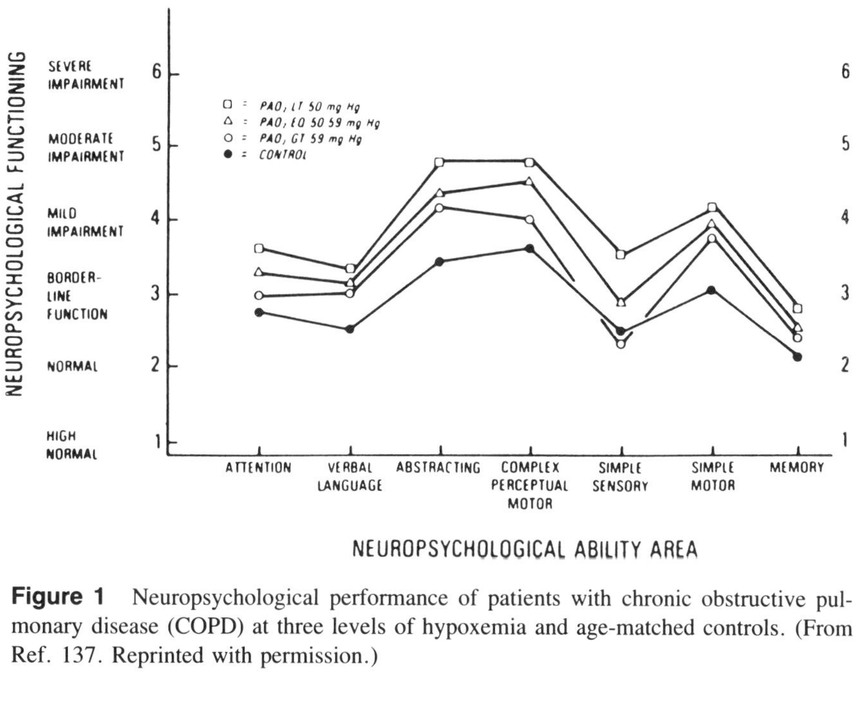

Figure 1 Neuropsychological performance of patients with chronic obstructive pulmonary disease (COPD) at three levels of hypoxemia and age-matched controls. (From Ref. 137. Reprinted with permission.)

normal control group and the three patient groups. Indeed, these data indicate that neuropsychological functioning is sensitive in general to the effects of hypoxemia and that the overall severity of the effects is related to the severity hypoxemia.

In addition, close inspection of Figure 1 also reveals that all neuropsychological functions are not equally sensitive to the effects of hypoxemia. In the typical case, mild hypoxemia has no significant effect on simple sensory skills; indeed, even severe hypoxemia produces only mild deficits. In contrast, mild hypoxemia results in marked deficits in abstraction/flexibility; additional hypoxemia results in even more disability. Other ability areas demonstrate intermediate patterns of response to hypoxemia.

The above-cited findings of Grant et al., supported by other reports (9,15), have implications for QL. If we assume that different aspects of QL depend on different skills, it follows that certain areas of life functioning will be more or less affected by different degrees of hypoxemia.

In summary, the evidence reviewed above indicates that COPD is a disease of the brain as well as the lungs.

Emotional Effects

Most studies of emotional problems in respiratory disease have been with patients having COPD.

Depression

By far, the most commonly reported emotional consequence associated with COPD is depression. Depressive symptoms, including pessimism, self-dislike, and feelings of sadness, have been reported in virtually every study of the psychological aspects of COPD as well as in reviews of the literature (16–22). Although the first results came from studies in North America, highly similar results have emerged from more recent studies in other countries (23–26).

Agle and Baum (27) reported "significant" depression in 74% of their patients, whereas Light et al. (22) and McSweeny et al. (28) both reported that 42% of their patients were primarily depressed. McSweeny et al. noted that an additional 7% had symptoms of depression combined with other psychiatric symptoms. Toshima et al. (29) and Yellowlees (30) reported a lower rate of depression in COPD: 16%. The differences between the results may reflect differences in patient samples and measurement methods. Nonetheless, the basic finding that COPD patients are at high risk for depression is consistent.

Part of the consistency may be due to the fact that several of the studies used a common instrument to assess emotional functioning, i.e., the Minnesota Multiphasic Personality Inventory (MMPI) (31). The MMPI includes a scale for measuring depression. Because physical complaints are often associated with depression, the MMPI depression scale contains several items that concern somatic manifestations, some of which occur in conjunction with COPD. Thus, the MMPI cannot be regarded as a "pure" measure of the depressed state. However, evidence from other studies, using other instruments, is quite consistent with the studies that do use the MMPI (23,25,26,28,29,32–40).

Of course, depression is common in many chronic diseases other than respiratory disorders. Friedman and Booth-Kewley (41) performed a meta-analysis of 101 studies concerned with the psychological aspects of various chronic diseases and found that depression was the most commonly reported psychological symptom. On the other hand, after reviewing the literature, Kaplan and his colleagues (17) concluded that COPD patients are more likely to experience depression than are patients with most other chronic diseases.

Different explanations exist for the causes of depression in COPD and the problem is undoubtedly multidetermined. Most analyses have focused on the psychosocial consequences of COPD, such as the loss of pleasurable activities, economic hardship, and difficulties in coping (16,18,26,42,43). Others have suggested that physiological factors, including the hypoxygenation of the limbic system and related brain mechanisms, might also be relevant factors (28,44). Labuhn (45) tested the relative importance of a variety of psychosocial, medical, and physiological factors in the development of depression in COPD patients using multivariate casual-modeling methods known as path analysis. The results of this study suggest that although physiological factors did play an important role in the development of depression, the depression that COPD patients experience is largely a reaction to their situation.

In a related study, Toshima et al. (39) found that the level of depression in COPD patients was significantly correlated with measures of functional status, including activities of daily living, exercise endurance, perceptions of self-efficacy, and social support. In contrast, correlations between depression and physiological measures, such as blood gases, were not generally significant. The investigators also interpreted their data as supporting the functional or situational explanation of depression in COPD.

Anxiety

Anxiety also appears to be common in COPD. Like depression, it is observed in almost all studies of the emotional sequelae of COPD irrespective of whether the MMPI is used or not (46). It is not difficult to imagine that anxiety and concern about one's bodily condition would be a frequent occurrence in COPD. As was the case with depression, the rates of anxiety disorders vary considerably from study to study. Agle and Baum (27), for example, reported disabling anxiety in 96% of their patients, while Yellowlees (30) reported that 34% of his patients suffered from excessive anxiety. At the lower end of the spectrum,

Karajgi et al. (47) reported that 16% of their COPD patients had an anxiety disorder whereas Light et al. (22) reported a rate of only 2%.

The concept of anxiety is related to somatic preoccupation, which is also commonly reported in COPD. McSweeny and his colleagues (28) reported somatic preoccupation in 8.7% of their patients in contrast to 0% in the demographically matched control group.

Other Emotional Disorders

Other emotional disorders, including hysterical disorders, suspiciousness, and aggressive behavior, have been reported in conjunction with respiratory disease, but the findings have been less reliable than for depression and anxiety. For example, some early studies suggested that hysterical disorders were common in respiratory disease, but later studies have not consistently confirmed these results (48). McSweeny et al. (28) found that 2.7% of their COPD patients exhibited primarily hysterical symptoms compared with 1.5% of the older healthy individuals. In addition, the MMPI hysteria scale, which is often used as the criterion of hysterical complaints in studies, contains a high number of somatic symptoms that could well be the product of genuine illness rather than personality characteristics. Thus, the presence of hysterical personality characteristics is likely to be overreported in studies that employ this instrument.

Although some patients with respiratory disorders are noted by clinicians to be angry, this does not appear to be a pervasive or unique problem. McSweeny et al. (28) failed to find unusual degrees of suspiciousness or anger, although relatives of the patients did report a moderately high degree of oppositional behavior.

Dyspnea and Emotional Distress

Several authors have commented on the relationship between dyspnea and emotional distress. Indeed, one study suggests that only 10% of the variance in chronic dyspnea can be accounted for by reduction in pulmonary function; much of the remaining variance is assumed to be psychological (49). The relationship of dyspnea to anxiety and panic is particularly well described. Anxiety and panic can lead to dyspnea, which can led to additional panic and fear. This downward cycle has been described as the "panic-dyspnea cycle" or, more colorfully, as the "vicious circle of dyspnea" (17,50). Make (50) notes that patients may avoid physical activity to exit the cycle, as indicated in Figure 2. This can lead to further deconditioning in these patients, which can, in turn, make them more susceptible to breathlessness, a situation that Haas and his colleagues (51) have described as the "dyspnea spiral."

Burns and Howell (48) examined what they described as "disproportion-

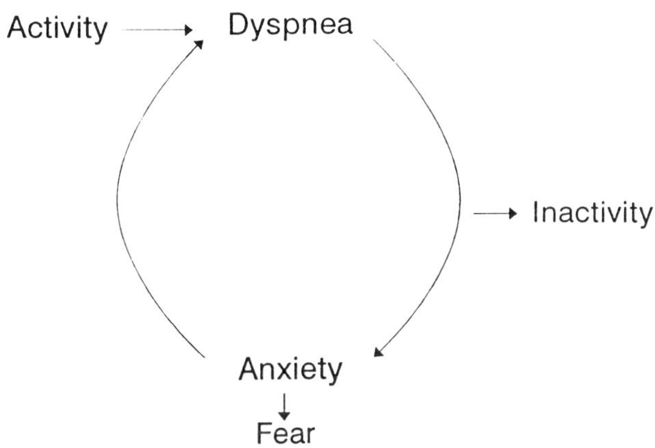

Figure 2 The vicious circle of dyspnea. Physical activity results in shortness of breath leading to anxiety, fear, and eventually additional dyspnea. (Adapted with permission from Ref. 50.)

ately breathless" (DB) patients and found that symptoms of breathlessness were more closely related to emotional status than degree of exertion. Consistent with other authors, Burns and Howell noted the usual relation of anxiety to dyspnea, but also found depressive affect to be an important explanatory variable. Furthermore, the DB patients had higher rates of emotional disorders, including depression and anxiety, than other patients. In addition, dyspnea improved with the resolution of emotional disturbance.

Dyspnea may also cause patients to restrict affective response, either deliberately or unconsciously, a condition Dudley et al. (52) described as the "emotional straitjacket." On the basis of his classic studies of the psychophysiology of breathing, Dudley suggested that the COPD patient learn to avoid the expression of strong emotions, including anger, to prevent the excessive oxygen uptake that occurs in conjunction with physiological arousal (52,53). Thus, breathless patients may not only suffer from emotional distress, they may not be able to express emotions in a normal fashion.

Since psychological factors play a major role in the development of dyspnea, psychological factors are also likely to play a major role in treating it successfully. Haas and his colleagues (51) suggest that exercise is the best treatment because it addresses psychological as well as physiological aspects: "It can provide an antidote to depression, provide a sense of mastery, involve social interaction and distraction, and achieve an improvement in aerobic conditioning." The treatment of dyspnea is discussed in more detail in a later section.

B. Social Role Functioning and Activities of Daily Living

General Activities

The performance of basic social roles and activities of daily living (ADL) is often used as a standard for the impact of disease entity on HRQL. A relatively early study by Barstow (54) reported "major changes" in the "style of living" manifested by the COPD patients. These included alterations in bathing, grooming, dressing, eating, sleeping, and mobility. She noticed, for example, that "the mode of dress was altered in favor of less restrictive clothing that was easily slipped on and off." Food intake was decreased by many of the patients because an overdistended stomach would interfere with diaphragmatic breathing. Sleep/rest difficulties received particular attention in Barstow's report. Disruptions of sleep because of cough, dyspnea, or restlessness were common. In addition, Barstow reported some sleep changes that were apparently related to endogenous depression.

Starting in the late 1970s, the availability of the Sickness Impact Profile (SIP), a measure of general HRQL, led to a series of studies on the effects of chronic illness with that instrument (55). An evaluation of COPD patients by McSweeny et al. (28) revealed a broad range of disturbances in sleep and rest and activities of daily living. COPD patients reported a much higher percentage of impairment than did control subjects in all categories of functioning except one, i.e., employment, presumably because the COPD and control groups both contained many elderly retired persons. The areas of functioning most severely affected were home management and sleep/rest. Eating and communication, on the other hand, seemed to be only moderately affected by the disease (Fig. 3). Additional results from the assessment to the viewpoint of relatives indicated that they regarded the patient's social role functioning as deficient; they expected less of the patients but still felt dissatisfied with the patients' performance of socially expected activities.

Prigatano and colleagues (38) also employed the SIP with COPD patients who were mildly hypoxemic. Their findings were quite similar to those obtained by McSweeny et al. with severely hypoxemic patients, although, as might be expected, the degree of impairment was proportionately less. One interesting exception was that Prigatano et al. did find significant differences in employment status between COPD patients and control, i.e., more employment in the control group, presumably because of the greater proportion of persons younger than 65 in the Prigatano et al. study.

A third study with the SIP was conducted by Bergner et al. (56) with three groups of COPD outpatients receiving home or office care. These patients, accordingly, would be less ill than those in the studies by McSweeny et al. and by Prigatano et al. Although they were less impaired than the patients in the other two studies, the overall level of impairment was still much higher

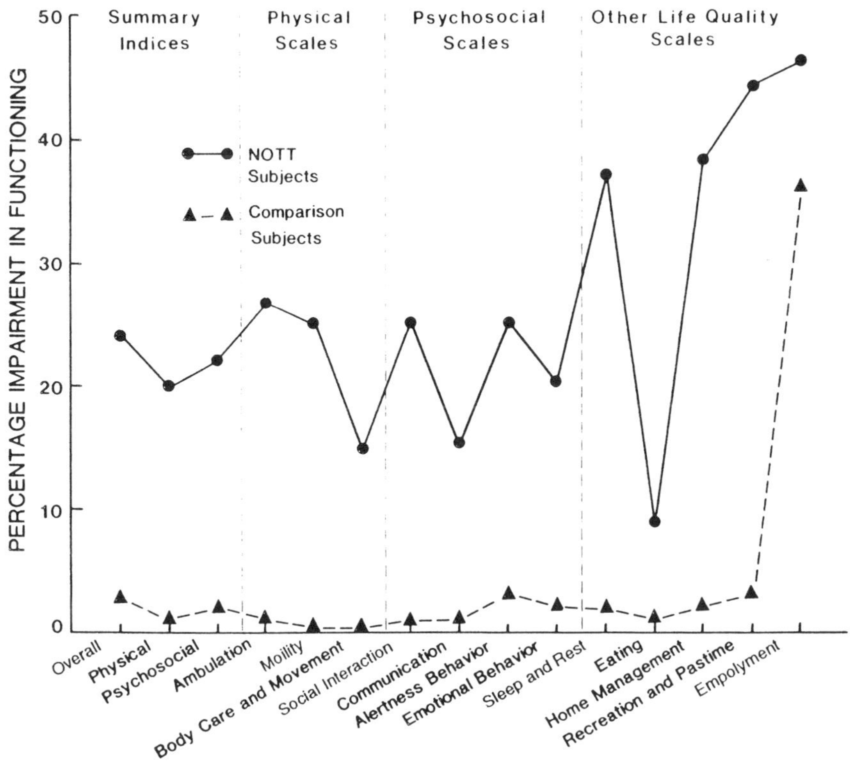

Figure 3 Mean Sickness Impact Profiles for patients with chronic obstructive pulmonary disease (COPD) and control subjects. Patients with COPD are significantly ($p < 0.001$) more impaired on all scales except employment using paired *t*-tests ($n = 66$). NOTT = Nocturnal Oxygen Therapy Trial. (From Ref. 28. Copyright, American Medical Association. Reprinted with permission.)

than expected relative to healthy individuals of a similar age and social standing.

Employing an Anglicized version of the SIP, Williams and Bury (25,26) studied 92 outpatients with COPD who, on average, were similar with respect to the severity of airways impairment and socioeconomic status to the patients in the study by Prigatano et al. Despite the differences in wording and in the location of study (the U.K. versus the U.S.), the results were virtually identical to those of Prigatano et al. and differed from those of McSweeny et al. only in terms of degree of impairment.

A second team from the United Kingdom, Jones et al. (23), employed the standard SIP to study 160 outpatients who, overall, were slightly less impaired in terms of lung function than the patients of Williams and Bury and

Prigatano et al. Interestingly, employment was not greatly impaired in the Jones et al. study, presumably, as noted above, because the patients were older than those in the Prigatano study (38). Jones et al. also found a correlation between QL as measured by the SIP and walking distance that was significantly higher than the correlation between spirometric (lung function) indices and walking distance.

Recent studies of COPD using the SIP have also been conducted in Holland and Sweden (57,58). The Dutch study is particularly interesting; it included patients at a relatively early stage of the disease. As might be expected, the SIP profile for these patients was much more similar to those for normal elderly individuals than to the profiles from most of the other studies with the SIP. Still, significant differences between the patients and normal elderly were found for the three summary indices (Overall, Physical, and Psychosocial) as well as for the specific indices of Communication, Emotional Behavior, Sleep/Rest, Eating, Home Management, and Employment. In keeping with the results of other studies, the authors found little relationship between SIP scores and lung function parameters.

Other studies of COPD and QL using measures other than the SIP have produced comparable results (24,29,32–36,59–70). A survey of 130 COPD patients by Hanson deserves some particular attention (71). Her questionnaire included 40 items assessing 11 areas, among which were several aspects of social role functioning and ADL, such as employment, self-care, home/personal business, marriage, care of grandchildren, and dependency on others. Hanson's results were consistent with those from the SIP-based studies in that she found a general negative effect of COPD across the different categories in her survey. However, her study was unique because her questionnaire allowed respondents to indicate a positive impact of COPD on different aspects of life as well as a negative impact. In fact, a few individuals did report positive effects, ranging from 28% for care of grandchildren to 40% for marriage. Perhaps there is some benefit in adversity or perhaps the respondents misunderstood the questions.

The patients in the studies described above were predominantly male. This is related to the fact that until recently, smoking, the major risk factor for COPD, was primarily a male activity. Sexton and Monro (72) studied 72 women with COPD and 40 demographically similar women who had no chronic illness. The two groups were compared with respect to their perceived health status, problems of daily living, amount of subjective stress, and life satisfaction. In comparison with their healthy controls, the female COPD patients were found to have lower perceived health status, more subjective stress, and less life satisfaction. They also reported more problems in daily living. Major problems included shortness of breath and fatigue, loneliness and depression, and restricted household and social activities. Thus, the results were quite consistent with those from the other studies of QL in COPD.

Sexual Functioning in Respiratory Disease

The impact of respiratory disease on sexuality depends on a complex web of factors including the specific disease and the medications used to treat it. Patients with diseases such as asthma and cystic fibrosis tend to be younger and typically are able to function sexually in a relatively normal pattern between episodic flareups in their conditions (73). Of course, life-threatening conditions, such as cystic fibrosis, often have a significant psychological impact on one's self-image as a sexual person and thus can have secondary effects on sexuality. Women with cystic fibrosis, for example, are discouraged from becoming pregnant because of the increased load that pregnancy places on the respiratory and other life support systems. Thus, they may feel that they are "less than complete" as women. Even less severe conditions, such as asthma, may have significant psychological effects on sexual self-image (73). Fortunately, most of the psychological problems associated with less severe forms of respiratory disease may be addressed by education and counseling (73,74).

A significant minority of persons with COPD suffer from sexual dysfunction. In an early study, Kass et al. (75) reported that 19% of their male COPD patients were impotent. Fletcher and Martin (76) reported that 30% of their male patients with COPD were impotent and that an additional 5% had ceased intercourse because of dyspnea. Frequency of intercourse for the remaining 65% of their patients fell to 16% of predisease levels.

Sexton and Monro (77) studied the impact of COPD on the spouse's life. They compared the subjective experiences of 45 wives of male COPD patients with those of 30 age-matched women whose husbands had no chronic illness. The patient's wives reported significantly fewer marital relations than did the comparison wives. Fifty-four percent of the COPD wives no longer engaged in sexual relations. Forty-eight percent of these wives, versus 15% of the controls, stated that they had no desire for sexual relations. The wives of the COPD patients also gave significantly lower ratings on their own health status, and this may account for their lack of sexual interest. However, health differences between these two groups of age-matched wives could also be due to stressors related to living with a COPD patient. The wives of COPD patients reported many difficulties with sleeping due to their husbands' breathing problems. They also had taken on many extra responsibilities and had given up many of their own social activities because of their husbands' illnesses.

Only limited data exist concerning sexual functioning in female COPD patients. Although it is probably safe to assume that several of the factors that affect sexual functioning in men affect sexual functioning in women as well, Pietropinto and Arora (78) concluded that women with COPD generally report fewer problems with sexual functioning. Several factors may account for this difference. Men typically take a more active role in sexual interactions, and male dysfunctions, such as erectile failure, may inhibit sexual interactions more and may be more difficult to treat than female dysfunctions (73).

The self-report study by Hanson (71) noted above dealt with sexual functioning in a mixed-sex (62% men, 38% women) sample. She found that among the 11 life areas assessed in her study, sexual functioning was the area most consistently rated as being negatively affected by COPD. Thus, Hanson's results are consistent with the findings from the studies of men and also suggest that COPD presents problems for sexual functioning for women as well as for men. Since Hanson did not report results separately for men and women, some doubt persists about this interpretation. Clearly, the sexuality of female COPD patients is a neglected area that is in need of further research.

One controversy in the area of sexuality and COPD concerns whether the problems are largely secondary to antecedent marital and sexual difficulties or to the more immediate physical effects of the disease. Based on a sample of 90 men and 10 women, Kass et al., concluded that the sexual problems associated with COPD patients were not primarily due to the effects of the disease. Rather, such problems were attributed to lifelong patterns of behavior. Another common problem was a wife who was angered by the level of support required by her husband (75).

Fletcher and Martin found results that contrast with those of Kass et al. They concluded:

> Data from this study suggest that sexual dysfunction and erectile impotence can accompany COPD in the absence of other known causes of sexual problems. Furthermore, sexual dysfunction tended to be worse in those subjects with more severe pulmonary function impairment as assessed by pulmonary function tests, blood gases, and exercise tests. (76, p. 420)

Fletcher and Martin (76) did note that although several of their subjects who were judged to be impotent by the criterion of nocturnal penile tumescence had high scores on some MMPI scales, only one of the 20 subjects clearly had psychogenic impotence. In the others, COPD was responsible for both the sexual dysfunction and the emotional disturbance; these two were either independently related to the COPD or at least some of the psychological distress was secondary to sexual failure brought on by the COPD.

COPD has some specific physical sequelae that are likely to contribute to sexual dysfunction. Semple et al. (79) have reported that chronic hypoxemia is associated with depression in testosterone levels, which could lower sexual drive and response. Patients with COPD fatigue more easily with exercise and may experience dyspnea in reaction to the physical demands of intercourse as well as the emotional response. Sexual activity may also result in bronchospasm in some COPD patients (80). In addition, some COPD patients may have unpleasant breath odor and dark, foul-smelling sputum, which may interfere with the social aspects of sexual interaction (81). Depression, which is common in COPD, is associated with decreased sexual interest and behavior (82). Finally, chronic disease is likely to affect one's self-image as a vital, sexually attractive person.

Advanced age has sometimes been implicated in some discussions of sexual difficulties associated with COPD. However, as Selecky (74) points out, recent surveys indicate that the majority of healthy persons remain sexually active into the ninth decade of life (83). Thus, age per se cannot be considered the major factor associated with impaired sexuality in the COPD patient.

Recently, several writers have described intervention programs for respiratory disease–related sexual dysfunction (74,80,81,84,85). Most programs provide information about sexuality in general, the specific sexual difficulties associated with pulmonary disease, and possible effects of medications. In addition, most programs attempt to correct myths and misconceptions and deal with the specific concerns of the participants. Many programs attempt to give patients and their partners the belief that they have "permission" to engage in sexual behavior. Specific suggestions for reducing the energy demands of intercourse are also usually included. In advanced cases of COPD, administration of bronchodilators prior to intercourse or using low-flow oxygen during intercourse may be useful (80,86). One educational program incorporates slide-tape programs to facilitate the learning process (87–89). Spica (85) noted that her program was "well received" by five COPD patients, but formal evaluations of the pulmonary disease sexual intervention programs appear to be lacking. On the other hand, most of the programs appear to be based on principles that are well established and have proven to be effective with other forms of sexual dysfunction.

In conclusion, respiratory disease, in the form of COPD, has a documented effect on sexuality in men and probably in women as well. Additional research is needed, including studies with women and with diseases other than COPD. In addition, more data on the mechanisms of sexual dysfunction in respiratory disease and formal outcome studies would be helpful in guiding the development of medical and educational intervention programs.

Hobbies and Recreational Activities

The effect of respiratory disease on other activities that bring enjoyment and meaning to one's life has been evaluated by several researchers, especially with respect to COPD. McSweeny et al. (28) noted that their patients reported severe restrictions in recreation and other leisure-time activities. The SIP results suggested a reduction of 40–50% in pleasurable activities, which is certainly an important aspect of QL. Indeed, the category of Recreation and Pastimes showed the greatest level of impairment relative to the other categories on the SIP (Fig. 3). Other data indicate that the relatives also recognize decrements in the free-time activities of the patients.

When respiratory disease is less severe, less severe reductions in the level of recreational activities (23,25,26,38,56–58) are observed. In general, a reduction of 15–40% in pleasurable activities was seen in the mildly hypoxic patients on the SIP. The Recreation and Pastimes section was the most impaired category on this test in three studies, and the second most impaired category in the fourth (23,25,26,38,58). As in the McSweeny et al. study, Prigatano and colleagues (38) found that the relatives were aware of the problem.

That there can be a significant loss of pleasurable activities in respiratory disease is relevant to theories of depression that suggest that the loss of reinforcers is a major contributory factor in the development of depression (90). Therefore, it is possible that helping patients to maintain old hobbies by adopting energy-saving strategies and to develop new, less energy-dependent ones might ameliorate the negative impact of severe respiratory disease on emotional status. In addition, this might partially explain the beneficial effects of exercise on emotional status noted previously.

II. Factors that Moderate Psychosocial Status in Respiratory Disease

A. Disease-Related and Physiological Factors

Both the specific disease process and disease severity are moderating factors in the impact of respiratory disease on psychosocial status and related aspects of QL. Others factors being equal, less severe respiratory disease generally results in less severe impairment in QL. This is apparent from reviews of the literature concerning respiratory disease as well as from studies that have examined the relationship of disease severity to QL. For example, a recent study found that adolescents with allergenic rhinoconjunctivitis experience limitations in activity, emotional difficulties, and other practical problems in everyday life (91). However, the impact of chronic rhinitis on HRQL is certainly less severe than the effects of COPD (92). In addition, late-stage COPD has a greater impact on HRQL and emotional status than does earlier-stage COPD (45,46).

The physiological factors related to the disease process account for some of the limitation in QL. Respiratory functioning itself has a significant impact on patients' functioning. When bronchodilators are used for symptomatic relief of breathing problems, temporary improvements in patients' functional capacity and emotional states are often seen (93). Treatment with oxygen may also result in improved functioning for some, though not all, patients with COPD (94–96).

Several investigators have examined the relation of exercise capability, pulmonary function variables, and other measures of the efficiency of the cardiopulmonary system in relation to QL (23,25,26,28,37,38,40,57). The relationship between traditional spirometric variables or blood gases and QL has been found to be statistically significant in most of the studies, but quite weak and probably of limited clinical significance. On the other hand, the relationship between exercise capability and QL is relatively robust (46). This suggests that the ability to engage in physical activity is an important determinant in one's QL. Data from an evaluation of a rehabilitation program also support the relationship between exercise capability and depression (39). Those patients who improved in emotional status also improved in terms of treadmill performance.

B. Demographic Characteristics

Age

The general decline in health status with advancing age is well known. The incidence of respiratory disease also varies at different times of life with certain diseases, such as asthma and chronic rhinitis, appearing relatively early and COPD appearing relatively late in life. Thus, it is difficult to assess independently the effects of age when considering respiratory disease in general. In addition, with respect to the effects of age on HRQL in the respiratory diseases of later life, the results are somewhat variable. Age was found to contribute significantly in a negative fashion to QL in studies of COPD patients by McSweeny et al. (28) and Williams and Bury (25,26), but not in studies by Prigatano et al. (38). Guyatt et al. (32) found that old patients reported fewer emotional problems than did young patients. While this finding is not consistent with the other studies of COPD, it does agree with the results of a study involving patients with several other chronic diseases (97). The reasons for the discrepant findings concerning the relationship of age to QL remain unclear.

Socioeconomic Factors

Several investigators have reported significant effects for socioeconomic status and education on QL in patients with respiratory diseases (25,26,28,38). In general, better-educated and more affluent patients fared better than those with lesser education and more limited resources.

For example, in a study of 163 COPD patients and their spouses, Young (98) found that patients' monetary savings and health insurance, as well as their personal resources (positive illness perceptions, knowledge of the illness, regimen compliance, and religion), predicted better adaptation. The 104 female COPD patients in Sexton and Monro's (72) study identified financial concerns as one of their major problems. Similarly, the COPD wives in Sexton and Monro's (77) earlier study had greater life satisfaction if they were satisfied with the amount of money that was available.

C. Psychological and Behavioral Factors

Psychological Assets and Social Support Resources

A number of investigators have studied patients' psychosocial assets and social support resources in relation to QL. Sandhu defined psychosocial assets as "those individual characteristics and social supports that allow coping with or modifying one's environment" (21). After reviewing the chronic illness literature, he concluded that psychosocial assets seem to "play a major, perhaps central, role in the patient's ability to cope adaptively." Sandhu noted that high assets correlate with positive outcome in medical treatment, whereas low assets typically are associated with a variety of poor outcomes, including increased morbidity and mortality.

Investigations among asthma and COPD patients indicate that those with stronger psychosocial assets require less medication, adapt to life changes more readily, respond more positively to group therapy, are less likely to be depressed, and have less dyspnea, better regimen compliance, and longer survival time (18,39,99,100).

The concept of psychosocial assets includes the psychological characteristics of the patient, such as emotional stability and coping style, as well as the amount of support the person receives from external sources. Thus, while COPD patients' psychosocial assets do predict outcomes that are relevant to QL, the impact of both the patients' internal psychological resources and external social supports must be considered.

Several investigators have attempted to study social support in relation to other factors that influence QL. Jensen (101) studied the impact of social support and various risk factors in COPD patients' symptom management. He found that social support and life stress predicted the number of hospitalizations better than did the patient's demographic characteristics, the severity of the illness, or previous hospitalizations. Labuhn (45) found that married COPD patients had better exercise tolerance than did single, widowed, or divorced patients, even after controlling for age, disease severity, and neuropsychological functioning. Marriage did not have a significant influence on patients' depressed mood states, but it indirectly contributed to patients' physical and psychosocial functioning through its impact on their exercise capacity.

Other studies provide evidence concerning personal social supports and the QL of COPD patients. Home interviews with COPD patients to assess their problems and coping strategies identified the presence of a supportive spouse as the most important factor for successful coping (42). In a study of female COPD patients, 95% of the married patients identified their husbands as important sources of support (72). The husbands helped with various household activities, treatments, and other things needed. About half of the women talked their problems over with their husbands and also turned to friends, relatives, and children for emotional support.

Young (98) found that community resources were not directly related to self-adaptation of the patients with COPD, but that they did impact significantly on the adaptation of the patients' spouses. Only 20% of Young's patients with COPD received assistance from persons other than their spouses, children, and parents; this may account for the greater importance of community support for the spouses in this study. About two-thirds of the spouses in Sexton and Monro's (77) study of male COPD patients said that they relied on their sons and daughters for help. Forty-six percent of these wives identified the physician as an important source of support. Thirty-seven percent also relied on friends and 34% relied on neighbors.

In a study of 126 COPD patients in which causal modeling techniques were used to examine the relative contributions of selected demographic, physical, and psychosocial factors to self-reported QOL, Anderson (102) concluded that the age, disease severity, and functional status of the patients were significant determinants of their self-reported QL. Three psychosocial variables—depression, self-esteem, and perceived social support—directly influenced the QL and also mediated (or buffered) the impact of the disease-related variables on the patients' QL.

Findings from the above studies have suggested that many patients with respiratory disease rely heavily on their immediate families for support, while family members may rely on each other as well as professional and community resources. It is important to consider the implications of these findings for patients who live alone as well as the QL of patients' families. Additional investigations are needed to examine the COPD family's social support needs in more detail, and to evaluate the effectiveness of interventions directed toward mobilizing supports.

Data from other studies of social support and chronic disease lend additional support to the importance of social support in understanding the variability in the effects of respiratory disease on QL (17).

Coping Strategies

The specific coping strategies that respiratory disease patients use to deal with the illness also affect their QL. Both cognitive and behavioral coping strategies are important. Fagerhaugh (103) discusses "routing" as a basic behavioral strategy that COPD patients can use to conserve energy while carrying out their daily activities. Routing includes planning the number and types of activities that are needed, making judgments about when to delete, postpone, or condense activities, and anticipating obstacles and planning solutions. Halcomb (104) emphasizes the changes in life-style that are necessary for COPD patients to improve their physical and mental well-being; patients need guidance in learning how to mobilize support resources and to deal with family and marital problems, as well as how to prevent and manage disease symptoms. Effective intervention should give the patient a sense of control over the environment. Stollenwerk (105) also suggests that COPD patients' spiritual resources be assessed for their potential as a coping resource. In a study of self care practices among COPD patients, she found that patients' values and spiritual beliefs affected their decisions regarding self-care, as well as their attitudes and emotional stability. Stollenwerk encourages professionals to become better aware of patients' values in order to assist individual patients to achieve their own goals.

Self-Efficacy and Mastery

Kaplan and his colleagues (17) have suggested that the concept of self-efficacy, originally described by Bandura (106), is important in understanding a patient's ability to cope adequately with the effects of respiratory disease and to benefit from pulmonary rehabilitation programs. They found that self-efficacy for walking was related to exercise capability even though it was not improved by rehabilitation or related to general HRQL or emotional status (40).

In patients with COPD, Moody et al. (35) found a significant relationship between the personality of mastery, as described by Guyatt et al. (62), and the general QL. Given the similarity of the concepts of mastery and self-efficacy, this finding from Moody and her colleagues appears to support the hypotheses of Kaplan et al. However, the importance of self-efficacy in the QL of COPD patients requires additional verification.

Family Functioning

Chronic pulmonary disease, like most chronic illnesses, has a negative impact on the family's functioning and QL as well as the patient's QL. Some of the problems that spouses of COPD patients experience have been discussed above. Interactions among family members in attempting to deal with the illness also influence the quality of the patient's adjustment (107).

Bruhn (108) points out the disintegrative effects on families of chronic illness. As duties and responsibilities are taken away from the ill person and are assumed by another, the ill person experiences a sense of loss, while the other family member is overburdened. This is the case in many families of patients with pulmonary disease (72–77). About one-third of female COPD patients reported that they felt lonely and depressed, despite the support given by their husbands and families. The major problems faced by wives of COPD patients were worry about their husband's physical condition, his negative attitudes and irritability, and coping with the loss of their own freedom. Less than one-third of the wives whose husbands had COPD shared problems with their husbands. Most were afraid that discussions of this type would bring on an attack of breathlessness in their husbands.

Patients with respiratory diseases and their family members often have different perceptions about the patients' capabilities and the problems posed by the illness. Guyatt et al. (32,62) had 36 pairs of COPD patients and their significant others complete identical questionnaires about problems posed by the illness. The COPD questionnaire included 108 items related to dyspnea, mastery, fatigue, sleep disturbance, emotional problems, social problems, and cognitive function. The patients identified more of the items as problematic than did their significant others, but the significant others attached greater importance to the problems they identified. Only 17 items were identified as problematic by equal numbers of patients and significant others, and correlations between the patients' and relatives' total scores were moderate in strength.

Guyatt et al. found that in patients with COPD, the severity of airflow limitation was not significantly related to the problems identified by the patients. These investigators emphasize the importance of the physician asking the patient and his/her family about their views of illness-related problems, rather than relying on physical manifestations of the disease. This seems to be good advice, because if patients and their family members do not share their perceptions of these problems, it will be difficult for them to find mutually acceptable solutions. Differing views and expectations can contribute to the isolation and depression of patients as well as to the subjective stress of spouses. A potential scenario is that the respiratory-disease patient and spouse may achieve a kind of shared life-style that limits the quality of life for both (77).

In general, research on family caregiving suggests that clinicians need to be very sensitive to the needs of spouse caregivers, particularly when the caregiver is elderly. While home care often is preferred by patients, spouses, and other family members, the caregiving role can be very demanding and place much physical, emotional, and financial strain on the caregiver (109,110). Spouse caregivers typically are middle-aged or elderly and most have at least one chronic illness (111). They may be at risk for exacerbations of their own illness if they do not receive adequate support for the caregiving role. In addition, up to one-third of spouse caregivers are employed and thus need to juggle caregiving responsibilities and work outside of the home (112). Even if the caregiver spouses do not experience acute physical health problems, they may break down under the emotional strain of caregiving. The burdens of caregiving in the home are becoming more recognized, and support services, e.g., respite programs, spouse support groups, and printed self-help materials, are becoming more available in communities and health care settings (110,111,113,114).

III. Psychosocial Interventions in Pulmonary Rehabilitation

A. Introduction

Given the abundance of evidence documenting the influence of psychosocial factors on the physical health and QL of patients with pulmonary diseases, most pulmonary rehabilitation programs now incorporate interventions aimed at improving patients' psychosocial outcomes as well as their physical health. However, while many clinicians and rehabilitation specialists are aware of the benefits their patients accrue from enhancement of their psychosocial assets, relatively few studies have systematically and rigorously tested the effects of psychosocial interventions in patients with pulmonary disease. The studies that have been conducted show that interventions that lessen patient distress and enhance their abilities to cope with pulmonary disease are psychologically beneficial and improve patients' adherence to exercise and medical regimens, potentially resulting in more favorable physiological outcomes. This section describes psychosocial interventions used in rehabilitation programs for pulmonary disease patients and reviews research documenting the effects of these interventions on patients' physical and psychosocial health.

B. Definition of Psychosocial Interventions

The term "psychosocial interventions" refers to any of a number of techniques designed to provide psychosocial support and improve patients' abilities to cope with and manage their disease. Psychosocially supportive interventions have as their goals: enhancing patients' HRQL, increasing adherence to behavioral and medical treatment regimens, and improving patients' physical health, as evidenced by symptomatic improvement, reduction in rehospitalization rate, and enhanced responsiveness to treatment.

Psychosocially supportive techniques include, but are not limited to, education of patients and family members as to the nature of the disease and the use of preventive and self-management strategies; counseling and therapy, whether group or individually oriented, of patients and family members; stress management and relaxation techniques; cognitive and behavioral modification techniques; and the provision of support to patients and their families. The techniques to be reviewed here fall into three categories: (1) psychotherapeutic and psychologically supportive approaches, which utilize individual or group therapy sessions to address the psychological needs of patients; (2) cognitive and behavioral modification techniques, which use techniques such as behavioral contracting, self-reinforcement strategies, desensitization, and guided mastery to reduce anxiety, enhance feelings of confidence and self-efficacy, and promote adherence to healthy behaviors; and (3) relaxation and stress management approaches, which include relaxation training, yoga, and meditation.

C. Psychotherapeutic and Psychologically Supportive Approaches

As noted above, a number of studies have documented a higher frequency of psychiatric morbidity, including depression and anxiety disorders, in COPD patients than in normals and in patients with other chronic diseases (17,22,27,28). Because of the benefits derived by patients with pulmonary disease from enhancement of their psychosocial assets, early psychosocial interventions focused on the use of psychotherapy and support groups in alleviating patients' psychological distress and enhancing the outcomes of rehabilitation (18,39,99,100). Individual and group psychotherapy programs were conducted in the context of pulmonary rehabilitation programs. They resulted in improvements in physical functioning, psychological adjustment, and symptom reduction. For example, Lustig et al. (115) found significant psychological improvement for patients enrolled in either a pulmonary rehabilitation program or psychotherapy sessions and concluded that rehabilitation programs should include a psychotherapeutic component for maximum benefit. Baum, Agle and colleagues (116,117) tested the effects of a rehabilitation program that included exercise, breathing retraining, vocational and social counseling, and group therapy sessions. They found that patients completing the program improved psychologically but without corresponding physiological improvement. Jensen (101) found that rates of hospitalization for COPD patients with high life stress and low social support who were assigned to either a pulmonary rehabilitation group or a self-help support group were lower than those for patients assigned to a wait-list control group.

Based on the findings in these early studies, Dudley et al. (18) proposed a comprehensive approach to psychosocial evaluation and treatment of COPD patients that includes a careful initial evaluation in which all aspects of patients' lives, including their psychological status, social interactions, family life, financial strains, and leisure time activities, are assessed. Dudley also recommended that patients receive psychiatric evaluation and treatment, where indicated, including psychopharmacological therapy as appropriate (118), and that rehabilitation programs include patient and family education about the disease and support for family members (18).

D. Cognitive and Behavioral Modification Approaches

Although studies of the effects of psychotherapy and psychological support in pulmonary disease patients showed benefits for such approaches, many of these studies used very small samples of patients, and most incorporated psychologically supportive techniques into a broader rehabilitation program involving exercise and physiological interventions. Thus, it is difficult to disentangle the effects attributable to the psychotherapeutic components of these programs from those resulting from other aspects of the programs.

Recently, the emphasis on psychodynamically oriented techniques to address the psychosocial needs of pulmonary disease patients in the rehabilitation context has been replaced by approaches that attempt to enhance patients' coping skills and sense of self-efficacy, or mastery, of the disease and its symptoms. The underlying principle of these approaches is that effective use of coping skills is a key factor in the positive outcomes observed in patients who participate in pulmonary rehabilitation programs. These approaches attempt to modify patients' cognitions and behaviors in order to deal more effectively with the demands imposed by the disease, increase feelings of master and control over the disease, and result in reduction of anxiety, better adherence to change in life-style, and more effective use of strategies in management of the disease.

Cognitive and behavioral techniques used to enhance coping skills include reinforcement of patients' adherence to life-style changes, e.g., the use of self-reinforcement in initiating and maintaining exercise and smoking cessation; methods for managing the disease and its symptoms, e.g., desensitization techniques to reduce the anxiety associated with dyspnea; and awareness of negative feelings and cognitions and their replacement with more positive ones, e.g., substituting positive, optimistic self-statements such as "I can learn to exercise, quit smoking," for negative, self-defeating ones.

Kaplan and Atkins (119) demonstrated the ability of cognitive and behavioral modification techniques to improve patients' adherence to exercise regimens. In their study, 75 COPD patients were randomly assigned to one of the following conditions:

1. *A behavior modification condition*, consisting of application of behavior modification techniques such as use of self-reinforcement to encourage daily walking; creating a behavioral contract specifying time of daily walk, and a reinforcer for achieving the walk; and relaxation techniques designed to enhance control over the anxiety associated with dyspnea.

2. *A cognitive modification condition*, in which the patient was taught to become aware of negative thoughts, feelings, and behaviors associated with exercise and replace them with positive cognitions.
3. *A cognitive-behavior modification condition*, which combined the use of behavioral and cognitive modification techniques.
4. *An attention control condition*, in which patients were provided with information about the importance of stress, support, and health history in managing chronic lung disease.
5. *A no-treatment control condition*, in which patients were given an exercise prescription and merely instructed to implement the walking program.

As shown in Figure 4, the greatest average increase in exercise tolerance was achieved for the cognitive-behavior modification group, followed by the cognitive group and the behavior modification group. The three experimental groups differed significantly from the two control groups, although the three treatment groups did not differ significantly from each other. The two control groups also did not differ significantly from each other.

Similar effects were found for patients' QL, as measured by the Quality of Well-Being Scale (Fig. 5). Patients in the three treatment groups showed increases in self-reported well-being over the 3-month intervention period, while the control groups showed declines in well-being. Again, the combination of the three treatment groups differed significantly from the combination of the two control groups.

Kaplan and colleagues attribute the improvements in exercise tolerance and well-being to increases in self-efficacy expectations gained through the performance and reinforcement of coping behaviors. In a related study, Toshima et al. (29) compared patients who were randomly assigned either to a program involving education, physical and respiratory therapy instruction, psychosocial support, and supervised exercise training or to a group receiving instruction and education regarding respiratory therapy, lung disease, and diet, but not exercise or support. Figure 6 shows that, 6 months after enrollment, patients participating in the comprehensive rehabilitation program showed significant increases in exercise endurance, while those in the education control group did not. In addition, these significant improvements were associated with increased self-efficacy, or greater patient confidence in their ability to walk various distances.

These findings are congruent with other research showing that COPD patients' feelings of mastery and control increase significantly following pulmonary rehabilitation and outpatient exercise programs (62,120), and that self-efficacy expectations are related to physiological status in COPD patients (40,121). Kaplan et al. (122) have also found that patient reports of self-effi-

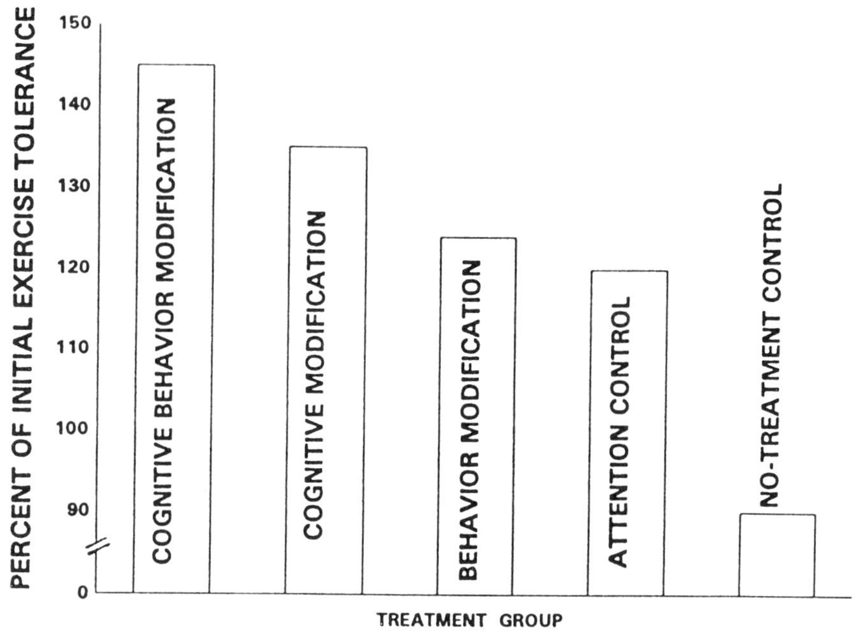

Figure 4 Exercise tolerance for three treatment and two control groups at 3 months as expressed in percent of baseline tolerance. (From Ref. 119. Reprinted with permission).

cacy expectations are a significant predictor of survival for patients with COPD.

Thus, behavioral and cognitive interventions within pulmonary rehabilitation programs have been found to increase adherence to exercise regimens, with resultant enhancement of exercise tolerance and self-reported well-being. These interventions appear to exert their effects by increasing patients' sense of self-efficacy, or feelings of control and mastery of their disease and its management, enhancing patients' ability to cope by making necessary life-style changes, and thereby improving their rehabilitation outcomes.

Another area in which cognitive and behavioral techniques have been applied in the management of pulmonary disease is dyspnea. Dyspnea is perhaps the most common and distressing symptom for patients with pulmonary disease. As noted earlier, it has long been acknowledged that certain emotional states, especially panic and anxiety, can increase dyspnea, and that a "vicious circle" can result in which panic triggers dyspnea, which in turn increases panic, and so on (117). Psychosocial interventions in this area have, as their goal, breaking this destructive cycle, allowing patients to experience a fuller emotional life without an increase in dyspnea.

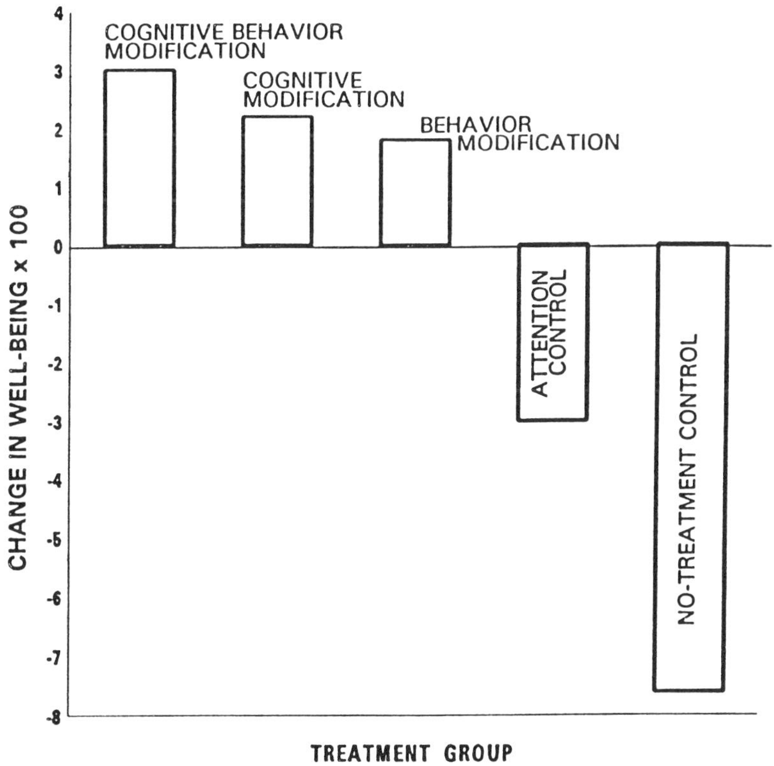

Figure 5 Mean change in Index of Well-Being scores (multiplied by 100). (From Ref. 119. Reprinted with permission.)

Recent research by Carrieri-Kohlman and colleagues has furthered our understanding of dyspnea and methods that can be used to break the anxiety-dyspnea cycle. These researchers have demonstrated that dyspnea has two distinct components: (1) an *affective* component, which is the distress and anxiety patients experience during an episode of breathlessness; and (2) a *sensory* component, which involves the intensity of the symptoms, or the degree of breathlessness experienced by the patient (123). Past research has primarily focused on the sensory, or intensity, component; however, recent studies show that COPD patients can distinguish between these two components of dyspnea (124,125). Furthermore, following repeated exercise testing dyspnea has been shown to decrease without concomitant physiological change. Presumably, the repeated exposure to exercise resulted in a "desensitizing" of the patient to the fear and anxiety associated with dyspnea (126). Exercise training also results in greater decrements in the anxiety and distress components of dyspnea than in

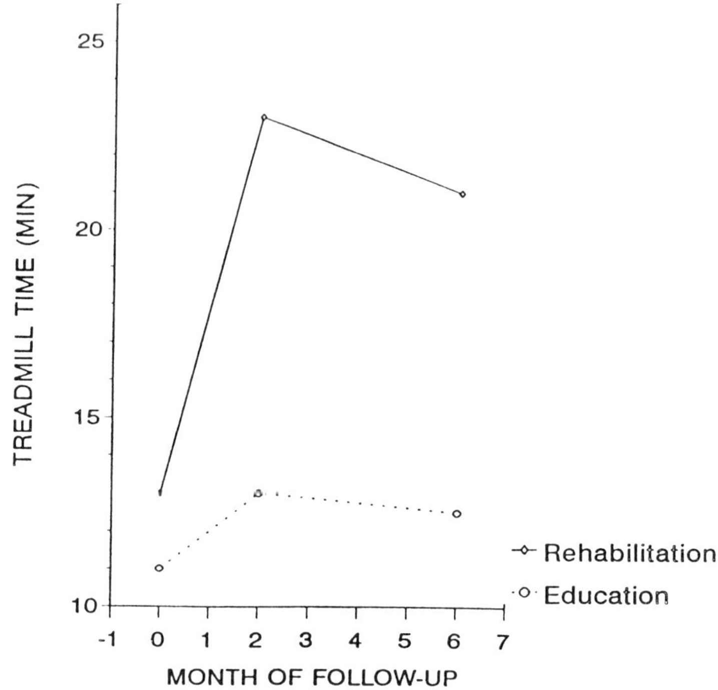

Figure 6 Treadmill time, by group and follow-up period. (From Ref. 29. Reprinted with permission.)

the intensity component, suggesting that relief of dyspnea following pulmonary rehabilitation may be partly attributable to decreases in anxiety resulting from repeated exposure to exercise (127). These observations, indicating that the degree of anxiety experienced by the individual affects the intensity of the symptom, suggest that attempts to decrease patients' anxiety should ameliorate the intensity of dyspnea.

A number of factors have been found to influence the anxiety and distress associated with dyspnea. Some, such as gender and cultural influences, are not easily amenable to intervention; others, such as social support, depression, self-efficacy, and a sense of control, can be influenced through psychosocial interventions (123). Figure 7 shows a model for decreasing the anxiety and distress associated with dyspnea based on enhancing self-efficacy and feelings of control and mastery (123). This model suggests that exposure of patients to greater-than-usual levels of dyspnea, e.g., via increasing exercise intensity, in a safe, monitored environment, should result in decreased anxiety and ultimately decreased intensity of dyspnea, as well as greater tolerance for exercise.

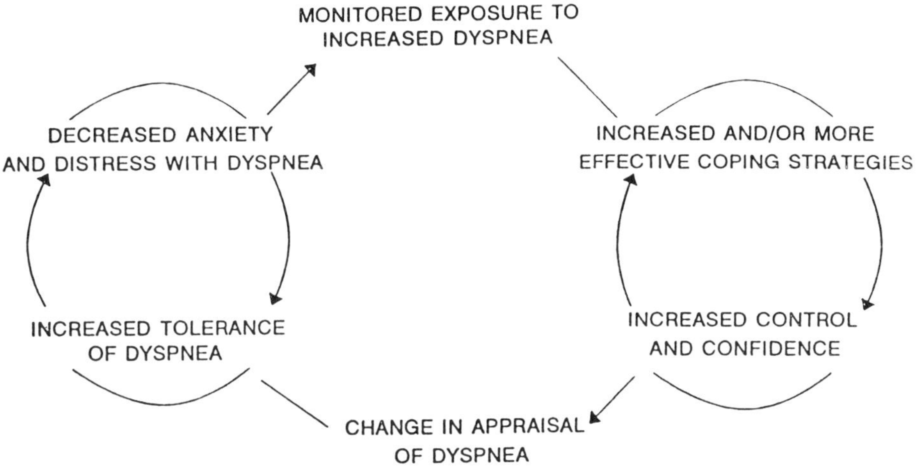

Figure 7 Suggested mechanism to decrease the anxiety and distress of dyspnea. (From Ref. 123. Reprinted with permission.)

This technique, called "desensitization," involving exposure of the patient to the symptom in small, graduated levels, can be combined with constant reinforcement and modeling of coping skills by the interventionist or therapist. When coupled with efforts directed at developing strategies for coping with dyspnea, the technique is called "guided mastery." Desensitization and, in particular, guided mastery techniques are hypothesized to increase patient confidence in dealing with dyspnea and to impart a greater sense of control. This heightened confidence should change the patient's appraisal of the threat imposed by dyspnea, increase his or her tolerance for breathlessness, and lead to decreased anxiety and distress, further decreasing the intensity of the symptoms. A detailed description of desensitization and guided mastery techniques to decrease the anxiety of dyspnea is presented in Carrieri-Kohlman et al. (123).

The use of relaxation techniques by patients with COPD decreases anxiety and the perception of dyspnea; also, enhancing patients' mastery or sense of control results in lowered anxiety and greater tolerance of a feared situation, such as breathlessness (128,129). Desensitization techniques have been shown to produce psychological and physiological benefits for COPD patients (116,126). Feelings of mastery and control, which are related to the level of dyspnea, have been shown to increase following participation in pulmonary rehabilitation programs (62,120).

Research is currently under way by Carrieri-Kohlman to identify optimal methods for helping patients cope with both the anxiety and sensory aspects of dyspnea, using guided mastery and other desensitization techniques. A randomized, controlled trial is comparing the effects of desensitization alone (monitored exercise training) with guided mastery (coached exercise training) on dyspnea intensity and anxiety. In 51 patients with COPD from this trial, dyspnea decreased with exercise training, and desensitization and guided mastery techniques proved to be equally effective in decreasing dyspnea outcomes (130–132).

E. Relaxation and Stress Management Approaches

Techniques such as relaxation training, hypnosis, yoga, and meditation have been studied in a variety of chronic illnesses, but few studies have examined the efficacy of these psychosocial techniques in patients with COPD (133). A study was made of the effects of progressive muscle relaxation training in 10 patients versus a control group that was instructed to relax, but given no specific techniques; the progressive relaxation group showed a statistically greater reduction in dyspnea and anxiety than did control subjects. These results suggest that relaxation training may be an efficacious psychosocial treatment for patients with COPD (134). Relaxation training has also been shown to decrease dyspnea in patients with COPD (128). Yoga techniques in these patients significantly increased their maximum work rate on a cycle ergometer and improved exercise tolerance; they also manifested quicker recovery following exertion, greater control over breathlessness, and greater improvement in their overall chest condition than did patients who received standard physiotherapy (135). Finally, although meditation may produce benefits in patients with pulmonary diseases, no data have as yet been provided to support its efficacy in these patients (136). Thus, while there is some evidence that yoga and meditative techniques can benefit COPD patients, more research is needed to establish their value as components of pulmonary rehabilitation programs.

IV. Conclusions

This chapter has attempted to review both the problems that psychosocial data bring to light when respiratory disease is studied and how psychosocial intervention might ameliorate these problems. It is clear that respiratory disease is not simply a disease of the lungs, but is also a disease of the brain as the organ of behavior. Thus, psychosocial factors should be considered when rehabilitative programs are developed and when they are evaluated. The measurement of psychosocial variables may assist in the determination of how successful a program is and help explain why a program is (or is not) successful on an individual or group basis. This recommendation is consistent with Engel's (3) conclusion that the science and profession of medicine is strengthened by the inclusion of psychosocial variables.

The rehabilitation process for patients with chronic pulmonary disease must incorporate an array of physical, psychological, and social components. Enhancing the patient's psychosocial resources, his or her ability to cope with the disease and its management, is a critical component of pulmonary rehabilitation. Given the benefits of enhanced psychosocial assets in pulmonary disease patients, the approach recommended by Dudley et al. (18,118,136), i.e., careful screening of patients with COPD for psychological problems, followed by referrals for appropriate psychological and pharmacological therapies, should be instituted as part of any structured rehabilitation program. In addition, psychosocial interventions utilizing cognitive and behavioral techniques have been shown to increase adherence to, and tolerance for, exercise and to decrease the anxiety and intensity of dyspnea. However, more research is needed to explore the efficacy of other types of psychosocial interventions, such as yoga and meditative techniques, that show promise but have not been adequately tested.

This chapter also indicates that research is needed along several lines: to determine the best approaches for special categories of patients with COPD, e.g., depressed patients, cognitively impaired patients, and ventilator-dependent patients; to determine the best methods for providing social support to patients and their families; to determine the advantages of comprehensive approaches to rehabilitation versus more precisely targeted techniques; to examine the benefits of standardized therapies versus individually tailored and stepped-care approaches; to identify which psychosocial interventions produce the best outcomes; and to identify those patients for whom specific interventions are most effective, so appropriate psychosocial interventions can be incorporated into pulmonary rehabilitation programs.

References

1. Kaplan RM. Behavior as the central outcome in health care. Am Psychol 1990; 45:1211–1220.
2. Engel GL. The need for a new medical model: a challenge for biomedicine. Science 1976; 196:129–136.
3. Engel GL. The clinical application of the biopsychosocial model. Am J Psychiatry 1980; 137:535–543.
4. Kaplan RM, Anderson JP. The general health policy model: update and application. Health Serv Res 1988; 23:203–235.
5. McSweeny AJ, Creer TL. Health-related quality of life assessment in medical care. Disease-a-Month 1995; 16:1–72.
6. Committee on the Accreditation of Rehabilitation Facilities (CARF). 1994 Standards for Organizations Serving People with Disabilities. Tucson, AZ: CARF, 1994.
7. DiCowden MA, Crossen BA, McSweeny AJ. Consensus statement: education and

training. In: Glueckauf RL, Frank RG, Bond GR, et al., eds. Health Care Reform and Psychological Practice in Rehabilitation and Health Care Settings. New York: Springer (in press).
8. Westlake EK, Kaye M. Raised intracranial pressure in emphysema. Br Med J 1954; 1:302–304.
9. Rourke SB, Grant I, Heaton RK. Neurocognitive aspects of chronic obstructive pulmonary disease. In: Casaburi R, Petty TL, eds. Principles and Practice of Pulmonary Rehabilitation. Philadelphia: WB Saunders, 1993:79–91.
10. Reitan RM, Wolfson D. The Halstead-Reitan Neuropsychological Test Battery: Theory and Clinical Interpretation, 2nd ed. Tucson, AZ: Neuropsychology Press, 1993.
11. Krop HD, Block AJ, Cohen E. Neuropsychologic effects of continuous oxygen therapy in chronic obstructive pulmonary disease. Chest 1973; 64:317–322.
12. Grant I, Heaton RK, McSweeny AJ, et al. Neuropsychologic findings in hypoxemic chronic obstructive pulmonary disease. Arch Intern Med 1982; 142:1470–1476.
13. Prigatano GP, Parsons OA, Wright EC, et al. Neuropsychological test performance in mildly hypoxemic patients with chronic obstructive pulmonary disease. J Consult Clin Psychol 1983; 51:108–116.
14. Grant I, Prigatano GP, Heaton RK, et al. Progressive neuropsychological impairment in relation to hypoxemia in chronic obstructive pulmonary disease. Arch Gen Psychiatry 1987; 44:999–1006.
15. Prigatano GP, Grant I. Neuropsychological correlates of COPD. In: McSweeny AJ, Grant I, eds. Chronic Obstructive Pulmonary Disease: A Behavioral Perspective. New York: Marcel Dekker, 1988:39–57.
16. Williams SJ. Chronic respiratory illness and disability: a critical review of the psychosocial literature. Soc Sci Med 1989; 28:791–803.
17. Kaplan RM, Eakin EG, Ries A. Psychosocial issues in the rehabilitation of patients with chronic obstructive pulmonary disease. In: Casaburi R, Petty TL, eds. Principles and Practice of Pulmonary Rehabilitation. Philadelphia: WB Saunders, 1993:351–365.
18. Dudley DL, Glaser EM, Jorgenson BN, et al. Psychosocial concomitants to rehabilitation in chronic obstructive pulmonary disease. Part I. Psychosocial and psychological considerations. Chest 1980; 77:413–420.
19. Greenberg GD, Ryan JJ, Bourlier PE. Psychological and neuropsychological aspects of COPD. Psychosomatics 1985; 26:29–33.
20. McSweeny AJ. Quality of life in relation to COPD. In: McSweeny AJ, Grant I, eds. Chronic Obstructive Pulmonary Disease: A Behavioral Perspective. New York: Marcel Dekker, 1988:59–95.
21. Sandhu HS. Psychosocial issues in chronic obstructive pulmonary disease. Clin Chest Med 1986; 7:629–642.
22. Light RW, Merrill EJ, Despars JA, et al. Prevalence of depression and anxiety in patients with COPD: relationship to functional capacity. Chest 1985; 87:35–38.
23. Jones PW, Baveystock CM, Littlejohns P. Relationships between general health measured with the Sickness Impact Profile and respiratory symptoms, physiologi-

cal measures, and mood in patients with chronic airflow limitation. Am Rev Respir Dis 1989; 140:1538–1543.
24. Dardes N, Chiappini, MG, Moscatelli B, et al. Quality of life of COPD patients treated by long-term oxygen. Lung 1990; 168 (Suppl):789–793.
25. Williams SJ, Bury, MR. "Breathtaking": the consequences of chronic respiratory disorder. Int Disabil Stud 1989; 11:114–120.
26. Williams SJ, Bury MR. Impairment, disability and handicap in chronic respiratory illness. Soc Sci Med 1989; 29:609–616.
27. Agle DP, Baum GL. Psychosocial aspects of chronic obstructive pulmonary disease. Med Clin North Am 1977; 61:749–758.
28. McSweeny AJ, Grant I, Heaton RK, et al. Life quality of patients with chronic obstructive pulmonary disease. Arch Itern Med 1982; 142:473–478.
29. Toshima MT, Kaplan RM, Ries AL. Experimental evaluation of rehabilitation in chronic obstructive pulmonary disease: short-term effects on exercise endurance and health status. Health Psychol 1990; 9:237–252.
30. Yellowlees PM. The treatment of psychiatric disorders in patients with chronic airways obstruction. Med J Aust, 1987; 147:349–352.
31. Dahlstrom WG, Welsh GS, Dahlstrom LE. An MMPI Handbook, rev. ed. Minneapolis: University of Minnesota, 1972.
32. Guyatt GH, Townsend M, Berman LB, et al. Quality of life in patients with chronic airflow obstruction. Br J Dis Chest 1987; 81:45–54.
33. Cox NJM, Hendricks JCM, Dijkhuizen R, et al. Usefulness of a medicopsychological questionnaire for lung patients. Int J Rehabil Res 1991; 14:267–272.
34. Moody L, McCormick K, Williams A. Disease and symptom severity, functional status, and quality of life in chronic bronchitis and emphysema. J Behav Med 1990; 13:297–306.
35. Moody L, McCormick K, Williams A. Psychophysiologic correlates of quality of life in chronic bronchitis and emphysema. West J Nurs Res 1991; 13:337–352.
36. Eakin EG, Sassi-Dambron D, Kaplan RM, et al. Clinical trial of rehabilitation in chronic obstructive pulmonary disease. J Cardiopulm Rehabil 1992; 12:105–110.
37. Niederman MS, Clemente PH, Fein AM, et al. Benefits of a multidisciplinary pulmonary rehabilitation program: improvements are independent of lung function. Chest 1991; 99:798–804.
38. Prigatano GP, Wright EC, Levin D. Quality of life and its predictors in patients with mild hypoxemia and chronic obstructive pulmonary disease. Arch Intern Med 1984; 144:1613–1619.
39. Toshima MT, Blumberg E, Ries AL, et al. Does rehabilitation reduce depression in patients with chronic obstructive pulmonary disease? J Cardiopulm Rehabil 1992; 12:261–269.
40. Toshima MT, Kaplan RM, Ries AL . Self-efficacy expectations in chronic obstructive pulmonary disease rehabilitation. In: Schwarzer R, ed. Self-Efficacy: Thought Control of Action. Washington, DC. Hemisphere, 1992.
41. Friedman HS, Booth-Kewley S. The "disease-prone personality": a meta-analytic view of the construct. Am Psychol 1987; 42:539–555.
42. Barstow RE. Coping with emphysema. Nurs Clin North Am 1974; 9:137–145.

43. Post L, Collins C. The poorly coping COPD patient: a psychotherapeutic perspective. J Psychiatry Med 1981–82; 11:173–182.
44. Katz IR. Is there a hypoxic affective syndrome? Psychosomatics 1980; 23:846–853.
45. Labuhn KT. An analysis of self-reported depressed mood in chronic obstructive pulmonary disease. (Doctoral dissertation, University of Michigan, 1984.) Diss Abstr Int 1984; 45:524B.
46. McSweeny AJ, Labuhn, KT. Quality of life in chronic obstructive pulmonary disease. In: Spliker B, ed. Quality of Life and Pharmacoeconomics in Clinical Trials, 2nd ed. New York: Raven Press (in press).
47. Karajgi B, Rifkin A, Doddi S, et al. The prevalence of anxiety disorders in patients with chronic obstructive pulmonary disease. Am J Psychiatry 1990; 147:200–201.
48. Burns BH, Howell JBL. Disproportionately severe breathlessness in chronic bronchitis. Q J Med 1969; 38:277–294.
49. Fuhs MF. Correlates of dyspnea in individuals with chronic obstructive pulmonary disorders. Doctoral dissertation, The Catholic University of America, Washington, DC, 1980.
50. Make B. COPD: management and rehabilitation. Am Fam Phys 1991; 43:1315–1324.
51. Haas F, Salazar-Schicchi J, Axen K. Desensitization to dyspnea in chronic obstructive pulmonary disease. In: Casaburi R, Petty TL, eds. Principles and Practice of Pulmonary Rehabilitation. Philadelphia: WB Saunders, 1993:241–251.
52. Dudley DL, Wermuth C, Hague W. Psychosocial aspects of care in the chronic obstructive pulmonary disease patient. Heart Lung 1973; 2:289–303.
53. Dudley DL. Psychophysiology of Respiration in Health and Disease. New York: Appleton-Century-Crofts, 1969.
54. Barstow RE. Coping with emphysema. Nurs Clin North Am 1974; 9:137–145.
55. Bergner M, Bobbitt RA, Carter W, et al. The Sickness Impact Profile: development and final revision of a health status measure. Med Care 1981; 12:787–805.
56. Bergner M, Hudson LD, Conrad DA, et al. The cost and efficiency of home care for patients with chronic lung disease. Med Care 1988; 26:566–579.
57. Schrier AC, Dekker FW, Kaptein AA, et al. Quality of life in elderly patients with chronic nonspecific lung disease seen in family practice. Chest 1990; 98:894–899.
58. Ström K, Boe J, Herala M, et al. Assessment of two oxygen treatment alternatives in the home. Int J Technol Assess Health Care 1990; 6:489–497.
59. Alonso J, Antó JM, González M, et al. Measurement of general health status of non-oxygen-dependent chronic obstructive pulmonary disease patients. Med Care 1992; 30 (Suppl):MS125–MS134.
60. Dompeling E, Van Grunsven PM, Molema J, et al. Early detection of patients with fast progressive asthma or chronic bronchitis in general practice. Scand J Prim Health Care 1992; 10:143–150.
61. van Schayck CP, Rutten-van Mölken MPMH, van Doorslaer EKA, et al. Two-year bronchodilator treatment in patients with mild airflow obstruction: contradictory effects on lung function and quality of life. Chest 1992; 102:184–1391.

62. Guyatt GH, Berman LB, Townsend M, et al. A measure of quality of life for clinical trials in chronic lung disease. Thorax 1987; 42:773–778.
63. Cottrell JJ, Paul C, Ferson S. Quality of life measures in COPD patients: how do they compare? Am Rev Respir Dis 1992; 145 (Suppl):A767.
64. Elliott MW, Simonds AK, Caroll MP, et al. Domiciliary nocturnal nasal intermittent positive pressure ventilation in hypercapnic respiratory failure due to chronic obstructive lung disease: effects on sleep and quality of life. Thorax 1992; 47:342–348.
65. Goldstein RS, Gort, EH, Brown DL, et al. A controlled trial of respiratory rehabilitation. Am Rev Respir Dis 1992; 145(Suppl):A767.
66. Guyatt GH, Townsend M, Keller JL, Singer J. Should study subjects see their previous responses? Data from a randomized control trial. J Clin Epidemiol 1989; 42:913–920.
67. Jaeschke R, Singer J, Guyatt GH. Measurement of health status: ascertaining the minimal clinically important difference. Controlled Clin Trials 1989; 10:407–415.
68. Kaplan RM, Atkins CJ, Timms R. Validity of a quality of well-being scale as an outcome measure in chronic obstructive pulmonary disease. J Chronic Dis, 1984; 37:85–95.
69. Anderson JP, Kaplan RM, Berry CG, et al. Interday reliability of function assessment for a health-status measure: The Quality of Well Being Scale. Med Care 1989; 27:1076–1083.
70. Kinsman RA, Yaroush RA, Fernandez E, et al. Symptoms and experiences in chronic bronchitis and emphysema. Chest 1983; 83:755–761.
71. Hanson El. Effects of chronic lung disease on life in general and sexuality: perceptions of adult patients. Heart Lung, 1982; 11:435–441.
72. Sexton DL, Monro BH. Living with a chronic illness: the experience of women with chronic obstructive pulmonary disease (COPD). West J Nurs Res 1988; 10:26–44.
73. Walbroehl GS. Sexual concerns of the patient with pulmonary disease. Postgrad Med 1992; 91:455–460.
74. Selecky, PA. Sexuality and the patient with lung disease. In: Casaburi R, Petty TL, eds. Principles and Practice of Pulmonary Rehabilitation. Philadelphia: WB Saunders, 1993:382–391.
75. Kass I, Updegraff K, Muffly RB. Sex in chronic obstructive pulmonary disease. Med Aspects Hum Sex 1972; 6:33–42.
76. Fletcher EC, Martin RJ. Sexual dysfunction and erectile impotence in chronic obstructive pulmonary disease. Chest 1982; 81:413–421.
77. Sexton DL, Monro BH. Impact of a husband's chronic illness (COPD) on the spouse's life. Res Nurs Health 1985; 8:83–90.
78. Pietropinto A, Arora A. Chronic pulmonary disease and sexual functioning. Med Aspects Hum Sex 1989; 23:78–82.
79. Semple PDA, Beastall GH, Watson WS, et al. Serum testosterone depression associated with hypoxia in respiratory failure. Clin Sci 1980; 58:105–106.
80. Conine TA, Evans JH. Sexual adjustment in chronic obstructive pulmonary disease. Respir Care 1981; 26:871–874.

81. Davis K. Sexual counseling for the patient with chronic lung disease (interview with HM Kravetz). Sex Med Today 1981; 5(3):10–15.
82. Timms RM. Sexual dysfunction and chronic obstructive pulmonary disease. Chest 1982; 81:398–399.
83. Brecher EM. Love, Sex and Aging. Boston: Little, Brown, 1984.
84. Keller S, Buchanan DC. Sexuality and disability: an overview. In: Nagler M, ed. Perspectives on Disability. Text and Readings on Disability. Palo Alto, CA: Health Markets Research, 1990:320–327.
85. Spica, MM. Educating the client on the effects of COPD on sexuality: the role of the nurse. Sex Disabil 1992; 10:91–101.
86. Lyons, HA . Sexual relations for male patients with chronic obstructive lung disease. Med Aspects Hum Sex 1977(Apr); 11:119–120.
87. Kravetz HM, Weiss M, Meadows R. Sexual Counseling for the Male Pulmonary Patient (slide-tape program). Prescott, AZ: HM Kravetz, 1980.
88. Kravetz HM. A Visit with Harry (slide-tape program). Prescott, AZ: HM Kravetz, 1981.
89. Kravetz HM. A Visit with Helen (slide-tape program). Prescott, AZ: HM Kravetz, 1982.
90. Costello CG. Depression: loss of reinforcers or loss of reinforcer effectiveness? Behav Ther 1972; 2:240–247.
91. Juniper EF, Guyatt GH, Dolovich J. Assessment of quality of life in adolescents with allergenic rhinoconjunctivitis: development and testing of a questionnaire for clinical trials. J. Allergy Clin Immunol 1994; 93:413–423.
92. McSweeny AJ. The psychosocial aspects of respiratory disease. Innovat Respir Dis 1995; 1 (in press).
93. Guyatt GH, Berman LB, Townsend M. Long-term outcome after respiratory rehabilitation. Can Med Assoc J 1987; 137:1089–1095.
94. Heaton RK, Grant I, McSweeny AJ, et al. Psychologic effects of continuous and nocturnal oxygen therapy. Arch Intern Med 1983; 143:1941–1947.
95. Heaton RK. Psychological effects of oxygen therapy for COPD. In: McSweeny AJ, Grant, I, eds. Chronic Obstructive Pulmonary Disease: A Behavioral Perspective. New York: Marcel Dekker, 1988:105–121.
96. Petty TL. Home oxygen in advanced chronic obstructive pulmonary disease. Med Clin North Am 1981; 65:615–627.
97. Casselith BR, Luck EJ, Strouse TB, et al. Psychosocial status in chronic illness: a comparative analysis of six diagnostic groups. N Engl J Med 1984; 311:506–511.
98. Young RF. Marital adaptation and response in chronic illness: the case of COPD. (Doctoral dissertation, Wayne State University, 1981.) Diss Abstr Int 1982; 42:4947A.
99. De Araujo G, Van Arsdel PP, Holmes TH, et al. Life change, coping ability and chronic intrinsic asthma. J Psychosom Res 1973; 17:359–363.
100. Pattison EM, Rhodes, RJ, Dudley, DL. Response to groups treatment in patients with severe chronic lung disease. Int J Group Psychother 1971; 21:214–255.

101. Jensen PS. Risk protective factors, and supportive interventions in chronic airway obstruction. Arch Gen Psychiatry 1983; 40:1203–1207.
102. Anderson, KL. Quality of life in chronic obstructive pulmonary disease. Dissertation completed at the Oregon Health Sciences University School of Nursing, May 1993.
103. Fagerhaugh S. Getting around with emphysema. In: Strauss AL, ed. Chronic Illness and Quality of Life. St. Louis: CV Mosby, 1975.
104. Halcomb R. Promoting self-help in pulmonary patient education. Respir Ther 1984; 14:49–54.
105. Stollenwerk R. An emphysema client: self care. Home Healthcare Nurse 1985; 3:36–40.
106. Bandura A. Self-efficacy: toward a unifying theory of behavioral change. Psychol Rev 1977; 84:191–215.
107. Litman TJ. The family as a basic unit in health and medical care: a social behavioral overview. Soc Sci Med 1974; 8:495–519.
108. Bruhn J. Effects of chronic illness on the family. J Fam Pract 1977; 4:1057–1060.
109. Archbold P, Stewart B. Family caregiving across the life span. Paper presented at the International Nursing Research Congress, American Nurses Association Council of Nurse Researchers. Washington, DC, October 1987.
110. Lubkin I. The family caregiver. In: Lubkin I, ed. Chronic Illness: Impact and Interventions, 2nd ed. Boston: Jones & Bartlett, 1990:200–217.
111. Crossman L, London C, Barry C. Older women caring for disabled spouses: a model for supportive services. Gerontologist 1981; 21(5):464–470.
112. Soldo B, Myllyluoma J. Caregivers who live with dependent elderly. Gerontologist 1983; 23:605–611.
113. Eisdorfer C, Cohen D. Management of the patient and family coping with dementing illness. J Fam Pract 1983; 12:831–837.
114. Mace NL, Babins PV. The 36-Hour Day. Baltimore: John Hopkins University Press, 1981.
115. Lustig FM, Haas A, Castillo R. Clinical and rehabilitation regime in patients with COPD. Arch Phys Med Rehabil 1972; 53:315–322.
116. Agle DF, Baum GL, Chester EH, et al. Multidiscipline treatment of chronic pulmonary insufficiency: psychologic aspects of rehabilitation. Psychosom Med 1973; 35:41–49.
117. Baum GL, Agle DF, Chester EN, et al. Multidiscipline treatment of chronic pulmonary insufficiency: functional status at one-year followup. In: Johnston RF, ed. Pulmonary Care. New York: Grune & Stratton, 1973:355–362.
118. Dudley DL, Glaser EM, Jorgenson BN, et al. Psychosocial concomitants to rehabilitation in chronic obstructive pulmonary disease. Part 3. Dealing with psychiatric disease (as distinguished from psychosocial or psychophysiologic problems). Chest 1980; 7:677–684.
119. Kaplan RM, Atkins CJ. Behavioral interventions for patients with COPD. In: McSweeny AJ, Grant I, eds. Chronic Obstructive Pulmonary Disease: A Behavioral Perspective. New York: Marcel Dekker, 1988:123–161.

120. Carrieri-Kohlman V. Education, coaching and patient identified strategies. Symposium on treatments for the relief of dyspnea. American Thoracic Society 1992 International Conference, Miami, FL, May 17–20, 1992.
121. Kaplan RM, Atkins CJ, Reinsch S. Specific efficacy expectations mediate exercise compliance in patients with COPD. Health Psych 1984; 3:223–242.
122. Kaplan RM, Ries AL, Prewitt LM, et al. Self-efficacy expectations predict survival for patients with chronic obstructive pulmonary disease. Health Psych 1994; 13:366–368.
123. Carrieri-Kohlman V, Douglas MK, Gormley JM, et al. Desensitization and guided mastery: treatment approaches for the management of dyspnea. Heart Lung 1993; 22:226–234.
124. Wilson RC, Jones PW. Differentiation between the intensity of breathlessness and the distress it evokes in normal subjects during exercise. Clin Sci 1991; 80:65–70.
125. Douglas M, Carrieri-Kohlman V, Gormley JM, et al. Differentiation among components of dyspnea in exercising patients with COPD. Am Rev Respir Dis 1992; 145:A766 (abstract).
126. Belman MJ, Brooks LR, Ross DJ, et al. Variability of breathlessness measurement in patients with chronic obstructive pulmonary disease. Chest 1991; 99:566–571.
127. Carrieri-Kohlman V, Douglas M, Gormley JM, et al. Exercise may result in greater decreases in anxiety and distress associated with dyspnea than in dyspnea intensity or perceived work of breathing. Am Rev Respir Dis 1992; 145:A765.
128. Gift AG, Moore T, Soeken K. Relaxation to reduce dyspnea and anxiety in COPD patients. Nurs Res 1992; 41:241–246.
129. Thompson SC. Will it hurt less if I can control it? A complex answer to a simple question. Psych Bull 1981; 90:89–101.
130. Gormley M, Carrieri-Kohlman V, Stulbarg MS. Dyspnea components decrease during treadmill treatment sessions in patients with chronic obstructive pulmonary disease (COPD). J Cardiopulm Rehabil 1992; 12:362 (abstract).
131. Carrieri-Kohlman V, Gormley JM, Douglas M, et al. Nurse monitoring is as effective as nurse coaching in decreasing dyspnea after exercise training. Am Rev Respir Dis 1993; 147:A531.
132. Carrieri-Kohlman V, Gormley JM, Douglas M, et al. Exercise training decreases dyspnea and the distress and anxiety associated with it: monitoring alone may be as effective as coaching (submitted for publication).
133. Sexton DL. Relaxation techniques and biofeedback. In: Hogkin JE, Petty TL, eds. Chronic Obstructive Pulmonary Disease: Current Concepts. Philadelphia: WB Saunders, 1987:99–112.
134. Renfroe KL. Effect of progressive relaxation on dyspnea and state anxiety in patients with chronic obstructive pulmonary disease. Heart Lung 1988; 17:408–413.
135. Tandon MK. Adjunct treatment with yoga in chronic severe airways obstruction. Thorax 1978; 33:514–517.
136. Dudley DL, Glaser EM, Jorgenson BN, et al. Psychosocial concomitants to reha-

bilitation in chronic obstructive pulmonary disease. Part 2. Psychosocial treatment. Chest 1980; 4:544–551.
137. Grant I, Heaton RK. Neuropsychiatric abnormalities in advanced COPD. In: Petty TL, ed. Chronic Obstructive Pulmonary Disease, 2nd ed, revised and expanded. New York: Marcel Dekker, 1985:355–373.

20

Cardiopulmonary Physical Therapy

CYNTHIA COFFIN ZADAI

Beth Israel Hospital
and Massachusetts General Institute
Boston, Massachusetts

The primary orientation of physical therapy (PT) in individuals with pulmonary impairments is to identify and deal with the pathophysiological processes that lead to, or have caused, movement dysfunction.

The management of the patient by the physical therapist consists of two essential elements: clinical evaluation and noninvasive testing that assess the patient's functional capacity at rest and during movement. The pulmonary patient is evaluated during a variety of functional activities, ranging from coughing, position change, bed mobility, and transfers, on the one hand, to the more demanding exercise activities, which include walking, stair climbing, and exercise to maximum capacity. The physiological responses of individual systems, e.g., neuromuscular and musculoskeletal, to changes in work and oxygen demand are used to diagnose and classify impairments related to movement dysfunction. Pulmonary impairments are generally categorized in terms of "functional" deficits, e.g., ventilatory pump impairments, airway protection deficits, gas exchange impairments, and so forth.

This chapter reviews the components of the PT evaluation, describes the process for program planning, and presents the methodology by which therapeutic interventions are chosen. It concludes with a discussion of some tools

Table 1 Summary of Physical Therapy Patient Interview

Assessment/questions	Details covered
General	Past medical history, allergies, current/past medication use, hospitalization Past surgical history, hospitalizations Family medical history, grandparents, parents, siblings, children
Specific	History of present illness to include onset of signs and symptoms (date, time, frequency) of: cough, temperature, congestion, chills, and/or sweats, dyspnea, pain, dizziness, nausea, pressure, lightheadedness, fainting
Functional activity history	Work history, perceived ambulatory ability, walking distance, assistive device use, stair climbing, independence in self-care, activities of daily living, exercise history, environmental affects (season, temperature, etc.), sleeping pattern
Social history	Support system/family, past/present social habits (ETOH, smoking), past/present living location, avocations

that are used to assess the outcome of treatment in terms of impairment and functional limitation.

I. Physical Therapy Examination

The pathological processes and injuries that can produce diseases and disorders of the pulmonary system cover a broad spectrum. They are illustrated, along with the impairments they may produce, in Table 2. Often the impairments they cause entail movement dysfunction. The impairments are assessed, categorized, and treated in terms of the "functional limitations," i.e. the restriction or inability to perform an action in the manner, or within a range, consistent with the purpose of an organ system (2). For example, decreased strength and endurance of ventilatory muscles may result from neuromuscular disease or chronic obstructive pulmonary disease (COPD) as the initiating mechanism, but the effect on the diaphragm and ventilatory pump is the focus of the PT assessment and treatment. Despite the wide variety of precipitating pathophysiological mechanisms, the effect of the impairment is to produce a deficit in performance that limits the functional movement of the ventilatory pump.

The results of the PT examination are used to group current and potential future impairments under four broad functional categories: ventilatory pump/

ventilation, airway maintenance/protection, gas exchange/respiration, and gas transport/oxygen delivery (Table 2). Since the pathophysiological mechanisms that lead to impairments often extend beyond more than one functional category, the therapeutic interventions have to address limitations across categories. In addition, the composite effect of the functional limitations is assessed in order to define the extent to which the patient can participate in the activities of daily living (ADL), the effect on his/her vocational and avocational aspects of life, and to measure the patient's perception of his/her general quality of life (QOL).

During the interview and observation phases of the examination (Table 1,3), the therapist determines whether the presenting problems are new or chronic and/or progressive. Areas that require objective testing are identified and the patient's current functional baseline is established. Also assessed is the patient's perception of the effects that the disability has on his/her daily life. The goals of treatment are best achieved if the patient perceives his/her limitations and is motivated to reverse the deficits.

Clinical assessment is performed in several positions (Table 4), i.e., sitting, 45° head up, side lying, supine, in order to look for changes brought about by an increase, or decrease, in the elastic and resistive loads on the ventilatory muscles and for changes in the ventilation/perfusion pattern (3,4). Also, simple clinical tests, such as sniff, cough, huff, swallow, Valsalva maneuver, and vocalization, are often done in the various positions to help in uncovering impairments in airway control, responses of the respiratory muscles to changes in load, and neuromuscular reflexes and coordination. Other objective measurements made in each position include tests of integrated neuromusculoskeletal and pulmonary function, i.e., respiratory rate, ventilatory volume, expiratory flow and inspiratory/expiratory forces, and cardiovascular and pulmonary function, i.e., heart rate, blood pressure, oxygen saturation, oxygen uptake, carbon dioxide production.

At the completion of the clinical assessment and observation at rest, the patient's response to activity is observed and monitored. Patients who are acutely ill and/or bedridden are evaluated during bed mobility, transfer, and self-care activities. Ambulatory patients are observed and monitored while changing from sit to stand, during low-level ambulation, while performing ADL, and during monitored exercise. Neuromusculoskeletal, cardiovascular, and pulmonary system performance responses are determined from rest to maximum exercise capacity. Values recorded throughout the assessment are related to normal values adjusted for age, sex, and size. Functional limitations that result from each impairment are described and the patient's potential for improvement is projected (Tables 5,6). This collective information forms the basis for the approach to therapy and for the prescription for exercise.

Finally, the assessment includes determination of the effects of the im-

Table 2 Pathologies/Pathophysiologies with Potential Pulmonary Impairments

Pathology/pathophysiology (1)	Impairment (1)	Measures of impairment
Ventilatory pump/ventilation		
Neuromuscular pathology, e.g., cervical or thoracic spinal cord injury, cerebrovascular accident, muscular dystrophy, polio, Guillain-Barré syndrome Musculoskeletal pathology, e.g., kyphoscoliosis, fractured ribs, flail chest Pulmonary pathology, e.g., hyaline membrane disease, obstructive airway disease, restrictive airway disease	Ventilatory muscle paralysis Decreased muscle strength/endurance Increased muscle fatigue Inefficient/ineffective thoracic pump motion Decreased chest wall compliance Obstructed airway with increased flow resistance Decreased lung/thorax compliance	Inspiratory muscle strength Expiratory muscle strength Vital capacity Forced expiratory volume/time Peak flow Maximum voluntary ventilation Observed coordinated pump motion RR/workload V_E/workload Measured response to exercise test
Airway maintenance/protection		
Neuromuscular pathology, e.g., cervical or thoracic spinal cord injury, polio, Guillain-Barré syndrome, etc. Airway pathology, e.g., asthma, chronic bronchitis, cystic fibrosis, bronchiectasis, foreign body aspiration, tumor	Loss of motor control/upper airway control Impaired swallowing Reduced cough pressures Smooth muscle spasm/increased resistance to airflow Mucus gland hypertrophy and hyperplasia Tracheal denudation; mucus stasis Obstruction/destruction of surface area Increased diffusion distance	Tongue deviation/control of purposeful actions Effective swallowing (elevation of trachea, effective airway occlusion) Low cough pressures Intact/effective cough/gag response Methylene blue test

Gas exchange/respiration		
Pulmonary pathology, e.g., hyaline membrane disease, emphysema, pneumonectomy, chronic bronchitis, bronchiectasis, pulmonary fibrosis, adult respiratory distress syndrome, cystic fibrosis	Loss of surface area Increased alveolar surface tension Retained volume/hyperinflation Destruction of surface area Obstruction of blood supply Increased diffusion distance Misdirected blood flow	Respiratory rate/activity V/Q, Pa_{O_2}, Pa_{CO_2}, at rest and with exercise Dead space/tidal volume Chest X-ray diffusing capacity V/Q scan Arteriogram
Cardiovascular pathology, e.g., congestive heart failure, pulmonary hypertension, tetralogy of Fallot, patent ductus arteriosus, pulmonary embolus		
Gas transport/oxygen delivery		
Cardiac pump pathology, e.g., congenital disorders, cardiomyopathy, connective tissue disorders, conduction disorders, valvular disease, obstruction to flow, inefficient pumping (stiff wall, high load), ineffective pumping	Decreased/absent pulmonary perfusion Ventilation/perfusion mismatch Mechanical obstruction/deviation of circulation Low/high perfusion pressures Increased resistance to blood flow Flow stasis Decreased oxygen-carrying capacity Loss of aerobic capacity Demineralization of bone Decreased muscle strength Decreased muscle endurance	Electrocardiogram Blood pressure, HR/activity Ventriculogram Cardiac catheterization Pulmonary capillary wedge pressure Coronary angiogram Thallium scan Doppler studies Exercise test response
Cardiovascular pathology, e.g., atherosclerosis, ischemic heart disease, hypertension, congestive heart failure, coronary vasospasm		
Hematological pathology, e.g., anemia, polycythemia		
Deconditioning: organ/system sequelae in response to bed rest or lack of physical conditioning		

Table 3 Physical Therapist's Observation and Assessment

Posture/response to position	Note signs and motions
Assess/supine/sitting/standing and response to position change	Observe for active muscle contraction: diaphragm, intercostals, abdominals, accessories, upper airway Symmetry of chest wall at rest/on motion, clavicle/scapular position, appropriate lateral and anterior/posterior ratios, vertebral curves, sternal position, subcostal angle, positional use of upper extremities, change in breathing at rest/activity
Thoracic/abdominal motion	Respiratory rate/range (infant, 40–50 breaths/min at rest, to 120 with activity; adult, 10–12 breaths/min at rest, to 60 with activity) Rhythm: inspiratory to expiratory ratio 1:2 at rest, 1:1 with activity including active contraction of abdominals on expiration Tidal breaths note: slight increase in anteroposterior diameter, symmetrical increase in lateral basal diameter, increased abdominal excursion at end-inspiration, note change from sitting to supine Note supraclavicular, subcostal, or intercostal retraction: note asymmetrical or paradoxical chest wall/abdominal motion: note pursed-lip breathing, stridor or grunting
Appearance	Skin: normal flesh tone versus loss of color, ruddy, cyanotic, or jaundiced; cool, clammy, dry Awake, alert, responsive
Head and neck	Facial expression, nasal flaring versus mouth breathing Mouth: assess for tongue control, dentures, swallowing, tracheal elevation, midline trachea, voice quality, effective cough/huff/sniff
Posture, transfers, gait	Categorize: lordosis, kyphosis, flatback, sway back, etc., base of support, limb symmetry, balance, strength, stability, note abnormality, need for assistance sit/stand, stand/walk, gait

Table 4 Body Positions and Treatment Options

Impairment category	Treatment techniques
Ventilatory pump/ventilation	
Decreased strength	Position to slightly increase load on muscle (lengthen muscle, provide resistance), facilitate with quick stretch
Decreased endurance	Position to decrease load on muscle and facilitate increased duration of contraction
Increased load	Position to decrease load, e.g., with increased abdominal girth Improve muscle mechanics, e.g., facilitate contraction with quick stretch, resistance
Inefficient/ineffective muscle contraction	Position to decrease or alternate use of accessories and increase use of diaphragm
Airway maintenance/protection	
Loss of airway/tongue control Impaired swallowing Inefficient/ineffective cough	Upright posture, head forward, facilitate tongue control, resistive exercise, tongue protraction/retraction, controlled swallow Upright posture, stabilize thorax for pain, splint supine or Trendelenburg posture for diaphragmatic weakness, quad cough techniques
Inefficient/ineffective mucociliary clearance	Segmental postural drainage positions
Gas exchange/respiration	
Decreased alveolar volume Decreased pulmonary perfusion Increased R→L shunt	Position segment with best V/Q relationship dependent Position to increase perfusion to best ventilated segment Position to increase ventilation as possible/consider prone
Gas transport/oxygen delivery	
Increased resistance to blood flow Flow stasis Systemic effects of bed rest/horizontal positioning	Position to increase/decrease venous return as appropriate Position upright as possible

Table 5 Normal Values Used in Pulmonary Physical Therapy

Measurements of ventilatory pump function	Normal values
Volume	
VC	75% of total lung capacity
V_T	10–15% of VC
Flow	
FEV_1	FEV_1:FVC = 80–100%
PEF (predicted)	PEF (L/sec) − 4.63 + 2.385[a] − 0.026A[b]
Rate	
RR	10–12 at rest, increase proportional to workload/oxygen demand
Strength	
MIP	Males: 103–124 cmH_2O[c]
	Females: 65–87 cmH_2O[c]
MEP	Males: 185–233 cmH_2O[c]
	Females: 128–152 cmH_2O[c]
Endurance	
MVV (predicted)	MVV = $FEV_1 \times 35$
MSVC	60% of MVV[d]

[a]Body surface area in square meters.
[b]Age in years. *Source:* Ref. 5.
[c]Mean values ± 2 SD. *Source:* Ref. 6.
[d]*Source:* Ref. 7.
VC, vital capacity; V_T, tidal volume; FEV_1, forced expiratory volume in 1 sec; RR, respiratory rate; MIP, maximum inspiratory pressure; MVV, maximum voluntary ventilation; MSCV, maximum sustainable ventilatory capacity; FVC, forced vital capacity; PEF, peak expiratory flow.

pairments on QOL and categorizing the patient according to his/her current level of functioning. In our outpatient clinic, we use a self-administered questionnaire to assess the patient's perception of his/her overall function and quality of life (9). Readministration of this questionnaire after a course of therapy is useful in highlighting areas of improvement or lack of change. Level of function is also determined based on the patient's performance in several categories, such as the maximum level of activity, symptoms elicited during activity, the ability to perform work-related tasks, or the level of independence in self-care. An American Lung Association Task Force on Comprehensive and Continuing Care (10) generated a description of five classes of functioning for patients with COPD (Table 7). This classification system relies on the findings during clinical evaluation and on measures of impairment that compare the particular individual with normal age-matched individuals.

Other instruments can be used to classify patients based on clinical obser-

Table 6 Normal Responses to Incremental Treadmill Exercise

Stage	Speed/grade (mph/%)	METs	HR (bpm)	SBP/DBP (mmHg)	V_E (L/min)	V_T(ml)	RR (bpm)
1	1.0/0	2.6	96 ± 15	140 ± 13/96 ± 8	18 ± 6	1153 ± 417	17 ± 4
2	1.5/0	3.1	98 ± 14	141 ± 12/93 ± 8	20 ± 5	1162 ± 450	19 ± 4
3	2.0/3.5	3.8	104 ± 13	145 ± 13/91 ± 7	24 ± 7	1270 ± 368	20 ± 4
4	2.0/7.0	4.7	110 ± 13	150 ± 13/87 ± 8	29 ± 9	1388 ± 394	22 ± 4
5	2.0/10.5	5.4	118 ± 14	155 ± 13/92 ± 11	33 ± 9	1468 ± 405	24 ± 3
6	3.0/7.5	6.2	126 ± 13	159 ± 21/87 ± 8	40 ± 12	1628 ± 456	25 ± 4
7	3.0/10.0	6.9	135 ± 15	168 ± 19/88 ± 9	46 ± 14	1776 ± 502	27 ± 6
8	3.0/12.5	7.9	144 ± 15	166 ± 19/91 ± 11	52 ± 17	1921 ± 502	28 ± 7
9	3.0/15.0	8.7	155 ± 14	169 ± 25/88 ± 10	61 ± 19	2153 ± 681	29 ± 7
10	3.4/14.0	9.2	162 ± 15	179 ± 21/86 ± 14	72 ± 25	2261 ± 700	33 ± 10

METs, metabolic equivalent (1 MET = 3.5 ml/min/kg O_2 uptake); HR, heart rate; SBP/DBP, systolic and diastolic blood pressure; V_E, minute ventilation; V_T, tidal volume; RR, respiratory rate; bpm, beats per minute.
Source: Data from Ref. 8. Reprinted with permission.

vation during physical activity coupled with standardized QOL measures and tests of functional capacity, e.g., symptoms during ADL, emotional functioning, and physical capacity function (11–13). Clinicians have also used a combination of the test scores obtained during the examination, e.g., distance walked in 6 min, the value obtained for the baseline dyspnea index, and the Specific Activity Scale Score, to classify the functional level of patients (11). A sum-

Table 7 American Lung Association Classification of Five Levels of Functioning for COPD Patients

I. Patient with recognized disease, no work restriction, is able to do what peers can do, continues usual life pattern
II. Patient with minimal or moderately restricted activity, is able to do productive work, has some difficulty keeping up with peers, has begun to modify life pattern
III. Patient with markedly restricted activity, is not homebound, may not be able to do productive work, but is able to care for self
IV. Patient with severely restricted activity, is not able to do productive work, is essentially homebound, but is able to care for self
V. Patient with very severely restricted activity, is homebound or in an institution, is not able to care for self

Source: Ref. 10.

mary of function is essential to establish the baseline, set realistic goals, and measure progress across the time course of treatment.

II. Program Planning and Treatment Intervention

All program planning is based on the assessment of the outcome of the individual patient. Treatment is directed toward reducing or reversing the specific impairments identified during the examination. Impairments are commonly listed as "problems" in the PT evaluation (14). Short-term goals are the measurable, objective, and subjective outcomes that are expected to result, directly or indirectly, from the PT intervention. Long-term goals are closely related to accomplishment of activities that will decrease limitations in mobility or improve the patient's level of function. Specific treatment interventions are selected for their ability to address each group of functional impairments previously identified, i.e., ventilatory pump, airway maintenance and protection, gas exchange, and gas transport or physiological conditions. Treatment techniques fall into categories that include body positioning, airway clearance, breathing exercises and strategies, and exercise conditioning (4,15–17). Commonly, multiple techniques within a single category or techniques from several categories are used to treat the impairments of a given patient. Impairments are addressed with respect to level of acuity, potential for resolution, and their effect on functional status; e.g., inability to ventilate at rest may preclude activities relating to self-care.

A. Body Positioning

Clinicians usually identify body positioning with postural drainage in the treatment of pulmonary patients who need to facilitate mucociliary transport (18,19). However, selection of body position is actually the initial step in any PT treatment program. Body position can be used in a variety of ways, depending on the impairment. One example is use of the prone position to improve ventilation/perfusion relationships. Another is positioning a C5–6 quadriplegic patient in the Trendelenburg position to increase the load on the diaphragm, thereby facilitating an improved force/frequency response and unloading the weaker, less-endurant, and less-efficient accessory muscles. The two major considerations for choice of position are: (1) the goal of treatment and (2) the physiological response of the patient to the position (4).

Selection of a body position is based on knowledge of normal lung volumes, ventilation mechanics, and perfusion patterns, how these are altered with change in position (Tables 8,9), the way in which the assumed body position will influence the pulmonary abnormalities of the particular patient, and the goals of treatment (Table 4). The patient with neuromuscular weakness is posi-

Table 8 Physical Characteristics, Lung Volumes,[a] and Vertical Lung Length[b] at Total Capacity

Subject	Age (years)	Height (cm)	Weight (kg)	D (cm)	Seated			Supine			Prone		
					TLC	FRC	RV	TLC	FRC	RV	TLC	FRC	RV
HD	31	177	79	19	7.06	3.59	1.56	6.50	2.60	1.30	6.58	2.78	1.38
GD	26	180	83	18	6.09	2.79	1.58	5.92	1.99	1.39	5.77	2.58	1.50
DT	32	167	73	20	5.65	2.81	1.25	5.37	1.94	1.31	5.49	2.06	1.34
					Seated			Right Lateral			Left Lateral		
					TLC	FRC	RV	TLC	FRC	RV	TLC	FRC	RV
GO	27	168	56	27	5.78	3.08	1.78	5.61	2.83	1.81			
GA	34	170	65	27	6.15	3.00	1.70	5.75	2.65	1.41			
KK	34	166	59	27	5.33	2.32	1.28	5.20	2.42	1.30	5.27	2.52	1.46
MW	34	181	81	29	7.33	3.03	1.82				7.20	2.86	1.70
BS	32	173	72	25	5.90	3.00	1.50				5.65	2.15	1.45

[a] Lung volumes were determined by the closed-circuit helium method and are expressed in liters.

[b] Vertical lung length was determined with radiographs taken in each posture studied in each subject, in the first three subjects being measured when they were supine, and in the remaining five when they were in the right or left lateral position.

D, vertical lung length; TLC, total lung capacity; FRC, functional residual capacity; RV, residual volume.

Source: From Ref. 20, with permission.

Table 9 Direct Hemodynamic Measurements,[a] Left Ventricular Dimensions, and Performance[b] in Normal Subjects at Rest

Parameter	Supine	Sitting
Heart rate (beats/min)	73 ± 4	84 ± 4
Pressure (mmHg)		
Brachial artery	96 ± 3	99 ± 4
Systolic	130 ± 5	132 ± 5
Diastolic	76 ± 3	82 ± 3
Pulmonary artery	13 ± 1	13 ± 1
Pulmonary capillary wedge	6 ± 1	4 ± 1
Left ventricular end-diastolic	8 ± 1	4 ± 1
Stroke index (ml/m^2)	50 ± 5	35 ± 3
Cardiac index ($L/min/m^2$)	3.5 ± 0.3	2.8 ± 0.2
Ejection fraction (%)	76 ± 2	72 ± 4
Volume (ml)		
End-diastolic	107 ± 10	85 ± 6
End-systolic	34 ± 4	32 ± 5
Stroke	76 ± 8	55 ± 5

[a]Means ± SE for 10 sedentary men.
[b]Means ± SE for seven normal subjects.
Source: Ref. 21. Reprinted with permission.

tioned by taking into account his/her physiological abnormalities and the prognosis for reducing the current level of impairment, e.g., the potential for retraining the muscles. If the pathological process has produced a fixed deficit, the patient can be positioned to enhance function, e.g., by placement of an abdominal binder on a C5–6 quadriplegic patient during sitting activities (22–24).

Positioning can also be used to retrain a functional activity, e.g., coughing in neuromuscular fixed deficits. If the neuromuscular disease is progressive, positioning could be chosen to facilitate retention of the patient's ventilatory muscle strength and endurance. For example, semirecumbent positions can decrease the ventilatory load below that of the supine position. Also, patients with acute obstructive disease of the airways may require immediate Trendelenburg positioning to clear the airway whereas those with chronic disease of the airways are apt to benefit from long-term use of multiple positions to keep airways open and to decrease the likelihood of recurrent airway infection/consolidation (4,15).

In essence, position selection is generally the initial step in any PT treatment program and is usually considered to be an essential and basic component of patient care. The physiological underpinnings of the choice of position include: (1) the work (force × distance) required of the ventilatory muscles, i.e., the diaphragm, intercostals, and accessories including abdominal muscles; (2) the "load" conditions, i.e., the lung/thorax compliance, airway resistance, abdominal resistance, metabolic oxygen demand; (3) the condition/ability of the ventilatory muscles to respond to the load; (4) the ventilation/ perfusion (V/Q) ratios; (5) the cardiovascular hemodynamics; and (6) the interplay among these variables as a result of the change in position and with respect to the desirable outcome (4,22,25).

B. Airway Clearance Techniques

Airway clearance techniques are often referred to collectively as "chest physical therapy" or "bronchopulmonary hygiene techniques." The PT literature generally groups these techniques into two categories: those used for mobilization of secretions and those used for clearance of secretions (15). Techniques for mobilization of secretions include manual procedures, such as percussion, shaking, and vibration, which are applied to the thorax to loosen secretions and to propel them centrally. In an unpublished study entailing bronchoscopy in anesthetized, intubated dogs, Kigin measured the movement of a bolus of radiopaque viscous secretion deposited below the carina in a lobar segment of the airways (26). A bolus of secretion was observed to move slowly cephalad while the dog was supine. The secretion was observed to "splatter" in the airway when the thorax was treated with "moderate and vigorous" percussion. In addition, the secretion bolus "elongated and moved en-mass in a cephalad direction" faster than the pretreatment mucociliary transport rate when the thorax was subjected to shaking and vibration. This observation is consistent with others directed at quantifying and qualifying the effects of manual techniques on the mobilization of secretions and choosing the proper technique for a particular impairment (27–35).

Both the quantity of secretions and the rate of mucociliary tracheal transport have been reported to increase when manual techniques are applied to individuals with impaired mucociliary transport (27–35). Mobilization of secretions from the peripheral to the central airways has been postulated to be necessary for effective secretion clearance with coughing. Increased volume of secretions per cough has been cited as evidence for improvement in the efficiency of clearing secretions and in decreasing the work of the ventilatory pump in accomplishing this task. For those patients subjected to airway clearance techniques, medications, e.g., bronchodilators, may be useful in ensuring adequate oxygenation and minimizing airway reactivity (15).

Undesirable side effects have been reported from the use of these techniques in individuals who have little or no retained secretions, bronchospastic airways, and the potential to become hypoxemic (35–37).

Techniques used for the clearance of secretions include invasive (suctioning) and noninvasive modalities [forced expiratory technique (FET), huffing, coughing, and quadriplegic coughing]. Patients in whom the neuromuscular system and cognition are intact are taught noninvasive modalities. Patients with cognitive deficits or physiological impairments that preclude the ability to clear secretions are suctioned; since this intervention is invasive and potentially harmful, it is usually reserved for mechanically ventilated or obtunded patients and is regarded as a choice of last resort.

Noninvasive techniques are commonly taught as a method of self-care to patients with chronic impairment. Effective coughing requires an increased inspiratory volume, the ability to control and close the upper airway, and an adequate abdominal force to generate successive compressive and expulsive force on expiration (38). Secretions have to be mobilized for coughing to be effective. Patients who cannot generate a significant expiratory force are assisted by positioning and quadriplegic coughing.

The FET maneuver is used in patients with small lung volumes, unstable airways, or hemoptysis who continue to retain secretions. The patient is encouraged to take progressive short inspirations that retain volume up to approximately 50% or more of vital capacity (VC); he/she then huffs air out, using short exhalations through an open airway, stopping before reaching residual volume (RV). Theoretically this technique "milks" the airways, progressively moving secretions centrally where they can be coughed out (38–45).

A lessening of impairment after airway clearance has been demonstrated by a variety of clinical indices. Most dramatically, clearing of the chest radiograph has occurred immediately post treatment (32). Other objective indices include improved arterial oxygenation and pulmonary function tests (45–48). Accompanying these changes are a decrease in adventitious breath sounds, an increase in aeration, and a decrease in dyspnea.

C. Breathing Exercises and Strategies

Breathing exercises and strategies are a part of the therapeutic approach in all four major pulmonary impairment categories. The category of physiological impairment directs the selection of the type and amount of a particular technique or strategy (Table 10). The therapeutic techniques are grouped according to those that address a reduction in lung volume, those that treat impaired strength and endurance of the ventilatory muscles, and those that attempt to correct inefficient patterns of breathing, which, in turn, decrease the efficiency of ventilation or entail a high oxygen cost of breathing during activity (16).

The initial group of breathing exercises (Table 11) was developed to in-

Table 10 Breathing Exercises/Strategies to Reduce or Correct Physiological Compromise

Physiological compromise	Breathing exercise/strategy
Group I	
Decreased intrathoracic-lung volume	Sustained maximal inspiratory maneuvers (SMI)
Decreased chest wall–lung compliance	Diaphragmatic breathing exercises
Increased flow resistance resulting in decreased lung volume	Segmental breathing exercises
VA/Q mismatch	
Group II	
Decreased lung-thorax compliance	Strength/endurance training
Decreased intrathoracic volume in neuromuscular or musculoskeletal impairments	Inspiratory resistance training (IMT)
	Isocapneic hypernea
Group III	
Increased work (elastic and flow resistive)	Diaphragmatic breathing exercises
Decreased compliance/increased resistance/load work; diaphragm/accessories	Pursed-lip breathing (PLB)
Change in length/tension/force generation, mechanical disadvantage	Paced breathing with exercise (PBE)
VA/Q mismatch	Exhale with exercise/activity (EWE)

Source: From Ref. 16, with permission.

crease lung volume, redistribute ventilation, and improve gas exchange. These exercises are commonly used to treat patients with thoracic or abdominal pain or with impairments of the ventilatory pump due to musculoskeletal deformities and/or neuromuscular abnormalities.

Exercise techniques to increase strength, endurance, and the efficiency of the ventilatory muscles have received considerable attention in the literature over the last decade and are addressed in other chapters (49–51). Physical therapists have commonly employed strength and endurance training of ventilatory muscles when strength and/or endurance is less than predicted with respect to sex and age (Table 5). The methods used range in complexity from inspiratory resistive or threshold loading to simple abdominal weighting, as in quadriplegic patients, using progressive resistive exercises. Outcome indicators for success in this group range from an increase in tidal volume and vital capacity to an increase in inspiratory force and improved cough.

The third group of breathing exercises is directed toward decreasing inefficiencies in the performance of the work of breathing and decreasing the sensa-

Table 11 Breathing Exercise Techniques

Techniques	Explanation
Sustained maximal inspiration (SMI)	Maximal inspiratory effort slowly inhaled through nose to total lung capacity—3 sec hold at maximum inspiration
Diaphragmatic breathing exercises	Incorporation of body position with tactile and verbal cueing and resistance to improve diaphragmatic recruitment/excursion during inspiration/expiration
Segmental breathing exercises	Incorporation of positioning with tactile and verbal cueing and resistance to enhance localized expansion of a specific lung segment to facilitate chest wall motion and increase ventilation

Source: From Ref. 16, with permission.

tion of dyspnea (Table 12). Patients who suffer chronically from dyspnea on exertion will often independently adopt breathing patterns that decrease the work of breathing and make them more comfortable (52). However, some patients may require instruction about suitable breathing patterns during activities such as ambulation, stair climbing, and self-care. Some patients adopt strategies that are maladaptive and need retraining using different techniques such as verbal instruction, tactile cueing, and constant repetition.

Increasing the patient's awareness of breathing during activity, objectively measuring symptoms during performance, as by visual analog scale (53), and cueing the patient for use of alternative patterns have all proven useful in decreasing dyspnea. Unfortunately, long-term compliance with these strategies has been difficult to achieve.

D. Mobilization and Exercise Conditioning

Prescription of exercise for patients with pulmonary impairment assumes that oxygen uptake and delivery are compromised. As a result, maximal and reserve capacity for responding to an increase in oxygen demand are decreased. The exercise assessment identifies and quantifies the existing and potential impairments.

Exercise as a treatment technique addresses many components of pulmonary impairment. Saltin et al. demonstrated that exercise reversed the multisystemic effects of deconditioning following bed rest, and Robinson and Kjeld-

Table 12 Breathing Strategies

Strategy	Explanation
Breathing retraining (BRT)	Can encompass the use of all techniques/devices that alter a patient's current breathing pattern; this includes all types of breathing exercises in group II and III, but is usually used in reference to those breathing exercises/strategies that alter the breath-to-breath tidal volume/rate in an effort to reduce oxygen consumption/work of breathing
Diaphragmatic breathing pattern	The incorporation of body position with tactile and verbal cueing and resistance to improve diaphragmatic recruitment/excursion during inspiration/expiration
Pursed-lip breathing exercises (PLB)	The expiratory phase of the breathing cycle is done through the patient's pursed lips; the expiratory phrase is usually passive, but a component of active expiration can be employed in certain instances
Paced breathing with exercises (PBE)	Encompasses low-frequency breathing techniques, but may refer to any change in respiratory rhythm or rate aimed at reducing dyspnea
Exhale with exercise/activity (EWE)	Used during activity/low-level exercise; body motion occurs only during the expiratory phase of the respiratory cycle; can be used alone or in conjunction with the above-listed techniques

Source: From Ref. 16, with permission.

gäard measured an increase in the ventilatory muscle strength and endurance in normals following exercise training (54,55). After use of upper-extremity exercise, patients with cystic fibrosis showed an increase in the endurance capacity of ventilatory muscles; Wolff et al. reported an increase in mucociliary transport in patients with cystic fibrosis during exercise (50,56). We have noted an increase in the total distance walked, a decrease in the rating of dyspnea, and an overall improved functional status in COPD patients who participate in exercise programs (57). These benefits were achieved with specific exercise prescriptions that addressed the documented level of performance or impairment in each individual or group of individuals; training techniques were directed specifically at the limitation.

The monitored and measured response to performance of activity establishes the baseline for evaluating the patient's exercise capacity and the potential for improving the observed abnormalities (Table 13). The exercise prescription is directed at reducing the measured impairment and using the variables of intensity, duration, and frequency to work toward goals. The mode of exercise is selected by the patient with the understanding that the exercise will be required daily for a lifetime. Access and interest are the major considerations. The individual prescription is based on the results of the exercise test. Those who can achieve 50–60% of predicted maximum oxygen uptake during maximal exercise testing are managed with aerobic exercise prescriptions using the guidelines for the normal population (58). Patients whose maximum predicted capacity values are reached during low-level activities, e.g., a respiratory rate of 55/min while climbing 10 stairs, are managed by using modified prescriptions directed at the impairment: if endurance is limited, the prescription focuses on prolonging duration; if strength is a limiting factor, a strengthening program using progressive resistance over the duration of exercise may be used. Prescriptions are modified as each impairment decreases. Outcome measures indicating improvement can include multiple indicators: longer distance walked in less time with a decrease in symptoms; increase in $\dot{V}O_2max$; or increased functional performance, e.g., less dyspnea during self-care, more stairs climbed in less time with decreased dyspnea, and so forth.

E. Classification of Function

Physical therapists practicing in rehabilitation settings usually classify function in terms of independence in the ability to perform self-care and activities of daily living (61). PT practitioners in the outpatient setting more often use a composite of impairment measures (distance walked, oxygen saturation, and PFTs) to indicate decrease in limitation and improvement in function and compare the results of the test to normative values. Patients have also been classified based on a system grouping such as that suggested by the American Lung Association (Table 7). More recently, PTs have begun integrating self-administered tests of functional limitation and disability into the initial evaluation of pulmonary-impaired patients (9,62). These tests consider aspects of emotional function, social role function, and ability to perform ADL. For example, COPD patients undergoing functional tests have been demonstrated to be more concerned with their perceived social limitations than with physical limitation; this finding is of particular interest to physical therapists, who are primarily focused on physical and movement limitations (63–65). Additional study with sessions of 15–20 min given by a trained research assistant during their hospitalization. Six months after discharge, 33.3% of subjects in the intervention group had quit compared to 21.4% in the control group. Because of the small sample size, the difference was not statistically significant.

Although smoking cessation interventions in patients with clinically evident COPD are effective, continued smoking by these patients despite respiratory symptoms probably reflects a high level of nicotine dependence. Therefore, patients with COPD may require intense interventions to maximize smoking cessation.

IV. Physician's Role in Smoking Cessation

Although the focus of this book is on pulmonary rehabilitation, the role of the physician and other health professionals in smoking cessation is considered within the broader context of preventing smoking-related diseases. Traditionally, the prevention of diseases has been categorized into three levels: primary, secondary, and tertiary. These levels provide a useful conceptual framework for discussing the role of the professional in preventing smoking-related diseases. Thus, the aim of *primary* prevention is to eliminate the initiation of cigarette smoking or to stop smoking before the onset of a smoking-related disease. In *secondary* prevention, the goal is to detect the presence of asymptomatic disease permitting prompt smoking cessation to prevent the occurrence of clinically evident disease. Finally, *tertiary* prevention involves smoking cessation in patients with established smoking-related diseases; smoking cessation interventions are part of a pulmonary rehabilitation program.

A. Primary Prevention

Physicians and other health professionals have many opportunities to intervene at the community level as well as with individual patients to prevent smoking-related diseases. Although individual patients usually comprise the most frequent context within which health professionals can effect smoking cessation, other contexts may have equal, or greater, impact for limiting the use of tobacco (50). Because social factors have a major influence on the initiation and maintenance of cigarette smoking, advocating private and public policies and changing societal norms that support nonsmoking are essential components in programs designed to prevent children and adolescents from starting to smoke (24) and for assisting smokers in their attempts to quit (51).

B. Secondary Prevention

The frequent contact of health professionals with smokers provides many opportunities to encourage, and to assist, individual patients with smoking cessa-

Table 13 Physiological Measures as Indicators of Impairment

Indicator	Measures
Ventilatory pump impairment	Achievement of predicted MVV, inability to maintain adequate MIP and/or development of discoordinated breathing, RR of 50–70, dyspnea
Maximum minute ventilation (V_E)	$35 \times FEV_1$ (actual) is rough MVV estimate; ventilation reaching or exceeding this value at minimum exercise intensities means poor probability for exercise conditioning
Maximum inspiratory pressure (mouth)	Critical level, 40–60 cmH_2O; below these values, ventilatory muscle training may need to precede or accompany exercise conditioning
Increased flow resistance	Development of bronchospasm or mucus mobilization, decreased FEV_1, change in ventilatory pattern and muscle use, dyspnea
Gas exchange impairment	Decreased Sao_2 or Pao_2, increasing $Paco_2$, dizziness, nausea, dyspnea, ECG abnormality
Oxygenation	Tolerable range for rest/exercise: $Sao_2 > 99\%$ to 85%, $Pao_2 > 104$ mmHg—(.42 × age) to 60 mmHg; inability to maintain within tolerable range indicates need for supplemental oxygen
Cardiovascular impairment	Rapid inappropriate increase in heart rate, no increase in heart rate with increase in workload, no increase or significant decrease in blood pressure with increase in workload, ECG abnormality, dyspnea, angina
Heart rate	(220—age) up to 60; after age 60, men plateau at 170, women, at 160; ability to reach 85% maximum predicted or greater without limitation means good probability for exercise conditioning
Deconditioning	Appropriate cardipulmonary response that quickly reaches predicted maximum cardiac values, symptom limitations (e.g., fear, weak extremities, lack of coordination)

MVV, maximum voluntary ventilation; FEV_1, forced expiratory volume in 1 sec; Sao_2, oxygen saturation; Pao_2, partial pressure of arterial oxygen; RR, respiratory rate.
Source: Ref. 3. Reprinted with permission.

this particular instrument has shown correlation between values recorded for dyspnea, on the one hand, and others that evaluate ADL performance, fatigue, embarrassment, depression, anxiety, and distance walked in 6 min, on the other. Consequently, measures of quality of life are now being incorporated by physical therapists into the initial evaluation and reevaluated following a course of either inpatient or outpatient rehabilitation (9).

III. Summary

The physical therapist's role in pulmonary rehabilitation is predominantly focused on identifying, measuring, diagnosing, and treating impairments that produce movement dysfunction and functional limitations. Assessment techniques quantify and qualify those impairments that are amenable to PT management. Treatment programs are designed to reduce systemic impairments that limit functional mobility and activity. Management techniques include positioning/postural drainage, mobilization and clearance of secretions, breathing exercises and strategies, and exercise conditioning. Patient improvement is demonstrated by using objective measures that reflect decreases in impairment and improved scores on functional assessment or quality of life.

References

1. Philosophical Statement on Physical Therapy (Position). APTA, 1983:HOD 06-83-03-05: Program 32, Alexandria, VA.
2. National Center for Medical Rehabilitation Research, National Institute of Child Health and Human Development: Report and Plan for Medical Rehabilitation Research. Bethesda, MD: NIH, 1991.
3. Zadai CC. Comprehensive physical therapy evaluation: identifying potential pulmonary limitations. In: Zadai CC, ed. Pulmonary Management in Physical Therapy. New York: Churchill-Livingstone, 1992:55–78.
4. Ross J, Dean E. Body positioning. In: Zadai CC, ed. Pulmonary Management in Physical Therapy. New York: Churchill-Livingstone, 1992:79–98.
5. Bass H. The flow volume loop: normal standards and abnormalities in chronic obstructive pulmonary disease. Chest 1973; 63:171–176.
6. Black LF, Hyatt RE. Maximal respiratory pressures: normal values and relationship to age and sex. Am Rev Respir Dis 1969; 69:696–702.
7. Rochester DF, Arora NS, Braun NMT, et al. The respiratory muscles in chronic obstructive pulmonary disease. Bull Eur Physiopathol Respir 1979; 15:951–975.
8. Weber KT, Janicki JS, eds. Cardiopulmonary Exercise Testing: Physiologic Principles and Clinical Applications. Philadelphia: WB Saunders, 1986.
9. Jette AM. Concepts of health and methodological issues in functional assessment. In: Granger L, Grisham G, eds. Functional Assessment in Rehabilitation Medicine. Baltimore: Williams & Wilkins, 1984.

10. American Lung Association. Report of the task force on comprehensive and continuing care for patients with COPD. New York: ALA, 1975.
11. Guyatt GH, Thompson PJ, Berman L, et al. How should we measure function in patients with chronic heart and lung disease? J Chronic Dis 1985; 6:517–524.
12. McSweeny AJ, Grant I, Heaton RK, et al. Life quality in patients with chronic obstructive pulmonary disease. Arch Intern Med 1982; 145:473–478.
13. Guyatt GH, Berman LB, Townsend M, et al. A measure of quality of life for clinical trials in chronic lung disease. Thorax 1987; 42:773–778.
14. Patrick, DF: Clinical decision making. In: Zadai CC, ed. Pulmonary Management in Physical Therapy. New York: Churchill-Livingstone, 1992:191–224.
15. Starr, JA. Manual techniques of chest physical therapy and airway clearance techniques. In: Zadai CC, ed. Pulmonary Management in Physical Therapy. New York: Churchill-Livingstone, 1992:99–133.
16. Levenson CR. Breathing exercises. In: Zadai CC, ed. Pulmonary Management in Physical Therapy. New York: Churchill-Livingstone, 1992:135–155.
17. Dean E, Ross K. Mobilization and exercise conditioning. In: Zadai CC, ed. Pulmonary Management in Physical Therapy. New York: Churchill-Livingstone, 1992:157–190.
18. Ciesla N. Postural drainage, positioning and breathing exercises. In: Mackenzie CF, Ciesla N, Imle PC, Klemic N, eds: Chest Physiotherapy in the Intensive Care Unit, 2nd ed. Baltimore: Williams & Wilkins, 1981:56.
19. Frownfelter DL. Postural drainage. In: Frownfelter DL, ed. Chest Physical Therapy and Pulmonary Rehabilitation. Chicago: Year Book Medical Publishers, 1987:271–287.
20. Kaneko K, Milic-Emili J, Dolovich MB, et al. Regional distribution of ventilation and perfusion as a function of body position. J Appl Physiol 1966; 21:767–777.
21. Thadani U, Parker JO. Hemodynamics at rest and during supine and sitting bicycle exercise in normal subjects. Am J Cardiol 1978; 41:52–59.
22. Tobin MJ. Respiratory muscles in disease. Clin Chest Med 1988; 9:263–286.
23. Braun NMT, Arora NS, Rochester DF. Force-length relationship of the normal human diaphragm. J Appl Physiol 1982; 53:405–412.
24. DeTroyer A, Pride NB. The respiratory system in neuromuscular disorders. In: Roussos C, Macklem PT, eds. The Thorax. Part B. New York: Marcel Dekker, 1985:1089–1121.
25. Rochester DF, Braun NMT. Determinants of maximal inspiratory pressure in chronic obstructive pulmonary disease. Am Rev Respir Dis 1985; 132:42–47.
26. Kigin CM. Observation of tracheal transport in intubated anesthetized dogs. Laboratory study performed at George Washington University Hospital, 1974.
27. Bateman J, Duant K, Newman S, et al. Regional lung clearance of excessive bronchial secretions during chest physiotherapy in patients with stable chronic airflow obstruction. Lancet 1979; 1:294–297.
28. Chopra S, Taplin G, Simmons D. Effects of hydration and physical therapy on tracheal transport velocity. Am Rev Respir Dis 1977; 115:1009–1014.
29. Mazzacco M, Owens G, Kirillof L, et al. Chest percussion and postural drainage in patients with bronchiectasis. Chest 1985; 88:360–363.

30. Cochrane G, Webber B, Clarke S. Effects of sputum on pulmonary function. Br Med J 1977; 2:1181–1183.
31. Denton R. Bronchial secretions in cystic fibrosis: the effects of treatment with mechanical percussion and vibration. Am Rev Respir Dis 1962; 86:41.
32. Mackenzie C. Physiological changes following chest physical therapy. In: Mackenzie C, Imle PC, Ciesla N, eds. Chest Physiotherapy in the Intensive Care Unit, 2nd ed. Baltimore: Williams & Wilkins, 1989:215–250.
33. Lorin M, Denning C. Evaluation of postural drainage by measurement of sputum volume and consistency. Am J Phys Med 1971; 50:215–219.
34. Sutton P, Lopez-Vidriero M, Pavia D, et al. Assessment of percussion, vibratory shaking and breathing exercises in chest physiotherapy. Eur J Respir Dis 1985; 66:147–152.
35. Campbell A, O'Connel J, Wilson F. The effect of chest physiotherapy upon the FEV_1 in chronic bronchitis. Med J Aust 1975; 1:33–35.
36. Newton D, Stevenson A. Effect of physiotherapy on pulmonary function. A laboratory study. Lancet 1978; 2:228–229.
37. Wollmer P, Ursing K, Midgren B, et al. Inefficiency of chest percussion in the physical therapy of chronic bronchitis. Eur J Respir Dis 1985; 66:233–239.
38. Irwin R, Rosen M, Braman S. Cough: a comprehensive review. Arch Intern Med 1977; 137:1186–1191.
39. Pryor J, Webber B, Hodson M. Evaluation of the forced expiration technique as an adjunct to postural drainage in treatment of cystic fibrosis. Br Med J 1979; 2:417–418.
40. Sutton P, Parker R, Webber B, et al. Assessment of the forced expiration technique, postural drainage and directed coughing in chest physiotherapy. Eur J Respir Dis 1983; 64:62–68.
41. Van Hengstrum M, Festen J, Beurskens C, et al. No effect of oral high frequency oscillation combined with forced expiration manouevers on tracheobronchial clearance in chronic bronchitics. Eur Respir J 1990; 3:14–18.
42. Clarke S. Management of mucus hypersecretion. Eur J Respir Dis 1987; 153 (Suppl 71):S136–S144.
43. Pavia D. The role of chest physiotherapy in mucus hypersecretion. Lung 1990; (Suppl 168):S614–S621.
44. Van Hengstrum M, Festen J, Beurskens C, et al. Convential physiotherapy and forced expiration technique manoeuvers have similar effects on tracheobronchial clearance. Eur Respir J 1988; 1:758–761.
45. Huber A, Eggleston P, Morgan J. Effect of chest physiotherapy in asthmatic children. J Allergy Clin Immunol 1974; 53:109 (abstract).
46. Feldman J, Traver G, Taussig L. Maximal expiratory flow after postural drainage. Am Rev Respir Dis 1979; 119:239–245.
47. Mackenzie C, Shin B, McAslan T. Chest physiotherapy: the effect on arterial oxygenation. Anesth Analg 1978; 57:28–30.
48. Mackenzie C, Shin B, Hadi F, et al. Changes in total lung/thorax compliance following chest physiotherapy. Anesth Analg 1980; 59:207–210.
49. Leith DE, Bradley M. Ventilatory muscle strength and endurance training. J Appl Physiol 1976; 41:508–516.

50. Keens TG, Krastins IR, Wannamaker EM, et al. Ventilatory muscle endurance training in normal subjects and patients with cystic fibrosis. Am Rev Respir Dis 1977; 116:853–860.
51. Belman MJ, Mittman C. Ventilatory muscle training improves exercise capacity in chronic obstructive pulmonary disease patients. Am Rev Respir Dis 1980; 121:273–280.
52. Jederlinic P, Muspratt JA, Miller MJ. Inspiratory muscle training in clinical practice: physiologic conditioning or habituation to suffocation. Chest 1984; 86:870–873.
53. Mahler DA, Weinberg DH, Wells CK, Feinstein AR. Measurement of dyspnea: contents, interobserver agreement, and physiologic correlates of two new clinical indexes. Chest 1984; 85:751–758.
54. Saltin B, Blomquist G, Mitchell JH, et al. Response to exercise after bedrest and after training. Circulation 1968; 38(Suppl VII):SVII1–78.
55. Robinson EP, Kjeldgäard JM. Improvement in ventilatory muscle function with running. J Appl Physiol 1982; 52:1400–1406.
56. Wolff RK, Dolovich MB, Obminski G, et al. Effects of exercise and eucapnic hyperventilation on bronchial clearance in man. J Appl Physiol 1977; 43:46–50.
57. Zadai CC, Bourgeois MC, Jette D. Unpublished clinical data utilizing 6-min walk tests, modified Borg Scale and the Functional status questionnaire pre- and post-exercise conditioning (9,59,60).
58. Pollock ML, Wilmore JH, Fox SM. Exercise in Health and Disease: Evaluation and Prescription for Prevention and Rehabilitation. Philadelphia: WB Saunders, 1984.
59. Guyatt GH. Use of the six-minute walk test as an outcome in clinical trials in chronic heart failure. Heart Failure 1987; Oct/Nov:211–217.
60. Borg GAV. Psychophysical bases of perceived exertion. Med Sci Sports Exerc 1982; 14:377–381.
61. Bergner M, Bobbitt RA, Pollard WE, et al. The Sickness Impact Profile: validation of a health status measure. Med Care 1976; 14:57–67.
62. Hyland ME. Quality-of-life assessment in respiratory disease: an examination of the content and validity of four questionnaires. Pharmac Econom 1992; 2:43–53.
63. McSweeny AJ, Grant I, Heaton RK, et al. Life quality in patients with chronic obstructive pulmonary disease. Arch Intern Med 1982; 142:473–478.
64. Guyatt GH, Berman LN, Townsend M, et al. A measure of quality of life for clinical trials in chronic lung disease. Thorax 1987; 42:773–778.
65. Guyatt GH, Thompson PJ, Berman LB, et al. How should we measure function in patients with chronic heart and lung disease? J Chronic Dis 1985; 6:517–524.

21

Therapeutic Exercise in Chronic Lung Disease

MICHAEL J. BELMAN

Cedars Sinai Medical Center
and UCLA School of Medicine
Los Angeles, California

Exercise is widely promoted as a means of improving physical endurance. It is recommended not only for the healthy, but also for individuals with various disabilities and diseases. Respiratory medicine has witnessed several decades of investigation directed not only at elucidating the pathophysiology of exercise in patients with chronic obstructive pulmonary disease (COPD), but also at examining the effects of exercise training in improving the functional capabilities of the individual. As was initially the case with coronary artery disease, many physicians of the mid-20th century discouraged patients with significant COPD from exercising. Although Dr. Alvin L. Barach, a pioneer in pulmonary medicine, had pleaded in the 1940s and 1950s for more physical exercise in patients with chronic lung disease, it was only in the late 1960s and early 1970s that his ideas were aggressively pursued (1). Currently, pulmonary rehabilitation programs in the United States and Europe, almost without exception, include a liberal measure of exercise training. The transfer of standard recommendations for exercise training from healthy subjects and even cardiac patients to pulmonary patients has not been easy. The exercise response in COPD presents some unusual, and in some cases unique, features that require rethinking of the traditional advice given to the normal subject and to individuals with heart disease. The purpose of this chapter is to review key features of the exercise pattern in COPD and to analyze the evidence that supports the use of exercise training in pulmonary rehabilitation.

It now appears that exercise training is a prerequisite to improving exercise tolerance. Those programs that offer only education do not improve exercise endurance. However, the proper amount of exercise is still unsettled; the intensity, frequency, and duration of exercise training vary greatly from clinic to clinic, and structured, high-intensity programs have not been shown to provide better results than more liberal, laissez-faire programs in which patients are encouraged to exercise to tolerance or ad libitum. In the past few years increasing attention has been paid to how the benefits obtained from the use of treadmills and cycle ergometers compare with the activities of daily living (ADLs). And because of the importance of breathlessness in compromising functional capability in lung disease, the effect of exercise training on minimizing dyspnea is also under close scrutiny.

I. Exercise Training as Part of Rehabilitation

Although exercise training has been used for the past three and a half decades, it is only recently that several randomized control studies have shown that exercise training is a critical component of a rehabilitation program (2–5). Toshima and Ries randomized 119 patients with COPD either to a comprehensive rehabilitation program including exercise reconditioning or, alternatively, to an education control program (2). The test group received education, physical and respiratory therapy, psychosocial support, and supervised exercise training for 8 weeks whereas the control group received twice-weekly classroom instruction in respiratory therapy, pharmacology, and diet, in addition to information about their lung disease, but did not exercise. Before and after the treatment and after an additional 6 months, both groups underwent extensive physiological and psychosocial tests. The major finding of this study was that at 8 weeks, the improvement in exercise endurance, measured by treadmill walking, showed a mean increase in treadmill time from 12.5 min to 23 min as compared to an insignificant change, i.e., from 12 to 13 min in the control group. At 6 months, the treated group maintained its advantage, i.e., treadmill endurance of approximately 21 min compared to 12 min in the control group. No difference in a quality of well-being scale, a measure of health-related quality of life, was noted. This well-designed, randomized, controlled study provides strong support for the idea that exercise therapy is an essential component of the pulmonary rehabilitation process.

A second randomized control study by O'Donnell et al. compared both exercise tolerance and dyspnea before and after an exercise program (3). The exercise included both upper- and lower-limb training, and patients were encouraged to exercise to tolerance without particular attention to target heart rates or metabolic rates. In contrast to the control group, which manifested little change in exercise capacity or breathlessness, the treated group showed a significant decrease in breathlessness during an incremental exercise test. Moreover, the slope of the relationship between breathlessness and minute ventilation decreased in the treated group along with a decrease in the ventilatory equivalent for oxygen. These changes represent a greater decrease in dyspnea than in minute ventilation as well as an improvement in breathing efficiency. The treated group also showed improvement in the performance of the 6-min walk, and breathlessness, measured by the transitional dyspnea index and the chronic respiratory questionnaire, decreased during ADL.

A third study focused on dyspnea and exercise in 20 patients randomized to treatment and control groups (5). Training followed a light schedule of biweekly training to tolerance. The study showed a decrease in dyspnea at the maximal treadmill workload and a decrease in the slope of the relationships between dyspnea and minute ventilation and dyspnea to oxygen consumption; the transitional dyspnea index also decreased in the control group. Thus, the studies by O'Donnell et al. and Reardon et al. showed both significant improvements in exercise capacity and clinically important reductions in dyspnea following pulmonary rehabilitation (3,5).

A more recent study reinforced the idea that exercise training is an important ingredient of an outpatient rehabilitation program (4). The patients exercised at home for 12 weeks for two half-hour sessions per day; the exercises included stretching, arm and leg cycling, and inspiratory muscle training. The maximal work rate and all components of the chronic respiratory questionnaire improved. However, even though exercise was found to be a critical component of the increase in endurance, this study found no correlation between increase in exercise capacity and the decrease in breathlessness.

II. Exercise Prescription

The American College of Sports and Medicine has made recommendations concerning the prescription of appropriate levels of exercise, and recent reviews have dealt with duration, intensity, and frequency (6,7). According to these recommendations, aerobic training calls for rhythmical, dynamic activity of large muscles performed 3–4 times a week for 20–30 min per session at an intensity corresponding to at least 50% of the maximal oxygen consumption. Alternative methods of regulating intensities use 60% of the maximum heart rate or 50% of the heart rate reserve. A program of aerobic training, as outlined above, is capable of inducing structural and physiological adaptations that provide the trained individual with improved endurance for performance of high-intensity activity. The characteristic physiological response is an increase in the $\dot{V}O_2max$, which is a result of an increase in both the maximum cardiac output and the arteriovenous difference in oxygen content. At comparable metabolic rates, the heart rate is slower and the minute ventilation is decreased at work rates above the anaerobic threshold.

The structural changes in the skeletal muscle of the trained limbs have been summarized elsewhere (8). In general, the oxidative enzymes and mitochondrial density increase in both the type 1 and type 2 muscle fibers. Myoglobin levels also increase. An increase in the density of muscle capillaries accounts for the reduction in the diffusion distance for oxygen between the red blood cells and the mitochondria in the muscle cell.

III. Lactic Acidosis

Lactic acid is produced during incremental exercise. When it appears in arterial blood depends on circulatory function and the level of fitness. The point at which the concentration of lactate in blood increases has been termed the "lactate threshold"; it precedes by approximately 150 ml of $\dot{V}O_2$ the increase in minute ventilation related to the increase in CO_2 output (9,10). This increase in ventilation can be detected by several indices of gas exchange, but recently, the use of the V-slope criterion has been emphasized (11). Using this index, the rate of rise in CO_2 output is plotted against O_2 uptake; whereas O_2 uptake remains linear at the onset of lactic acid production, CO_2 output increases, so a breakpoint can be discerned. This inflection point was originally termed the "anaerobic threshold"; other investigators have since preferred the term "ventilation threshold."

The difference in terminology reflects difference in concept: whereas Wasserman et al., the original proponents, feel that the appearance of lactic acid indicates a transition to anaerobic glycolysis because of tissue hypoxia, others consider that the increase in blood lactic acid during exercise does not necessarily imply anaerobiosis but, instead, may simply reflect an imbalance between lactate production, on the one hand, and its utilization, on the other (12,13). Nonetheless, in patients with COPD, even those with moderately severe disease, lactic acid and anaerobic thresholds can be determined (14). However, the peak lactate levels will be lower in patients with COPD because of their overall reduction in exercise capacity (14,15). The lactic acid probably arises from working limb muscles and not the ventilatory muscles since it is the patients who reach the highest work rates who show the highest blood lactate levels (15). Conversely, patients with very severe obstructive disease, in whom respiratory muscle work is high, have low blood lactate levels, and their lactate levels during isocapnic hypernea are only marginally increased (16).

The reliability of the V-slope criterion in detecting metabolic acidosis in these patients is debatable (Fig. 1) (14,17). In a recent study, not only was there considerable interobserver variability in V-slope detection, but a considerable number of patients with exercise-induced metabolic acidosis did not manifest inflection points. Conversely, inflection points were found in patients without metabolic acidosis. This finding detracts from the value of the V slope in detecting metabolic acidosis in patients with COPD.

IV. Exercise Prescription in COPD

Two approaches to exercise prescription in patients with COPD are in current use: the first entails a highly structured approach that is directed at achieving specific exercise intensities to induce aerobic training responses; the second uses a looser, more informal approach in which patients are encouraged to exercise to tolerance or ad libitum without specific targets or goals.

CO_2 output is the major drive to ventilation during exercise (18). Based on the following well-known formulation, Casaburi and Wasserman suggested

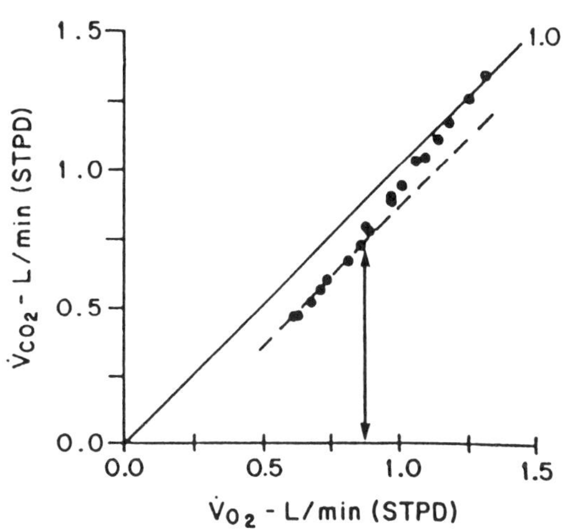

Figure 1 Carbon dioxide output ($\dot{V}CO_2$) plotted against oxygen uptake ($\dot{V}O_2$). When the anaerobic threshold is reached, $\dot{V}CO_2$ accelerates compared with $\dot{V}O_2$. The infection point marking this acceleration is shown by the arrows. (Reproduced with permission from Ref. 14.)

that aerobic training in patients with COPD would reduce CO_2 output and the ventilatory stimulus.

$$\dot{V}_E = \frac{k\ \dot{V}CO_2}{PaCO_2}(1 - V_D/V_T)$$

where $\dot{V}_E$ is expired minute ventilation, $\dot{V}CO_2$ is carbon dioxide output, $PaCO_2$ is partial pressure of arterial CO_2, and V_D/V_T is the ratio of the physiological dead space to tidal volume; *k* is a constant.

The lactic acid produced during exercise is buffered mainly by bicarbonate with the generation of carbonic acid, which dissociates to CO_2 and H_2O. The CO_2 produced by the buffering of lactic acid must be excreted by the lungs in addition to CO_2 produced by muscle metabolism during exercise. Exercise training delays the rise in blood lactate. Thus, any delay in lactic acid production will, by reducing the CO_2 load, decrease the ventilatory requirements during exercise. The effect of aerobic training and reduction in $\dot{V}_E$ during exercise has been well documented in normal subjects. At high levels of work near peak $\dot{V}O_2$, large reductions of 30–40 L/min in $\dot{V}_E$ can be achieved in normal individuals (15).

With this rationale in mind, a study was conducted in which high-intensity and low-intensity training was performed in patients with COPD and the effects on lactate production were examined in considerable detail (15). Training was performed on a calibrated cycle ergometer 5 days a week for 8 weeks. The major results of this study were in the high-intensity group, which showed a reduction in the peak $\dot{V}CO_2$ and in the maximal ventilatory equivalent for oxygen ($\dot{V}_E/\dot{V}O_2$). At a high work rate, constant load test, the high-intensity trained group showed significant reductions in blood lactate, $\dot{V}_E$, $\dot{V}CO_2$, $\dot{V}O_2$, and the ($\dot{V}_E/\dot{V}O_2$). In addition, the heart rate at comparable work rates was reduced. These findings confirm the development of a true aerobic training effect (Fig. 2). On the other hand, the group who trained at low intensity showed smaller changes in these variables even though the total work performed was similar. In this group, although the decrease in lactate was significant (10%), the decrements in $\dot{V}_E$, $\dot{V}CO_2$, and $\dot{V}O_2$, were not. Furthermore, a significant increase in endurance during high-intensity, single-stage work rate was seen in the high-intensity-trained group (6.6–11.4 min), but was not seen in the low-intensity-trained group (6.9–7.5 min). A significant relationship was found between the decrease in minute ventilation during exercise and the decrease in blood lactate ($r = 0.73$, delta $\dot{V}_E = 2.46$ L/min per mEq lactate). The slope of the $\Delta\dot{V}_E/\Delta$ lactate relationship in these patients (Fig. 3) was considerably lower than that found in a previous study on normal subjects in whom the $\dot{V}_E$ decreased by 7.2 L/min for each mEq decrease in lactate.

This study clearly shows that: (1) during exercise, lactic acidemia occurs

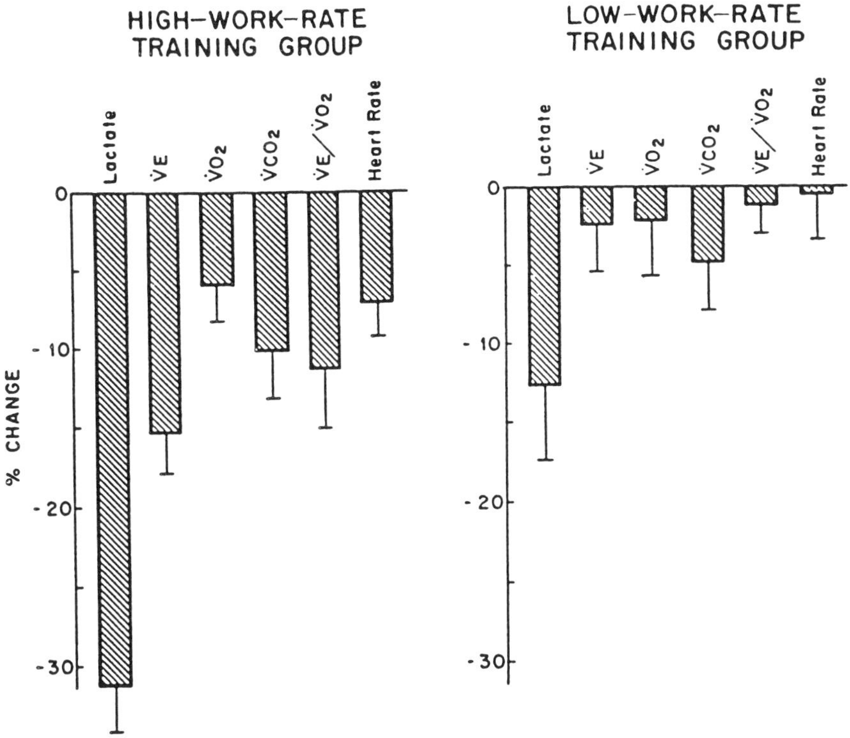

Figure 2 Changes in physiological responses to identical exercise tasks in high and low work rate training group. (Reproduced with permission from Ref. 15.)

in patients with mild to moderate COPD, and in some instances, this may develop at low work rates (unloaded cycling); (2) both high- and low-intensity training reduce the increase in lactate, but the effect is considerably greater in patients who undergo high-intensity training; and (3) although lactate levels and $\dot{V}_E$ are lower after training in patients with COPD, the decrease in ventilation in patients is only about one-third of the decrease seen in normal subjects. The reason for this difference is attributed to the decrease in the ventilatory response of patients with COPD to the lactic acidosis of exercise; therefore, a decrease in lactic acid after training elicits a smaller decrease in $\dot{V}_E$. The study did not attempt either to quantify dyspnea or the health-related quality of life.

This study clearly shows the development of an aerobic training response. However, it has some limitations with respect to its applicability to the usual candidates for pulmonary rehabilitation: the patients were relatively young (49 years old on average), the obstructive disease was mild ($FEV_1 = 56\%$ of predicted; $FEV_1/FVC = 58\%$). These values are better than those generally found

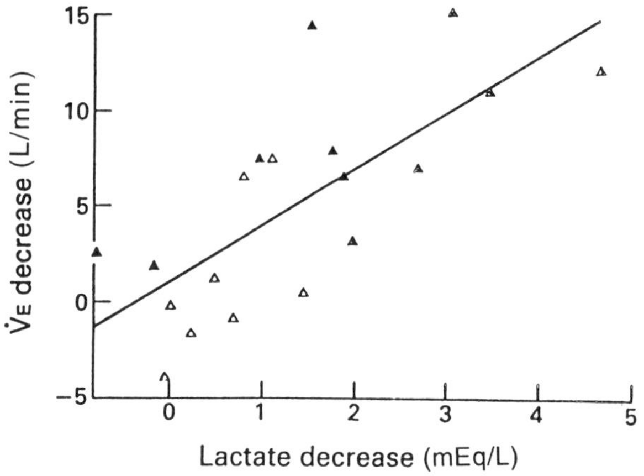

Figure 3 Relationship between the decrease in ventilation and the decrease in arterial lactate resulting from a program of exercise training. The test was at a high, constant work rate. ▲, high work rate trained group; △, low work rate trained group. Solid line is obtained by linear regression. $\Delta\dot{V}_E = 2{\cdot}84$, Δlactate $= 1{\cdot}19$. (Reproduced with permission from Ref. 15.)

in most rehabilitation programs (5,19). Moreover, before the training, the patients were relatively unfit as shown by the pretraining lactate threshold, i.e., at values for $\dot{V}O_2$ less than 1 L/min. It is not surprising, therefore, that they responded dramatically to the exercise program. Similar studies in a more severely affected group of patients would be helpful before the exercise recommendations of this report can be generalized (20).

V. Exercise Training to Tolerance

Exercise testing and training directed at manipulation of blood lactate involves complex measurements and contrasts sharply with exercising to tolerance (19). Even though the latter method does not decrease blood lactate, patients with severe COPD—some of them with extreme hypercapnia—can be exercised safely with impressive gains in submaximal exercise endurance and decrements in minute ventilation and breathlessness (21). This is particularly striking in the study of Niederman et al., in which the greatest percentage improvements were seen in those patients with the lowest FEV_1s and low pretraining exercise endurances (22). In this study, the training was done without emphasis on intensity, patients being allowed to choose their own exercise level. Exercise sessions were conducted three times a week for 2 hr for a total of 9 weeks. During each session, the time was divided among cycling, treadmill walking, and lifting weights. The most impressive gains were in cycle endurance, which increased from 129.5 to 726.1 watt/min. Similar results were obtained by Holle et al., who showed large increases in treadmill endurance (23).

High-intensity training has resulted in results comparable to those above obtained by exercising to tolerance (24,25). Thus, large gains in endurance were achieved through high-intensity training that involved achievement of maximum levels of ventilation (24,25). However, the investigators were quick to point out that their results do not imply that a high-intensity training regimen is necessary for patients with COPD. In fact, both high-intensity and low-intensity training accomplished similar gains in endurance and both approaches appear to be effective in the moderate to severely affected patient (26). As a corollary, there seems to be no intrinsic benefit to recommending training at almost maximal ventilatory capacity. High-intensity exercise may also be disadvantageous because of the higher risk of injury and because the discomfort of extreme exercise may reduce compliance with exercise programs (27). The results of studies that compare high-intensity training to those that used unstructured approaches are summarized in Table 1.

VI. Reductions in Minute Ventilation Without Change in the Anaerobic Threshold

Two studies, in addition to those cited above, demonstrate that reduction in ventilation may occur even in the absence of changes in the anaerobic threshold (3,5). Although no measurements of blood lactate were made, the exercise intensities were generally so low as to make it unlikely that the protocols would generate aerobic training responses. Nevertheless, in both studies, reductions in ventilation occurred at comparable oxygen consumptions, presumably because of an increase in the efficiency of breathing or a decrease in anxiety (3). Thus, a wide variety of training regimens seem to produce improvements in exercise endurance. Indeed, a recent review of the literature on exercise training showed that despite a wide variety of training protocols, 31 of 32 training programs increased endurance (7).

VII. Strength Training

Although the emphasis on training has concentrated on endurance activities, recent evidence supports an important role for peripheral muscle strength. One-third of patients with COPD implicate muscle fatigue as the limiting factor during exercise (28). Muscle fatigue was the limiting factor even in patients

Table 1 Exercise Training in COPD

	Casaburi 1991 (15)	Punzal 1991 (24)	Niederman 1991 (22)	Reardon 1994 (5)	Wijkstra 1994 (4)	Strijbos 1989 (35)
Number of patients	9	57	24	10 trained, 10 control[a]	28 trained, 15 control[a]	30 trained, 15 control[a]
FEV_1/FVC	58%	44%	50%	40%	39%	36%
Intensity	High, above AT	1. V_{Emax} 2. at AT	Unstructured Laissez-faire	Unstructured	75% Wmax	Not given
Frequency	5/week	Daily TM	3/week	12 × 3 hr	12 min BID	2 × week
Duration	8 weeks IP 45′ cycle	Supervised 2/week × 4 and then 1/week × 4 free daily unsupervised walking	9 weeks 20′ or cycle, TM, UE	6 weeks	12 weeks	12 weeks
Test	Cycle endurance 6.6–11.4 min AT ↑	Treadmill endurance 12.1–22.0 min	Cycle endurance 5.0–12.0 min 12-min walk ↑	Cycle endurance 5.7–7.7 min		
Peak Vo_2	10% ↑	10% ↑	19% ↑	NS	Wmax ↑ 10%	Wmax ↑
Psychosocial	Not measured	Breathlessness ↓ Fatigue ↓	Depression ↓ Disability ↓	Breathlessness ↓ Breathlessness/V_{Emax}	CRQ dyspnea ↓	Borg dyspnea ↓ Borg leg fatigue ↓

[a]Control group: Changes not significant. IP = inpatient; AT = anaerobic threshold; TM = treadmill; NS = not significant; CRQ = chronic respiratory questionnaire.

with marked reduction in FEV_1. A weight-lifting program in these patients, coupled with arm- and leg-strengthening exercises, resulted in gains in strength in arms and legs, increase in cycle ergometer endurance, and a decrease in symptoms as measured by the Chronic Respiratory Questionnaire (29). Thus, strength training is an important component of overall training regimens.

VIII. Upper-Extremity Exercise and Training

Activity of the upper limbs aggravates impaired diaphragmatic function in patients with COPD (30). During arm work, the stabilizing effect of the shoulder-to-shoulder girdle on the thorax is lost and the inspiratory load is shifted onto the diaphragm and muscles of expiration. In these circumstances, although the diaphragm is required to assume a greater load, it is ill prepared to do so. The net result in many patients with severe COPD is a greater limitation of arm exercise than of leg exercise, accompanied by an earlier onset of dyspnea (Fig. 4). Performance of many ADL requires arm work, an important requirement for patients with COPD. The specificity of arm training is emphasized by the findings of Lake et al., who randomized patients to one of three groups (31): a control group who received no training; a group that received upper-limb training only; and a group that underwent combined upper- and lower-limb training. Upper-limb training included cycle ergometry with varying resistances, throwing a ball against a wall with the arms above the horizontal, passing a beanbag over the head, and arm exercise with ropes and pulleys. Lower-limb exercise was tested by cycle ergometry and a 6-min walk distance. Training was continued for 1 hr, three times a week, for 8 weeks. The results showed that limb training was limb-specific: only in the group that trained with the upper extremity did upper-extremity endurance increase whereas walk distance improved only in the lower-limb-trained group; the combination-trained group showed improvements in both upper- and lower-limb endurance. A modified quality-of-life questionnaire showed significant changes only in the group that received combined upper- and lower-limb training.

Other studies have confirmed the value of arm training in increasing arm endurance and in decreasing the metabolic cost of arm exercise (32,33). The improved endurance, in conjunction with the reduced metabolic cost, is indicative of improved mechanical efficiency of movement of the arms and possibly breathing muscles during arm activity. However, another study revealed that even though patients who underwent the upper-extremity training improved their performance on an arm cycle ergometer, they did not improve performance in arm ADL (34).

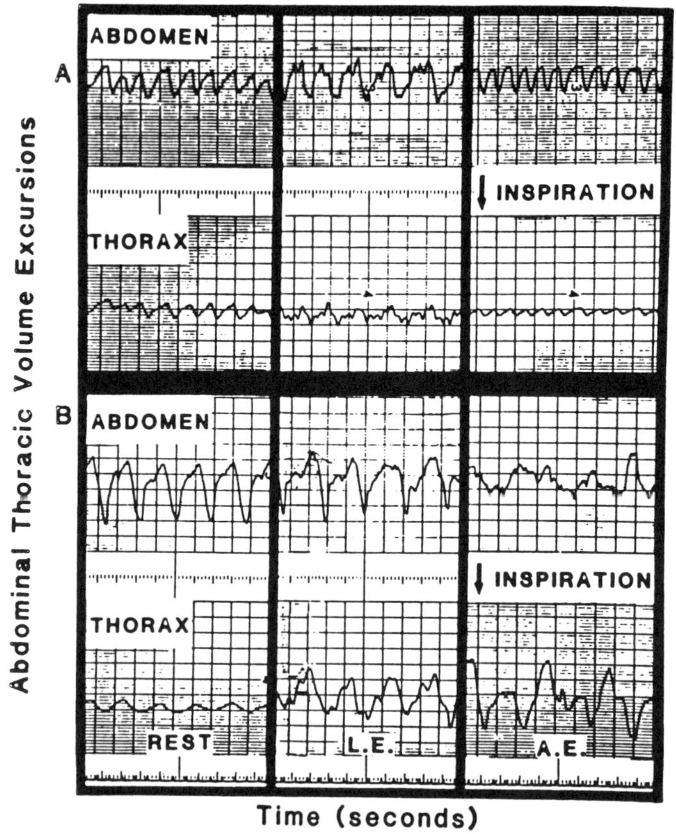

Figure 4 Tracing of abdominal and thoracic excursions. (A) Excursions in a patient with synchronous thoracoabdominal movements at rest during leg exercise (LE) and arm exercise (AE). (B) The synchronous pattern observed at rest and during LE changed to dyssynchronous during AE. Full inward retraction during inspiration is seen in the last two breaths of the arm exercise tracing. (Reproduced with permission from Ref. 30.)

IX. Dyspnea

Dyspnea, or breathlessness, is a major symptom in patients with lung disease and is often the reason for stopping exercise or ADL. It has repeatedly been shown that exercise training decreases breathlessness (3–5,35). Several mechanisms have been examined as possible causes of the decrease in dyspnea in COPD patients postrehabilitation: (1) improvement in pulmonary function; (2) improvement in ventilatory muscle function; (3) a true aerobic training effect;

or (4) increased tolerance of desensitization to dyspnea. Of these four, the first three have not withstood scrutiny as major influences (15,36,37). However, the last, involving psychological factors, is still plausible.

That psychological factors play a role in the genesis of dyspnea in COPD has been repeatedly emphasized (38–40). Both anxiety and depression influence dyspnea. Dyspnea is also affected by attitudes and beliefs. Over 20 years ago, Agle and co-workers showed that relief of dyspnea in COPD was associated with amelioration of depression and anxiety (41). More recent work has suggested that tolerance to dyspnea may be altered favorably in COPD so that higher levels of work can be performed with less dyspnea (42–44). This type of evidence suggests that in a medically controlled environment in which patients are given support and encouragement, patients with dyspnea can learn to overcome the anxiety and apprehension associated with their dyspnea. Progressive exercise may lead to a decrease in the unrealistic fear of activity and dyspnea. This desensitization, i.e., increased tolerance to dyspnea, may be a key component of the improved endurance after exercise. Further investigation is necessary to clarify mechanisms of this increased tolerance to dyspnea.

Much of the early work in exercise training was conducted by pulmonary specialists who focused on pulmonary function testing, arterial blood gases, hemodynamic indices, and measurements of gas exchange. However, since these indices have generally proved to be of little clinical relevance, increasing attention is now directed at measures of functional capacity, including performance of ADLs and relief of breathlessness. In addition, quality-of-life measures are being applied to COPD patients with the understanding that the health-related aspect of the quality of life (HRQL) is of the greatest importance to these patients. These indices of function provide a measure of the impact of an individual's health on his or her ability to participate in and enjoy daily life (40). It is important to underscore that they correlate poorly with indices of pulmonary function and arterial blood gases (Fig. 5), and the effectiveness of exercise training can be assessed only in terms of functional outcomes rather than physiological measurements.

X. Summary

Sporadic visits to the doctor, followed by changes in oral or inhaled bronchodilators and by the addition of steroids, often do little to relieve symptoms and function in the patient disabled with COPD. As in other chronic diseases, the management of these patients is facilitated by a team approach in conjunction with general rehabilitation principles. The rationale and practical implementation of such a program have recently been outlined by the American Associa-

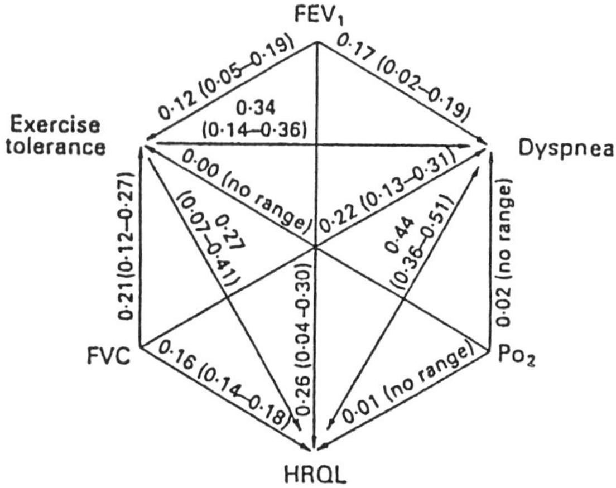

Figure 5 Squared correlation coefficients (R^2) between health-related quality of life (HRQL), dyspnea scale, pulmonary physiological parameters, demographic characteristics, and psychological states. R^2 can be viewed as an estimate of the proportion of the variability in HRQL or dyspnea that is explained by measures of pulmonary function, oxygenation, and exercise tolerance. The numbers represent the median of the R^2 values and the ranges are in parentheses. (Reproduced with permission from Ref. 40.)

tion of Cardiopulmonary Rehabilitation. The programs are multifaceted and include exercise training as a key component.

However, uncertainty persists about the optimal method of training. Two main approaches to exercise training can be delineated: one emphasizes the detailed definition of the impaired physiology and relies on therapeutic measures targeted to specific defects. In contrast are the unstructured programs, which use treadmill and free-range walking and cycling. However, both the high-intensity structured programs and the low-intensity programs improve endurance for walking. Upper-extremity training is of additional benefit for improving arm endurance although definitive proof of improved performance of ADLs is still lacking.

Programs with as little as two to three sessions per week of light exercise have proved successful. Moreover, since they obviate the need for complex testing and training, these programs can be implemented at relatively low cost. Future research will concentrate on delineating the essential components of rehabilitation that reliably and significantly improve important functional outcomes. A recent conference sponsored by the NIH has summarized key findings of past studies and emphasized important courses for future action (45).

References

1. Barach AL, Bickerman HA, Beck G. Advance in the treatment of nontuberculous pulmonary disease. Bull NY Acad Med 1952; 28:353–384.
2. Toshima MT, Ries AL. Experimental evaluation of rehabilitation in chronic obstructive pulmonary disease: short-term effects on exercise endurance and health status. Health Psychol 1990; 9:237–252.
3. O'Donnell DE, Webb KA, McGuire MA. Older patients with COPD: benefits of exercise training. Geriatrics 1993; 48:59–66.
4. Wijkstra PJ, Van Altena R, Kraan J, Otten V, Postma DS, Koeter GH. Quality of life in patients with chronic obstructive pulmonary disease improves after rehabilitation at home. Eur Respir J 1994; 7:269–273.
5. Reardon J, Awad E, Normandin E, Vale F, Clark B, ZuWallack RL. The effect of comprehensive outpatient pulmonary rehabilitation on dyspnea. Chest 1994; 105:1046–1052.
6. American College of Sports Medicine. The recommended quantity and quality of exercise for developing and maintaining cardiorespiratory and muscular fitness in healthy adults. Med Sci Sports Exerc 1990; 23:265–274.
7. Casaburi R. Exercise training in chronic obstructive lung disease. In: Casaburi R, Petty TL, eds. Principles and Practice of Pulmonary Rehabiliation. Philadelphia: WB Saunders, 1993:204–224.
8. Holloszy JO, Coyle EF. Adaptations of skeletal muscle to endurance exercise and their metabolic consequences. J Appl Physiol 1984; 56:831–838.
9. Wasserman K, Beaver WL. Anaerobic threshold and respiratory gas exchange during exercise. J Appl Physiol 1973; 35:236–243.
10. Wasserman K, Beaver WL, Whipp BJ. Gas exchange theory and the lactic acidosis (anaerobic) threshold. Circulation 1990; 81:II14–30.
11. Beaver WL, Whipp BJ. A new method for detecting anaerobic threshold by gas exchange. J Appl Physiol 1986; 60:2020–2027.
12. Davis JA. Anaerobic threshold: review of the concept and directions for future research. Med Sci Sports Exerc 1985; 17:6–18.
13. Brooks GA. Anaerobic threshold: review of the concept and directions for future research. Med Sci Sports Exerc 1985; 17:22–31.
14. Sue DY, Casaburi R. Metabolic acidosis during exercise in patients with chronic obstructive pulmonary disease. Chest 1988; 94:931–938.
15. Casaburi R, Patessio A, Ioli F, Zanaboni S, Donner CF, Wasserman K. Reductions in exercise lactic acidosis and ventilation as a result of exercise training in patients with obstructive lung disease Am Rev Respir Dis 1991; 143:9–18.
16. Belman MJ, Mittman C. Ventilatory muscle training improves exercise capacity in chronic obstructive pulmonary disease patients. Am Rev Respir Dis 1980; 121:273–280.
17. Belman MJ, Epstein LJ, Doornbos D, Elashoff JD, Koerner SK, Mohsenifar Z. Noninvasive determinations of the anaerobic threshold. Reliability and validity in patients with COPD. Chest 1992; 102:1028–1034.

18. Casaburi R, Wasserman K. Exercise training in pulmonary rehabilitation. N Engl J Med 1986; 314:1509–1511.
19. Ries AL. Position paper of the American Association of Cardiovascular and Pulmonary Rehabilitation. Scientific basis of pulmonary rehabilitation. J Cardiopulm Rehabil 1990; 10:418–441.
20. Belman MJ, Mohsenifar Z. Reductions in exercise lactic acidosis and ventilation as a result of exercise training in patients with obstructive lung disease. Am Rev Respir Dis 1991; 144:1220–1221.
21. Foster S, Thomas HM. Pulmonary rehabilitation in COPD patients with elevated PCO_2. Am Rev Respir Dis 1988; 138:1519–1523.
22. Niederman MS, Clemente PH, Fein AM, et al. Benefits of a multidisciplinary pulmonary rehabilitation program. Improvements are independent of lung function. Chest 1991; 99:798–804.
23. Holle RHO, Williams DV, Vandree JC, Starks GL, Schoene RB. Increased muscle efficiency and sustained benefit in an outpatient community hospital based pulmonary rehabilitation program. Chest 1988; 94:1161–1168.
24. Punzal PA, Ries AL, Kaplan RM, Prewitt LM. Maximum intensity exercise training in patients with chronic obstructive pulmonary disease. Chest 1991; 100:618–623.
25. Carter R, Nicotra B, Clark L, et al. Exercise conditioning in the rehabilitation of patients with chronic obstructive pulmonary disease. Arch Phys Med Rehabil 1988; 69:118–122.
26. McGavin CR, McHardy GJR. Physical rehabilitation for the chronic bronchitic: results of a controlled trial of exercises in the home. Thorax 1977; 32:307–311.
27. Belman MJ, Gaesser GA. Exercise training below and above the lactate threshold in the elderly. Med Sci Sports Exerc 1991; 23:562–568.
28. Killian KJ, LeBlanc P, Martin DH, Summers E, Jones NL, Campbell EJM. Exercise capacity and ventilatory, circulatory, and symptom limitation in patients with chronic airflow limitation. Am Rev Respir Dis 1992; 146:935–940.
29. Simpson K, Killian K, McCartney N, Stubbing DG, Jones NL. Randomised controlled trial of weightlifting exercise in patients with chronic airflow limitation. Thorax 1992; 47:70–75.
30. Celli BR, Make BJ. Dyssynchronous breathing during arm but not leg exercise in patients with chronic airflow obstruction. N Engl J Med 1986; 314:1485–1490.
31. Lake FR, Henderson K, Briffa T, Openshaw J, Musk AW. Upper-limb and lower-limb exercise training in patients with chronic airflow obstruction. Chest 1990; 97:1077–1082.
32. Couser JI, Martinez FJ, Celli BR. Pulmonary rehabilitation that includes arm exercise reduces matabolic and ventialtory requirements for simple arm elevation. Chest 1993; 103:37–41.
33. Martinez FJ, Vogel PD, Dupont DN, Stanopoulos I, Gray AW, Beamis JF. Supported arm exercise vs unsupported arm exercise in the rehabilitation of patients with severe chronic airflow obstruction. Chest 1993; 103:1397–1402.
34. Ries AL, Ellis BE, Hawkins RW. Upper extremity exercise training in chronic obstructive pulmonary disease. Chest 1988; 93:688–692.

35. Strijbos JH, Sluiter HJ, Postma DS, Gimeno F, Koeter GH. Objective and subjective performance indicators in COPD. Eur Respir J 1989; 2:666–669.
36. Smith K, Cook D, Guyatt GH, Madhavan J, Oxman AD. Respiratory muscle training in chronic airflow limitation: a meta-analysis. Am Rev Respir Dis 1992; 145:533–539.
37. Belman MJ, Kendregan BK. Physical training fails to improve ventilatory muscle endurance in patients with chronic obstructive pulmonary. Chest 1982; 81:440–443.
38. Dudley DL, Glaser EM, Jorganson PN. Psychosocial concomitants to rehabilitation in chronic obstructive pulmonary disease. Chest 1980; 77:413–420.
39. Morgan AD, Peck DF, Buchanan DR. Effects of attitudes and beliefs on exercise tolerance in chronic bronchitis. Br Med J 1983; 286:171–173.
40. Curtis JR, Deyo RA, Hudson LD. Health related quality of life among patients with chronic obstructive pulmonary disease. Thorax 1994; 49:162–170.
41. Agle DP, Baum GL, Chester EH, Wendt M. Multidiscipline treatment of chronic pulmonary insufficiency. 1. Psychologic aspects of rehabilitation. Psychosom Med 1973; 41–49.
42. Belman MJ, Brooks LR, Ross DJ, Mohsenifar Z. Variability of breathlessness measurement in patients with chronic obstructive pulmonary disease. Chest 1991; 99:566–571.
43. Levine S, Weiser P, Gillen J. Evaluation of a ventilatory muscle endurance training program in the rehabilitation of patients with COPD. Am Rev Respir Dis 1986; 133:400–406.
44. Carrieri-Kohlman V, Gormley JM, Stulbarg MS. Monitored exercise and coached exercise decrease dyspnea intensity. Ann Behav Med 1993; 15:S168 (abstract).
45. Cole, TM, Fishman AP. Workshop on Pulmonary Rehabilitation Research. A Commentary. NIH Workshop Summary held April 26–28, 1993, in Rockville, Maryland. Am J Phys Med Rehabil 73(2):132–133, 1994.

22

Respiratory Muscle Training

BARTOLOME R. CELLI and HARMEET S. GILL

Tufts University School of Medicine
and St. Elizabeth's Medical Center
Boston, Massachusetts

Maintenance of ventilation depends on the ability of the respiratory pump to move air in and out of the gas exchange portion of the system, the lung. The respiratory muscles constitute a vital link in the pump. Their contraction, during portions of the breathing cycle, changes the anatomical configuration of the thorax and displaces its components so that air moves in and out (1–3). This article reviews the effect of training on respiratory muscles, without losing sight of their special relationship with the other components of the pump: the respiratory centers, the conducting nerves, and the ribcage and abdomen. All these links must function synchronously to guarantee effective ventilation at a low energy cost.

Most of what is known about training and the respiratory muscles relates to patients with chronic airflow obstruction (CAO), because CAO is the condition that afflicts most of the patients in whom training is considered, and for which most of the data has been obtained. Many of the concepts are nevertheless applicable to patients with other pulmonary (restrictive interstitial disease, lung cancer, and lung transplant) and nonpulmonary (chest wall disorders, neuromuscular diseases, pre- and postoperative treatment) conditions. We review the limited data that has been obtained from patients undergoing weaning from mechanical ventilation with the hope that we can stimulate more research in this vital area.

I. Anatomical and Mechanical Considerations

The diaphragm is the best-studied respiratory muscle (2). Normally, it exerts its inflating action on the ribcage by three mechanisms: (1) by using the abdomen as a fulcrum against which it leans, exerting an expanding action on the ribcage, (2) by the vertical and downward orientation of its muscle fibers and the curvature of its shape, and (3) by transmitting the increase in abdominal pressure during contraction to the ribcage, through its zone of apposition (2–5).

The hyperinflation of CAO causes the fibers to become horizontal and the curvature of the diaphragm to decrease. By altering the mechanisms detailed above, flattening of the diaphragm decreases its capacity to generate pressures (6). Recent evidence suggests that the diaphragm adapts to the chronic changes of CAO by shortening the optimal length of its fibers. Under these conditions, each bundle generates its maximal tension for that new length (7,8). If this is correct, the decreased diaphragmatic pressure-generating capacity in patients with CAO is due to mechanical derangement or to contractile dysfunction of the muscle, and not to simple length tension changes.

The external intercostal, the parasternal part of the internal intercostal, and the scalene are essential muscles of respiration, which means that they are active even during quiet breathing in normals (9). Their functional importance increases with the hyperinflation of CAO since they appear to undergo less marked shortening and are at less of a mechanical disadvantage than the diaphragm (10). Other respiratory muscles are called "accessory" inspiratory muscles because they are inactive during quiet breathing in normal subjects. Because of their anatomical arrangement, the accessory muscles may be inspiratory in action under certain circumstances. The sternomastoid, subclavian, pectoralis minor and major, serratus anterior, upper and lower trapezius, and latissimus dorsi hold an extrathoracic anchoring point and a ribcage insertion. If they are fixed on their extrathoracic anchoring point, they may exert a pulling force on the ribcage (11). Except for the sternomastoid and pectoralis, the respiratory function of these muscles has not been fully studied. They are probably inactive during quiet breathing in normal subjects but may participate in ventilation during strenuous circumstances. This may explain the common observation that normal subjects brace their arms after fatiguing exercises.

Three recent studies confirm this observation. Banzett et al. showed that normal volunteers could sustain a higher ventilatory target if their arms were braced on a table than if they were unsupported at the sides (12). Maestro et al. showed that normal volunteers achieved lower work loads when cycling with the arms elevated versus supported on the ergometer handle (13). We have shown that unsupported arm exercise is more limiting than leg exercise in patients with severe chronic obstructive pulmonary disease (COPD). We believe that this is due to derecruitment of these muscles from their ventilatory contribution during unsupported arm activity (14). As we discuss later, these muscles become more important in patients with poorly functioning diaphragms. Understanding their function opens a therapeutic avenue through techniques different from generalized ventilatory muscle training.

The abdominal muscles are considered muscles of expiration. Inasmuch as they oppose diaphragmatic contraction by helping generate abdominal pressure, they are also inspiratory in action. By contracting during expiration, they decrease end-expiratory lung volume, a position in which the chest wall stores elastic energy that assists in the subsequent inspiratory effort (15). We have recently shown that with severe airflow obstruction, there is progressive recruitment of the abdominal muscles of exhalation (16). These observations have recently been confirmed by Ninane et al. using needle electrodes electromyograms (EMG) in patients with different degrees of airflow obstruction (17). It is unclear why patients with the most severe CAO would choose a breathing strategy that compromises already obstructed airways even more. The best explanation is that by recruiting accessory muscles during inspiration and abdominal muscles during expiration, the patients may shift work away from an overworked and inefficient diaphragm.

II. Composition, Metabolism, Blood Flow, and Coordination of the Respiratory Muscles

The diaphragm and other respiratory muscles are composed of striated muscle fibers. The fibers can be of three types: Type I, or slow-twitch oxidative (SO), have well-developed oxidative enzyme systems and are fatigue-resistant. Type II-A, or fast-twitch oxidative glycolytic (FOG), have well-developed oxidative and glycolytic enzyme systems. They are more resistant to fatigue than the fast-twitch glycolytic fibers but not as much as type I-SO fibers. Finally, some fibers possess a well-developed glycolytic enzyme system and have a fast-twitch response to a stimulus. They constitute the fast-twitch glycolytic fibers (FG), or type II-B, and are best suited for fast, powerful activities not requiring endurance. The actual composition of most of the accessory muscles remains unknown. The human diaphragm contains approximately 55% type I or II-A (fatigue-resistant) fibers, perhaps reflecting the enduring work it has to perform through an individual's life (18).

During quiet breathing only a fraction of the fibers (mostly type I fibers) are activated. With progressive efforts (loads) more fibers are recruited. Training involves the loading of muscles so that the fibers may hypertrophy (strength) or change their composition to one that is more fatigue-resistant (endurance).

The state of blood flow and energy supply is very important to achieve good training effect because imbalances in energy supply and demand result in fatigue. Most of what is known about energy and the respiratory muscles concerns the diaphragm. Like the heart, diaphragmatic perfusion occurs preferentially during relaxation and decreases during contraction. The diaphragm is supplied by a well-developed system that is arranged to minimize the decrease in blood flow during inspiration. Two factors determine the contracting compromise of the diaphragm during breathing. The duration of contraction or duty cycle, which can be expressed as the ratio of inspiratory time to total cycle time (TI/TTOT), and the load, which can be described by the relation of the pressure needed to perform the ventilatory effort, as a function of the maximal pressure that the muscle can generate. The latter relationship have been defined as Pdi/Pdi_{max} for the diaphragm or PI/Pi_{max} for the sum of the inspiratory pressure measured at the mouth. The product of both ratios is the tension time index (TTi). The TTi has been shown to relate to electromyographic and other signals of muscle fatigue (19).

Training should attempt to modify the above-mentioned factors: decrease PI, increase P_{imax}, or decrease contraction time. On the other hand, the possibility exists that excessive overload (of already loaded muscles) may lead to more dysfunction and perhaps overt fatigue. Finally, if overt fatigue is present, the best therapeutic avenue is rest, so that the muscle may recover. The ideal therapeutic tool for patients with a weak, compromised respiratory muscle system is a combination of resting and training.

III. Neural Control, Coordination

The diaphragm and the other respiratory muscles are innervated by a wide array of motor neurons that range from cranial nerve 11 (C-11) to lumbar roots L-2 to L-3. The respiratory cycle is regulated by a complex series of centrally organized neurons. This complex arrangement maintains rhythmical breathing that usually goes unnoticed, but can be voluntarily overridden by cortical connections. Since we use primarily the diaphragm, the scalene, and some intercostals to breathe quietly, the system functions without problems. Some of the respiratory muscles serve other purposes. Upper-torso and shoulder girdle muscles participate in positioning of the upper chest and upper extremity, while the diaphragm and muscles of the abdomen partake in the generation of sound (speech, singing), cough, defecation, and parturition.

It has been postulated that the automatic and voluntary ventilatory pathways are different, and that the respiratory and tonic functions of these muscles are driven from different central nervous areas and integrated at the spinal level (20, 21). In patients in whom some of these muscles are participating in respiration to perform nonventilatory work, they must maintain a high degree of coordination. Either because of the load, or because of competing central integration, muscle function may become dyscoordinated and result in dysfunction. We have shown this to occur in patients with CAO who perform unsupported arm exercise. This type of exercise leads to early fatigue of the muscles involved in arm positioning and to dyssynchrony between ribcage and diaphragm-abdomen. This could also be caused by competing outputs of the various driving centers that control rhythmical respiratory and tonic activities of the accessory ventilatory muscles and the diaphragm (14). This dyssynchrony may be perceived as dyspnea. Its occurrence has been observed in normal subjects made to breathe against resistive loads and in patients with CAO breathing during voluntary hyperventilation (22). Likewise, it has been observed in patients immediately after disconnection from ventilators, but before eviendence of contractile fatigue. This suggests that the dyssynchrony is a consequence of the load and not an indication of fatigue itself (23). Whatever the reason, this breathing pattern is innefective and is associated with respiratory muscle dysfunction.

From this review it is clear that training may involve several different approaches and that perhaps simply associating it with strength or endurance is too limiting and simplistic.

IV. Effect of Systemic Training on Respiratory Muscle Function

A. Leg Exercise Conditioning

Exercise conditioning diminishes dyspnea and improves exercise performance and quality of life. There are no studies of patients in the process of weaning that have systematically analyzed the consequence of leg conditioning on the ability to wean. Table 1 shows two randomized studies of patients with COPD in which control groups were included. There were no changes in strength of quadriceps and minute ventilation, but there was a significant increase in 12-min walking distance and peak oxygen uptake (24,25). The study by Sinclair and Ingram showed a significant increase in forced vital capacity. It is only speculative whether this improvement was due to improved respiratory muscle strength.

Numerous studies have used the untreated patients as their own control. Most of them show increased exercise endurance, but the mechanisms responsible for the improvement remain debatable. Some have shown a drop in heart

Table 1 Controlled Studies of Patients with Chronic Airflow Obstruction

Author	No. patients	Duration	Course	Results
Cockroft	18 T	Daily	16 weeks	↑ 12 MW. ↑ Vo_2
	16 C	NT	NT	No change
Sinclair	17 T	Daily	40 weeks	↑ FVC. ↑ 12 MW
	16 C	NT	NT	No change

T = treated; C = controls; 12 MW = 12-min walk test; FVC = forced vital capacity; Vo_2 = peak oxygen uptake; NT = no treatment.

rate at similar work level, a hallmark of training effect; perhaps this effect was due to a decrease in the lactate level during the exercise (26,27). Other studies have not found changes in maximum oxygen uptake or decreases in heart rate or lactate at similar work rate. The study by Belman and Kendregan is interesting because the patients had muscle biopsy specimens taken from the trained limbs. They found no decrease in heart rate for the same work load as represented by $\dot{V}O_2$ and no change in the muscle biopsy enzyme content (28). Nevertheless, they observed improved exercise endurance. They concluded that the improvement was not due to improved cardiovascular or local muscle performance, and the actual reason for the improvement could not be determined.

None of these studies evaluated respiratory muscle function specifically, but it is reasonable to assume a lack of effect since, in most of the studies in which it was measured, no changes were observed in FVC, a test that depends on respiratory muscle strength.

B. Arm Exercise

Much less information exists about the effects of arm training on respiratory function, even though many of the shoulder girdle muscles have a dual (respiratory and postural) function. Tangri and Wolf used a pneumobelt to study seven patients with COPD and showed that they developed an irregular and rapid pattern of breathing with unsupported arm activities (tying shoes, brushing teeth) (29). After the exercise, they breathed deeper. We have documented dyssynchronous thoracoabdominal motions during arm exercise in patients with severe airflow obstruction and shown that they are not due to diaphragmatic fatigue (14).

We have also evaluated ventilatory muscle function during simple arm elevation, arm exercise, and before and after training. Thus, Martinez et al. evaluated the metabolic and respiratory consequences of simple arm elevation to a 90° angle at shoulder level in patients with CAO (16). The results showed a significant increase in $\dot{V}O_2$, $\dot{V}CO_2$, $\dot{V}E$. Using continuous recording of endoesophageal (Ppl), abdominal (Pg), and transdiaphragmatic (Pdi) pressures, we noted that arm elevation increased diaphragmatic and abdominal muscle use and decreased the contribution of the inspiratory muscles of the ribcage. This shift is also present during unsupported arm exercise. We postulated that this shift is due to the recruitment of some of the muscles of the shoulder girdle to help position the arm, with a decrease in their contribution to ventilation. From this analysis it follows that arm training, aimed at allowing the arms to perform more work or to decrease the ventilatory requirement for the same work, could result in improved capacity to perform activities of daily living. Perhaps it could also improve the inspiratory muscle function of those muscles of the shoulder girdle that have a dual function.

Several studies have shown that the addition of arm training to regular leg exercise results in improved task-specific performance (Table 2). One of the studies included six patients who underwent upper-limb exercises only, and there were no differences in pulmonary function, maximal inspiratory and expiratory pressures, and respiratory muscle endurance compared to controls (30). In contrast, Keens et al. studied a group of cystic fibrosis patients using upper-extremity exercise consisting of swimming and rowing. They observed increases in maximum sustained ventilatory capacity that were similar to those achieved by hyperventilatory isocapneic respiratory muscle training and significantly greater than the maximum sustained ventilatory capacity in untreated controls (31).

In a very important study, Ries et al. randomized patients to two forms of arm exercise, gravity resistance exercise (GR), which was low-resistance and highly repetitive, and proprioceptive neuromuscular facilitation (PNF), which involved lower-frequency, progressive resistance training. The control group received the educational component of the program and all patients underwent training in walking. With upper-extremity training, there was improvement in exercise tolerance with a decrease in the perception of effort for the task (32). The authors observed no improvement in respiratory muscle function as measured by the time that the patients could tolerate a resistive breathing run.

In summary, arm exercise improves performance in arm activities and leads to a drop in the metabolic and ventilatory requirements (33,34). Although some studies indicate an improvement in respiratory muscle endurance, more research is needed in this important area.

C. Coordination

As discussed earlier, the breathing apparatus is complex; even more complex is the neuromuscular array responsible for generation of pressures during ventilation. In patients with COPD, as the diaphragm becomes impaired, more and

Table 2 Controlled Studies of Arm Exercise in Patients with Chronic Obstructive Lung Disease

Author	No. patients	Duration	Course	Type	Results
Keens	7 arms	1.5 hr qd	4 wk	Swimming Canoeing	↑ VME (56%)
	4 VMT	15 min qd	4 wk	VMT	↑ VME (52%)
	4 control	NT	NT	VMT	↑ VME (22%)
Belman	8 arms	20 min 4×/wk	6 wk	Arm ergometry	↑ Arm end No ΔPFT
	7 legs	20 min 4×/wk	6 wk	Cycle ergometry	↑ Leg end No ΔPFT
Lake	6 arms	1 hr 3×/wk	8 wk	Several types	No change PImax, VME
	6 legs	1 hr 3×/wk	8 wk	Walking	No change PImax, VME
	7 arms and legs	1 hr 3×/wk	8 wk	Combined	No change PImax, VME
Ries	8 gravity resistance	15 min qd	6 wk	Low resistance High repetition	↑ Arm end
	9 neuro-muscular facilitation	15 min qd	6 wk	Weight lifts	↑ Arm end
	11 controls	NT	6 wk	Walk	No change
Epstein	13 arm	30 min qd	8 wk	UAE	↓ $\dot{V}O_2$ and VE for arm elevation ↑ PImax
	10 VMT	30 min qd	8 wk	VMT	↑ PImax and VME

VMT = ventilatory muscle training; VME = ventilatory muscle endurance; PFT = pulmonary function tests; PImax = maximal inspiratory pressure; Leg end = leg exercise endurance; VE = minute ventilation; Vo_2 = oxygen uptake; Arm end = arm endurance; UAE = unsupported arm exercise.

more accessory muscles increase their contribution to ventilation even during quiet breathing. The system is further stressed during exercise when, in many patients, $\dot{V}E$ may exceed MVV.

Patients with COPD stop exercising because of dyspnea. Recent evidence indicates that dyspnea relates better to respiratory muscle function than to airflow obstruction (16,35–37). It has been shown that dyspnea increases as the ratio between the pressure needed to ventilate and the maximal pressure that the muscles can generate (Pbreath/PImax) increases. Dyspnea worsens in proportion to the duration of the inspiratory contraction (T_I/T_{TOT}) and respiratory frequency. Since these are also the factors that are associated with electromyographic (EMG) evidence of respiratory muscle fatigue, changes in any of them may explain the increased exercise performance observed after training. Finally, dyspnea may relate to recruitment of accessory ribcage and neck muscles, especially if their contraction is dyssynchronous with the diaphragm (38).

With the above in mind, it seems reasonable to postulate treatment goals that may improve respiratory muscle performance by using systemic (legs or arms) exercise or even specific (ventilatory muscle) training. They are:

1. Reduction in inspiratory forces during breathing
2. Shortening of inspiratory time
3. Increase in maximal inspiratory pressures
4. Decrease in respiratory frequency
5. Better coordination among the different respiratory muscles

It does not seem as if decreased load is an achievable goal since most rehabilitation patients are fully treated. Indeed, in most studies, systemic training does not change pulmonary function. It may be through the last two mechanisms (decrease in respiratory frequency and/or better coordination of different respiratory muscles) that systemic training in COPD may improve exercise endurance and, perhaps, respiratory muscle function. In contrast, ventilatory muscle training may have its beneficial effects through its increase in strength.

Casciari et al. studied 22 patients with COPD (FEV_1/FVC less than 0.50) before, during, and after 9 weeks of rehabilitation that included exercise on a treadmill 3 times weekly. At the end of 6 weeks, 12 of the patients continued to exercise and served as controls. In contrast, the experimental group (10 patients) exercised and underwent breathing retraining. Although there were no changes in pulmonary function, all patients improved their exercise performance and their peak $\dot{V}O_2$. The patients whose breathing was retrained manifested a significantly larger increase in $\dot{V}O_2$ and in exercise endurance. Analysis of these results shows an increase in tidal volume and a drop in respiratory rate at rest and at end-exercise (39). Cherniack postulated that in patients with COPD, the efficiency of the respiratory muscles is decreased and that retraining may improve their efficiency (40). We have recently studied some of these factors. Work of breathing, as determined by the pressure time integral of the excursions of the continuously recorded Ppl, was measured before and after rehabilitation in 16 patients with COPD. In these patients, there were no changes in pulmonary function, but there was a significant decrease in $F \int Pes^{dt}$ at exercise isotime after rehabilitation (Table 3). This decrease was mostly due

Table 3 Work of Breathing, Exercise Endurance, and Maximal Transdiaphragmatic Pressure Before and After Pulmonary Rehabilitation

	Endurance time (sec)	F ∫ Pes^{dt} ($CmH_2O \cdot min^{-1}$)	Pdimax (CmH_2O)
Prerehab	434	288	48
Postrehab	512*	219*	52

*$p<0.05$.
F ∫ Pesdt = work of breathing as estimated by the pressure time index calculated from continuous recording of endoesophageal pressure (Ppl); Pdimax = maximal transdiaphragmatic pressure.

to a decrease in respiratory frequency (41). Finally, retraining in breathing techniques or pursed-lip breathing that decreases breathing frequency increases tidal volume and arterial oxygen saturation and decreases dyspnea.

In summary, the evidence that systemic training improves some aspects of respiratory muscle function is limited but important. This limited information underscores the need for more systematic research in patients undergoing exercise training in whom more aspects of respiratory muscle functions are better analyzed.

V. Respiratory Muscle Training: Specific Strength and Endurance Training

It has been almost 20 years since Leith and Bradley first demonstrated that, like their skeletal counterparts, the respiratory muscles of normal individuals could be specifically trained to improve their strength or endurance (42). Following that observation, multiple studies have shown that a training response will occur if there is enough of a stimulus. As discussed earlier, an increase in inspiratory muscle strength (and perhaps endurance) should result in improved respiratory muscle function by decreasing the P_{breath}/PI_{max}. Since reduced inspiratory muscle strength is evident in patients with COPD, considerable efforts have been made to define the role of respiratory muscle training in these patients.

A. Strength Training

To achieve this goal, a high-intensity, low-frequency stimulus is needed: inspiratory muscles are trained by performing inspiratory maneuvers against a closed glottis or shutter. Several studies have shown an increase in maximal inspiratory pressures when the respiratory muscles have been specifically trained for strength. Lecoq et al. studied nine patients (some of whom had COPD) and after 4 weeks showed a 50% increase in PI_{max} (43). Reid and Warren observed a 53% increase in six COPD patients after 5 weeks of training (44). Both groups noticed a smaller, but significant, increase in expiratory muscle pressure.

It is important to point out that respiratory muscle strength has been shown to increase as a by-product of the endurance training achieved with the use of resistive loads. It is then possible that some of the observed benefits reported after endurance training may relate to the achieved increased strength.

B. Endurance Training

This is achieved by low-intensity, high-frequency training. The programs that have been used are of three types: flow-resistive loading, threshold loading, and voluntary isocapneic hyperpnea.

Flow-Resistive Training

In this training, the load has consisted mainly of decreasing the size of the inspiratory breathing hole. The load will increase provided frequency, tidal volume, and inspiratory time are held constant. Although most studies in patients with COPD have shown an improvement in the time that a given respiratory load can be maintained (ventilatory muscle endurance), the results have to be interpreted with caution since endurance can be increased with changes in the pattern of breathing. Threshold loading has been shown to result in muscle training by assuring that at least the inspired pressure is sufficiently high to ensure training; this result is independent of inspiratory flow rate. When threshold devices are used, the breathing pattern (T_I and respiratory rate) is not as critically important.

Threshold Training

Many studies of threshold training have been uncontrolled. It is difficult to interpret the results as an outcome of the training. The controlled studies summarized in Table 4 have shown an increase in the endurance time that the ventilatory muscles could tolerate a known load (45–57). In response to an inspiratory load, some studies have shown a significant increase in strength (45–48,54–57) and a decrease in dyspnea (47,57). In the studies in which systemic exercise performance was evaluated, walking distance decreased minimally (45,46,53,54,57). From the studies by Larson and Lisboa, it is clear that the pressure required to achieve some training has to exceed 30% of maximal inspiratory pressure (46,57).

In summary, extensive data indicate that ventilatory muscle training, by

Table 4 Controlled Trials of Ventilatory Muscle Resistive Training in COPD

Author	No. of pts.	Type	Frequency	Duration	Results
Pardy	9	RB	bid	8 wk	↑ VME, ↑ 12 MW
	8	PT	3 × /wk	8 wk	No change
Larson	10	RB	qd 30% PImax	8 wk 30 min	↑ PImax, ↑ ET ↑ 12 MW
	12	RB	qd 15% PImax	8 wk 30 min	No Δ in PImax, ET, or 12MW
Harver	10	RB	bid	8 wk 15 min	↑ PImax, ↓ dyspnea
	9	Sham	bid	8 wk 15 min	No change in PImax, dyspnea
Belman	8	RB	qd	6 wk	↑ VME, ↑ PImax
	9	RB low intensity	qd	6 wk	↑ PImax
Chen	7	RB	qd	4 wk (30 min)	↑ VME
	6	Sham	qd	4 wk (30 min)	No ΔVME
Bjerre	14	RB	qd	6 wk (45 min)	↑ VME, no Δ exercise
	14	Sham	qd	6 wk (45 min)	No Δ VME or exercise
Falk	12	RB	qd	12 mo	↑ VME (45 min)
	15	Sham	qd	12 mo	No ΔVME
Noseda	12	RB	qd	8 wk	↑ VME (30 min)
	13	Breathing exercises	qd	8 wk	No ΔVME
Jones	7	RB	qd	10 wk	↑ ET
	6	Sham	qd	10 wk	↑ ET
	8	Exercise	qd	10 wk	↑ ET
Weiner	12	RB/ex	3 × /wk	6 mo	↑ ET ↑ PImax, ↑ VME
	12	Ex	3 × /wk	6 mo	↑ ET
	13	C	NT	6 mo	No change
Wanke	21	RB and ergometry	4 × /wk	8 wk	↑ PImax ↑ ET
	21	ergometry	4 × /wk	8 wk	No ΔPImax ↑ ET
Lisboa	10	RB 30% PImax	qd	5 wk	↑ PImax ↑ ET ↑ dyspnea
	10	RB 15% PImax	qd	5 wk	No changes in PImax ET and dyspnea

RB = resistive breathing; PT = physical therapy; VME = ventilatory muscle endurance; PImax = maximal inspiratory pressure; bid = twice daily; qd = once daily; ET = leg exercise endurance.

means of resistive breathing, improves ventilatory muscle strength and endurance and has marginal effects on overall exercise performance. It is not clear whether this effort results in decreased morbidity or mortality or offers any other clinical advantage. In many of the studies, compliance was low, with up to 50% of patients failing to complete the studies (46).

Ventilatory Isocapneic Hyperpnea

Ventilatory isocapneic hyperpnea is a training method by which patients maintain high levels of ventilation over time (15 min, 2 or 3 times daily). The concentrations of O_2 and CO_2 in the breathing circuit are held constant. The results of an uncontrolled study showed that after 6 weeks of training, the patients with COPD not only increased their maximal sustained ventilatory capacity, but also increased arm and leg exercise performance (55). Two controlled studies also reported increases of maximal sustainable ventilatory capacity in COPD patients trained for 6 weeks, but their exercise endurance was better than that in the control group (58,59).

It seems that respiratory muscle training increases the strength and the capacity of the muscles to endure a respiratory load. There is debate as to whether it also results in improved performance of exercise or the activities of daily living. From the respiratory muscle factors that may contribute to ventilatory limitation in COPD, it seems logical to predict that increases in strength and endurance should help respiratory muscle function, but this is perhaps important only with respect to the capacity of the patients to handle inspiratory loads, e.g., in acute exacerbations of their disease.

VI. Ventilatory Muscle Training in the Patient in Intensive Care

There are few data on this important subject. It is apparent that as soon as a patient is left to breathe on his/her own (as during any form of weaning), his/her respiratory muscles are being retrained.

There is very little experience with ventilatory muscle training in patients recovering from ventilatory failure. Belman reported improvement in two patients (60). In a larger but also uncontrolled study, Aldrich et al. recruited 30 patients who had been in stable chronic respiratory failure for at least 3 weeks and who had failed repeated weaning attempts (61). They excluded patients with active infections or unstable cardiovascular, renal, or endocrine problems, as well as those with gross malnutrition (albumin < 2.5 g/dl) and/or neuromuscular disease. The patients were intermittently trained by having them breathe through one inspiratory resistor while they spontaneously breathed or were supported 2–8 breaths per minute by synchronized mandatory ventilation. In these patients, PI_{max} improved from -37 ± 15 to -46 ± 15 cmH_2O and vital capacity increased from 561 ± 325 to 901 ± 480 ml. Of the 30 patients, 12 were weaned after 10–46 days of training (40% success). Because the study is uncontrolled and selective, these findings may not apply to most patients recovering from respiratory failure. Compared to other series, the success rate in the study by Aldrich et al. is not much different from those reported in weaning facilities that have not used ventilatory muscle training (62). In spite of these encouraging reports, more rigorous studies are needed before ventilatory muscle training can be recommended as a form of treatment for patients with respiratory failure.

Finally, it is important to note that ventilatory muscle training, especially with resistive or threshold loading, may be deleterious. It has been shown that breathing at high PI/PI_{max} or prolonged T_I/T_{TOT} may induce muscle fatigue (19). Since both these factors are inherent in this form of training, it is possible that a sufficiently intense program may actually precipitate fatigue.

VII. Breathing Retraining

There are other, less conventional forms of training that are conceptually solid and may offer new avenues of treatment. As we have seen, the ventilated patient has a high ventilatory drive (63). This increased drive may result in a pattern of rapid, shallow breathing that may be deleterious to adequate ventilation and gas exchange. Interventions designed to change the breathing pattern could prove useful.

A. Feedback

In a recent study, Holliday and Hyers studied 40 patients after 7 days of mechanical ventilation. The patients were randomized to conventional weaning or weaning accompanied by EMG feedback training using the surface EMGs of frontalis muscle, the intercostals, and the diaphragm as indicators of respiratory activity. Using feedback signals, the investigators encouraged relaxation and breathing using larger tidal volumes. The mean ventilator days for the biofeedback group decreased while VT and mean inspiratory flow increased significantly. The authors concluded that breathing retraining resulted in a more efficient breathing pattern, which, in turn, decreased dyspnea and anxiety and allowed for quicker weaning time in the treated patients (64).

We have recently studied some of these factors. Work of breathing, as determined by the pressure time integral of the excursions of the continuously recorded Ppl, was determined before and after rehabilitation in 16 patients with COPD. In these patients, there were no changes in pulmonary function, but F $\int Pes^{dt}$ at the exercise isotime decreased significantly after rehabilitation (Table 5). This drop was mostly due to a decrease in respiratory frequency (65). Fi-

Table 5 Controlled Trials of Ventilatory Isocapneic Hyperpnea in Patients with COPD

Authors	No. of patients	Type	Frequency	Duration	Results
Ries	5	VIH	45 min	6 wk	↑ MSVC ↑ Exercise endurance
	7	Walking	45 min	6 wk	↑ Exercise endurance
Levine	15	VIH	15 min	6 wk	↑ MSVC ↑ Exercise endurance ↑ ADL
	17	IPPB	15 min	6 wk	↑ ADL ↑ Exercise endurance

VIH = ventilatory isocapneic hyperpnea; MSVC = maximal sustainable ventilatory capacity; ADL = activities of daily living; IPPB = intermittent positive-pressure breathing.

nally, retraining in breathing techniques or pursed-lip breathing, techniques that decrease breathing frequency, have been shown to increase tidal volume and arterial oxygen saturation and to decrease dyspnea (66).

B. Yoga

There are other ways to alter ventilatory patterns to more effective ones. Yoga is a philosophical doctrine that includes control of posture and voluntary control of breathing. The latter includes slow, deep breaths with apnea at the end of inspiration and of expiration and/or utilization of rapid abdominal maneuvers. The breathing rate may be brought down to 4–6 breaths per minute.

Stanescu et al. compared the breathing pattern of eight well-trained yoga practitioners with eight controls matched for sex, age, and height. The yoga group had a pattern of breathing characterized by larger tidal volume and slower breathing frequency. They also had a lower ventilatory response to CO_2 rebreathing (67). Although the mechanism by which this occurs is not clear, one possibility is habituation to chronic overstimulation of stretch receptors. Since ventilation is automatically controlled by structures in the upper medulla and brainstem and voluntarily by the cortex, sustained slow, deep breathing may become a "learned" reflex. Whatever the mechanism, it may have applications. Tandon studied patients with CAO trained in yoga breathing and compared them with controls. The patients were able to control their dyspnea better, and this seemed to improve their exercise tolerance (68).

C. Postural Changes

It is known that musculoskeletal tone and contraction may be determined by habitual positioning. Over the last few years, increasing attention has been given to the voluntary inhibition of those patterns. This has been particularly useful for artists (69,70). Recently, Austin and Asubel demonstrated improved peak expiratory flow rate, maximal voluntary ventilation, and maximal inspiratory and expiratory pressures in normal subjects who underwent lessons in proprioceptive musculoskeletal education compared to controls (71). These lessons, per se, have not been systematically evaluated in patients with lung disease. Nonetheless, breathing retraining (pursed-lip breathing and diaphragmatic breathing) constitutes forms of therapy that resemble the above-discussed techniques.

D. Pursed-Lip Breathing

Pursed-lip breathing slows the breathing rate and increases tidal volumes. It also shifts the pattern of recruitment of the ventilatory muscles from one that is predominantly diaphragmatic to one that recruits more the accessory muscles of the ribcage and abdominal muscles of exhalation (66,72). Perhaps this shift may contribute to the relief of dyspnea that has been reported by patients when this breathing technique is adopted.

In summary, there are more unresolved questions than absolute facts in the area of training and respiratory muscle function. A wealth of information remains to be gained if systematic scientific analysis is applied to answer those questions.

References

1. Roussos CH, Macklem PT. The respiratory muscles. N Engl J Med 1982; 307:786–797.
2. Rochester DF. The diaphragm: contractile properties and fatigue. J Clin Invest 1985; 75:1397–1402.
3. Celli BR. Respiratory muscle function. Clin Chest Med 1986; 7:567–583.
4. Mead J. Functional significance of the area of apposition of diaphragm to ribcage. Am Rev Respir Dis 1979; 119:31–32.
5. Tobin M. Respiratory muscles in disease. Clin Chest Med 1988; 9:263–286.
6. Sharp JT. Therapeutic considerations in respiratory muscle function. Chest 1985; 88(2):118–123.
7. Supinsky GS, Kelsen SG. Effects of elastase-induced emphysema on the force-generating ability of the diaphragm. J Clin Invest 1982; 70:978–988.
8. Farkas G, Rooussos C. Adaptability of the hamster's diaphragm to emphysema and/or exercise. J Appl Physiol 1982; 53:1263–1271.

9. DeTroyer A, Estenne M. Coordination between ribcage muscles and diaphragm during quiet breathing in humans. J Appl Physiol 1984; 57(3):899–906.
10. Farkas GA, Decramer M, Rochester DF, et al. Contractile properties of intercostal muscles and their functional significance. J Appl Physiol 1985; 59(2):528–535.
11. Celli BR. Arm exercise and ventilation. Chest 1988; 93:673–674.
12. Banzett R, Topulos G, Leith D, Natios C. Bracing arms increases the capacity for sustained hyperpnea. Am Rev Respir Dis 1983; 133:106–109.
13. Maestro L, Dohnage T, Avendano MA, Goldstein R. Influence of arm position in ventilation during incremental exercise in healthy individuals. Chest 1990; 98(2):113S.
14. Celli BR, Rassulo J, Make B. Dyssynchronous breathing during arm but not leg exercise in patients with chronic airflow obstruction. N Engl J Med 1986; 314:1485–1490.
15. DeTroyer A, Sampson M, Sigrist S, et al. How the abdominal muscles act on the ribcage. J Appl Physiol 1983; 54(2):465–469.
16. Martinez F, Couser J, Celli B. Factors influencing ventilatory muscle recruitment in patients with chronic airflow obstruction. Am Rev Respir Dis 1990; 142:276–282.
17. Ninane V, Rypens F, Yernault JC, DeTroyer A. Abdominal muscle using during breathing in patients with chronic airflow obstruction. Am Rev Respir Dis 1992; 146:16–21.
18. Sieck GC. Diaphragm muscle: structural and functional organization. Clin Chest Med 1988; 9:195–210.
19. Bellemare F, Grassino A. Evaluation of diaphragmatic fatigue. J Appl Physiol 1982; 53:1196–1206.
20. Moltke E, Skouby AP. The influence of tonic neck reflexes on the activity of some muscles of the trunk in patients with asthma and emphysema. Acta Med Scand 1963; 173:299–305.
21. Sant'Ambrogio G, Widdicombe J. Respiratory reflexes acting on the diaphragm and inspiratory intercostal muscles of the rabbit. J Physiol 1965; 180:766–779.
22. Sharp JT. The inspiratory muscles in emphysema. Clin Chest Med 1983; 4:421–432.
23. Tobin M. The respiratory muscles in disease. Clin Chest Med 1988; 9:263–286.
24. Sinclair DJ, Ingram CG. Controlled trial of supervised exercise training in chronic bronchitis. Br Med J 1980; 1:519–521.
25. Cockroft AE, Saunders MJ, Berry G. Randomized controlled trial of rehabilitation in chronic respiratory disability. Thorax 1981; 36:200–203.
26. Paez PN, Phillipson EA, Mosangkay M, et al. The physiological basis of training patients with emphysema. Am Rev Respir Dis 1967; 95:944–953.
27. Mohsenifar Z, Horak D, Brown H, et al. Sensitive indices of improvement in a pulmonary rehabilitation program. Chest 1983; 83:189–192.
28. Belman M, Kendregan BA. Exercise training fails to increase skeletal muscle enzymes in patients with chronic obstructive pulmonary disease. Am Rev Respir Dis 1981; 123:256–261.
29. Tangri S, Wolf CR. The breathing pattern in chronic obstructive lung disease

during the performance of some common daily activities. Chest 1973; 63:126–127.
30. Lake FR, Hendersen K, Briffa T, et al. Upper limb and lower limb exercise training in patients with chronic airflow obstruction. Chest 1990; 97:1077–1082.
31. Keens TG, Krastins B, Wannamaker EM, et al. Ventilatory muscle endurance training in normal subjects and patients with cystic fibrosis. Am Rev Respir Dis 1977; 116:853–860.
32. Ries AL, Ellis B, Hawkins RW. Upper extremity exercise training in chronic obstructive pulmonary disease. Chest 1988; 93:688–692.
33. Epstein S, Breslin E, Roa J, Celli B. Impact of unsupported arm training (AT) and ventilatory muscle training (VMT) on the metabolic and ventilatory consequences of unsupported arm elevation (UAE) and exercise (UAEX) in patients with chronic airflow obstruction (CAO). Am Rev Respir Dis 1991; 193:81.
34. Make BJ, Gilmartin M. Rehabilitation of ventilator assisted individual. Clin Chest Med 1986; 7:679–691.
35. Cherniack NS, Altose M. Mechanisms of dyspnea. Clin Chest Med 1987; 8:207–214.
36. Killian KJ, Gandevia SC, Summers W, et al. Effect of increased lung volume on perception of breathlessness effort and tension. J Appl Physiol 1984; 57:686–691.
37. Ward ME, Eidelman D, Stubbing DG, et al. Respiratory sensation and pattern of respiratory muscle activation during fatigue. J Appl Physiol 1988; 65:2181–2189.
38. Breslin E, Garroutte B, Kohlman-Carrieri V, Celli B. Correlations between dyspnea, diaphragm and sternomastoid recruitment during inspiratory resistance breathing in normal subjects. 1990; 98:298–302.
39. Casciari R, Fairshter R, Harrison A, et al. Effects of breathing retraining in patients with chronic obstructive pulmonary disease. Chest 1981; 79:393–398.
40. Cherniack R. The oxygen consumption and efficiency of the respiratory muscles in health and emphysema. J Clin Invest 1959; 38:494–499.
41. Benditt J, Pollock M, Breslin E, et al. Comprehensive pulmonary rehabilitation decreases the work of breathing during leg cycle ergometry in patients with severe chronic airflow obstruction (CAO). Am Rev Respir Dis 1990; 141(2):A509.
42. Leith DE, Bradley M. Ventilatory muscle strength and endurance training. J Appl Physiol 1976; 4:508–516.
43. Lecoq A, Delhez L, Janssens S, et al. Reentrainement de la fonction motrice ventilatoire chez des insuffisants respiratoire chroniques. Acta Tuberc Pneumol Belg 1970; 61:63–69.
44. Reid WD, Warren CP. Ventilatory muscle strength and endurance training in elderly subjects and patients with chronic airflow limitation: a pilot study. Physiol Can 1984; 36:305–311.
45. Pardy R, Livingston R, Despas P, et al. Inspiratory muscle training compared with physiotherapy in patients with chronic airflow limitation. Am Rev Respir Dis 1981; 123:421–425.
46. Larson JL, Kim MJ, Sharp JT. Inspiratory muscle training with a pressure threshold breathing device in patients with chronic obstructive pulmonary disease. Am Rev Respir Dis 1988; 138:689–696.

47. Harver A, Mahler D, Daubenspeck J. Targeted inspiratory muscle training improves respiratory muscle function and reduces dyspnea in patients with chronic obstructive pulmonary disease. Ann Intern Med 1989; 111:117–124.
48. Belman M, Shadmehr R. Targeted resistive ventilatory muscle training in chronic obstructive pulmonary disease. J Appl Physiol 1988; 65:2726–2735.
49. Chen H, Dukes R, Martin B. Inspiratory muscle training in patients with chronic obstructive pulmonary disease. Am Rev Respir Dis 1985; 131:251–255.
50. Bjerre-Jempsen K, Secher N, Kok-Jensen A. Inspiratory resistance training in severe chronic obstructive pulmonary disease. Eur J Respir Dis 1981; 62:405–411.
51. Falk P, Eriksen AM, Kolliker K, et al. Relieving dyspnea with an inexpensive and simple method in patients with severe chronic airflow limitation, Eur J Respir Dis 1985; 66:181–186.
52. Noseda A, Carpiaux J, Vandeput N, et al. Resistive inspiratory muscle training and exercise performance in COPD patients. A comparative study with conventional breathing retraining. Bull Eur Physiopathol Respir 1987; 23:457–463.
53. Jones DT, Thomson RA, Sears MR. Physical exercise and resistive breathing training in severe chronic airways obstruction. Are they effective? Eur J Respir Dis 1985; 67:159–166.
54. Weiner P, Azgad Y, Ganam R. Inspiratory muscle training combined with general exercise conditioning in patients with COPD. Chest 1992; 102:1351–1356.
55. Belman M, Mittman C. Ventilatory muscle training improves exercise capacity in chronic obstructive pulmonary disease patients. Am Rev Respir Dis 1980; 121:273–280.
56. Wanke Th, Formanek D, Lahrmann H, et al. Effects of combined inspiratory muscle and cycle ergometer training on exercise performance in patients with COPD. Eur Respir J 1994; 7:2205–2211.
57. Lisboa C, Munoz V, Beroiza T, Leiva A, Cruz E. Inspiratory muscle training in chronic airflow limitation: comparison of two different training loads with a threshold device Eur Respir J 1994; 7:1266–1274.
58. Ries AL, Moser KM. Comparison of isocapneic hyperventilation and walking exercise training at home in pulmonary rehabilitation. Chest 1986; 90:285–289.
59. Levine S, Weiser P, Gillen J. Evaluation of a ventilatory muscle endurance training program in the rehabilitation of patients with chronic obstructive pulmonary disease. Am Rev Respir Dis 1986; 133:400–406.
60. Belman MJ. Respiratory failure treated by ventilatory muscle training (VMT): a report of two cases. Eur J Respir Dis 1981; 62:391–393.
61. Aldrich TK, Karpel JP, Uhrlass RM, et al. Weaning from mechanical ventilation: adjunctive use of inspiratory muscle resistive training. Crit Care Med 1989; 17:143–147.
62. Scheinhom DJ, Ho C. Avoiding home mechanical ventilation; the regional weaning center. Proceedings of International Conference on Pulm. Rehab. and Home Vent., 1991; 3:A35.
63. Sasson C, Tee T, Mahutte CK, Light RW. Airway oclussion pressure: an important indicator for successful weaning in patients with chronic obstructive pulmonary disease. Am Rev Respir Dis 1987; 135:107–113.

64. Holliday JE, Hyers TM. The reduction of weaning time from mechanical ventilation using tidal volume and relaxation feedback. Am Rev Respir Dis 1990; 141:1214–1220.
65. Benditt J, Pollack M, Breslin E, Celli B. Comprehensive pulmonary rehabilitation decreases the work of breathing during leg cycle ergometry in patients with severe CAO. Am Rev Respir Dis 1990; 141:A-509.
66. Roa J, Epstein S, Breslin E, Shannon T, Celli B. Work of breathing and ventilatory muscle recruitment during pursed lip breathing. Am Rev Respir Dis 1991; 143:A77.
67. Stanescu D, Newery B, Veriter C, Marechal C. Pattern of breathing and ventilatory response to CO_2 in subjects practicing hatha-yoga. J Appl Physiol 1991; 51:1625–1629.
68. Tandon M. Adjunct treatment with yoga in chronic severe airways obstruction. Thorax 1973; 33:514–517.
69. Alexander FM. The Resurrection of the Body: The Essential Writings of F Matthas Alexander. Selected and introduced by Edward Maisel. New York: Dell, 1974.
70. Jones F. Voice production as a function of head balance in singers. J Psychol 1972; 82:209–215.
71. Austin JH, Asubel P. Enhanced respiratory muscular function in normal adults after lessons in proprioceptive musculoskeletal education without exercises. Chest 1992; 102:486–490.
72. Breslin EH. The pattern of respiratory muscle recruitment during pursed lip breathing. Chest 1992; 101:75–78.

23

Nutrition in Pulmonary Rehabilitation

ROBERT M. ROGERS and MICHAEL DONAHOE

University of Pittsburgh School of Medicine
Pittsburgh, Pennsylvania

In pulmonary rehabilitation, the assessment and treatment of altered nutritional states is often oversimplified or ignored. While this may reflect lack of knowledge regarding the potential importance of nutritional factors in disease outcome, equally important is the clinician's frustration with the limited options to treat the problems of undernutrition and obesity in patients with pulmonary disease.

Practical clinical approaches, based on sound scientific inquiry, are lacking. In theory, optimal nutritional status should help to maximize the patient's state of health, respiratory muscle function, and overall sense of well-being, and possibly improve disease outcome. To date, the therapeutic benefit of intervention programs for pulmonary patients as an isolated treatment goal has been difficult to demonstrate. Despite this limitation, a great deal of practical clinical knowledge has been gained regarding nutrition and particularly chronic obstructive pulmonary disease (COPD). Therefore, this review focuses on this particular patient population since work on other populations of patients with pulmonary disease is limited. First, the pathophysiological effects of malnutrition are addressed, followed by a discussion of screening techniques for selection of patients likely to benefit from nutritional intervention. Finally, therapeutic approaches for these patients are discussed.

I. Pathophysiology of Malnutrition

A. Metabolism and Gas Exchange

The total ventilatory requirement of the patient with pulmonary disease is linked to the tissue metabolic rate through tissue carbon dioxide production. This tight linkage of metabolism and ventilation establishes an integral relationship between nutritional therapy and the respiratory system.

The total daily metabolic rate can be measured as three individual components: basal energy expenditure (BEE), diet-induced thermogenesis, and the energy expenditure associated with activity.

BEE is that component measured at rest under fasting conditions and is typically assessed in clinical medicine by indirect calorimetry studies. The BEE makes up approximately 80% of total energy expenditure. A number of prediction models, including the Harris-Benedict (HB) equation, and disease-specific models have been utilized to estimate the BEE component (1,2). These models use anthropometric parameters, i.e., height, weight, age, to estimate lean tissue mass, as basal metabolic rate is normally determined by the size of the metabolically active lean tissue compartment (3).

Unlike normal individuals, basal metabolic rate in patients with COPD does not correlate directly with indicators of lean tissue mass, so traditional prediction models for patients with COPD are less accurate than for normals (4). For example, in malnourished COPD patients, resting metabolism is higher than in normally nourished COPD patients and controls when compared to predicted values (Table 1). This behavior contrasts with the normally reduced metabolic rate usually observed in malnutrition and has been attributed to an increase in the oxygen cost of breathing (5).

Under normal conditions, the energy expenditure necessary to support the ventilatory system is a small fraction (1–2%) of overall total energy require-

Table 1 Comparison of Resting Metabolic Rate Measurements Determined in Two Investigations of COPD Patients

Investigator	Type	REE/HB	REE	1.3×REE
Donahoe, 1989 (5)	WS COPD	105 (19)	1622 (240)	2108
	WL COPD	119 (12)	1409 (210)	1831
Schols, 1991 (4)	WS COPD	110 (11)	1539 (177)	2000
	WL COPD	118 (17)	1490 (218)	1937

WS COPD = weight-stable COPD patients; WL COPD = weight-losing COPD patients; REE/HB = resting energy expenditure/Harris-Benedict predicted energy expenditure; REE = resting energy expenditure; 1.3×REE = total daily energy requirements estimated as 1.3×REE.

ments (5,6). However, malnourished COPD patients utilize a greater fraction of their total tissue metabolism to support the metabolic needs of the respiratory muscles (5). The augmented energy cost of ventilation has been found to correlate best with the RV/TLC ratio, reflecting the degree of hyperinflation ($r = 0.72$).

Despite this knowledge, the finding of relative hypermetabolism alone cannot explain the weight loss seen in COPD patients, as total energy requirements necessary for metabolic balance are not significantly different between weight-stable and weight-losing patients (Table 1). Furthermore, some investigators have reported that weight loss is not uniformly associated with hypermetabolism (7). Other disorders characterized by moderate hypermetabolism, e.g., hyperthyroidism, are not invariably associated with weight loss since patients augment their caloric intake to meet energy needs. Therefore, patients with COPD appear to have either a limitation on their ability to augment caloric intake or an inability to utilize nutrients properly.

Energy requirements associated with physical activity should be increased in patients with COPD due to the increased work of breathing. Therefore, total daily energy requirements should also be increased. A single investigation of total daily energy requirements of patients with COPD living in a chamber found values comparable to those of normal subjects (8). The investigators hypothesized that the increase in metabolic requirements of the respiratory muscles were offset by restricted activity secondary to the severe lung disease. As a result, total energy requirements of the COPD subjects were not increased. However, it is also possible that the chamber restricted physical activity. No data are currently available to estimate "free living" total energy requirements in these patients.

The thermogenic component of energy expenditure represents the energy expenditure associated with dietary intake. Provision of any form of caloric intake increases energy metabolism. Under normal conditions, this small change in CO_2 production exerts only a minor effect on minute ventilation. However, in the patient with COPD, nutritional support could theoretically increase alveolar ventilation sufficiently to contribute to the meal-associated dyspnea that occurs in these patients. The magnitude of this ventilatory stimulus depends on the total caloric intake and, possible, on the substrate composition.

Comparison of an isocaloric (1.7 $\times$ resting energy expenditure) high-carbohydrate formula (53% of total calories) and a high-fat formula (55% of total calories) during enteral or parenteral nutrition in patients with COPD suggested that resting energy expenditure (REE) increased >10% on both diets although the increase was slightly greater for the carbohydrate-based diet (9); in the control population, the increase in resting energy expenditure for the carbohydrate and fat-based diets was 8% and 9%, respectively. In a population of patients with respiratory failure who were given continuous feeding, CO_2

production ($\dot{V}CO_2$) increased by a mean of 15% in subjects fed a caloric intake of 1.0 times REE, 33% in subjects fed a caloric intake of 1.5 times REE, and 54% in subjects fed 2.0 times the measured REE (10). In a study of diet-induced thermogenesis in COPD patients following a standardized meal ($0.3 \times$ REE with noncontinuous feeding), energy expenditure increased by approximately 15% within 30 min of the ingested meal. However, this change was not significantly different from normal (11). Oxidation of an isocaloric amount of fat compared to a carbohydrate fuel source will decrease CO_2 production for a given ATP synthesis. However, the benefit of shifting fat to carbohydrate ratios in favor of carbohydrates in patients with COPD, when calories are supplied in keeping with energy demands, remains unproven.

It has been suggested that protein administration influences the ventilatory demand by changing the ventilatory drive. Protein administration, following a period of nutritional deprivation, is associated with increased ventilatory responses to hypoxia and hypercapnia (12). It is postulated that branched-chain amino acids play an important role in mediating the effect of protein on respiratory drive (13,14). Dietary intake of amino acids may influence central nervous system neurotransmitters through competitive transport of substrate at the blood-brain barrier. The magnitude of this effect and the potential role for manipulation of dietary protein intake as a therapeutic tool are unclear. Attempts to utilize branched-chain amino acids in postoperative patients have not been beneficial (15,16). Whether these findings are important to the chronic administration of protein in patients with pulmonary disease is unclear.

In summary, patients with COPD have a unique relationship between energy metabolism, lean tissue mass, and ventilatory demand. Although individual substrates have variable effects on metabolism and gas exchange, the primary focus must be directed at selection of caloric support that is appropriately adjusted to the energy demands of the patient.

Energy requirements of underweight COPD patients may be poorly estimated by available prediction models, suggesting a role for indirect calorimetry. An element of resting hypermetabolism is evident in some patients with COPD, but the limited data currently available do not resolve whether total daily energy requirements are abnormal in these patients. Furthermore, resting hypermetabolism does not appear to be the sole explanation for the weight-losing process in these patients. The potential beneficial effects of nutritional intake must be weighed against the ventilatory stress to the gas exchange process. Administration of calories in excess of energy requirements may result in excess CO_2 production, which can be deleterious (10,17). The clinical impact of increasing CO_2 production will be greatest in the patient with a high degree of ventilatory insufficiency (high dead space fraction).

B. Respiratory Muscle Function

The adverse effects of malnutrition on respiratory muscle function occur primarily in the patient with undernutrition and progressive muscle wasting. Protein-calorie malnutrition (PCM) in the nonstressed animal results in a progressive reduction in body weight and skeletal muscle mass. This change in peripheral skeletal muscle with PCM is paralleled by a proportional reduction in the dimensions of diaphragm muscle of animals (18–20) and humans (21,22).

Under conditions of PCM, the rate of degradation of muscle protein exceeds that of muscle protein synthesis, resulting in net muscle catabolism. This catabolic process appears, at least initially, to preferentially affect specific muscle fibers. Thus, in a rat model of protein-calorie deprivation designed to produce a weight loss of approximately 25% of baseline, there was no significant change in fiber frequency following PCM but there did occur a statistically significant reduction in fast-twitch diaphragm muscle fiber size; in contrast, the slower-twitch fibers did not undergo significant change (20). These results are consistent with previous studies that suggested sensitivity of fast-twitch fibers to protein-calorie deprivation in rat and hamster models (18,19). However, a shift in the relative slow:fast-twitch muscle fiber dimensions is not specific for malnutrition since similar changes occur as part of the aging process and in disuse atrophy (23,24).

The greater sensitivity of fast-twitch fibers to PCM may relate to differences in the sensitivity of muscle fiber types to circulating, or locally produced, hormonal factors. The rat diaphragm changes during PCM were paralleled by changes in circulating insulin-like growth factor (IGF-1) (20). A deficiency of this growth factor in relation to peripheral skeletal muscle atrophy has been described (25,26). Thyroid hormone also appears to play an important role in the regulation of muscle structure and function although its exact relationship to specific fiber types is unclear (27). The effect of corticosteroids on diaphragm muscle structure appears to be identical to that of PCM, suggesting that this factor may also be contributory (28).

The effects of undernutrition are recognized to be greater in underactive muscles, implicating neural activation as an important factor (29). Blood flow and cellular metabolism may serve to regulate fiber dimensions. Although the mechanism is still unclear, both human and animal models confirm that fast-twitch fibers are predominantly affected by PCM.

Intracellular electrolytes, including magnesium and phosphate, and intracellular energy stores are abnormal in malnourished patients with COPD (30–32). Reductions in phosphate, magnesium, and calcium are recognized to affect adversely the performance of respiratory muscles, especially with respect to strength parameters (33–35). For patients with COPD, phosphate levels in serum may not be representative of intracellular levels of phosphate (31). Hypophosphatemia in these patients may occur secondary to malnutrition and/or to a renal phosphate leak caused by drug therapy.

In patients with COPD, biopsies of both intercostal and quadriceps muscles have shown a decrease in energy stores as manifested by reduced concentrations of ATP and phosphocreatine (36). The forearm muscles of patients with stable COPD manifest an abnormal increase in the concentration of intracellular organic phosphate and an abnormal decrease in pH with increasing levels of work (37). These studies suggest an abnormal oxidative capacity of peripheral muscles in these patients. These biochemical and intracellular electrolyte changes would be expected to contribute to a decrease in muscle power.

PCM is associated with characteristic neurophysiological changes. In isolated muscle strips of both rat and hamster diaphragm, low stimulation frequencies elicit a small fraction of the maximal tetanic force generated at higher stimulation frequencies (18,19). Protein-calorie deprivation reduces generation of force primarily at the high stimulation frequencies, thereby shifting the force/frequency curve and increasing the ratio of low:high-frequency force generation. The reduction in force generation at a given frequency may be explained solely by the reduction in muscle bulk since the tension per unit of muscle cross-sectional area or per unit weight of the animal is similar in undernourished and control animals (19). During acute starvation, a shift in the force-frequency relationship of the diaphragm has been described to occur in animal models in as short an interval as 4 days (38).

Compared to normally nourished controls, the sternocleidomastoid demonstrates a reduction in maximal force, a slower maximal relaxation rate, and a shorter time to fatigue in malnourished patients with COPD (39). These changes reverse with nutritional therapy. Similar changes have been demonstrated for the human diaphragm in the setting of PCM (40).

Attempts to correlate nutritional status with parameters of inspiratory muscle function in patients with COPD have led to conflicting results (41,42). The same is true for results from patients with cystic fibrosis (43–45).

The pattern of physiological change in muscle function described for PCM is similar to the pattern described for high-frequency respiratory muscle fatigue (46,47). These changes can be induced in respiratory muscles during high-intensity exercise, resistive or threshold loading, and sustained hyperventilation. Many other factors can influence muscle function in patients with pulmonary disease, including the length-tension relationship, tissue oxygenation, acid-base parameters, and pharmacological therapy (48).

The ability to isolate the influence of nutritional status on respiratory muscles in clinical disorders is limited by the multiple factors that impact on the measurement variable. For example, inspiratory muscle strength correlates with expiratory muscle strength and with the operating length of the diaphragm. Because the expiratory muscles are not "disadvantaged" by the hyperinflation of COPD, a reduction in the strength of these muscles, along with a concomitant reduction in inspiratory muscle strength, suggests a myopathic process (41). In contrast, inspiratory muscle strength is influenced by both the lung volume and myopathic process, so the respective roles of each in diminishing inspiratory muscle strength are not easy to dissociate.

In summary, PCM is associated with characteristic changes in skeletal muscle structure and function. Although the reduction in muscle strength is not specific for malnutrition, it does appear to be sensitive to energy balance and to respond to nutritional intervention.

What are the implications of these changes for subjects with pulmonary disease? Muscle fibers are recruited for activity according to the intensity of the stimulus. Fast-twitch oxidative fibers are generally active only during maximal contractile activity. Undernutrition may exert a minimal adverse influence on basal activities of skeletal muscle but play a greater role during activities that require maximal force output (49). However, patients with high inspiratory impedance, i.e., COPD, are obliged to use a greater fraction of maximal output at baseline, suggesting the possibility of greater involvement of all types of muscle fibers. Therefore, malnutrition, with the associated fast-twitch fiber atrophy and reduction in maximal twitch strength, may play a greater role in the pulmonary patient with high respiratory impedance.

C. Host Defenses

T-cell function, complement activity, and humoral immunity are altered in malnourished states. However, the most significant and consistent change occurs in cell-mediated immunity. These changes are believed to explain the increased rate of infection characteristic of severe states of PCM. Such evidence suggests that immunological tests can be used as a functional assessment of nutritional status. The most common clinical tools used in the immunological assessment of nutritional status are delayed cutaneous hypersensitivity and total lymphocyte counts.

II. Nutritional Screening

The primary goal of nutritional screening is to identify patients at high risk of complications secondary to an abnormal nutritional status and to identify patients who would benefit from intervention. Effective screening tools must be safe, cost-effective, widely applicable, yet accurate in predicting adverse sequelae.

Nutrition screening begins with a careful history of the patient's diet, which includes assessment of nutritional, medical, socioeconomic, and other pertinent details in relationship to adequate nutrient intake. The dietitian plays a critical role in this component of nutritional assessment and therapy. Diet intake can be assessed by a number of methods, e.g., a 24-hr recall, or a history of usual food intake, or a food frequency questionnaire. Each of these methods suffers, in varying degrees, from biases in measurement and inaccuracies in reporting.

Anthropometric measurements are utilized to assess body composition and, indirectly, nutritional status. These tools include measurements of body weight, height, skinfold, and skeletal frame. A brief weight history that includes parameters such as recent weight loss or gain and usual body weight are important to identify patients at risk of nutritionally related complications.

The measured body weight can be referenced to accepted norms to determine the percentage ideal body weight (%IBW). Two commonly used standards are the Metropolitan Life Insurance Tables and the Dietary Guidelines for Americans (5,6). The use of weight standards to assess nutritional status has significant limitations: common standards utilize populations that are skewed demographically, often excluding the elderly and minorities; the Metropolitan Tables are based on a sample of 19- to 59-year-old, mostly white, middle-class, insured individuals. An attempt is currently underway to establish a data base in the third National Health and Nutrition Examination Survey (NHANES III) of nutritional indices in the U.S. population that utilizes a more diverse population.

Body weight, although an incomplete assessment of lean body mass, provides a risk-free, widely applicable, nutritional assessment tool that should be an integral part of any pulmonary rehabilitation program. Further, it represents the only nutritional assessment parameter in patients with COPD that is clearly associated with an increased mortality rate (<90% of ideal weight predicted by the Metropolitan Tables) (50).

Since the primary goal of nutrition intervention is maintenance or repletion of lean body mass (LBM), measurement of this factor is a useful outcome parameter. LBM, which includes the muscles of respiration, can be measured either once or serially to monitor ongoing changes.

One approach to determination of LBM involves the use of anthropometric measurements, which assess the size of skinfolds, skeletal breadths, and circumferences at various body sites. These measurements need to be applied by a skilled technician using standardized techniques to minimize observer error.

As with body weight, individual measurements can be compared to a group norm utilizing traditional measurement sites such as the triceps skinfold (TSF) and mid-arm circumference (51). Measurement sites can be monitored serially during a pulmonary rehabilitation program to monitor the effects of therapy. Skinfold measurements assume that the distribution of total body fat is uniform. This assumption may be false, particularly for the elderly, who may centralize and internalize adipose tissue in the trunk (52).

Regression equations based on measurement at different anatomical sites are available to predict body density, which, in turn, can be used to calculate total body fat (51,53,54). Based on the assumption of a two-compartment model, lean mass is determined as the difference between anthropometric fat mass and total body weight. Although the populations that were used to develop the regression equations did vary demographically, they did not include patients with lung disease.

Skinfold measurements are complementary to measurements of body weight in the serial assessment of body composition. A recent examination of patients with COPD who were experiencing an exacerbation of disease demonstrated that the majority of patients gained weight during therapy. Although this might initially be interpreted as favorable, anthropometric studies suggest the weight gain was primarily in body fat and was accompanied by a decrease in muscle strength (55). Thus, the anthropometric measurements served to identify an adverse nutritional effect in patients with COPD; this effect is not evident if only the body weight is monitored.

An alternative approach for estimating LBM depends on bioelectrical impedance analysis (BIA). The technique has the advantages of being easy to use, noninvasive, and relatively low in cost. BIA measures the total body impedance to a nondetectable current that is delivered by electrodes placed on a hand and foot on the same side. The theoretical basis for use of BIA in the estimation of body composition is the assumption that the human body is a series of connected cylinders in which impedance is related to the length and area of the cylinders (56). The current is conducted by body water and electrolytes. Because the water and electrolytes of the body are concentrated in the LBM, a mathematical relationship exists between the length (or height) of the person, resistance to current flow, and the size of the LBM.

This method has been well validated in normal populations but has not been validated in the ill, obese, or malnourished. Moreover, even though the relationship between body fluid and electrolytes to impedance is generally accepted, the constancy of the relationship between fluid and electrolytes and lean body mass is not. In the patient with pulmonary disease, edema, malnutrition, or therapeutic steroids may influence body fluids status without affecting LBM change. In patients with COPD, values for LBM determined by anthropometric measurements are higher than those found by BIA (57,58). Despite these limitations, BIA estimates of lean tissue mass seem to have important prognostic implications for the patient with COPD; this information is not provided by simple anthropometric measurements (59).

Based on the 12-min walking test, individuals with a normal body weight (%IBW ≥ 90%) but a low lean tissue mass determined by BIA (< 60% of predicted ideal body weight) seem to have a lower exercise tolerance than do underweight patients (≤ 90% IBW) with a normal lean tissue mass. These observations suggest that more detailed analysis of body composition might provide greater insights into the relationship between functional and nutritional status in these patients.

The hepatic secretory proteins include albumin, prealbumin, transferrin, and retinol-binding protein. These proteins are often assessed in a comprehensive nutritional assessment program as an indication of visceral protein stores. A number of clinical trials have shown that patients with COPD generally do not manifest decrements in these parameters (39,60–62).

A major goal of nutritional rehabilitation in patients with COPD is to optimize the immune response in this infection-prone population. The total lymphocyte count affords evidence concerning nutritional status and is related to immunocompetence. It has been reported that the total lymphocyte count increases significantly in patients with COPD and recent weight loss who are given supplemental feeding (63). However, even though the level of circulating lymphocytes is influenced by dietary intake, it is also influenced by other body constituents, which may complicate interpretation.

Urinary metabolites, such as creatinine and 3-methylhistidine, which are metabolites derived from skeletal muscle, have been used as part of comprehensive nutritional assessments in hospital and research settings. Both measurements require precise collections of urine for 24 hr and rigid control of protein in the diet. In practice, other measures of LBM are more appropriate for the rehabilitation setting.

Nutritional status can also be assessed indirectly by certain measurements of functional status, such as muscle function and delayed cutaneous hypersensitivity. Measurement of handgrip strength has been utilized in surgical populations to predict outcome more precisely than other indices of nutritional status, such as albumin (64). Handgrip strength is an inexpensive and simple method of assessing muscle function and is easily measured in the outpatient setting. It can also be used serially to confirm strength changes resulting from nutritional intervention and exercise.

A logical goal of pulmonary rehabilitation is to improve respiratory muscle function. Provision of adequate substrate with restoration of muscle mass should produce measurable changes in respiratory muscle strength. Several investigators have reported improvement in respiratory pressures along with weight gain in underweight patients with COPD (65–68). Serial measurement of inspiratory and expiratory pressures can be used to monitor nutritional progress in pulmonary rehabilitation.

For pulmonary rehabilitation programs, regular screening of body weight is indicated. The use of anthropometrics or BIA to measure body composition can be helpful in identifying individuals with specific depletion of LBM and to monitor the adequacy and effects of an intervention. Functional assessment, including parameters of muscle strength (handgrip and respiratory muscle), are complimentary to the assessment of body composition. Synthesis of these physiological and historical findings is then used to identify the specific nutritional problems of the individual patient and to develop a comprehensive care plan. Based on these data and observations, appropriate interventions can be implemented and evaluated.

The patient with COPD is often afflicted with other medical conditions that call for alternate diet therapy. These include cardiac disease, diabetes, and hypertension. Conflicting diet therapies may be indicated, i.e., sodium restriction and calorie supplementation in an underweight patient with COPD who is also hypertensive. In this instance, close collaboration between the dietitian and physician is required to prioritize the goals and nutritional interventions.

III. Nutritional Therapy

A. The Underweight Patient

Weight loss occurs in up to 50% of patients with chronic obstructive lung disease who require hospitalization (69,70). Openbrier and colleagues (71) first called attention to the association of weight loss and emphysema. Numerous studies report an association between mortality and weight loss in COPD (66,72,73). In one series, approximately 26% of patients enrolling in a pulmonary rehabilitation program were malnourished (74).

Recognition of the relationship between weight loss and early mortality has prompted investigators to evaluate the role of nutritional support in these patients. These investigations have typically utilized standard oral nutritional support in malnourished patients with COPD who were judged to be primarily "stable," without evidence of infection or disease exacerbation (39,60–62,65–68). The patients have been selected using a variety of entry criteria, which usually incorporate a history of weight loss and/or a reduction in percentage of ideal body weight.

Controlled, inpatient investigations designed to provide nutrient support adjusted to 1.7 times REE and protein at 1.5 g/kg body weight (approximately a 150:1 nonprotein calorie:nitrogen ratio) have resulted in weight gain, nitrogen retention, and improvement in the physiological indices of muscle strength (65–68). These investigations used indirect calorimetry to enhance the accuracy of estimates of energy requirements.

The benefit from altering fat:carbohydrate ratios in providing nonprotein calories to patients with COPD remains to be proven. At rest, both normocapnic and hypercapnic patients appear to maintain a constant P_{CO_2} after a carbohydrate load (63). Immediately after an isocaloric feeding of fat or carbohydrate, exercise tolerance has been reported to be slightly less in the carbohydrate-loaded patient than in the fat-loaded patient (75,76). Despite these findings, long-term administration of a diet consisting of approximately 55% carbohydrates, at a level as high as 2 × REE, does not result in measured changes in REE, dyspnea indices, or blood P_{CO_2} (77).

Clinical trials in outpatient settings have found it difficult to provide adequate nutritional support for extended periods under these "uncontrolled" conditions (60,61). Weight gain in the outpatient setting has been minimal, and positive therapeutic benefits have been difficult to demonstrate.

The difficulty with nutritional supplementation of patients with COPD is attributable to various factors. Malnourished patients with COPD often develop a variety of symptoms in relation to meals that appear to limit caloric intake (Table 2). Attempts to circumvent these difficulties have met with only limited success. In our experience, success with the various therapeutic strategies depends largely on the motivation of patient and counselor.

The high frequency of gastrointestinal symptoms, including bloating and early satiety, has long been noted (78). These symptoms are often attributed to an associated high incidence of peptic ulcer disease in COPD, to side effects of patient medications, e.g., theophylline compounds, or to the abnormal position of the diaphragm with respect to the stomach that accompanies hyperinflation of the lungs.

A second important factor that might limit caloric intake is "meal desaturation" (79). Arterial desaturation during meals occurs primarily in patients who are hypoxemic at rest. This finding may contribute to meal-related dyspnea and is likely to respond to an increase in supplemental oxygen during meals.

Some studies have suggested that calorie intake in patients with COPD is adequate in the outpatient setting (69). However, measurement of caloric intake during a stable patient interval need not reflect intake during intercurrent illness. Long-term follow-up of patients undergoing nutritional intervention suggests that weight loss occurs in a "step decline" fashion (66). During an exacerbation of disease, when caloric intake is likely to be limited, marked weight loss occurs and subsequently stabilizes as the disease exacerbation subsides.

Two successful outpatient studies have been associated with positive energy and nitrogen balance and have produced the expected improvements in measured parameters of strength (68,80) (Fig. 1). Improvements in walking distance, dyspnea, and quality of life have also been reported. However, the results have been inconsistent and the magnitude of positive effects has been

Table 2 Summary of Symptoms and Counseling Strategies for Nutritional Therapy in Chronic Obstructive Pulmonary Disease[a]

Complaint	Estimated frequency (%)	Recommendations
Anorexia	73	Eat high-calorie food first. Have favorite foods available. Try more frequent meals and snacks throughout the day. Instruct patients to push themselves. Add margarine, butter, mayonnaise, sauces, and gravies to add calories.
Early satiety	87	Eat high-calorie foods first. Limit liquids in meal; sip an hour after meals. Cold foods can give less of a sense of fullness than hot foods.
Dyspnea	73	Rest before meals. Use bronchodilators before meals. Use secretion clearance strategies if indicated. Eat more slowly. Use pursed-lip breathing between bites. Use tripod position for meals. Have readily prepared meals available for periods of increased shortness of breath. Evaluate for meal desaturation; refer for oxygen evaluation if necessary.
Fatigue	60	Rest before meals. Have readily prepared meals available for periods of increased fatigue or illness. Have patient try to eat larger meals when he or she is less tired.
Bloating	80	Treat shortness of breath early to prevent air swallowing. Eat smaller, more frequent meals. Avoid rushed meals. Avoid gas-forming foods individual to patient.
Constipation	50	Incorporate exercise as tolerated. Instruct patient in high-fiber foods and adequate fluids. Refer for medical evaluation for stool softener.
Dental problems	30	Instruct patient in use of soft, high-caloric density foods. Facilitate use of dental services as appropriate.

[a]Estimated frequency based on a survey of 19 malnourished COPD patients.
Source: Adapted from Ref. 84.

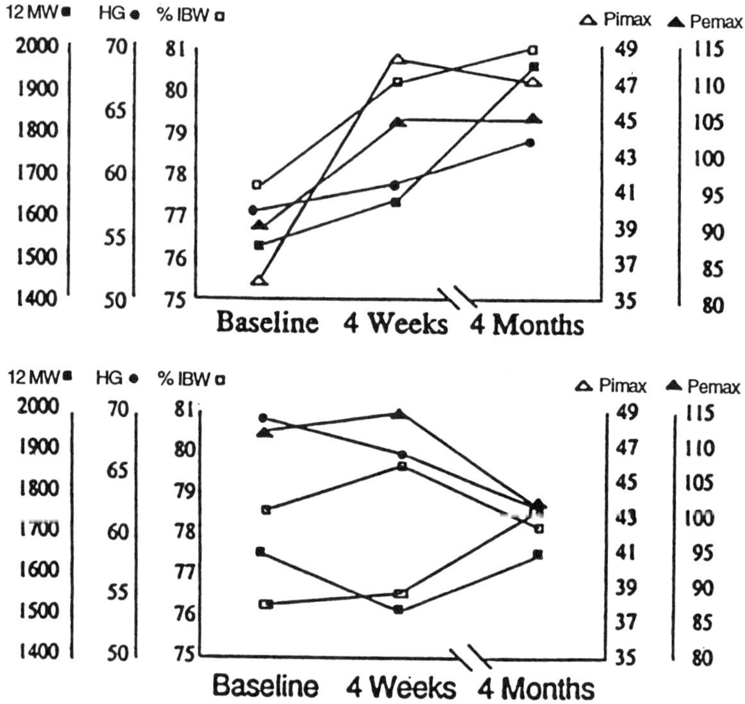

Figure 1 Comparison of physiological parameters in patients with COPD who participated in a nutritional intervention program (top) and controls (bottom). The baseline-to-4-week period was a nutritional intervention conducted in the inpatient setting followed by an outpatient follow-up (4 weeks–4 months). 12 MW = 12-min walk (feet); HG = handgrip strength in kg-force; %IBW = % ideal body weight; Pimax = maximum inspiratory pressure; Pemax = maximum expiratory pressure. (Adapted from Ref. 68, with permission.)

slight. To date, no study has reported significant improvements in morbidity or mortality.

Our experience with an aggressive outpatient nocturnal enteral feeding regimen has shown that this form of intervention is safe in these patients. However, this form of "forced" feeding results primarily in expansion of body fat mass without improvement in physiological indices.

There may be a potential role for the use of anabolic agents, i.e., growth hormone and androgens, in these patients. In a rat model of malnutrition (Fig. 2), growth hormone restores diaphragmatic function to normal following a period of protein-calorie deprivation. This same effect is not seen with simple restoration of protein and calorie intake. The use of growth hormone supplementation in a population of underweight patients with COPD was also effective in improving muscle strength in a nonrandomized investigation (81). However, at present, the use of anabolic agents, including growth hormone, must be restricted to the research environment.

All reported investigations have examined nutritional intervention without regard to other aspects of pulmonary rehabilitation. The expectation that nutritional therapy administered as an isolated intervention will significantly alter the course of patients with COPD may be unrealistic. At present, nutritional intervention should be viewed as complementary to the other components of a comprehensive rehabilitation program. There is strong evidence that the presence of ongoing weight loss is a poor prognostic indicator. Identification of the weight-losing patient suggests that the disease is unstable and indicates the need for modification of the treatment plan, if possible.

Modest weight gain, if achieved, enhances the prospect for improved muscle function and possibly for improved exercise tolerance. This can generally be accomplished by a dietary counseling program; occasionally nutritional supplements may be necessary. Clearly, specific electrolyte abnormalities or deficiencies should be corrected. At this time, aggressive nutritional support programs, such as the use of parenteral or enteral feeding, cannot be justified

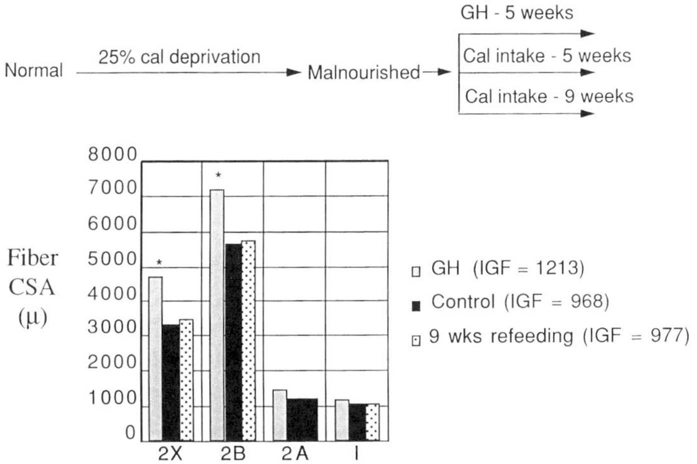

Figure 2 Comparison of the cross-sectional area of rat diaphragm muscle fiber types following a period of calorie deprivation and subsequent nutritional repletion in the presence and absence of growth hormone. CSA = fiber cross-sectional area (μ); 2X, 2B, 2A = type II muscle fibers; I = type I muscle fibers; control = malnourished animal following calorie deprivation; GH = malnourished animal following growth hormone supplementation; 9 wk refeeding = malnourished animal following 9 weeks of refeeding. $*p < 0.05$ compared to control and 9 wk refeeding. (Adapted from Ref. 20, with permission.)

in patients with COPD. Excessive weight gain, especially of body fat, would exert a deleterious effect in these patients and should be avoided.

B. The Obese Patient

Obesity (greater than 20% over ideal body weight) is also frequently seen in patients with COPD and may represent their most common nutritional disorder. Data from 153 patients in a Veterans Administration (VA) pulmonary clinic revealed a high incidence (37.2%) of obesity (>120% midpoint of the Metropolitan Tables) (82). In this population, two-thirds either maintained or gained weight in the year prior to the evaluation.

That obesity has a detrimental effect on respiratory function has been assumed but has not attracted as much attention as have undernutrition and COPD. It is logical that a metabolically inactive, added mass of fat will increase the work done by the compromised respiratory system, particularly during weight-bearing activities (83). Therefore, reductions in body fat mass should be beneficial to this patient population.

Obesity is notoriously resistant to treatment. Current recommendations for treatment are comprehensive in scope, including careful assessment and long-term, multidisciplinary intervention. Studies of these interventions in patients with pulmonary disease are lacking. While a variety of commercial weight loss programs and traditional nutritional counseling are available as interventions, the use of these in pulmonary rehabilitation has not been explored. Obesity therapy in pulmonary patients is often further complicated by the patients' limited exercise capacity. However, an exercise component should be an integral component of any pulmonary rehabilitation program.

Selection of patients for weight control programs must proceed with caution. Openbrier compared nutritional patterns of normal weight and underweight patients with COPD and found 70% of the normal-weight patients (90–110% IBW) were losing weight (unpublished doctoral thesis). In preliminary data, we found 22% of obese and 34% of normal-weight patients in a VA clinic population had documented weight loss of 5 lb or more in the previous year (82). These findings suggest a careful review of weight history is indicated for patients before they start weight reduction. Factors such as fluctuations in weight or appetite, loss of weight during exacerbations, or weight gain associated with prolonged use of steroids must be taken into account when deciding on a treatment plan.

IV. Conclusions

The problem of an abnormal nutritional state in patients who enroll in a pulmonary rehabilitation program remains a difficult issue for the clinician. Effective treatment strategies for both the underweight and obese patient are limited. However, the multidisciplinary model of effective pulmonary rehabilitation should provide the ideal environment to incorporate effective nutritional therapy into a comprehensive treatment plan.

Weight loss in the patient with COPD is an adverse prognostic variable, and greater understanding of its pathophysiology will benefit long-term outcomes. Although current studies have focused on nutritional therapy as an isolated therapeutic goal, future studies must include integrated rehabilitation programs that entail not only nutritional assessment, but also exercise and programs designed to prevent wasting. The problem of treating obesity in patients with lung disease remains unexplored.

References

1. Moore J, Angelillo V. Equations for the prediction of resting energy expenditure in chronic obstructive pulmonary disease. Chest 1988; 94:1260–1263.
2. Harris J, Benedict F. A Biometric Study of Basal Metabolism in Man. Washington, DC: The Carnegie Institute, 1919:1–266.
3. Roza A, Shizgal H. The Harris-Benedict equation reevaluated: resting energy requirements and the body cell mass. Am J Clin Nutr 1984; 40:168–182.
4. Schols A, Soeters P, Mostert R, Saris W, Wouters E. Energy balance in chronic obstructive pulmonary disease. Am Rev Respir Dis 1991; 143:1248–1252.
5. Donahoe M, Rogers R, Wilson D, Pennock B. Oxygen consumption of the respiratory muscles in normal and malnourished patients with chronic obstructive pulmonary disease. Am Rev Respir Dis 1989; 140:385–391.
6. Cherniak R. The oxygen consumption and efficiency of the respiratory muscles in health and disease. J Clin Invest 1959; 38:494–499.
7. Congleton J, Green J, Muers M. Basal metabolic rate, weight loss and decline in FEV_1 in COPD. Monaldi Arch Dis Chest 1993; 48:539–540.
8. Hugli O, Schutz Y, Leuenberger P, Fitting J. The daily energy expenditure of COPD patients in confined and free-living conditions. Am Rev Respir Dis 1991; 143:A453 (abstract).
9. Goldstein S, Askanazi J, Weissman C, Thomashow B, Kinney J. Energy expenditure in patients with chronic obstructive pulmonary disease. Chest 1987; 91:222–224.
10. Talpers S, Romberger D, Bunce S, Pingleton S. Nutritionally associated increased carbon dioxide production. Chest 1992; 102:551–555.
11. Hugli O, Frascarolo P, Schutz Y, Jequier E, Leuenberger P, Fitting J. Diet-induced thermogenesis in chronic obstructive pulmonary disease. Am Rev Respir Dis 1993; 148:1479–1483.
12. Zwillich C, Sahn S, Weil J. Effects of hypermetabolism on ventilation and chemosensitivity. J Clin Invest 1977; 60:900–906.
13. Soreide E, Skeie B, Kirvela O, et al. Branched-chain amino acid in chronic renal failure patients: respiratory and sleep effects. Kidney Int 1991; 40:539–543.

14. Takala J. Total plasma clearance of intravenous essential amino acids: evidence of abnormal metabolism of amino acids in chronic renal failure. J Parent Ent Nutr 1983; 7:146–150.
15. Delafosse B, Bouffard Y, Bertrand O, Viale J, Annat G, Motin J. Effects of protein intake on pulmonary gas exchange and ventilatory drive in postoperative patients. Anesthesiology 1989; 70:404–407.
16. Abbott W, Bistrian B, Blackburn G. The effect of dextrose and amino acids on respiratory function and energy expenditure in morbidly obese patients following gastric bypass surgery. J Surg Res 1986; 41:225–235.
17. Askanazi J, Elwyn D, Silverberg P, Rosenbaum S, Kinney J. Respiratory distress secondary to a high carbohydrate load: a case report. Surgery 1980; 87:596–598.
18. Lewis M, Sieck G, Fournier M, Belman M. Effect of nutritional deprivation on diaphragm contractility and muscle size. J Appl Physiol 1986; 60:596–603.
19. Kelsen S, Ference M, Kapoor S. Effects of prolonged undernutrition on structure and function of the diaphragm. 1985; 58:1354–1359.
20. Lanz J, Donahoe M, Rogers R, Ontell M. Effects of growth hormone on respiratory muscle recovery from malnutrition. J Appl Physiol 1992; 73:801–805.
21. Thurlbeck W. Diaphragm and body weight in emphysema. Thorax 1978; 33:483–487.
22. Arora N, Rochester D. Effect of body weight and muscularity on human diaphragm muscle mass, thickness, and area. J Appl Physiol 1982; 52:64–70.
23. Klitgaard H, Mantoni M, Schiaffino S, et al. Function, morphology and protein expression of ageing skeletal muscle: a cross-sectional study of elderly men with different training backgrounds. Acta Physiol Scand 1990; 140:41–54.
24. Russell D, Leiter L, Whitwell J, Marliss E, Jeejeebhoy K. Skeletal muscle function during hypocaloric diets and fasting: a comparison with standard nutritional assessment parameters. Am J Clin Nutr 1983; 37:133–138.
25. Turner J, Rotwein P, Novakofski J, Bechtel P. Induction of mRNA for IGF-I and -II during growth hormone–stimulated muscle hypertrophy. Am J Physiol 1988; 255:E513–517.
26. Devol D, Rotwein P, Sadow J, Novakofski J, Bechtel P. Activation of insulin-like growth factor gene expression during work-induced skeletal muscle growth. Am J Physiol 1990; 259:E89–95.
27. Miyashita A, Suzuki S, Suzuki M, et al. Effect of thyroid hormone on in vitro contractility of the canine diaphragm. Am Rev Respir Dis 1992; 145:1456–1462.
28. Ferguson G, Irvin C, Cherniack R. Effect of corticosteroids on respiratory muscle histopathology. Am Rev Respir Dis 1990; 142:1047–1052.
29. Goldberg A. Influence of insulin and contractile activity on muscle size and protein balance. Diabetes 1979; 28(Suppl):18–24.
30. Fiaccadori E, Coffrini E, Ronda N, et al. Hypophosphatemia in the course of chronic obstructive pulmonary disease. Chest 1990; 97:857–868.
31. Fiaccadori E, Coffrini E, Fracchia C, Rampulla C, Montagna T, Borghetti A. Hypophosphatemia and phosphorus depletion in respiratory and peripheral muscles of patients with respiratory due to COPD. Chest 1994; 105:1392–1398.

32. Fiaccadori E, Canale SD, Coffrini S, et al. Muscle and serum magnesium in pulmonary intensive care unit patients. Crit Care Med 1988; 16:751–760.
33. Dhingra S, Solven F, Wilson A, et al. Hypomagnesemia and respiratory muscle power. Am Rev Respir Dis 1984; 129:497–498.
34. Aubier M, Viires N, Piquet J, et al. Effects of hypocalcemia on diaphragmatic strength generation. J Appl Physiol 1985; 58:2054–2061.
35. Aubier M, Murciano D, Lecocguic Y, Jacquens Y, Squara P, Pariente R. Effect of hypophosphatemia on diaphragmatic contractility in patients with acute respiratory failure. J Appl Physiol 1985; 58:2054–2061.
36. Gertz I, Hedenstierna G, Hellers G, Wahren J. Muscle metabolism in patients with chronic obstructive pulmonary disease. Clin Sci Mol Med 1977; 52:395–403.
37. Tada H, Kato H, Musawa T, et al. ^{31}P nuclear magnetic resonance evidence of abnormal skeletal muscle metabolites in patients with chronic lung disease and congestive heart failure. Eur Respir J 1992; 5:163–169.
38. Dureuil B, Viires N, Veber B, et al. Acute diaphragmatic changes induced by starvation in rats. Am J Clin Nutr 1989; 49:738–744.
39. Efthimiou J, Fleming J, Gomes C, Spiro S. The effect of supplementary oral nutrition in poorly nourished patients with chronic obstructive pulmonary disease. Am Rev Respir Dis 1988; 137:1075–1082.
40. Fraser I. Effects of refeeding on respiration and skeletal muscle function. Clin Chest Med 1986; 7:131–139.
41. Rochester D, Braun N. Determinants of maximal inspiratory pressure in chronic obstructive pulmonary disease. Am Rev Respir Dis 1985; 132:42–47.
42. Byrd R, Hyatt R. Maximal respiratory pressures in chronic obstructive lung disease. Am Rev Respir Dis 1968; 98:848.
43. Lands L, Desmond K, Demizio D, Pavilanis A, Coates A. The effects of nutritional status and hyperinflation on respiratory muscle strength in children and young adults. Am Rev Respir Dis 1990; 141:1506–1509.
44. O'Neill S, Leahy F, Pasterkamp H, Tal A. The effects of chronic hyperinflation, nutritional status, and posture on respiratory muscle strength in cystic fibrosis. Am Rev Respir Dis 1983; 128:1051–1054.
45. Szeinberg A, England S, Mindorff C, Fraser I, Levison H. Maximal inspiratory and expiratory pressures are reduced in hyperinflated, malnourished, young adult male patients with cystic fibrosis. Am Rev Respir Dis 1985; 132:766–769.
46. Aubier M, Murciano D, Lecocguic Y, Viires N, Pariente R. Bilateral phrenic stimulation: a simple technique to assess diaphragm fatigue in humans. J Appl Physiol 1985; 58:58–64.
47. Esau S, Bellemare F, Grassino A, Permutt S, Roussos C, Pardy R. Changes in relation rate with diaphragmatic fatigue in humans. J Appl Physiol 1983; 54:1353–1360.
48. Roussos C, Campbell E. Respiratory muscle energetics. In: Fishman A, ed. Handbook of Physiology. Section 3: The Respiratory System. Baltimore, MD: Williams & Wilkins, 1986; 481–509.
49. Gray-McDonald K, Gibbons L, Shapiro S, Martin J. The effect of nutritional state

on exercise performance in patients with chronic obstructive pulmonary disease. Am Rev Respir Dis 1989; 139:1435–1438.
50. Wilson D, Rogers R, Wright E, Anthonisen N. Body weight in chronic obstructive pulmonary disease: the National Institutes of Health Intermittant Positive Pressure Breathing Trial. Am Rev Respir Dis 1989; 139:1435–1438.
51. Lohman T. Anthropometry and body composition. In: Lohman T, ed. Anthropometric Standardization Reference Manual. Champaign, Il: Human Kinetics Books, 1988.
52. Baumgartner R. Body composition in elderly persons: a critical review of needs and methods. Prog Food Nutr Sci 1993; 17:223–260.
53. Durnin J, Womersley J. Body fat assessed from total body density and its estimation from skinfold thickness: measurements on 481 men and women from 16 to 72 years. Br J Nutr 1974; 32:77–97.
54. Visser M, Heuvel EVD, Deurenberg P. Prediction equations for the estimation of body composition in the elderly using anthropometric data. Br J Nutr 1994; 71:823–833.
55. Mancino J, Donahoe M, Lebow H, Rogers R. The effects of COPD exacerbations on body composition and nutritional status. Am Rev Respir Dis 1993; 147:A199.
56. Segal K, Loan MV, Fitzgerald P, Hodgdon J, Itallie TV. Lean body mass estimation by bioelectrical impedance analysis: a four-site cross validation study. Am J Clin Nutr 1988; 47:7–14.
57. Mancino J, Donahoe M, Rogers R, Openbrier D. Determination of lean body mass in patients with chronic obstructive pulmonary disease. Am Rev Respir Dis 1990; 141:A34.
58. Schols A, Wouters E, Soeters P, Westerterp K. Body composition by bioelectrical impedance analysis compared with deuterium dilution and skinfold anthropometry in patients with chronic obstructive pulmonary disease. Am J Clin Nutr 1991; 53:421–424.
59. Schols A, Soeters P, Dingemans A, Mostert R, Frantzen P, Wouters E. Prevalence and characteristics of nutritional depletion in patients with stable COPD eligible for pulmonary rehabilitation. Am Rev Respir Dis 1993; 147:1151–1156.
60. Otte K, Ahlburg P, D'Amore F, Stellfeld M. Nutritional repletion in malnourished patients with emphysema. J Parent Ent Nutr 1990; 13:152–156.
61. Lewis M, Belman M, Dorr-Uyemura L. Nutritional supplementation of ambulatory patients with chronic obstructive pulmonary disease. Am Rev Respir Dis 1989; 135:1062–1068.
62. Knowles J, Farbarne M, Wiggs B, Chan-Yan C, Pardy R. Dietary supplementation in respiratory muscle performance in patients with COPD. Chest 1988; 93:977–983.
63. Fuenzalida C, Petty T, Jones M, et al. The immune response to short-term nutritional intervention in advanced chronic obstructive pulmonary disease. Am Rev Respir Dis 1990; 142:49–56.
64. Hunt D, Rowlands B, Johnston D. Hand grip strength—a simple prognostic indicator in surgical patients. J Parent Ent Nutr 1985; 9:701–704.
65. Goldstein S, Thomashow B, Kvetan V, Askanazi J, Kinney J, Elwyn D. Nitrogen

and energy relationships in malnourished patients with emphysema. Am Rev Respir Dis 1988; 138:636–644.
66. Wilson D, Rogers R, Sanders M, Pennock B, Reilly J. Nutritional intervention in malnourished patients with emphysema. Am Rev Respir Dis 1986; 134:672–677.
67. Whittaker J, Ryan C, Buckley P, Road J. The effects of refeeding on peripheral and respiratory muscle function in malnourished chronic obstructive pulmonary disease patients. Am Rev Respir Dis 1990; 142:283–288.
68. Rogers R, Donahoe M, Costantino J. Physiologic effects of oral supplemental feeding on malnourished COPD patients: a randomized controlled study. Am Rev Respir Dis 1992 146:1511–1517.
69. Hunter A, Carey M, Larsh H. The nutritional status of patients with chronic obstructive pulmonary disease. Am Rev Respir Dis 1981; 124:376–381.
70. Fiaccadori E, Canale SD, Coffrini E, et al. Hypercapnic-hypoxemic chronic obstructive pulmonary disease (COPD): influence of severity of COPD on nutritional status. Am J Clin Nutr 1988; 48:680–685.
71. Openbrier D, Irwin M, Rogers R, et al. Nutritional status and lung function in patients with emphysema and chronic bronchitis. Chest 1983; 83:17–22.
72. Renzetti A, McClement J, Litt B. The Veterans Administration Cooperative Study of Pulmonary Function. Mortality in relation to respiratory function in chronic obstructive pulmonary disease. Am J Med 1966; 41:115–129.
73. Vandenburgh E, Woestigne KVD, Gyselen A. Weight changes in the terminal stages of chronic obstructive lung disease. Am Rev Respir Dis 1967; 96:556–565.
74. Braun S, Keim N, Dixon R, Clagnaz P, Anderegg A, Shrago E. The prevalence and determinants of nutritional changes in chronic obstructive pulmonary disease. Chest 1984; 86:558–563.
75. Efthimiou J, Mounsey P, Benson D, Madgwick R, Coles S, Benson M. Effect of carbohydrate rich versus fat rich loads on gas exchange and walking performance in patients with chronic obstructive pulmonary disease. Thorax 1992; 47:451–456.
76. Brown S, Wiener S, Brown R, Marcarelli P, Light R. Exercise performance following a carbohydrate load in chronic airflow obstruction. J Appl Physiol 1983; 58:1340–1346.
77. Donahoe M, Rogers R, Mancino J. Energy balance in malnourished COPD patients. Am J Respir Crit Care Med 1995 (abstract) (in press).
78. Browning R, Olsen A. The functional gastrointestinal disorders of pulmonary emphysema. Mayo Clin Proc 1961; 36:537–543.
79. Schols A, Mostert R, Cobben N, Soeters P, Wouters E. Transcutaneous oxygen saturation and carbon dioxide tension during meals in patients with chronic obstructive pulmonary disease. Chest 1991; 100:1287–1292.
80. Efthimiou J, Fleming J, Spiro S. Sternomastoid muscle function and fatigue in breathless patients with severe respiratory disease. Am Rev Respir Dis 1987; 136:1099–1105.
81. Pape G, Friedman M, Underwood L, Clemmons D. The effect of growth hormone on weight gain and pulmonary function in patients with chronic obstructive pulmonary disease. Chest 1991; 99:1495–1500.
82. Donahoe M, Mancino J, Rogers R, Costantino J, Lebow H. Clinical factors do

not predict weight loss in patients with chronic obstructive pulmonary disease. Am Rev Respir Dis 1991; 143:A453.
83. Swinburn C, Cooper B, Mould H, Corris P, Gibson G. Adverse effect of additional weight on exercise against gravity in patients with chronic obstructive airways disease. Thorax 1989; 44:716–720.
84. Openbrier DR, Donahoe M, Rogers RM. Eating patterns and factors associated with weight loss in patients with COPD. Am Rev Respir Dis 1989; 139:A194 (abstract).

24

Habilitation of the Child with Chronic Pulmonary Failure

VIRGINIA SIMSON NELSON

C. S. Mott Children's Hospital
University of Michigan Medical Center
Ann Arbor, Michigan

Continued medical and technological advances are resulting in higher survival rates for medically fragile infants and children, with a significant number of these requiring long-term mechanical ventilation. This growing incidence of ventilator-assisted children, combined with the pressures of increasing hospital costs and subsequent need to find cost-effective alternatives, is resulting in earlier discharge from hospitals. Earlier discharge, in turn, places additional responsibility on the families and community resources to maintain these children in their homes. Who makes the decision for long-term ventilation? On what information is this based? In what stage of the illness or how soon after the injury is this decision made? Are any choices given to the family (or the child or adolescent), or are the issues even fully explained to them? While our rehabilitation team fully supports long-term ventilation in many cases, families (and children when they are old enough) must understand what this means to them. They must have a complete understanding of the medical situation; they must be able to perform (or direct) all daily care; they must be fully aware and accepting of the risks inherent in home ventilation.

This chapter reviews causes of ventilatory failure in children, making the decision for home ventilation, goals of home mechanical ventilation, options and methods for long-term ventilation in children, approaches to facilitate oral communication in children using trach positive-pressure ventilation, habilitation (and rehabilitation) in the hospital, and transition from hospital to home, community, and school.

I. Causes of Ventilatory Failure in Children

There are several ways to classify the types of chronic ventilatory failure in children. Which system is used depends on the number of patients followed and the preferences of the professionals involved. The physician may classify patients one way, while the speech/language pathologist may use another classification. One convenient classification system of causes of ventilatory failure is: (1) neuromuscular dysfunction or "bellows failure," e.g., myopathy, spinal cord injury (SCI); (2) lung disease, e.g., bronchopulmonary dysplasia (BPD); (3) central hypoventilation, e.g., congenital central hypoventilation syndrome (CCHS); (4) airway problems, e.g., tracheomalacia, bronchomalacia; (5) mixed.

As with any classification system, questions arise about where to place certain patients. Where does the child with respiratory failure and myelodysplasia fit—neuromuscular or central hypoventilation? What about the child with respiratory failure due to a traumatic brain injury (TBI)? Does he/she have central hypoventilation or neuromuscular dysfunction? The answers to these questions may not be important, but must be consistent if statistics about the population are to be reported or comparisons across various populations are to be made.

Another classification system is: (1) disorders of respiratory muscles, e.g., myopathy; (2) central nervous system (CNS) dysfunction, e.g., SCI, central hypoventilation, TBI; (3) airway and pulmonary problems, e.g., BPD, tracheomalacia. Still other classification systems may be used, depending on the purposes for classifying patients, e.g., medical or communication needs.

Which type of respiratory failure predominates in any given clinic or geographical area depends on resources for long-term ventilation, philosophy of who should be provided with long-term ventilation, and the expertise of the professionals treating these children; e.g., a pulmonologist will probably see more children with lung disease while a physiatrist will probably treat more children with neuromuscular diseases, as well as demographic factors.

II. Experience with Long-Term Mechanical Ventilation

Children have been provided with the option for long-term mechanical ventilation at Mott Children's Hospital at the University of Michigan since 1978 (1). Prior to the current program, there was a Polio Respiratory Center treating

Table 1 Reasons for Ventilator Use[a]

Condition	% of patients
Neuromuscular or "bellows failure"	70
Lung disease	15
Airway problems	8
CCHS	7

[a]$N = 89$.

children and adults during the years of polio epidemics, but this program ended when these epidemics ceased with the availability of polio vaccine. A total of 89 children were treated in the 15 years ending in March 1993 (an additional 25 have been treated since then). The male:female ratio was 1.8:1, reflecting the large number of children in this group with spinal cord injuries. Eighty-six percent of the children were still alive at the time statistics were analyzed, with only 7% weaned from the ventilator. Children were first mechanically ventilated at ages ranging from birth to 21 years, with a median of 4.4 years and a mean of 7.2 years. Twenty-four percent of these children were initially ventilated at birth. Reasons for ventilator use are shown in Table 1.

The large percentage with neuromuscular problems reflects the fact that the Pediatric Home Ventilator Program was started by a physiatrist and did not have a pulmonologist as part of the core team for the first 10 years. Diagnoses of the children in this program are shown in Table 2.

The other category includes children with cancer (3%), skeletal dysplasia (3%), myelodysplasia (2%), and VACTERL syndrome (2%). Children were ventilated in a variety of ways: intermittent positive pressure through a trache-

Table 2 Diagnoses[a]

Diagnosis	% of patients
SCI	34
Myopathy	21
BPD	8
CCHS	7
SMA	4
Other, including:	26
Cancer	3
Dwarfism	3
Myelodysplasia	2

[a]$N = 89$.

ostomy (71%), bilevel positive pressure through a tracheostomy (12%), bilevel positive pressure through a face mask (11%), and negative pressure (6%). Twenty-eight percent used supplemental oxygen at least part of the time. Mechanical ventilation was used an average of 19 hr/day, with a range of 10–24 hr/day. Fifty-seven percent of the children used mechanical ventilation 24 hr/day.

III. Decision for Home Ventilation

The decision for home mechanical ventilation starts when either chronic or acute respiratory failure is diagnosed in the child. Unfortunately, for many children this is a sudden event and there is no time for discussion with the parents about their wishes or even time to explain the situation. For those with a chronic condition that will eventually lead to respiratory failure (such as Duchenne muscular dystrophy), a full discussion of the practical, ethical, and legal issues can be held. In such cases, parents (and children if they are capable) must understand the disease process, daily care needs, financial implications, and the risks of home ventilation, and they must fully accept the responsibilities required by home ventilation. While there may no longer be the option for long-term hospitalization for children who are ventilator users, families must still know that there are risks at home that are increased, e.g., only one caregiver present when an emergency occurs, no available backup equipment, and others that are decreased, e.g., infection. Professionals must understand and teach families the impact of the degree of ventilator dependence, the type of mechanical ventilation, and the diagnosis on risks and outcome. Whether a child has a pulmonary or neuromuscular disorder, a static or progressive condition, and coexisting medical problems, have an impact on the risks of home mechanical ventilation as well as on the overall outcome.

There are no controlled studies that prove that children develop better at home than in the hospital when they are ventilator users, but those who work in this field can share many anecdotal reports about the dramatic developmental gains made as soon as the child is discharged from the hospital to his/her home. Parents must understand this, but they must also understand the effect on the family of having a ventilator-assisted child at home (2,3).

Once the decision for home ventilation has been made, families must begin preparations for home care. While medical stability is being achieved, parents must begin training so that they become the experts in their child's care. They must understand the disease process and complications; total daily care; tracheostomy management, if applicable; ventilator use, maintenance, and troubleshooting; cardiopulmonary resuscitation; developmental stimulation; how to access community resources including schools and Children's Special

Health Care Services; and how to advocate for their child in all settings. They must learn how to access financial resources, including private money, insurance, governmental money, and "creative" funding. Necessary equipment must be obtained and environmental changes must be made to accommodate the child's needs. Community resources must be arranged, including home nursing, primary care physician, psychosocial services, equipment and supply vendors, emergency services, and school.

IV. Goals of Home Mechanical Ventilation

The obvious goal of long-term mechanical ventilation is maintenance of life. This is achieved through the provision of adequate oxygenation and the achievement of normal carbon dioxide levels. But this is not enough. Ventilation must provide for optimal health, growth and development, and stamina. Thus, the best ventilation is not necessarily the least, but rather that level necessary to optimize the child's quality of life.

V. Ventilation Options

Long-term mechanical ventilation of children may be done in a variety of ways, with the choice of the method depending on many factors, including: (1) age of the child; (2) diagnosis; (3) experience of the treating physicians; and (4) availability of equipment and its maintenance.

Basic options are negative pressure and positive pressure. The former is delivered by the iron lung or tank respirator, cuirass or chest shell, and pulmowrap. Rate and pressure may be set and all of these may be used in a patient with a tracheostomy, although one is not required. The advantage of negative-pressure ventilation is that tracheostomy, nasal mask, and mouthpiece are not required and the equipment is relatively easy to service. But the iron lung is large and relatively nonportable (the portable model weighs approximately 100 lb); does not work well with decreased lung compliance; requires assistance for use even for adults; and positioning of the child is difficult. A cuirass must be custom-made for small children and those with chest deformities or severe scoliosis. It also does not work well in patients with decreased lung compliance, is difficult to don independently, and has no internal battery. Whether the advantages outweigh the limitations must be decided on a case-by-case basis.

Home positive-pressure ventilation may be delivered by mask, mouthpiece, or tracheostomy. It may be continuous positive airway pressure (CPAP) or pressure support, bilevel positive-pressure ventilation (BLPPV), or intermittent positive-pressure ventilation (IPPV). BLPPV is indicated for respiratory support for the child who can initiate a breath. It improves functional residual capacity, augments tidal breathing with pressure support, improves pulmonary hygiene by providing constant pressure to keep alveoli open, and rests respiratory muscles. It cannot be used in children who have no respiratory effort or in small babies who are too weak to trigger a breath, and it requires an external battery and alarms. The machine used for BLPPV is smaller and lighter in weight than those used for IPPV and it is easier to learn to use.

IPPV is indicated for those who need full respiratory support, although it may also be used by those who have respiratory effort. Machines may be small enough to fit on a wheelchair ventilator tray, although for those who are ambulatory, these machines are difficult to move without the use of some type of mobile device such as a cart or heavy-duty wheeled walker with a large enough tray to accommodate the machine.

Long-term positive-pressure ventilation may be delivered by mask, mouthpiece, or tracheostomy. Which option is used is often dictated by the experience and expertise of the treating physicians. Masks are commercially available or may be custom-made from a variety of materials. Currently, no commercial infant masks are available. Skin irritation may limit mask use even with the alternation of various masks, and patients rarely tolerate long-term 24 hr daily use because of skin breakdown. Orthodontic problems may be increased with long-term use of masks in young children, although data are not yet published on this (Steinberg B, Nelson VS, unpublished data, 1995). The main advantages of mask or mouthpiece use are noninvasiveness, the simplification of care needs, and decreased bacterial colonization of the lower respiratory tract (4). But limitations include lack of direct access to the trachea for suctioning and inability to use in patients with severe oral motor dysfunction. Indications for chronic mask ventilation in children are increasing as more experience is gained (5,6).

VI. Ventilation Methods

Various ventilator parameters can be adjusted until respiratory goals are reached. For BLPPV, inspiratory and expiratory pressures (IPAP and EPAP, respectively) may be varied and oxygen may be added. A backup rate (BUR) may be added, although not all ventilator models allow this. A BUR is useful for the child who has occasional periods of apnea that necessitate a delivered breath rate.

IPPV machines allow the setting of rate, delivered volume, oxygen concentration, inspiratory and expiratory pressures and times, and mode (assist, control, and synchronized intermittent mandatory ventilation). For children on full-time ventilation, settings may be varied depending on wake-sleep cycle or other factors. Minute ventilation is determined by standard methods with other factors being determined by the child's clinical status. We have found that low rates and large delivered volumes minimize atelectasis and promote optimal speech. Delivered volumes of 10–20 cm^3/kg body weight are used initially and adjusted to achieve adequate exhaled volumes, oxygenation, and carbon dioxide levels.

VII. Facilitating Oral Communication

In addition to achieving respiratory goals, attention must be paid to communication in those children ventilated through a tracheostomy. To promote this, cuffless tracheal tubes ("trach tubes") should be used whenever possible to allow the leakage of air over the vocal cords for the production of sound. This is a different system than the closed system used in the hospital setting, but its efficacy in adults has been well documented by Bach and Alba (7). If cuffed trach tubes are initially used, children may have difficulty tolerating the switch to a cuffless tube, even with very slow changes. In larger children, we have found it best to initially use a cuffed tube with the cuff deflated. The cuff can be inflated if an emergency situation occurs, but the child does not usually have an opportunity to become accustomed to the cuff being inflated. Once the situation is stable, the cuffed tube is changed to an uncuffed one of the same size.

Volumes must be increased to allow for air leakage, and the trach tube should be the smallest possible tube that permits adequate ventilation. Large delivered volume, low rate, and long inspiratory time encourage optimal speech production by allowing more time for speaking, which occurs on inspiration (8). A one-way speaking valve may also be used to promote the flow of air over the vocal cords during expiration (9), but this should be used only with an uncuffed trach tube and after airway pressures have been measured and indicate adequate space for the escape of air around the trach tube and past the vocal cords. To assess inner tracheal pressures, attach a manometer to the trach tube and measure inspiratory and expiratory pressures generated during normal tidal breathing. For the child who has no respiratory effort, the manometer can be connected in line with the ventilator tubing. Normal pressures range from 5 to 8 cmH_2O for expiration and -5 to -8 cmH_2O for inspiration. Values greater than 10 or -10 cmH_2O, respectively, indicate increased resistance, and bronchoscopy may be indicated to rule out obstruction. Elevated inspiratory pressures are more consistent with tracheo- or bronchomalacia, while elevated expiratory pressures usually indicate the presence of granulation tissue (10). The one-way speaking valve should not be used with increased resistance. Use of the valve in line with the ventilator should only be in situations where the child is observed since the valve increases pressures at the alveolar level if obstruction occurs in the trachea or larynx.

For the child who must use a cuffed trach tube, a talking trach may be tried. This is a tube with a supplementary source of air that is released above the cuff and allows air to flow upward over the vocal cords to produce sound. Disadvantages of this include the difficulty in keeping the small supplemental channel free of secretions and the necessity to have an additional air source, which must be turned on whenever the child wants to talk. These tubes are also not available in small sizes.

For the child with severe oral motor dysfunction, alternative communication systems may be used. These include pointing (eye or hand), signing, or various computer-based systems. Discussion of these is beyond the scope of this chapter.

VIII. Rehabilitation/Habilitation and Transition to the Community

Preparing the ventilator-assisted child and family for entry (or reentry) into the community is a complex process that requires extensive education of the child and family and planning that incorporates the family and community providers (11,12). Education and planning can begin while medical stability is being achieved. Medical stability includes all facets, not just respiratory. Adequate nutrition, which can be maintained at home, needs to be established. Medications, ventilation, and other procedures need to be stable, with no changes in the week or so prior to discharge. Parents and child need to be psychologically ready to return home.

Families need to be experts in their child's care and need to demonstrate their ability to manage all aspects for at least 24–48 consecutive hours without assistance. This can be achieved by teaching parents all necessary information and giving them progressive responsibility as they learn the care. Children should be transitioned to equipment to be used at home prior to hospital discharge so they and their families are familiar with their "own" equipment. The daily schedule to be used at home should likewise be used in the hospital prior to discharge. A "trial run" overnight pass at home, if possible, is critical to increasing the likelihood of success. If a home stay is not possible, the child may stay at a hotel or, if necessary, in the hospital without nursing or other assistance being used. This pass is very helpful for increasing family confidence and finding gaps in knowledge or planning.

Successful transition to home is also enhanced by training of community people like home nurses and school personnel. For children returning to school, inservice training of classmates and teachers by members of the hospital team can be very helpful in easing the transition. A video of the child may be shown and questions answered, with emphasis on the fact that the child has many of the same capabilities as his/her classmates. For the child who now needs computers to enhance capabilities, this may be a way to attract other children who may see the chance to play a computer game and not the disability.

Although ventilator-assisted children may have many of the same needs and participate in many of the same activities as normal children, they also have special needs. A home ventilator clinic may be helpful in assisting with specialized needs. Family and sibling support groups may also be helpful, both for support and to organize advocacy efforts. We have also found that Vent Camp, an overnight camp for children who are ventilator users, is also very successful in providing respite for families and a camping experience for children who are excluded from other camps. Here they are children first and can experience many things while practicing skills learned in therapy. They are "regular kids," which is the goal professionals have for children who are ventilator-assisted.

References

1. Nelson VS, Carroll JC, Hurvitz EA, Dean JM. Home mechanical ventilation: parameters of change in 15 years of experience. Dev Med Child Neurol 1994; 36(Suppl 70):35.
2. Engel L, Warschausky SA, Nelson VS. Assessing family adaptation to ventilator-dependent children. Arch Phys Med Rehabil 1989; 70:A20.
3. Engel L, Warschausky SA, Nelson VS. A model of the psychology of adjustment to ventilator dependency in pediatric patients. Arch Phys Med Rehabil 1989; 70:A23.
4. Niederman MS, Ferranti RD, Zeigler A, et al. Respiratory infection complicating long-term tracheostomy. Chest 1994; 85:39–44.
5. Brown RW, Grady EA, Van Laanen CJ, et al. Invasive bi-level positive airway pressure (BLPAP) home ventilation for chronic respiratory failure in children. American Thoracic Society/American Lung Society Annual Meeting, Boston, May 1994.
6. Brown RW, Grady EA, Van Laanen CJ, et al. Home use of bi-level positive airway pressure (BLPAP) ventilation for chronic respiratory failure in children. American Association for Respiratory Care Annual Meeting, Denver, December 1994.
7. Bach JR, Alba AS. Tracheostomy ventilation: a study of efficacy with deflated cuffs and cuffless tubes. Chest 1990; 97:679–683.
8. Driver LE, Nelson VS, Kurcz KB, et al. A team approach to managing ventilator-assisted children. ASHA 1993; 35:166.
9. Fornataro-Clerici L, Zajac DJ. Aerodynamic characteristics of tracheostomy speaking valves. J Speech Hearing Res 1993; 36:529–532.
10. Driver LE, Nelson VS. A team approach to managing ventilator-assisted children. American Speech Language Hearing Association Annual Meeting, Anaheim, CA, November 20, 1993.

11. Engel L, Warschausky S. Bridging the gap between inpatient and outpatient care for ventilator-assisted children. Annual Meeting of the American Psychological Association, San Francisco, August 1991.
12. Warschausky S, Nelson VS, Engel L. Challenges and solutions for interdisciplinary planning for home care of the ventilator-assisted child. Annual Meeting of the American Academy for Cerebral Palsy and Developmental Medicine, San Diego, October 1992.

Part Four

THE VENTILATOR-DEPENDENT PATIENT

25

Failure to Wean

The Chronic Ventilator-Dependent Patient

NICHOLAS S. HILL

Brown University
and Rhode Island Hospital
Providence, Rhode Island

Dependence on chronic mechanical ventilation is a phenomenon of modern technology. Although a sizable population of patients became dependent on mechanical ventilation during the poliomyelitis epidemics of the 1930s–1950s, the increasing use of invasive positive-pressure ventilation and the proliferation of intensive care units since the 1960s have given rise to a much larger population of patients who fail to wean from mechanical ventilation following bouts of acute respiratory failure. In addition, patients with slowly progressive neuromuscular diseases, chest wall deformities, or chronic obstructive pulmonary disease (COPD) may gradually deteriorate and become dependent on at least intermittent ventilatory support before developing acute respiratory failure. As is so often the case with increasing applications of technology, widespread support of chronically ventilator-dependent patients places enormous strains on human and financial resources, outstripping knowledge about optimal application, and raising complicated ethical issues. This chapter considers the types of patients who become chronically ventilator-dependent, the technologies available, approaches to rehabilitation, options for placement, and ethical issues.

I. Characteristics of Ventilator-Dependent Patients

A. Definitions

No consensus appears in the literature on the duration that a patient must be mechanically ventilated to be considered chronically dependent, or how many hours per 24-hr period the ventilator must be in use. A number of authors have used the description "prolonged" for mechanical ventilation that is used for as little as 1 or 2 days (1,2). For practical purposes, however, this analysis defines chronic ventilator dependency according to the guidelines used in the Health Care Finance Administration Demonstration Trial for Chronic Ventilator Units: use of at least 6 hr of mechanical ventilation daily for at least 21 days (3).

B. Failure to Wean

Those who fail to wean after bouts of acute respiratory failure constitute an important source of chronically ventilator-dependent patients. The composition of this population depends heavily on the site in question; most centers report a preponderance of COPD patients and variable numbers of postsurgical patients. In addition, the aggressiveness of medical support and the nature of attempts at weaning are likely to be important determinants of eventual success in weaning. Although much has been learned about the science of weaning over the past several decades, weaning the difficult-to-wean patient remains largely an art (4). The availability of not only highly experienced physicians, but also skilled nurses and respiratory therapists, facilitates weaning in these challenging patients. Accordingly, specialized weaning units, either contained within acute care facilities or free-standing, have been forming throughout the United States. Some of these report highly favorable success rates in weaning (5,6).

In previous decades, a number of physiological parameters were proposed to serve as guidelines to weaning, e.g., maximal inspiratory pressure exceeding -25 to -30 cmH_2O, tidal volume > 10 ml/kg, and minute volume < 10 L/min (7). These parameters were useful in postoperative patients with little underlying lung disease. But, they fared poorly as predictors of success in weaning when applied to chronically debilitated medical patients. More recently, other methods have been proposed to help in predicting the likelihood of success in weaning. Morganroth et al. (8) proposed a scoring system that took into account not only ventilator factors, such as positive end-expiratory pressure (PEEP), F_{IO_2}, and compliance, but also medical factors, including cardiac, nutritional, infectious disease, and functional status. Tobin et al. (9) observed that patients who failed attempts at weaning developed a rapid, shallow breathing pattern; subsequently, they proposed the rapid, shallow breathing index as a simple means of assessing likelihood of weaning success (10).

Insights gained from these studies have led specialized weaning units to adopt a multidisciplinary approach aimed at optimizing the overall medical and functional status of the patient (11), and to explore ways in which breathing pattern on the ventilator could be altered to improve efficiency. Examples of the latter approach include inspiratory muscle training (12), use of tidal volume and relaxation feedback, and use of the pressure support mode. Among patients who remained ventilator-dependent for at least a week, Holliday and Hyers (13) decreased the duration of weaning from 32.6 to 20.6 days by adjusting tidal volumes and using relaxation feedback to increase tidal volume and breathing efficiency, i.e., an improved tidal volume/diaphragm electromyographic ratio. Also, pressure support ventilation was recently shown to reduce the frequency of weaning failures more than did synchronized intermittent mandatory ventilation (SIMV) and t-piece weaning (14). The reason for the greater effectiveness of pressure support ventilation is that it probably restores respiratory muscle coordination more effectively because, unlike SIMV or t-piece weaning, it can be used to titrate the amount of ventilatory assistance breath by breath; it is also more comfortable, reducing anxiety and the need for sedation. Thus, specific techniques used to wean patients may be important determinants of the duration of weaning or eventual rate of weaning success.

A complete discussion of weaning techniques is beyond the scope of this chapter, but in the author's experience, specific techniques are of less overall importance than meticulous medical care of the patient. Most patients who remain ventilator-dependent 21 days after a bout of acute respiratory failure have multiple complicating conditions. They are often elderly, malnourished, deconditioned, and recovering from major surgery or episodes of sepsis or pneumonia. Left ventricular or neurological function may be severely compromised, and patients are usually frightened, anxious, and depressed. Weaning is often not even a consideration until infection is controlled, nutritional deficits corrected, a physical conditioning program initiated, and other pertinent conditions appropriately treated. With careful attention to these problems, patients' respiratory muscle strength, endurance, and efficiency often gradually improve. Concurrently, the work of breathing gradually decreases as airway obstruction and secretions respond to treatment, catabolic states subside as sepsis resolves, and dead space diminishes as lung injury heals. As the imbalance between supply and demand for ventilatory work that leads to chronic ventilator dependency (15) is corrected, many difficult-to-wean patients eventually wean regardless of the specific weaning technique used.

C. Factors Associated with Inability to Wean and Mortality in Mechanically Ventilated Patients

Some studies that have examined survival rates after mechanical ventilation for acute respiratory failure are listed in Table 1. These are mainly retrospective,

Table 1 Survival Outcomes After Mechanical Ventilation for Acute Respiratory Failure

Author	Year	Type[a]	No. of pts	Min dur vent[b]	Survival (%) Discharge	Survival (%) 1 yr	% weaned
Davis (2)	1980	T	100	>48 hr	44	40	
Witek (16)	1985	C	100	—	50	33	
Gillespie (1)	1986	T	327[d]	>24 hr	54	44	
Papadakis (17)	1987	V	78	—	24	—	
Spicher (18)	1987	T	250	>10 days	39	29	
Elpern (19)	1989	T	95[c]	>3 days	33	16	
Menzies (20)	1989	T	104	—	—	34	75
Gracey (21)	1992	T	383	>1 hr	43	30	

[a]T = tertiary care; C = community hospital; V = veterans hospital.
[b]Minimum duration on ventilator to be eligible for study.
[c]Patients >60 years.
[d]COPD patients.

with entry criteria varying from no minimum duration of ventilation to at least 29 days; also, the patient populations differ substantially among them. Despite these limitations, it is apparent that patients requiring mechanical ventilation for acute respiratory failure have high mortality rates, with only 40–50% surviving to hospital discharge, and an average of 30% alive a year later. The more favorable survival rates in the Gracey study (21) may have been related to a high percentage of surgical patients (83%). In the Elpern study (19), poor survival rates were observed in patients over 60 years old; only 16% were alive after 1 year.

Factors associated with poor survival are listed in Table 2. These include premorbid incapacity, left ventricular dysfunction, low serum albumin, and multiorgan system failure (1). Certain diagnoses also portend a poor prognosis, e.g., recent cardiopulmonary arrest, acute pulmonary edema (18), cancer (23), and AIDS. Patients with COPD have lower hospital mortality rates than do those with other diagnoses, but tend to have higher postdischarge mortality rates (1). Fewer studies have sought factors associated with failure to wean than for mortality (Table 2). Not surprisingly, they overlap with those that predict mortality, including the level of serum albumin, dyspnea, and the functional status. In addition, abnormalities in a number of pulmonary functions predict failure to wean (Table 2).

Because few studies have examined weaning rather than survival rates, it is difficult to determine the frequencies of chronic ventilator dependence. Gillespie et al. (1) found a relatively high rate of "ventilator dependence" during

Table 2 Factors Associated with Mortality and Weaning Failure in Chronically Ventilated Patients

Mortality	Failure to wean
Advanced age	Low FEV_1
Low FEV_1	Low albumin
Low serum albumin	Poor functional status
Hypercapnea	Dyspnea
Cor pulmonale	Low maximal inspiratory pressure force
History of left ventricular failure	Low tidal volume
Dyspnea	Rapid respiratory rate
Poor functional status	
Multiple organ system failure	

Source: Adapted from Ref. 20.

hospitalization among COPD patients (43%); they did not define the duration of dependence. Gracey et al. (21) found that 13% of 783 patients receiving mechanical ventilation for more than a week remained ventilator-dependent beyond 29 days. Menzies et al. (20), also studying COPD patients, found that 58% of 95 patients remained ventilator-dependent after 2 weeks, and only 13% after 45 days. After a year, only 3% continued to receive mechanical ventilatory assistance. On the other hand, Make et al. (24) surveyed hospitals and home respiratory care companies in Massachusetts for patients who had been ventilator-dependent for more than 3 weeks and found that although 33% of the patients had died a year later, 81% of the survivors were still ventilator-dependent. However, this survey included patients in chronic care facilities and at home, and was probably not as representative of patients recovering from bouts of respiratory failure in acute care hospitals.

Thus, most studies indicate that the rate of ventilator dependence falls progressively as time passes after an episode of acute respiratory failure. This attrition is related partly to eventual weaning and partly to mortality. In any case, it may be anticipated that only a small proportion of patients mechanically ventilated for acute respiratory failure will require long-term ventilatory support extending beyond a few months.

D. Ventilator Dependence After Progression of Chronic Respiratory Failure

In patients with chronic respiratory failure, chronic ventilator dependence may develop after a bout of acute respiratory failure because of disease progression rather than inability to wean. Although precise statistics on the incidence of this type of patient are unavailable, their ailments fall into several large categories, e.g., slowly progressive neuromuscular disorders, chest wall deformities, central hypoventilatory disorders, and severe COPD (25). Among the common neuromuscular disorders leading to chronic respiratory failure are the postpolio syndrome, muscular dystrophies such as Duchenne or limb-girdle, and amyotrophic lateral sclerosis. Kyphoscoliosis with an angle of curvature exceeding 130° and thoracoplasty for treatment of prior tuberculosis predispose to development of respiratory failure, as do the obesity-hypoventilation syndrome and severe obstructive sleep apnea. The onset of respiratory failure in these patients (as indicated by daytime CO_2 retention) is usually heralded by symptoms of chronic hypoventilation including morning headache, daytime hypersomnolence, restless sleep, and nightmares. Numerous studies have now demonstrated that nocturnal ventilation in these patients effectively reduces daytime CO_2 retention and improves symptoms (26).

E. Scope of the Problem

Estimates of total numbers of chronically ventilator-dependent patients are difficult to make because of the turnover of the population: relatively few patients remain ventilator-dependent permanently, and new patients continually enter the population while others are weaning or dying. In addition, no central agency maintains statistics on such patients. However, a few attempts have been made to ascertain numbers of patients and costs. In their 1984 survey, Make et al. (24) estimated that 6800 patients were ventilator-dependent for more than 3 weeks in the entire United States, based on an extrapolation from the 147 patients they identified in Massachusetts. In 1990, the American Association of Respiratory Care (AARC) commissioned the Gallup Organization to survey 300 respiratory care department managers and 100 pulmonary specialists about the number of patients in their hospitals who required more than 6 hr of mechanical ventilation for more than 30 days (27). Based on an extrapolation, they estimated that there were more than 11,000 ventilator-dependent hospitalized patients in the United States at an estimated cost of \$800/patient/day, or a total cost of \$9 million daily. They also found that among Medicare-Medicaid patients, who made up 60% of the total, reimbursement rates covered only 46% of costs. In addition, the lack of chronic care facility beds caused an average delay of 35 days in discharge from acute care facilities, adding \$27,000/patient to the cost of acute care.

In 1990, Goldberg and Frownfelter (28) also reported a rate of ventilator dependency almost identical to that determined by the AARC. In a survey of acute and chronic care facilities and home care companies, they identified 453 ventilator-dependent individuals in Illinois, a number that extrapolates to 11,000 for the entire United States, assuming an Illinois population of 11.5

million. They also identified a lack of community services and financial constraints as barriers to discharge from acute care facilities.

Other investigators have reported large discrepancies between the cost of caring and reimbursement rates for chronically ventilator-dependent patients. In 1987, Gracey et al. (29) and Douglass et al. (30) estimated an average hospital loss of $20,000 and $23,000, respectively, per hospitalized patient mechanically ventilated for more than 2 or 3 days. A year later, after the Health Care Financing Administration (HCFA) had introduced two new diagnosis-related groups (DRGs 474 and 475) for mechanically ventilated patients, a large discrepancy persisted, partly because the DRGs required a primary respiratory diagnosis and 75% of mechanically ventilated patients had a nonrespiratory primary diagnosis (31).

Partly in response to these reimbursement problems, the Medicare Catastrophic Coverage Act of 1988 established five ventilator demonstration units to track the actual costs of caring for ventilator-dependent patients (3). Criteria for admission to the units included the need for ventilator assistance for at least 6 hr per 24-hr period for at least 3 weeks, and the potential for weaning or rehabilitation, with the aim of returning patients home or to an alternative chronic care facility. The project was initiated by HCFA in 1991, and the initial data collection was completed in 1994; the results are not yet available. Nonetheless, the project has highlighted the need for additional chronic care facility beds for chronically ventilated patients, since several of the units reported a dearth of such beds when patients who had been unable to go home were ready for discharge (5,6). In summary, current evidence demonstrates that acute care hospitals are inadequately reimbursed for a large number of chronic ventilator-dependent patients whose discharges to chronic care facilities are often delayed because of a shortage of available beds and to home by a lack of community resources.

II. Modes of Mechanical Ventilation for Chronic Ventilator-Dependent Patients

Two fundamental modes of mechanical ventilation are used for chronic ventilator-dependent patients: invasive and noninvasive. Invasive refers to the delivery of mechanical ventilation via an artificial endotracheal airway, usually a tracheostomy tube. Noninvasive refers to a variety of techniques that assist ventilation without requiring an invasive airway. Equipment and principles of application are discussed briefly in the following sections; invasive mechanical ventilation is discussed in more detail in another chapter.

A. Invasive Positive-Pressure Mechanical Ventilation

Invasive mechanical ventilation for acute respiratory failure is usually initiated via a translaryngeal endotracheal tube. Because this tube interferes with speech and swallowing and traumatizes the larynx and upper airway, replacement by a tracheostomy tube is recommended within 3 weeks (32). However, even after tracheostomy placement, the presence of an artificial invasive airway adds substantially to the risk of complications and complexity of care for patients who are chronically ventilator-dependent (33). The circumvention of natural airway defenses by a foreign body increases the risk of infection and serves as a source of chronic irritation that generates airway secretions. This increases the risk of stomal and respiratory tract infections as well as mucous plugging. In addition, airway trauma from suctioning or from tube manipulations in the stoma may cause hemorrhage, and pressure from the tube on the tracheal wall may give rise to tracheoesophageal fistulas, particularly if the cuff is kept inflated.

To minimize the likelihood of complications, the tracheostomy requires daily care, including humidification, cleaning, dressing changes, and suctioning. If the cuff must be kept inflated, pressure should be kept at no higher than the minimum pressure necessary to prevent air leaking (34). The tube must be replaced every few weeks to months by a skilled caregiver who should also inspect the site for early detection of possible complications. These requirements add to the complexity of care for patients and caregivers, who must be adequately trained in carrying out these tasks and in handling potential emergencies if the tracheostomy tube plugs or dislodges.

Accordingly, use of invasive mechanical ventilation should be limited to patients with respiratory failure who cannot be safely or successfully managed using noninvasive ventilation. These include patients with inadequate airway protection due to neurological or anatomical impairment or inability to mobilize secretions due to inadequate cough. Patients dependent on continuous mechanical ventilation who would be at risk for respiratory arrest after brief disconnection are also candidates for invasive mechanical ventilation, even though some of these patients can be managed using noninvasive techniques as long as they have intact upper airway function (35).

For patients who meet the above criteria, a permanent tracheostomy should be placed, and mechanical ventilation provided by a portable positive-pressure ventilator. The preferred type of ventilator is a portable volume ventilator such as the PLV-100 or 102 (Lifecare, Inc., Boulder, Co), LP-10 (Aequitron, Inc., Minneapolis, MN), or Companion 2801 (Puritan-Bennett, Inc., Topeka, KS). The ventilator should be adjusted to maintain arterial blood gases in the desired range using the assist/control mode, an appropriate tidal volume (8–12 ml/kg), and an adequate backup rate (10–14/min). In patients unable to trigger the ventilator, the rate must be adjusted to maintain the desired arterial

P_{CO_2}, and further adjustments may be necessary if metabolic demands change. Sufficient oxygen is administered to maintain adequate oxygenation; a humidifier should also be used. For paraplegic or quadriplegic patients, the ventilator and a suction machine can be attached to a wheelchair to optimize mobility (36). For patients who are dependent on continuous mechanical ventilation, a backup battery or generator and backup ventilator are mandatory. These ventilator systems are adequate for ventilatory assistance in chronic care facilities or in the home as long as caretakers are adequately trained in their use.

Recently, bilevel positive-airway pressure systems (BiPAP, Respironics, Inc., Murrysville, PA) have been introduced for use in noninvasive ventilation (see below). It has been reported anecdotally that these have been used to support patients receiving invasive mechanical ventilation. Since they are pressure-limited systems and lack sophisticated alarms, they must be used with extreme caution in this circumstance. Unless adequate monitoring and alarm systems are added, the use of these systems should be restricted to patients with stable airway function who are capable of at least some unassisted spontaneous breathing.

Proper airway management is another important technical aspect of invasive mechanical ventilation. Many different tracheostomy tubes are available, and selection should be based on the patient's risk of aspiration and the desire to optimize speech and eating via the oral route. Obviously, if the patient is dependent on continuous mechanical ventilation and has severe impairment of speech and swallowing functions, use of a standard single-lumen, cuffed tracheostomy tube is appropriate. However, the need for continuous ventilatory assistance does not preclude restoration of speech and swallowing if upper airway function is intact. The Communitrache (Implant Technologies) consists of two channels, one used to ventilate the lungs, and the other to direct air through the larynx. The patient modulates the flow of compressed air through the upper channel using a thumb-operated port. Although the device works quite well in occasional patients, in the author's experience, most critically ill patients have difficulty in modulating the airflow and are unable to use the device effectively.

Another option is to partially deflate the tracheostomy cuff, allowing a sufficient air leak through the larynx to permit speech (37). Ventilator tidal volume is increased to compensate for the leak while the patient is closely monitored, because the leak may vary with position. The Passy-Muir valve (38), a unidirectional valve that is inserted in-line between the ventilator tubing and tracheostomy tube, may be used in combination with a deflated cuff to direct all exhaled air through the larynx and improve the efficiency of speech. The above maneuvers entail risks such as hypoventilation and aspiration, especially in neuromuscular patients, and should be done in consultation with a speech therapist. Further discussion of methods for facilitating swallowing and speech is provided in Section IV.

As patients recover from acute respiratory failure, the need for invasive mechanical ventilation may diminish. Patients may wean for portions of the day and recover upper airway function. The possibility of replacing invasive methods of ventilatory support by noninvasive methods should be considered as these improvements occur. This approach may facilitate extubation and allows more convenient and less costly provision of chronic ventilatory support to patients who fail to wean completely (39,40). Comparisons of some properties of invasive and noninvasive ventilation are listed in Table 3.

III. Techniques of Noninvasive Ventilation

A. Noninvasive Positive-Pressure Ventilation

Although the technology for administration of noninvasive positive-pressure ventilation (NPPV) has been available for decades (41), chronic use in the United States was limited mainly to a few rehabilitation centers (42), largely because of the lack of convenient, comfortable, commercially available masks (or interfaces). With the introduction of the nasal continuous positive airway pressure (CPAP) mask for treatment of obstructive sleep apnea (43), investigators began connecting CPAP masks to standard volume-limited portable ventilators and quickly found that the technique was an effective way to assist ventilation, particularly at night (44–46). Use of nocturnal nasal ventilation was associated with improved nocturnal gas exchange, amelioration of daytime symptoms, and prolongation of survival in patients with chronic respiratory

Table 3 Comparison of Noninvasive and Invasive Ventilation

	Invasive	Noninvasive
Easy to use	+ +	+ + + +
Comfort	+	+ +
Cost	+ + +	+
Portability	+ +	+ + +
Complexity		
Suctioning	+	–
Trache care	+	–
Reliability	+ +	+
Complications		
Hemorrhage	+	–
Infection	+	–
Nasal ulceration	–	+
Gastric distention	–	+

failure due to neuromuscular disease or chest wall disorders (47–52). In addition, the technique had advantages in convenience and portability over other forms of noninvasive ventilation. Also, as long as upper airway function was intact, it eliminated many of the shortcomings of invasive PPV, including interference with speech and swallowing, cosmetic disadvantages, and the need for tracheostomy care and suctioning.

These advantages have now made NPPV the preferred mode of administering intermittent ventilatory assistance to patients with chronic respiratory failure who have adequate upper airway function. Use of the technique requires selection of a positive-pressure ventilator, which may be either volume-limited or pressure-limited. Volume-limited portable ventilators that may be used include those listed above for invasive positive-pressure ventilation. Although these have been shown to be effective and reliable (48) the more recent bilevel positive airway pressure devices, for patients requiring only nocturnal NPPV, such as the BiPAP S/T (Respironics, Inc., Murrysville, PA), have a number of advantages (53). These devices cycle between adjustable inspiratory (IPAP) and expiratory positive airway pressures (EPAP). The advantages of bilevel systems include simplicity of operation, portability (weight of approximately 6 kg for the BiPAP versus 15 kg for volume-limited portable ventilators), and lower cost (53). Currently available bilevel devices lack builtin alarms, but this is an advantage in patients requiring only nocturnal ventilation, because overly sensitive alarms may needlessly interfere with sleep. However, the lack of alarms is a disadvantage in patients dependent on continuous ventilation; these ventilators should not be used in such patients unless adequate alarm systems are added.

Mask (or interface) selection is also critical for the successful application of NPPV. Most patients with chronic respiratory failure using NPPV prefer standard nasal CPAP masks such as those provided by Respironics, Inc., Lifecare, Inc, Healthdyne, Inc., and Rescare, Inc. Because these masks compress the nasal bridge and may cause discomfort, some patients prefer nasal pillows (Adam Circuit, Puritan-Bennett, Inc.) that consist of pledgets inserted into each nostril. Nose masks can also be custom-fitted using commercially available kits (Lifecare, Inc.). Oronasal masks are also available (Vital Signs, Inc., Totowa, NJ), but in the author's experience, these are less well tolerated by patients with chronic respiratory failure, who prefer the mouth unfettered. The use of custom-fitted mouth interfaces and mouthpieces held in place by lip seals should be considered in patients in whom air leaks excessively through the mouth during use of nasal masks, but adaptation may be more difficult than to nasal masks because of difficulty in swallowing saliva and more aerophagia (35). Oronasal masks have been used more often for treatment of acute than chronic respiratory failure (54).

The major limitations of NPPV include difficulty on the part of the pa-

Table 4 Problems Encountered During Noninvasive Positive-Pressure Ventilation and Possible Remedies

Problem	Remedy
Mask intolerance	Try different masks, loosen straps
Nasal bridge ulceration	Artificial skin, nasal "pillows"
Nasal congestion	Nasal steroids, decongestants
Nasal dryness	Nasal saline, humidification
Excessive air pressure	Lower IPAP or V_T
Persistent hypoventilation	Increase IPAP, V_T or rate
Air leaking through mouth	Chinstrap, oronasal mask, or mouthpiece

tient in adapting and failure to improve gas exchange, possibly related to excessive air leakage through the mouth (Table 4) (55). Although occasional patients using PPV may adapt quite readily, sometimes within a few nights, most require weeks to months before they are able to sleep through the night (51,56). A minority, perhaps up to 20%, fail to adapt successfully and must be considered for alternative approaches. Failure to adapt is usually caused by mask discomfort or poor tolerance of air pressure. Because nasal masks commonly cause ulceration of the nasal bridge, strap tension should be kept at a minimum at all times; if ulceration should occur, artificial skin such as Duoderm (Bristol Meyers, Inc.) may be useful. Patients also commonly complain of congestion or dryness of the nose and mouth. To relieve these complaints, instillation of nasal saline, inhalation of steroids, or the oral administration of decongestants may be helpful. Air leaking through the mouth occurs almost universally during application of NPPV via nasal masks. This may be associated with sleep arousals (57) and in some patients may negate efficacy of the technique. In dealing with such leaks, bilevel ventilators can be useful to increase flow rates to compensate for the leaks; volume-limited ventilators can also compensate if tidal volumes are adjusted upward sufficiently. Use of chinstraps does not eliminate mouth leaking, but may ameliorate it. Switching to oronasal or mouth interfaces can be helpful when other methods fail. Periodic nocturnal monitoring is advisable in patients receiving NPPV, particularly if daytime hypoventilation fails to improve or deteriorates after a period of stability.

If patients who are candidates for noninvasive ventilation refuse NPPV or fail to adapt to it despite an adequate trial, then other noninvasive ventilators should be tried before invasive ventilation is considered. Several of these alternative ventilators are classified as "body ventilators," referring to devices that mechanically assist ventilation by exerting pressure on body surfaces or by altering body position. Although these ventilators may be effective in appropriately selected patients, they should be regarded as second-line choices for most patients with chronic respiratory failure because they are more inconvenient and less effective than NPPV (26).

Negative-pressure ventilators assist ventilation by intermittently applying subatmospheric pressure to the thorax and abdomen. First designed over 150 years ago (58), they became the main form of chronic mechanical ventilation during the first half of the present century for patients with respiratory failure due to paralytic poliomyelitis. The prototype negative-pressure ventilator, the "iron lung," saw extensive use during this time and proved to be effective and reliable. Modifications designed to enhance portability and convenience led to the development of the raincoat, or Numowrap (Lifecare, Inc.), and chest shell ventilators, which are also somewhat less efficient than the iron lung (58). Although these ventilators are still used occasionally, they are more cumbersome and time-consuming to apply than NPPV and considerably less portable. In addition, because they may induce obstructive sleep apnea and severe oxygen desaturation during sleep (59,60), their use has been largely supplanted by NPPV. Significant obstructive sleep apnea contraindicates the use of negative-pressure ventilation. Therefore, because obstructive sleep apnea occurs commonly in patients with neuromuscular and chest wall disorders (61), polysomnography is mandatory in these patients before use of negative-pressure ventilation is initiated.

The intermittent abdominal pressure respirator (pneumobelt) and rocking bed both work by displacing the abdominal viscera, thereby assisting motion of the diaphragm (62,63). The pneumobelt consists of an inflatable rubber bladder within a corset that is tightened firmly around the abdomen. With bladder inflation, the abdominal viscera are compressed, forcing the diaphragm cephalad and assisting exhalation; when the bladder is deflated, gravity returns the abdominal viscera and diaphragm to their original positions, assisting inhalation. Because pneumobelt function depends on gravity, it requires a sitting angle of at least 30°, and its nocturnal use is limited to patients who can adapt to sleeping in the sitting position (64). It is best used as a daytime adjunct to other forms of noninvasive ventilation, permitting freedom of the hands and face, and providing cosmetic advantages because it can be hidden under clothing (65).

The rocking bed works in a similar fashion, utilizing gravitationally induced motion of the abdominal viscera to assist the diaphragm (63). Consisting of a mattress that the user lies on supine, the bed rocks through an arc of approximately 40° via a fulcrum located at hip level. When the head rocks down, gravity forces the abdominal viscera and diaphragm cephalad, assisting exhalation, and when the head rocks up, the abdominal viscera slide caudad, assisting inhalation. Because efficacies of both the pneumobelt and rocking bed depend on compliance of the abdominal viscera and chest wall, the devices function poorly in patients with severe kyphoscoliosis or excessive obesity

(66). On the other hand, both are capable of supporting ventilation in patients with virtually complete respiratory muscle paralysis as long as body habitus is relatively normal (67).

Considering that both the pneumobelt and rocking bed act to assist diaphragm motion, they are particularly useful in patients with diaphragmatic paralysis (68) and may be useful in a variety of neuromuscular conditions characterized by diaphragmatic weakness. In the past, the rocking bed had been used to support patients with respiratory muscle paralysis due to poliomyelitis, sometimes for decades (69). Currently, the rocking bed is used only occasionally, while the pneumobelt has been used as a convenient way of providing daytime mechanical ventilation to patients with high cervical cord lesions (70). Neither ventilator is appropriate for use in patients with acute respiratory failure, however.

Two other adjuncts to mechanical ventilation may be useful in special circumstances. Glossopharyngeal breathing was first described during the 1950s in a patient with poliomyelitis who learned the technique spontaneously (71). It consists of gulping motions of the tongue that force boluses of air into the lungs. By repeating these boluses, the subject can achieve normal resting levels of minute ventilation or can augment single breaths to achieve tidal volumes as large as 2 L to assist with coughing. As long as upper airway function is adequate, the technique can be used to support ventilation for hours, even when lower respiratory muscles are severely weakened or paralyzed. This provides patients with periods of "free time" from mechanical ventilation and a safety margin in the event of power failure or ventilator disconnection. In recent years, the technique has been taught mainly to patients with high cervical cord lesions, postpoliomyelitis patients, and occasional patients with other neuromuscular conditions that are well suited to the technique (72).

Diaphragmatic pacers consist of surgically implanted electrodes and receivers, usually in the supraclavicular area, that stimulate the phrenic nerves; they are powered by external radio transmitters. They require a functional diaphragm and phrenic nerves and have been used primarily in patients with high cervical cord lesions or central hypoventilatory disorders (73). Because the transmitter is compact, very portable, and provides freedom from more cumbersome mechanical devices, some patients with high cervical cord lesions prefer pacers. However, these advantages are countered by the tendency to induce obstructive sleep apnea, necessitating continued use of a tracheostomy, and high overall costs (74). Accordingly, current use is limited mainly to pediatric patients who are unable to tolerate other noninvasive forms of mechanical ventilation (32).

The above discussion outlines the ventilator techniques and equipment available to ventilator-dependent patients, but specific choices depend on many considerations. Simplicity, convenience, portability, and cost are all important, but, ultimately, the severity of the patient's impairment, intactness of the upper airway, patient comfort, and physician preference will be the determining factors. As stated earlier, noninvasive ventilators are usually preferred by patients and caregivers over invasive because of their convenience, cost, and comfort advantages, as long as upper airway function is adequate (40). However, some clinicians prefer invasive ventilation if the patient is dependent on mechanical ventilation most of the time (75), whereas others prefer noninvasive ventilation even if the patient is dependent on mechanical ventilation continuously (35,70). Since no studies have compared efficacy and safety of the two approaches directly, either may be considered acceptable as long as it is managed by knowledgeable and experienced clinicians.

A more complete discussion of the various indications for noninvasive mechanical ventilation can be found elsewhere (26, 55). In general, NPPV is preferred in patients with neuromuscular disorders or chest wall deformities who develop symptomatic chronic respiratory failure and have intact upper airway function. Patients with obstructive sleep apnea who continue to hypoventilate despite a trial of nasal CPAP and those with central hypoventilation are also good candidates. Indications for chronic noninvasive ventilation for patients with severe stable COPD are currently unclear, but evidence is accruing to suggest that the subset with marked CO_2 retention and nocturnal oxygen desaturations may respond favorably (76).

In contrast to those patients who can be managed by chronic noninvasive ventilation, those patients who develop chronic ventilator dependency after a bout of acute respiratory failure are almost always managed at the outset by invasive mechanical ventilation. Their subsequent course, i.e., rapidity of recovery, likelihood of survival or weaning, institution of noninvasive ventilation if they fail to wean entirely, and eventual placement, depends largely on the nature of medical treatment and attention they receive. It is likely, although not proven in controlled studies, that a coordinated rehabilitative approach to these patients helps speed their recovery and assures return to an optimal level of function. The following sections describe such an approach in patients who fail to wean, focusing on restoration of functional status and optimization of placement, ideally a return to the patient's home.

IV. Rehabilitation of the Ventilator-Dependent Patient

The rehabilitation needs of ventilator-dependent patients vary widely, depending on the nature of the underlying illness and whether they are recovering from a bout of acute respiratory failure. Patients with slowly progressive neuromuscular disorders who initiate nocturnal noninvasive ventilation in the home may have few rehabilitation needs, having gradually adapted to their illnesses over many years. At the other extreme, a patient recovering from a bout of severe acute respiratory failure who has been unable to wean has an artificial airway, the need for continuous ventilatory support, and total dependence on caregivers. These latter patients present a great challenge in rehabilitation, but even if they are unable to wean entirely from mechanical ventilation, they may be able to return home with a surprising degree of functional recovery. Achieving such ends requires an appropriate patient, a coordinated team effort by health care professionals, and achievable goals. Usually, it is best accomplished in a specialized unit, either within an acute care institution or at an outside chronic ventilator unit (5,6). The overriding goal should be to optimize the patient's medical, psychological, and functional status, achieving the highest level of functioning with the least medical intervention.

A. The Team Approach

As outlined by Make et al. (11,36) and others (77–79), the chronic ventilator unit should be staffed by a team of medical professionals with expertise in the various areas that require rehabilitation (Table 5). Ideally, these professionals should have specific expertise in patients with respiratory failure.

Well-trained nursing personnel are critical to the success of the program. Nurses spend more time at the bedside of these often highly complicated patients than any other member of the team and become adept at assessing patient needs, even when patients are unable to communicate effectively. They become sensitive to patient pain, anxiety, fear, need for repositioning, and bladder and bowel functions. Highly skilled nurses also aid in minimizing complications such as self-extubations or bed sores. They are also often the first to detect signs of deterioration, such as changes in vital signs, and communicate these problems to other members of the team. More than any other team member,

Table 5 Members of the Specialized Ventilator Unit Team

Experienced nursing staff
Respiratory therapists
Physicians
Pulmonologist
Physiatrist
Physical and occupational therapists
Nutritionist
Speech therapist
Psychologist
Social services
Discharge coordinator

highly skilled nurses can optimize patient comfort and confidence in caregivers, crucial factors in reducing anxiety and enhancing recovery of function.

Respiratory therapists also serve crucial functions as members of the team. Their responsibilities center more on respiratory aspects of the patient's care, including provision and maintenance of appropriate ventilatory therapy, adjusting the ventilator to optimize patient comfort, and monitoring patient responses to the ventilator. Depending on the unit, respiratory therapists may be responsible for intubations, drawing of arterial blood gases, suctioning, and weaning of the patient under physician supervision. In some units, these responsibilities may be carried out by nursing personnel or may be shared by nurses and therapists.

Physicians serve as team leaders in the units, overseeing all medical aspects of care, writing orders and guidelines, and helping to coordinate care administered by other members of the team. In some units, a nurse coordinator or therapist may undertake many of the coordination responsibilities, such as organizing group meetings or trips into the patient's home. The physician, usually a pulmonary specialist or rehabilitation physician (physiatrist), assesses the patient's medical status and overall progress daily and is ultimately responsible for deciding when the patient is sufficiently rehabilitated to be discharged to a chronic care facility or home.

Physical and occupational therapists assess patients' physical limitations and devise a therapy plan aimed at optimizing strength, endurance, and coordination. In severely debilitated patients, this may begin with simple range-of-motion exercises, eventually leading to the patient walking without assistance. Occupational therapists may instruct patients in energy conservation measures or provide mechanical aids to overcome functional limitations. Some units have chest therapists who can prescribe breathing exercises to optimize respiratory muscle function and administer chest physiotherapy to patients with difficulty mobilizing secretions.

Nutritionists assess nutritional deficiencies and caloric needs, prescribe an appropriate diet, and monitor adequacy of nutritional supplementation. They assure that appropriate proportions of carbohydrates, lipids, and proteins are administered and make certain that special diets are provided, such as low-protein diets in patients with hepatic encephalopathy.

Speech therapists assess limitations in communication and may suggest devices to improve communication, such as letter boards, mouthing of words, or talking tracheostomies in patients who are tracheally intubated and ventilator-dependent. They also aid in the assessment of swallowing function, helping to decide when patients are able to eat by mouth.

Psychologists and psychiatrists help patients cope with the many stresses encountered during ventilator dependency. Often, however, this kind of help is very difficult to provide to patients who are severely ill, suffering from side effects of medication, and whose ability to communicate is severely compromised. Psychiatrists may be helpful in suggesting appropriate medications for treatment of anxiety, depression, or psychosis.

Social workers and home care coordinators help in determining availability of insurance benefits and financial needs. They also coordinate communications with outside agencies, including home respiratory therapy companies, visiting nurse associations, and referrals to chronic care facilities. Therapists from home respiratory services companies should be involved in the rehabilitation process well before patients are to be sent home so that they are fully aware of the individual patient's needs.

Members of the team should make an effort to communicate with one another as often as possible, and periodic group meetings, sometimes involving the patient and family, should be held as needed, usually weekly or biweekly.

B. Rehabilitation Program for the Chronic Ventilator-Dependent Patient

Evaluation and Plan

The first step in implementing rehabilitation of the chronic ventilator-dependent patient is to assess patient needs and to list goals and specific plans for reaching them (11,36). Because individual needs vary so much, each plan must be carefully tailored to the needs of the particular patient. Some patients require intermittent mechanical ventilatory assistance but have minimal other rehabilitation needs. Others, such as the elderly hospitalized patient with multiple medical problems recovering from a bout of acute respiratory failure, pose large challenges to the rehabilitation team, consuming large amounts of time and resources. In these cases, it is important, at the start of the rehabilitation process, to identify specific goals for improvement and to assess progress at periodic team meetings. A list of such goals should include the following.

Medical Stabilization

Stabilization of medical problems should be a paramount goal in patients who have become ventilator-dependent after an episode of acute respiratory failure. These patients are usually recovering from an acute crisis such as pneumonia, exacerbation of COPD, major surgery, acute neurological disease such as a stroke or polyneuropathy, or a number of other acute medical conditions. They are often elderly with underlying diabetes, renal, or heart disease. Their rehabilitation program progresses poorly unless their medical problems are controlled and treatment optimized. Ongoing infections must be aggressively diagnosed and eradicated. Airway disease is treated with optimal bronchodilator and anti-inflammatory regimens; airway secretions are managed appropriately. Fluid and electrolyte imbalances are corrected, and other acute problems, such as cardiac ischemia or arrhythmias and gastrointestinal bleeding, are controlled. Proper management of these problems allows the rehabilitation program to proceed.

Simplification of the Ventilator Regimen

Many patients who remain ventilator-dependent after bouts of acute respiratory failure will ultimately wean when the acute medical conditions and other factors that contribute to their respiratory failure respond to appropriate therapy. Weaning, however, should not be the major focus of the rehabilitation plan (36). Rather, the patient's capacity for weaning should be tested periodically as the rehabilitation program progresses, but the focus should be on optimizing the bodily functions of the patient, even if that implies continued use of the ventilator. Should weaning from mechanical ventilation become the major focus, the patient who is unable to wean completely is perceived by himself and others as a failure, even when other aspects of the rehabilitation program succeed. In addition, incessant and inappropriate weaning efforts may contribute to patient malaise and fatigue, impeding progress with rehabilitation. On the other hand, some free time from the ventilator, even a few hours, may add to patient self-esteem and facilitate other aspects of rehabilitation (36).

An important goal of ventilator management should be to use the simplest ventilator that satisfies the patient's needs. This means that patients should be switched to portable ventilators as soon as feasible, and, when possible, noninvasive forms should be substituted for invasive forms of mechanical ventilation. Noninvasive ventilation may lead to earlier extubation and eliminates the need to care for, and the complications associated with, a tracheostomy. It is less costly once the patient leaves the acute care setting, and more convenient, particularly if NPPV is used (80). However, it must be used cautiously in patients with compromised upper airway function, secretion problems, or weakened cough, and in those needing continuous ventilatory assistance (79).

Although simplicity and convenience are particularly important considerations when planning discharge to home, safety concerns should not be ignored. Patients with little capacity for spontaneous breathing should use ventilators with adequate alarms and an alternative power source, and a backup ventilator should be available. Portable volume ventilators are usually preferred for these patients; they are set in the assist/control mode, since the synchronized intermittent mandatory ventilation (SIMV) mode may add to ventilatory work (81). For patients capable of several hours of ventilator-free time, the simplicity, portability, and lower cost of bilevel positive airway pressure systems are advantageous, particularly in patients receiving NPPV (51). For patients unable to ambulate, installation of the ventilator on a wheelchair may greatly enhance independence.

Physical Reconditioning

Muscular deconditioning afflicts virtually all patients recovering from prolonged bouts of respiratory failure. Deconditioning is characterized not only by weakness and poor endurance, but also by muscle incoordination and inefficiency. Commonly associated conditions, such as advanced age or neuromuscular disease, complicate matters even more. Deconditioning affects most skeletal muscles, but its effects are very apparent on the respiratory system, leading to inefficient breathing patterns (9) and inability to wean. Physical therapy aimed at reversing muscle deficiencies plays an important role in patient rehabilitation. The physical therapy program is tailored to the individual, beginning with passive range-of-motion exercises in severely disabled patients, and progressing as tolerated to active limb exercises, sitting, transfers, and eventually walking without assistance. Obviously, coexisting neuromuscular disease may limit the ability of physical therapy to achieve these goals, and inability of patients to cooperate may also impede progress.

Functional recovery of the respiratory muscles often accompanies recovery of other muscles, but exercises specifically directed at the respiratory muscles may also be useful (82). Therapists may teach diaphragmatic breathing exercises to improve respiratory muscle coordination, and inspiratory resistance devices may be used to improve diaphragmatic muscle strength in an effort to expedite weaning (12). Biofeedback techniques have also been used to enhance respiratory muscle coordination and efficiency (13) and may speed weaning. However, as emphasized above, complete weaning from the ventilator may not be an achievable goal, and optimization of function despite ventilator dependence may be a more appropriate goal.

Patients with physical limitations affecting hand or upper-extremity function may be aided by occupational therapy that teaches use of specially designed appliances such as elongated eating utensils or braces. Such adaptations may be particularly useful for patients who plan to go home, reducing dependence on caregivers. Other aspects of the occupational therapy plan might include energy conservation, pacing techniques, work simplification measures, and assistance with planning ahead before performing tasks.

Nutritional Repletion

Nutritional deficiencies are common in patients who have been ventilator-dependent for long periods and may contribute to muscular deconditioning, impairment of immunity, reduced ventilatory responses, and failure to wean (83). The acute illness may lead to a sustained catabolic state, with negative nitrogen balance. Synthetic functions, such as albumin production, are also adversely affected. Low levels of albumin in serum have been associated with inability to wean and mortality (20). Iron utilization may also be abnormal and, in combination with other nutritional deficiencies and phlebotomy, renders patients anemic.

The nutritional assessment should consist of a comparison between actual and ideal body weight, measurements of serum prealbumin and albumin, hematocrit, blood sugar, prothrombin time, and other nutritional factors as dictated by specific findings. In addition, daily caloric requirements should be determined, either by using the Harris-Benedict equation (84) or, more accurately, by direct measurement of oxygen consumption. These calculations should be used to prescribe dietary composition and caloric targets. In chronically ventilator-dependent patients, the following guidelines are helpful: approximately 50–60% of calories are usually derived from fat; protein content is determined by whether or not restoration of lean body mass is desired; and carbohydrate content is kept proportionately small, so that the respiratory quotient is maintained <1 and CO_2 production is minimized (85). As nutritional repletion progresses, caloric intake, body weight, and indexes of synthetic function, such as serum albumin levels, should be monitored.

Enteral nutrition is preferred over parenteral, unless gastrointestinal problems preclude use of the enteral route (86). Most patients who become ventilator-dependent after a bout of acute respiratory failure are fed using tubes inserted via the nose or mouth, or via percutaneous gastric or jejunostomy tubes. However, once the patient has a tracheostomy, eating by mouth should be encouraged unless swallowing problems or recurrent aspiration occurs. Feeding by the oral route boosts patient morale and increases feelings of independence (87). Unfortunately, swallowing problems are very common in chronic ventilator-dependent patients with tracheostomies, even in those without underlying neurological disorders. Among nine patients ventilated via a tracheostomy tube for 3 or more weeks, seven had swallowing abnormalities, including impaired laryngeal elevation and rotation and cricopharyngeal spasm (88). These abnormalities, thought to be related to traction by the tracheostomy tube, predisposed to abnormal pooling in the valleculae and piriform sinuses, and even gross aspiration. Consultation with a speech therapist may be helpful in evaluating these swallowing problems and determining the appropriateness of oral feedings.

Optimization of Communication

The ability to communicate is usually severely compromised in patients who develop chronic ventilatory dependency following a bout of acute respiratory failure. Not only are patients recovering from severe debilitating illness that leaves them withdrawn, exhausted, and perhaps cognitively impaired, but also, because the tracheostomy cuff is usually kept inflated, the inability to phonate increases barriers to communication, forcing them to mouth or write words or to use a communication board. Patients and staff often become frustrated, tending to limit communication to the bare essentials, so fears and emotional needs of the patient are never addressed. This contributes to the patient's sense of isolation, fueling feelings of anger and despair, and exacerbating depression.

Efforts to optimize communication may reverse many of these adverse consequences and should begin as soon as the patient is stabilized on the ventilator. Communication boards and coaching in mouthing words are helpful, and some patients may be able to communicate in writing, but many are limited by weakness, tremors, and impediments such as intravenous lines. Because the return of speech is usually so uplifting for patients, enhancing self-esteem and alleviating feelings of isolation and depression, optimization of communication and measures to facilitate speech are priorities during rehabilitation. A speech therapist should monitor the patient and recommend appropriate measures depending on patient capabilities.

Once the patient's overall condition has stabilized, efforts should be made to facilitate speech. Patients with neuromuscular disorders that impair bulbar function or cognition may be incapable of intelligible speech, but phonation is usually possible in others. The Communitrache (see description above) may restore speech to some entirely ventilator-dependent patients, but most patients have difficulty controlling the airflow and prefer other techniques. Another option for patients who have no time free from the ventilator is to create an air leak around a partially deflated tracheostomy cuff with or without a Passy-Muir valve (38) (discussed above).

The greatest strides in restoring speech are usually made if the patient is able to wean off the ventilator for at least an hour or 2. The tracheostomy cuff is deflated during these periods as long as aspiration is not excessive. Speech is then possible if the patient occludes the tracheostomy tube orifice with a finger during exhalation, forcing air through the larynx, or if the tracheostomy tube is capped. Use of a fenestrated tracheostomy tube reduces airflow resistance related to the tube, thereby making capping more tolerable, but some patients still have difficulty in tolerating capping. Use of a smaller tracheostomy tube or a Passy-Muir speaking valve may alleviate this discomfort by reducing inspiratory resistance. Any of these techniques permits vocalization in patients with chronic tracheostomies, but their use assumes that the cuff can be deflated and that the risk of aspiration is not excessive. Patients who have gross aspiration, such as occurs after massive stroke, have few options for preservation of speech, consisting of the Communitrache or electronic voice box. Conversely, if the patient has intact upper airway function and is able to wean from the ventilator for several hours daily, switching to noninvasive ventilation using a nasal mask should be contemplated, so that the tracheostomy can be eliminated entirely.

Psychological Support

Chronic ventilator dependency, particularly during recovery from acute respiratory failure, is extremely stressful psychologically. Numerous factors contribute to psychological deterioration, including the stress of the acute illness, the use of mind-altering drugs for sedation and analgesia, the pain of repeated procedures, the loss of security that is associated with the unfamiliar environment, and the inability to communicate anxieties and fears. Prospects for survival are often uncertain, and patients feel loss of control over their environment. Sleep deprivation is also nearly universal, related to frequent interruptions and high noise levels in the environment: high noise levels have been recorded in a chronic ventilator unit, and in most patients, the high levels correlate strongly with sleep arousals (89,90).

In response to these stresses, patients frequently experience fear, anxiety, anger, and depression. In addition, cognitive impairments are quite common, including deficits in memory, orientation, and verbal and abstract reasoning (91). These emotional problems and cognitive deficits interfere with the rehabilitative effort, particularly if discharge home is a consideration. Motivation and coping skills are important qualities if patients are to be discharged home (87); severe depression or cognitive impairment precludes such placement unless there is an unusually strong support system in the home.

Measures that can reduce psychological stress in ventilator-dependent patients include removing as much monitoring equipment from the patient's room as possible, placing orienting devices like clocks, calendars, and family artifacts near the bedside, minimizing nocturnal noise and interruptions, and using private rooms with windows (92). Input from psychological counselors and psychiatrists may also be useful in helping patients to cope with the many psychological stresses and in making recommendations regarding appropriate use of psychotropic medications. However, psychological counseling may be limited by communication problems, and few studies have explored the issue of whether chronic ventilator-dependent patients benefit from counseling. Judicious use of sedative and psychotropic medication may be helpful in allowing patients to cope with chronic ventilator dependency, particularly during weaning in dyspneic patients, but great care must be taken to avoid excessive use (92).

In the author's experience, the greatest psychological boost occurs when patients regain the ability to eat by mouth, speak, and care for themselves, even if complete weaning is not possible. The return of hope and self-esteem associated with these improvements serves as a stronger elixir than any psychotrope. Patients are also often buoyed by the prospect of returning home, which serves as a strong motivating factor. However, returning home while dependent on a ventilator, particularly if a permanent tracheostomy is necessary, raises many other psychological and coping issues, not only for patients, but also for their caregivers. Some of these issues are addressed in subsequent sections.

Optimal Placement

When it becomes apparent that a patient who is chronically ventilator-dependent has stabilized in an acute care setting, placement planning should begin. The major considerations in determining placement options include financial resources of the patient, degree of ventilator dependency, ability of the patient to care for himself, family support and the need for additional caretakers, and the availability of chronic care facilities if home is not a realistic option. Social workers should begin exploring personal financial resources, insurance benefits, and other private sources of funding such as the Muscular Dystrophy Association or centers for independent living that are found in some areas. Practitioners should wean the patient to the least amount of ventilation necessary. The need for only nocturnal rather than continuous mechanical ventilation, and the elimination of a tracheostomy, if possible, greatly reduce caretaker demands. Nursing staff and respiratory therapists should encourage the patient to take on as many daily activities as possible, including eating, bathing, using a bathroom, and suctioning. This not only improves the patient's sense of independence, but also reduces caretaker demands.

Unfortunately, many patients have few personal financial resources, large caregiver needs that cannot be met by third-party payers, and inadequate family support, so discharge home is not a consideration. Such patients require placement in chronic ventilator facilities. Although recent changes in reimbursement have led to a burgeoning of private, free-standing, for-profit chronic ventilator units (see below), few of these centers take patients who have no prospect of weaning or eventually returning home. Thus, to relieve congestion at acute care facilities and avoid stays of up to years, there is still a need for more chronic ventilator beds in many states and for improved reimbursement for care of patients at home (28).

Placement Options for the Ventilator-Dependent Patient

Acute Care Facilities

As noted above, patients who become chronically ventilator-dependent in acute care hospitals may be difficult to place elsewhere, particularly if they have limited financial and family resources and the need for highly skilled nursing care. Such patients are usually very debilitated, often elderly, with end-stage conditions such as severe emphysema, severe congestive heart failure, or neurological impairment such as occurs after a stroke or after anoxic damage related to a cardiac arrest. In past years, in many hospitals, such patients would be cared for in an intensive care unit where they might occupy a bed for months before the inevitable complications led to their eventual demise. More recently, partly related to changes in medical ethics (see below), such patients have been transferred to general medical floors, where they receive supportive care, i.e., fluids, nutrition, and continued ventilator support, but no heroic measures. Some acute care hospitals have also established specialized respiratory care units (5,6,93), where patients who are chronically ventilator-dependent, but still have some prospect for weaning or outside placement, are sent to receive intensive respiratory rehabilitation.

These units have different roles depending on the institution, varying from mainly weaning and rehabilitation units in some institutions (5,6), to multipurpose units that not only wean chronically ventilator-dependent patients but also manage acute respiratory conditions (39) and serve as intensive care step-down units when ICU bed shortages occur (author's institution). In either case, nursing staff and respiratory therapists become highly skilled at the care of ventilator patients in such units, improving efficiency and lowering cost of care compared to intensive care units (ICUs) (93). More data on these units should be forthcoming when results of the recent HCFA-sponsored ventilator unit demonstration project are analyzed.

Specialized Chronic Ventilator-Dependent Units

The realization that the lack of beds in chronic care facilities for chronic ventilator patients has led to long stays in acute care hospitals (27), often in suboptimal settings such as ICUs or general medical wards, has spawned the development of specialized chronic ventilator-dependent units. Descriptions of such units first began appearing during the early 1980s (94). These units have usually been located within acute care institutions, but have also served as regional referral centers; they apply rehabilitation principles, as described above, to the care of chronic ventilator-dependent patients. Results of a number of analyses of such units are summarized in Table 6. Admission criteria were not given for the Indihar study (94). In the other reports, patients were admitted to the units if they were ventilator-dependent, otherwise medically stable without the need for invasive monitoring, and candidates for rehabilitation.

Weaning rates differed markedly between the units, but this was probably related to differences in patient populations and priorities of the units. Patients in the Make study (95) were ventilator-dependent for longer periods prior to their admission than were patients in the other studies; the longer periods of ventilator dependence made weaning less likely. Also, the main goal in this unit was to rehabilitate patients; no concerted effort was made to wean patients entirely. On the other hand, weaning rates in the Gracey (5) and Criner (6) studies, and survival rates in all of the studies, were very high, particularly in view of the much poorer survival rates reported for all patients with acute

Table 6 Outcomes and Costs in Specialized Chronic Ventilator-Dependent Units

Author	Year	No. of pts	% Male	Diagnosis		% Weaned	Survival (%)		Costs	% Home
				% COPD	% surgical		At discharge	1 year		
Indihar (94)	1984	182	47	57	—	—	61	—	38% less[a]	24
Make (95)	1989	46	52	50	—	4	87	82		83
Gracey (5)	1992	61	49	46	66	87	95		$604[b]	70
Criner (6)	1993	58	47	21	28	71	93	71	—	—

[a]Home costs 38% less than hospital.
[b]Daily hospital cost.

respiratory failure (Table 1). In addition, a high percentage of these patients were eventually discharged home, and costs were up to 38% less than in an ICU (94). Although these remarkably favorable findings support the wider use of specialized units for chronic ventilator-dependent patients, controlled studies will be necessary to determine how much patient selection influences success rates.

For-Profit Hospitals Specializing in Chronic Ventilator Care

Over the past decade, for-profit hospitals specializing in subacute or chronic care have proliferated. For example, Vencor, Inc., a corporation that owns free-standing hospitals devoted mainly to chronic respiratory and ventilator care, has increased from 14 hospitals 3 years ago to 34 hospitals nationwide today and continues to expand rapidly. Other multihospital organizations, such as Mediplex Rehab (Sun Health, Inc.), have a more generalized rehabilitation focus, but also accept chronic ventilator-dependent patients. This rapid expansion has been fueled by Medicare rules that allow DRG-exempt status for hospitals with a rehabilitation focus and average lengths of stay exceeding 25 days (in the case of subacute centers). Most of these centers screen patients carefully, selecting those who have adequate insurance coverage and the potential for weaning or rehabilitation. They also incorporate a team approach as outlined earlier, maintaining skilled nurses, respiratory therapists, physical and occupational therapists, nutritionists, and relatively few physicians on their full-time staffs. Presumably, they are able to maintain profitability by providing chronic ventilator beds for patients transferred from acute care hospitals after coverage provided by DRGs has run out and by keeping costs below Medicare reimbursement rates. At present, there are no published data on the numbers or outcomes of patients treated in these for-profit centers, so cost-effectiveness, success rates, and overall impact on the care of ventilator-dependent patients cannot be assessed.

Home

Eventual discharge home is a desirable outcome for chronic ventilator-dependent patients, but as discussed above, technical and financial resource limitations are often prohibitive. Discharge home should be considered only for motivated patients with adequate financial resources and caregiver needs that can be adequately met (87). The more free time the patient has from the ventilator and the more independent in performing activities of daily living, the more promising the outlook for returning home. In addition, a large and supportive family willing to take on the bulk of caretaking responsibilities greatly increases the likelihood of success. Patients with minimal abilities for self-care and a need for continuous ventilatory assistance are usually poor candidates for home discharge unless several family members are available to help or the patient has unusually large financial resources to pay partially for round-the-clock caregivers. The costs of providing skilled caregivers to support such a patient at home may well exceed $100,000 yearly, and few third-party payers are willing to provide such support. In the author's experience, a single devoted family member, even if highly motivated and assisted by part-time caregivers, rarely succeeds in satisfying the great demands required of caregivers. Psychological stress and sleep deprivation usually limit home stays for such patients to no more than a few weeks.

Patients who are being considered for discharge home should undergo a thorough evaluation and training program to facilitate the transition home and to optimize the likelihood of success. The program is usually initiated several weeks before the planned discharge date, and progress is monitored by periodic meetings between staff, patient, and family. A home respiratory care company is contacted early during the process so that home therapists and the patient become familiar with each other before discharge. Training sessions should be scheduled so that patients and caregivers can acquire a thorough knowledge of the operation and maintenance of ventilators, oxygen equipment, humidifiers, and suctioning machines, and the proper care of tracheostomies. Nurses should review principles of patient hygiene and feeding, and caregivers should meet with other members of the rehabilitation team to learn about aspects of nutrition or physical therapy, as dictated by patient need. Particular attention should be paid to familiarizing patients and caregivers with potential problems, and mock emergencies should be staged so that in the event these occur in the home, they can be handled without inducing panic.

Prior to discharge, evaluation of the home should be performed by the home respiratory care company and an occupational therapist so that alterations in the living space can be made, if necessary. Such alterations might include conversion of a first-floor room into a bedroom, reorientation of furniture to accommodate equipment or a wheelchair, installation of handles in bathrooms, and, if time permits, installation of wheelchair ramps or widening of doors as necessary. As the discharge date nears, the patient, family, and other caregivers are encouraged to take on more responsibilities, and to assume primary care of the patient for a night or two in the hospital prior to discharge. If possible, before the discharge date, a trial night at home might also be useful in detecting potential problems.

Prior to the patient's arrival at home, the home respiratory care company should place all of the necessary equipment in the home. This should include backup ventilators and batteries or emergency generators for patients who have limited free time from the ventilator. In addition, emergency numbers should be provided and emergency plans thoroughly rehearsed. During the initial period at home, frequent visits from home respiratory therapists and nurses will be necessary as the patient and family adjust to the new situation. Despite the many steps and careful planning required before ventilator-dependent patients are discharged home, many can make the transition successfully and can be supported at home for years. Also, as noted previously, the process is much less complicated if the patient is receiving only noninvasive ventilation nocturnally and is capable of self-care.

Outcomes of Home Mechanical Ventilation

Data on outcomes of home mechanical ventilation in the United States are quite limited. The Center for Home Mechanical Ventilation at National Jewish Center for Immunology and Respiratory Diseases in Denver, Colorado, has collected information on several hundred of such patients by surveying home respiratory therapy companies. Among 453 patients surveyed as of late 1993, 79% were adults, and of these, 58% had neuromuscular disease, 9% each had a chest wall disorder or sleep apnea, and only 20% had obstructive airway disease. Most patients had been ventilator-dependent for 3 years or less, and only 21%, mainly neuromuscular or kyphoscoliosis patients, had been using their ventilator at home for more than 6 years (Make BJ, personal communication).

This experience mirrors that reported by a number of groups from France, where large extended families have facilitated delivery of mechanical ventilation in the home (Table 6). Most of these patients received positive-pressure ventilation via a tracheostomy, and, as might be anticipated, patient age, oxygenation, and diagnosis were found to be important predictors of outcome (20). In some studies, age < 65 years and $Pa_{O_2} > 55$ torr on room air imparted a favorable prognosis (97), and in all studies, patients with restrictive chest wall disorders fared much better than those with obstructive diseases. In one of the larger series reported (Table 7, Fig. 1), Robert et al. (97) found that patients with respiratory failure due to poliomyelitis had almost a 90% 10-year survival, whereas patients with obstructive diseases had only a 25% survival at 5 years. These investigators also found that patients with obstructive diseases had less comfort in terms of quality of life and reduction of dyspnea than did patients with restrictive lung disease; they also spent more time, per day, on the ventilator (96).

These findings have led some investigators to discourage the use of chronic ventilator support in patients with COPD. However, Muir et al. (102) recently reported more favorable results in 259 COPD patients treated with home mechanical ventilation via a tracheostomy (Table 7), with 44% still alive at 5 years. These authors point out that this survival rate approximates that of patients in the Nocturnal Oxygen Therapy Trial and suggest that these data "should lead to a review of the value of permanent tracheostomy in advanced COPD" (102). However, with the recent increased interest in noninvasive ventilation, trials in COPD patients that compare oxygen supplementation alone

Table 7 Survival of Patients Receiving Home Mechanical Ventilation

Author	Year	Method	No. of pts	Survival (%) 5 year Restrictive	5 year COPD	10 year Restrictive	10 year COPD
Gerard (96)	1981	Trache	150	—	—	85	35
Robert (97)	1983	Trache	222[a]	84	25	58	—
Bertrand (98)	1985	Trache	118	—	—	50	20
Dudeffant (99)	1985	Trache	60	77	42	—	—
Splaingard (100)	1985	Tank	40	76	—	61	—
Ordonneau (101)	1986	Trache	—	86	54	—	—
Muir (102)	1994	Trache	259	—	44	—	20

[a]Restrictive survival extrapolated from polio, kyphoscoliosis, myopathy, and tuberculosis groups; COPD from obstructive and bronchiectasis groups.
Trache = positive-pressure ventilation via tracheostomy; Tank = negative-pressure ventilation via iron lung.

versus noninvasive ventilation plus oxygen supplementation are of more immediate interest.

Studies on long-term outcomes of NPPV are few, largely because widespread use of the modality is a recent development. Bach et al. (35) reported success using NPPV administered via a mouthpiece in 66 patients with postpolio respiratory insufficiency, some with no measurable vital capacity. These patients had been using NPPV for an average of 14.5 years, and only seven had died at the end of the follow-up interval. More recently, Leger et al. (103) reported several years' follow-up in 276 patients treated with nasal NPPV for chronic respiratory insufficiency due to a variety of etiologies. The experience paralleled that previously reported for patients with tracheostomies, in which those with restrictive lung disease fared better than those with obstructive diseases, even though gas exchange improved and the frequency of hospitalization fell in both groups (Fig. 1).

Although no randomized, prospective trials have demonstrated improved survival with NPPV in patients with neuromuscular disease, Vianello et al. (52) found that four of five patients with Duchenne muscular dystrophy who declined ventilatory assistance died over a 2-year period, whereas all five similar patients who received NPPV survived. On the other hand, a French multicenter group (104) recently used a randomized, prospective design to test the hypothesis that initiation of "prophylactic" nasal NPPV prior to the onset of CO_2 retention or symptoms in patients with Duchenne muscular dystrophy would retard the relentless progression of the disease. Instead of proving the hypothesis, the

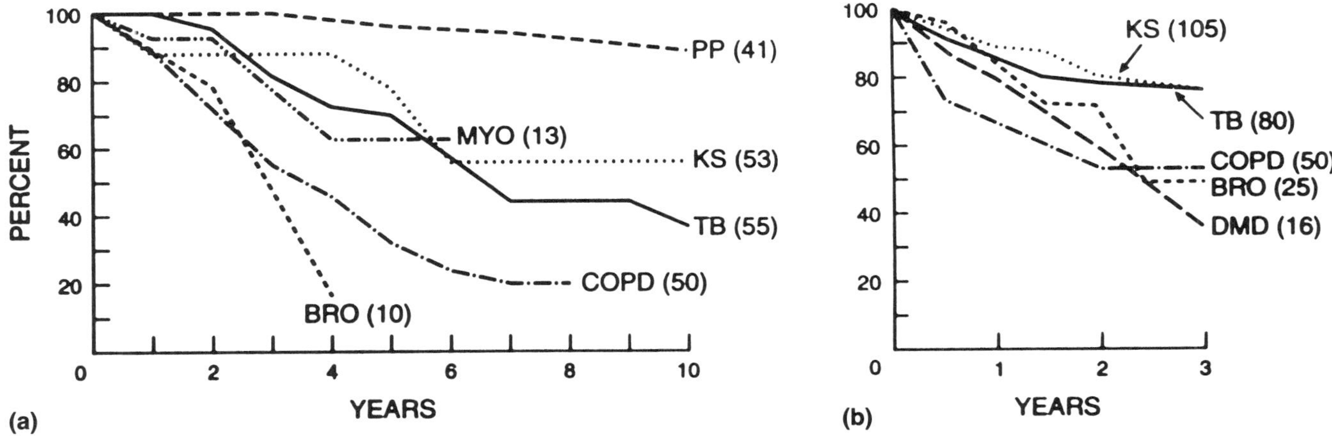

Figure 1 (a) Survival after tracheostomy in 222 patients with chronic respiratory failure of various etiologies followed for up to 10 years. (Redrawn from Ref. 97 with permission.) (b) Likelihood of continuing noninvasive positive-pressure ventilation in 276 patients with chronic respiratory failure followed for up to 3 years. (Redrawn from Ref. 103 with permission.) BRO = bronchiectasis; COPD = chronic obstructive pulmonary disease; DMD = Duchenne muscular dystrophy; KS = kyphoscoliosis; MYO = myopathy; PP = postpolio syndrome; TB = history of tuberculosis.

investigators were forced to terminate the trial early because of excess mortality in the NPPV group. Although they were unable to explain this unexpected finding, the authors speculated that patients had a false sense of security while using NPPV and delayed excessively in seeking help for infections. Although most evidence still supports the use of NPPV when patients have developed symptomatic CO_2 retention, this study does underline the importance of randomized, prospective trials in evaluating clinical practice.

A number of long-term studies on patients using alternative noninvasive ventilators have reported favorable survival rates for patients with neuromuscular diseases. In 40 patients primarily with muscular dystrophy treated with tank-type, negative-pressure ventilators, Splaingard et al. (100) reported a 10-year survival rate of 61% (Table 7). Mohr and Hill (105) and Curran and Colbert (106) reported on eight and 23 patients with Duchenne muscular dystrophy, respectively, who were ventilated initially with negative-pressure ventilators. Both groups found that home ventilation extended survivals well beyond the onset of respiratory failure, but that patients still experienced a progressive deterioration of their underlying disease, eventually requiring either tracheostomy for better access to the airway, or dying. Although no studies have directly compared outcomes from the use of the different ventilatory modes in the home, at the present time, convenience, cost, and efficacy considerations make NPPV the preferred mode (40,80).

Although home mechanical ventilation in patients with neuromuscular disease is clearly successful in improving gas exchange and symptoms, and almost certainly prolongs survival in selected patients, the practice takes a toll in other ways. Robins Miller et al. (107,108) surveyed patients with Duchenne muscular dystrophy receiving home mechanical ventilation and their families. Although most patients rated themselves as somewhat or very satisfied with their lives, most families registered dissatisfaction with recreational and vocational aspects of their own lives, felt isolated from friends, and considered their own quality of life to be worse than it had been before the initiation of mechanical ventilation. Most families felt they had been inadequately prepared by health care practitioners. Echoing these concerns, Oppenheimer (109) recently identified a number of obstacles to living with a ventilator at home. Chief among these were inadequate advance planning, lack of caregiver preparation and support, unnecessarily complex care, deficient medical and psychological follow-up, and a dearth of community support services. Many of these obstacles reflect the inadequate funding for home support services provided by health insurers in most areas despite the evidence that home mechanical ventilation is usually less costly than care in an institution. As a consequence, although placement in the home may be the preferred destination for most chronically ventilator-dependent patients, it proves to be a realistic option for only a minority.

C. Ethical Considerations

Ethical concerns relating to the management of ventilator-dependent patients have received much attention in the recent literature, including publication of the proceedings of an NIH-sponsored Workshop on Withholding and Withdrawing Mechanical Ventilation (110), and an official statement by the American Thoracic Society (111). Although numerous difficult ethical dilemmas are encountered when dealing with individual patients, certain general principles have been elucidated to aid in decision making. First, patients have the preeminent right to make decisions regarding their care. Thus, a competent patient has the right to refuse intubation and mechanical ventilatory assistance. If the patient is incompetent to make this decision, then it falls on the next of kin to serve as surrogate decision makers. For this reason, all persons, particularly those at risk for respiratory failure, are encouraged to discuss advance directives with family members before a crisis arises. Most states recognize living wills that state the patient's desire to avoid artificial life support in the event of irreversible complications. They also recognize durable powers of attorney that leave specific instructions and designate the next of kin who will serve as surrogates in the event that the patient cannot participate in the decision making.

Dilemmas arise when a decision-incompetent patient without advance directives remains dependent on mechanical ventilation with little prospect for weaning or restoration to a tolerable quality of life. In the eyes of ethicists, withdrawing ventilatory support in such a situation is tantamount to withholding it in the first place. In either case, it is incumbent on medical providers and family to anticipate the patient's desires and decide how hopeless the situation must be before care is terminated. When in doubt, the decision may be made to continue ventilatory support, but to initiate no further heroic measures should complications ensue. One unresolved issue is the right of patients or families to demand further care when it is deemed futile by health care providers (112). Such demands undoubtedly prolong death for many patents and inflate medical costs. Nonetheless, most providers are reluctant to refuse care in such circumstances except to withhold cardiopulmonary resuscitation in the event of a terminal arrest.

Based on the above principles, health care providers are advised to initiate discussions regarding advance directives with all patients at risk for respiratory failure. Patients should be informed of their rights, prognosis, and likelihood of weaning should they receive ventilatory support. They should receive complete and realistic information on living with a tracheostomy and, if that is a consideration, should be encouraged to contact tracheostomized patients to gain first-hand knowledge. Their families should be involved in the decision making, particularly if mechanical ventilation at home is a possibility. With the advent of noninvasive ventilation, some patients may opt for noninvasive ventilatory assistance, but stop short of endotracheal intubation. By using the above approach, providers prepare patients and their families for the future, easing emotional burdens and crises as the patient's respiratory failure progresses.

V. Conclusions

Although precise numbers are not available, each year thousands of patients in the United States become dependent on mechanical ventilation for periods exceeding 3 weeks, leading to enormous expenditure of financial and other resources in acute care hospitals. This is a dynamic population, with most patients eventually weaning or dying, but a substantial minority remain ventilator-dependent for long periods of time. Advances in weaning techniques, such as use of particular ventilator modes or biofeedback, may reduce numbers slightly. Programs aimed at the rehabilitation of ventilator-dependent patients probably afford the best hope of returning these individuals to their highest level of function, ideally in their own home. Such programs may be offered in specialized chronic-ventilator-dependent units within acute care hospitals or free-standing, for-profit weaning facilities that have been expanding rapidly in recent years.

These rehabilitation programs use a team approach with nurses, respiratory therapists, physicians, physical and occupational therapists, nutritionists, speech therapists, psychologists, and social services workers all coordinating their efforts. The team works to optimize the patient's medical status, muscle strength, endurance, communication, and nutritional and psychological states. The ventilator regimen is simplified as much as possible, and if the patient can be freed from the ventilator for even a few hours daily or, preferably, use noninvasive ventilation, this greatly facilitates care and increases the likelihood of returning home. Unfortunately, financial, family, and community resources are often inadequate for patients who need high levels of care, rendering discharge to home impossible. Chronic care beds for patients who have little prospect for weaning or rehabilitation are also lacking in many states, so these patients may remain in acute care hospital beds, sometimes for years. Since third-party payer reimbursement rates for these patients are inadequate, this places financial strains on acute care hospitals, and because little attention may be paid to the rehabilitation of these patients, care may be suboptimal.

Advances in medical technology have reaped wonderful benefits in terms of illness cured and lives saved. However, each advance is accompanied by new costs and problems. In the case of ventilator care, the minority of patients who fail to wean after initiation of ventilatory assistance for acute respiratory failure poses a major problem. Often, in the past, these patients have been placed on mechanical ventilation with too little forethought about ethical issues like the prospects for weaning or restoring an acceptable quality of life. In the future, efforts must be directed at preparing patients better for the possibility of ventilator dependence, encouraging those who wish to avoid ventilator dependence to provide advance directives, creating more rehabilitation programs for those with the potential for weaning or discharge home, and providing more financial and caretaker support for home care. In this way, the quality of life of these patients can be improved, the number of institutionalized patients reduced, and ultimately, the costs of caring for these patients lowered.

References

1. Gillespie DJ, Marsh HM, Divertie MB, Meadows JA. Clinical outcome of respiratory failure in patients requiring prolonged mechanical ventilation. Chest 1986; 90(3):364–369.
2. Davis H, Lefrak SS, Miller D, Malt S. Prolonged mechanically assisted ventilation. JAMA 1980; 243(1):43–45.
3. Health Care Financing Administration. Chronic Ventilator-Demonstration: Technical Advisory Panel. Washington, DC: HCFA, 1990.
4. Milic-Emili J. Is weaning an art or science? Am Rev Respir Dis 1986; 134:1107–1108.
5. Gracey DR, Viggiano RW, Naessens JM, Hubmayr RD, Silverstein MD, Koenig GE. Outcomes of patients admitted to a chronic ventilator-dependent unit in an acute-care hospital. Mayo Clin Proc 1992; 67:131–136.
6. Criner GJ, Kreimer DT, Pidlaoan L. Patient outcome following prolonged mechanical ventilation (MV) via tracheostomy. Am Rev Respir Dis 1993; A874.
7. Sahn SA, Lakshminarayan S, Petty TL. Weaning from mechanical ventilation. JAMA 1976; 235:2208–2212.
8. Morganroth ML, Morganroth JL, Nett LM, Petty TL. Criteria for weaning from prolonged mechanical ventilation. Arch Intern Med 1984; 144:1012–1016.
9. Tobin JM, Pérez W, Guenther SM, et al. The pattern of breathing during successful and unsuccessful trials of weaning from mechanical ventilation. Am Rev Respir Dis 1986; 134:1111–1118.
10. Yang KL, Tobin M. A prospective study of indexes predicting the outcome of trials of weaning from mechanical ventilation. N Engl J Med 1991; 324:1445–1450.
11. Make B, Gilmartin M, Brody JS, Snider GL. Rehabilitation of ventilator-dependent subjects with lung diseases. Chest 1984; 86(3):358–365.
12. Aldrich TK, Karpel JP. Inspiratory muscle resistive training in respiratory failure. Am Rev Respir Dis 1985; 131:461–462.
13. Holliday JE, Hyers TM. The reduction of weaning time from mechanical ventilation using tidal volume and relaxation biofeedback. Am Rev Respir Dis 1990; 141:1214–1220.
14. Brochard L, Rauss A, Benito S, et al. Comparison of three methods of gradual

withdrawal from ventilatory support during weaning from mechanical ventilation. Am J Respir Crit Care Med 1994; 150:896–903.
15. Marini JJ. Weaning from mechanical ventilation. Am Rev Respir Dis 1988; 138:1043–1046.
16. Witek TJ, Schachter EN, Dean NL, Beck GJ. Mechanically assisted ventilation in a community hospital. Arch Intern Med 1985; 145:235–239.
17. Papadakis MA, Browner WS. Prognosis of noncardiac medical patients receiving mechanical ventilation in a veterans hospital. Am J Med 1987; 83:687–692.
18. Spicher JE, White DP. Outcome and function following prolonged mechanical ventilation. Arch Intern Med 1987; 147:421–425.
19. Elpern EH, Larson R, Douglass, P, Rosen RL, Bone RC. Long-term outcomes for elderly survivors of prolonged ventilator assistance. Chest 1989; 96:1120–1124.
20. Menzies R, Gibbons W, Goldberg P. Determinants of weaning and survival among patients with COPD who require mechanical ventilation for acute respiratory failure. Chest 1989; 95:398–405.
21. Gracey DR, Naessens JM, Krishan I, Marsh HM. Hospital and posthospital survival in patients mechanically ventilated for more than 29 days. Chest 1992; 101(1):211–214.
22. Stauffer JL, Fayter NA, Graves B, Cromb M, Lynch JC, Goebel P. Survival following mechanical ventilation for acute respiratory failure in adult men. Chest 1993; 104(4):1222–1229.
23. Snow RM, Miller WC, Rice DL, Ali MK. Respiratory failure in cancer patients. JAMA 1997; 241:2039–2042.
24. Make B, Dayno S, Gertman P. Prevalence of chronic ventilator-dependency. Am Rev Respir Dis 1986; 132:A167.
25. Strumpf DA, Millman RP, Hill NS. The management of chronic hypoventilation. Chest 1990; 98:474–480.
26. Hill NS. Noninvasive ventilation: does it work, for whom, and how? Clin Comment 1993; 147:1050–1055.
27. Milligan S. AARC and Gallup estimate numbers and costs of caring for chronic ventilator patients. AARC Times 1991; 150:30–36.
28. Goldberg AI, Frownfelter D. The ventilator-assisted individuals study. Chest 1990; 98:428–433.
29. Gracey DR, Gillespie D, Nobrega F, Naessens JM, Krishan I. Financial implications of prolonged ventilator care of Medicare patients under the prospective payment system. Chest 1987; 91:424–427.
30. Douglass PS, Bone RC, Rosen RL. DRG payment for long-term ventilator patients. Chest 1987; 91:412–417.
31. Douglass PS, Bone RC, Rosen RL. DRG payment for long-term ventilator patients—revisited. Chest 1988; 93:629–631.
32. Moxham J, Shneerson JM. Diaphragmatic pacing. Am Rev Respir Dis 1993; 148:533–536.
33. Stauffer JL, Olsen DE, Petty TL. Complications and consequences of endotracheal intubation and tracheostomy: a prospective study of 150 critically ill patients. Am J Med 1981; 70:65–76.

34. Floretti OG, Gammage GW. Complications of ventilatory support. In: Kirby RR, Banner JM, Downs JB, eds. Clinical Applications of Ventilatory Support. New York: Churchill Livingstone, 1990:337–360.
35. Bach JR, Alba AS, Bahatiuk G, Saporito L, Lee M. Mouth intermittent positive pressure ventilation in the management of post-polio respirtory insufficiency. Chest 1987; 91:859–864.
36. Make BJ, Gilmartin ME. Rehabilitation and home care for ventilator-assisted individuals. Clin Chest Med 1986; 679–691.
37. Bach JR, Alba AS. Tracheostomy ventilation: a study of efficacy with deflated cuffs and cuffless tubes. Chest 1990; 97:679–683.
38. Manzano JL, Lubillo S, Henriquez D, Martin JC, Perez MC, Wilson DJ. Verbal communication of ventilator-dependent patients. Crit Care Med 1993; 21:512–517.
39. Udwadia ZF, Santis GK, Stevan MH, Simonds AK. Nasal ventilation to facilitate weaning in patients with chronic respiratory insufficiency. Thorax 1992; 47:715–718.
40. Bach JR. A comparison of long-term ventilatory support alternatives from the perspective of the patient and care giver. Chest 1993; 104:1702–1706.
41. Barach AL. The treatment of anoxia in clinical medicine. Bull NY Acad Med 1950; 26:370–383.
42. Alba A, Khan A, Lee M. Mouth IPPV for sleep. Rehab Gaz 1981; 24:47–49.
43. Sullivan CE, Berthon-Jones M, Issa FO, Eves L. Reversal of obstructive sleep apnea by continuous positive airway pressure applied through the nose. Lancet 1981; 1:862–865.
44. Bach JR, Alba A, Mosher R, Delaubier A. Intermittent positive pressure ventilation via nasal access in the management of respiratory insufficiency. Chest 1987; 94:168–170.
45. Kerby GR, Mayer LS, Pingleton SK. Nocturnal positive pressure ventilation via nasal mask. Am Rev Respir Dis 1987; 135:738–740.
46. Ellis ER, Bye PTP, Bruderer JW, Sullivan CE. Treatment of respiratory failure during sleep in patients with neuromuscular disease. Am Rev Respir Dis 1987; 1135:148–152.
47. Carroll N, Branthwaite MA. Control of nocturnal hypoventilation by nasal intermittent positive pressure ventilation. Thorax 1988; 43:349–353.
48. Leger P, Jennequin J, Gerard M, Robert D. Home positive pressure ventilation via nasal masks in patients with neuromuscular weakness and restrictive lung or chest wall disease. Respir Care 1989; 34:73–79.
49. Heckmatt JZ, Loh L, Dubowitz V. Nighttime nasal ventilation in neuromuscular disease. Lancet 1990; 335:579–581.
50. Gay PC, Patel AM, Viggiano RW, Hubmayr RD. Nocturnal nasal ventilation for treatment of patients with hypercapneic respiratory failure. Mayo Clin Proc 1991; 144:1234–1239.
51. Hill NS, Eveloff SE, Carlisle CC, Goff SG. Efficacy of nocturnal nasal ventilation in patients with restrictive thoracic disease. Am Rev Respir Dis 1992; 145:365–371.
52. Vianello A, Bevilaqua M, Salvador V, et al. Long-term nasal intermittent positive

pressure ventilation in advanced Duchenne's muscular dystrophy. Chest 1994; 105:445–449.
53. Strumpf DA, Carlisle CC, Millman RP, Smith KW, Hill NS. An evaluation of the Respironics BiPAP bi-level CPAP device for delivery of assisted ventilation. Respir Care 1990; 35:415–422.
54. Meduri GU, Abou-Shala N, Fox RC, Jones CB, Leeper KV, Wunderink RG. Noninvasive face mask mechanical ventilation in patients with acute hypercapneic respiratory failure. Chest 1991; 100:445–454.
55. Meyer TJ, Hill NS. Noninvasive positive pressure ventilation to treat respiratory failure. Ann Intern Med 1994; 120:760–770.
56. Strumpf DA, Millman RP, Carlisle CC, et al. Nocturnal positive-pressure ventilation via nasal mask in patients with severe chronic obstructive pulmonary disease. Am Rev Respir Dis 1991; 144:1234–1239.
57. Meyer TJ, Pressman MR, Benditt J, McCool DF, Millman RP, Hill NS. Mouth leaking during nocturnal nasal ventilation: effect on sleep quality. Am J Respir Crit Care Med 1995; 151:A423.
58. Woollam CHM. The development of apparatus for intermittent negative respiration. Anaesthesia 1976; 31(5):666–685.
59. Bach JR, Penek J. Obstructive sleep apnea complicating negative pressure ventilatory support in patients with chronic paralytic restrictive ventilatory dysfunction. Chest 1991; 99:1386.
60. Hill NS, Redline S, Carskadon MA, Curran FJ, Millman RP. Sleep-disordered breathing in patients with Duchenne muscular dystrophy using negative pressure ventilators. Chest 1992; 102:1656–1662.
61. Smith PEM, Edwards THT, Calverley PMA. Oxygen treatment of sleep hypoxemia in Duchenne muscular dystrophy. Thorax 1989; 44:997–1001.
62. Adamson JP, Lewis L, Stein JD. Application of abdominal pressure for artificial respiration. JAMA 1959; 169:1613–1617.
63. Plum F, Whendon DG. The rapid-rocking bed: its effect on the ventilation of poliomyelitis patients with respiratory paralysis. JAMA 1951; 245:235–241.
64. Yang G-FW, Alba A, Lee M, Khan A. Pneumobelt for sleep in the ventilator user: clinical experience. Arch Phys Med Rehabil 1989; 70:707–711.
65. Hill NS. Use of rocking beds, pneumobelt, and other noninvasive aids to ventilation. In: Tobin MJ, ed. Principles and Practice of Mechanical Ventilation. New York: McGraw-Hill, 1994.
66. Hill NS. Clinical applications of body ventilators. Chest 1986; 90:897–905.
67. Bach JR, Alba AS. Total ventilatory support by the intermittent abdominal pressure ventilator. Chest 1991; 99:630–636.
68. Abd AG, Braun NMT, Baskin MI, O'Sullivan MM, Alkaitis DA. Diaphragmatic dysfunction after open heart surgery: treatment with a rocking bed. Ann Intern Med 1991; 111:881–886.
69. Sternberg L, Sternberg D. Life from the Seesaw. Boston: Dodd-Mead, 1986.
70. Bach JR, Alba AS. Noninvasive options for ventilatory support of the traumatic high level quadraplegic. Chest 1990; 98:613–619.
71. Dail CW, Affeldt JE, Collier CR. Clinical aspects of glossopharyngeal breathing. JAMA 1953; 158:445–449.

72. Bach JR, Alba AS, Bodofsky E, Curran FJ, Schultheiss M. Glossopharyngeal breathing and noninvasive aids in the management of post-polio respiratory insufficiency. Birth Defects 1987; 23:99–113.
73. Glenn WWL, Brouillette RT, Dentz B, et al. Fundamental considerations in pacing of the diaphragm for chronic ventilatory insufficiency: a multicenter study. PACE 1988; 11:2121–2127.
74. Bach JR, O'Connor K. Electrophrenic ventilation: a different perspective. J Am Paraplegia Soc 1991; 14:9–17.
75. Branthwaite MA. Noninvasive and domicillary ventilation: positive pressure techniques. Thorax 1991; 46:208–212.
76. Meecham-Jones DJ, Paul EA, Wedzicha JR. Nasal pressure support ventilation with supplemental oxygen therapy compared with oxygen therapy alone in stable hypercapnic COPD—a randomized controlled study. Am J Respir Crit Care Med 1994; 149:A292.
77. Banaszak EF, Travers H, Frazier M, Vinz T. Home ventilator care. Respir Care 1981; 26(12):1262–1268.
78. O'Donahue WJ, Giovannoni RM, Goldberg AI, et al. Long-term mechanical ventilation. Guidelines for management in the home and at alternate community sites. Chest 1986; 90:1S–37S.
79. Hill NS. Home care of ventilator-assisted and ventilator-dependent patients. J Cardiopulm Rehabil 1988; 11:462–472.
80. Bach JR, Intintola P, Alba AS, Holland IF. The ventilator-assisted individual. Cost analysis of institutionalization vs rehabilitation and in-home management. Chest 1992; 101:26–30.
81. Kacmarek RM, Stanek KS, McMahon K, et al. Increased work of breathing during synchronized intermittent mandatory ventilation (SIMV) in home care ventilators. Am Rev Respir Dis 1988; 137(4, part 2):64.
82. Rondinelli RD, Hill NS. Rehabilitation of the patient with pulmonary disease. In: Delisa JA, ed. Rehabilitation Medicine Principles and Practice. Philadelphia: Lippincott, 1988.
83. Wilson DO, Rogers RM, Hoffman RM. Nutrition and chronic lung disease. Am Rev Respir Dis 1985; 123:1347–1365.
84. Roza AM, Shizgal HM. The Harris-Benedict equation re-evaluated: resting energy requirements and the body cell mass. Am J Clin Nutr 1984; 40:168–182.
85. Askenazi J, Weissman C, Rosenbaum H, Hyman AI, Milic-Emili J, Kinney JM. Nutrition and the respiratory system. Crit Care Med 1982; 10:163–172.
86. Frankel DL. Nutrition. In: Delisa JA, ed. Rehabilitation Medicine Principles and Practice. Philadelphia: Lippincott, 1988.
87. Gilmartin M. Transition from the intensive care unit to home: patient selection and discharge planning. Respir Care 1994; 39:456–480.
88. Hungerpiller J, Leonard C, Criner G. Swallowing function in trached patients requiring prolonged mechanical ventilation. Chest 1989; 96:296S.
89. Meyer TJ, Eveloff SE, Bauer MS, Schwartz WA, Hill NS, Millman RP. Adverse environmental conditions in the respiratory and medical ICU settings. Chest 1994; 105:1211–1216.
90. Aaron J, Carskadon M, Meyer T, Hill N, Millman RP. Environmental noise is a

a cause of sleep disruption in a respiratory intensive care unit. Am J Respir Crit Care Med 1995 (abstract).

91. Isaac L, Hungerpiller J, Criner G. Neuropsychologic deficits in chronic ventilator-dependent patients. Chest 1989; 96:255S.
92. Criner GJ, Tzovnakis, A, Kreimer DT. Overview of improving tolerance of long-term mechanical ventilation. Crit Care Clin 1994; 10:845–866.
93. Elpern EH, Silver MR, Rosen RL, Bone RC. The noninvasive respiratory care unit. Patterns of use and financial implications. Chest 1991; 99:205–208.
94. Indihar JF, Walker NE. Experience with a prolonged respiratory care unit—revisited. Chest 1984; 86:616–620.
95. Make BJ. Long-term management of ventilator-assisted individuals. The Boston University experience. Respir Care 1989; 31:303–313.
96. Gerard M, Robert D, Salamand J, Buffat J, Chemorin, Bertoye A. Étude de la survie chéz 150 insuffisants respiratoires chroniques tracheotomises traités par la ventilation assistée a domicile. Lyon Med 1981; 245(8):555–558.
97. Robert D, Gerard M, Leger P, et al. La ventilation méchanique a domicile définitive par trachéostomie de l'insuffisant respiratoire chronique. Rev Fr Mal Respir 1983; 11:923–936.
98. Bertrand A, Milane J, Dufranc P. Traitement au long cours de l'insuffisance respiratoire chronique par ventilation endotrachéale à domicile chez 118 patients trachéotomisés. Rev Mal Respir 1985; 2:91–95.
99. Dudeffant P, Manier G, Gbikpi-benissan G, Cardinaud JP. Devinir des insuffisants respiratories chroniques traités à domicile par trachéostomie et ventilation assistée. Rev Mal Respir 1985; 2:145–150.
100. Splaingard ML, Frates RC, Jefferson LS, Rosen CL, Harrison GM. Home negative pressure ventilation: report of 20 years of experience in patients with neuromuscular disease. Arch Phys Med Rehabil 1985; 66:239–243.
101. Ordonneau J, Chailleux E, Chollet S, et al. Actuarial survival rate in 99 tracheostomized patients with chronic pulmonary insufficiency treated by pulmonary mechanical ventilation at home. Eur J Respir Dis 1986; 69(Suppl 146):383–388.
102. Muir JF, Girault C, Cardinaud JP, et al. Survival and long-term follow-up of tracheostomized patients with COPD treated by home mechanical ventilation. Chest 1994; 106:201–209.
103. Leger P, Bedicam JM, Cornette A, et al. Nasal intermittent positive pressure. Long-term follow-up in patients with severe chronic respiratory insufficiency. Chest 1994; 105:100–105.
104. Raphael JC, Chevret S, Chastang C, Bouvet F. French multicenter trial of prophylactic nasal ventilation in Duchenne muscular dystrophy. Lancet 1994; 343:1600–1604.
105. Mohr CH, Hill NS. Long-term follow-up of nocturnal ventilatory assistance in patients with respiratory failure due to Duchenne-type muscular dystrophy. Chest 1990; 97:91–96.
106. Curran FJ, Colbert AP. Ventilator management in Duchenne muscular dystrophy and post poliomyelitis syndrome: twelve years' experience. Arch Phys Med Rehabil 1989; 70:180–185.
107. Robins Miller J, Colbert AP, Schock NC. Ventilator use in progressive neuro-

muscular disease: impact on patients and their families. Dev Med Child Neurol 1988; 30:200–207.
108. Robins Miller J, Colbert AP, Osberg JS. Ventilator dependency: decision-making, daily functioning, and quality of life with Duchenne muscular dystrophy. Dev Med Child Neurol 1990; 32:1078–1086.
109. Oppenheimer EA. Home mechanical ventilation: obstacles to living at home. IVUN News 1994; 8:2–3.
110. Hyers TM. NIH Workshop on Withholding and Withdrawing Mechanical Ventilation. Am Rev Respir Dis 1989; 140(2, part 2):S1–S46.
111. American Thoracic Society. Withholding and withdrawing life-sustaining therapy. Ann Intern Med 1991; 115:478–485.
112. Osborne ML. Physician decisions regarding life support in the intensive care unit. Chest 1992; 101:217–224.

26

Ventilator Dependency as Seen by the Patient/Client

IRA E. HOLLAND

Concepts of Independence, Inc.
New York, New York

The last major polio epidemic struck Boston during the summer of 1955, only a few weeks before the availability of the Salk vaccine. As a result of this epidemic, hundreds of people died or were disabled.

During this summer, at the age of 15, I was employed as a camp counselor on Cape Cod. In August, two youngsters from Boston arrived at the camp to escape the city for a few weeks. Shortly after their arrival, they became ill and evidently exposed me to the polio virus.

I. Onset and Acute Stage

Within a week, I had become acutely ill. The inability to walk, bouts of nausea, and muscle spasms accompanied by a high fever resulted in my transport by ambulance from the camp to a local hospital on the Cape. A spinal tap was performed confirming the diagnosis, necessitating my transfer to Haynes Memorial Hospital in Boston.

My breathing was becoming more difficult, necessitating my being placed into an Emerson Iron Lung. After I spent many hours struggling to remain alive, the tank was sealed, and I experienced the extraordinary relief of air rushing to fill my lungs. My first thought was that death, which seemed so imminent, had been postponed.

The tank ventilator was opened each day to determine if I could breathe on my own. I remember attempting to pull, to strain, desperately attempting to draw the next impossible breath. After continuing this futile effort for a minute or two, I felt as though I would suffocate. It was becoming rapidly apparent that my breathing dependency would continue permanently.

II. Rehabilitative Process

In November 1955, I was transferred to Goldwater Memorial Hospital on Roosevelt Island, New York. I was transported in the iron lung by means of a large, generator-equipped moving van. This transfer was accomplished after a 9-hr ordeal, while I remained within the body of the iron lung. During this period, I had to endure a dual ordeal: the deafening roar of the sirens generated by the police escort provided by the four states that we traveled through, and the life-sustaining generator. This odyssey ultimately ended with the humiliation at being met by my parents and younger brother, who were surrounded by a mob of newspaper photographers at the entrance to the hospital. I was "unloaded" at the Goldwater Memorial Hospital Respiratory Center, which was, at the time, a part of the March of Dimes network. Within the next 30 min, I was transferred from the iron lung, within whose "body" I had lived for the past 3 months, into yet another tank respirator so that my initial ventilator could be returned to Boston. During this transfer, I had the first glimpse of my now atrophied body. I was startled at the sight of myself. It was as though I was looking at a body other than my own.

The transformation to "quadriplegic" was now complete. I could neither move nor breathe—my life was wholly dependent on that large yellow machine. Although a relatively brief period had elapsed, it appeared that I had been living this nightmare for longer than I could remember.

My ventilator dependency was becoming a more frightening part of my everyday reality. My awareness of the inherent risks and threats to my life as a direct result of my reliance on a ventilator was becoming more apparent. The simple action of being bathed or toileted required elaborate measures to maintain my ventilation. To allow the tank to be opened, my head was encased in a plastic dome, which permitted the delivery of positive pressure, so that I might continue to breathe. It was my hope that some machine would soon be developed that would free me from my imprisonment.

During this period, I had frequent sessions with the physical therapists. In the course of these treatments, the therapists administered chest percussion and used a new device that permitted them to deliver very deep breaths, via a mask, while the tank was left open. These therapists, the precursors of respiratory therapists, became my connection to developments that were occurring in the world of ventilatory support. It was from these therapists that I first learned of a new company that was introducing a "portable" ventilator. As explained to me, the new ventilator would permit assisted breathing in the wheelchair for periods up to 5 hr using a single battery. This news held open the prospect of eventually leaving the iron lung completely. I was determined to use whatever new equipment became available to enhance my independence and separation from the iron lung.

The months passed quickly: my former high-school friends had returned to their studies, and autumn had turned the enormous old oaks and maples outside my window to brilliant reds and yellows. The colors served to remind me that time had stopped for myself. My former school friends came to visit me, but after we exchanged hellos, there was not much left to say. I lay in bed with the "new chest ventilator device." Although for me it was release from the confinement of the iron lung, for these adolescents who came to visit and who knew me in what seemed to me to be another world I was as trapped or confined as ever. I don't know who was more uncomfortable, but I determined that it would never happen again. I never asked my former friends to return. Their discomfort at my paralysis and ventilator dependency only served to make me more aware of how uncomfortable the rest of the world was with me. I began to think, on the one hand, about my wish to die quickly and be finished with it, and, on the other, about the desire to continue and to attempt to find a way of becoming functional.

I remember at this juncture that I began to focus on the complexity of my mechanical ventilator support. Although I had learned glossopharyngeal breathing (frog breathing), which could sustain me for a short period, I still felt extremely vulnerable. To help me come to terms with this sense of vulnerability, I needed a goal toward which I could direct myself, to help me move beyond the emotional confines of my ventilator dependency. The opportunity of a college experience appeared to afford me this stimulus.

The essential first step of identifying a goal and of "coming to terms," indicated that I, as a ventilator-dependent individual, had started the ongoing process of determining what degree of risk would be acceptable while I was attempting to accomplish something that I felt was important. I think that this process is one that must continue as long as one lives as a ventilator-dependent person.

When one first becomes ventilator-dependent, there are extended periods during which the individual focuses on the fact that life is inexorably tied to a machine. These periods when one concentrates on this thin line of mortality are eventually precluded by the ongoing momentum of activities and desires that fill one's daily life.

The experience of being able to attend a university, to participate in the pursuit of courses, to meet and to interact with other people—most of whom are not disabled—and to take on the responsibility of completing a program of study is of great importance. The advent of small portable ventilators in the 1960s and 1970s provided me with a new sense of independence. I was no longer tied to an electrical outlet; although the batteries were heavy and the power consumption was exorbitant, I finally could make brief excursions into the world outside of the institution.

I was graduated with honors from Long Island University in 1973. The fact that I had completed this venture made me ecstatic. This accomplishment encouraged me to think about new goals and directions, which included the possibility of leaving the institution.

As I prepared to reenter the world I had left 21 years earlier, I began the process of recruiting my first personal care assistants. I resorted to classified advertisements in the newspapers and had potential candidates trained with the assistance of the respiratory staff at Goldwater Memorial Hospital. The focus of my training program was on the use of ventilatory support, assisted coughing, personal needs, and, most important, the manner in which my attendants would maximize my functional capabilities.

I chose an apartment on Roosevelt Island, a relatively spacious, sunny, and accessible home. I was looking for a two-bedroom apartment as I was married to Victoria. Vicki was also postpolio, ventilator-dependent, and used a wheelchair. We had met many years before at Goldwater and had lived as patients within the confines of the respiratory center. We married in 1968 while continuing to live in the hospital; the decision was not very well thought out, and subsequently I regretted the lack of forethought. Despite what we considered to be "extensive and comprehensive discussions," there were just too many problems and irreconcilable differences. I am now firmly convinced that for my own personal needs and peace of mind, marriage between two quadriplegics does not promote marital bliss. Rather, I believe that the frustrations and anxieties of disabilities are enhanced by such a union.

Vicki and I lived together for 11 years, until her death in 1979. After her death, I was again on my own. I began moving aggressively toward reestablishing my independence and self-assertiveness.

For the first few years at home, I lacked a sense of personal direction. Perhaps this was due, in part, to the fact that I had spent so many years confined in the hospital. Initially I felt that I needed space and time to unwind, to "find myself and a sense of purpose." In some respects, the process that I underwent in establishing a new direction was similar to that which I went through when I first began dealing with my ventilator. There is a tendency for severely disabled individuals, especially those using mechanical ventilatory support, to drift back into the protected environment of an institution. To elude this tendency, one must push continually to attempt to accomplish tasks that become increasingly difficult. As the severely disabled individual pursues this struggle, he/she is attempting to compete with able-bodied people who do not need caregivers to "process them" for a day's work. This unremitting need to compete adds yet another level of frustration to an already complex life-style.

In 1980, I suffered a bout of an upper respiratory infection that necessitated my returning to Goldwater. I was placed in the iron lung for treatment. It was later determined that the chest (cuirass) ventilator I was using was limited in effectiveness. This information reinforced an impression that I had held for a lengthy period, i.e., that the cuirass, which had served me since 1956, was now inadequate. After my recovery, I spoke with Dr. Augusta Alba regarding an alternative for ventilatory assistance. Dr. Alba recommended that I utilize the Puritan-Bennett lip seal with Velcro straps. This device proved to be very comfortable and quite satisfactory with respect to maintaining adequate nocturnal ventilation. The Puritan-Bennett lip seal, in conjunction with the Maxivent, proved to be an ideal mechanism for supporting sleep.

III. Employment

Having completed college in 1973, I chose to direct my efforts toward issues with which I had a working familiarity. To accomplish this goal, I utilized the management skills I had developed over the years in dealing with the complexities of disability and the discipline of independent living.

A management career is an opportune direction for a disabled person. The decision to move in that direction is prompted by the fact that independent living is really an ongoing exercise in management-type decisions. Virtually every aspect of every day is comprised of an ongoing decision-making process. For me, surrounded by personal care assistants and often confronted by a seemingly endless stream of problems seeking solutions, management intervention was the only appropriate course of action.

As a management consultant to providers of home care services, I am in a unique position to offer support, direction, and perspective on ventilatory assistance to an industry that is an integral component of my everyday life.

In 1978, I initiated a consulting relationship with Thompson Respiratory Products, Inc. This opening wedge enabled me to provide input in the areas of product development and marketing. My many activities expanded in 1979 when I began a relationship with Paramedical Specialties, Inc., a local home care provider. My work with Paramedical was primarily in the areas of inservice training and the planning of discharge for ventilator-dependent patients who were trying to leave hospitals or rehabilitation centers for life in their own homes.

In 1983, Thompson Respiration Products, Inc., was acquired by the Puritan-Bennett Corporation. Consequently, I became a consultant to the Portable Ventilator Division of this large international manufacturer of ventilator products. For more than 11 years, I served as a consultant, working with engineers, physicians, administrators, and many hundreds of ventilator-assisted individuals across the United States and in Europe, Japan, and other parts of the world. I evaluated the marketplace and analyzed equipment, providing Puritan-Bennett with detailed analyses that would permit the manufacture of improved ventilatory equipment. When Puritan-Bennett stopped manufacturing portable ventilators in 1994, I turned my attention to the Aequitron Medical Corporation after evaluating it and determining that Aequitron was the manufacturer with the best perspective on the portable marketplace. Aequitron manufactures the LP6+ and the LP10. Both are portable volume ventilators that perform with great reliability.

With Puritan-Bennett out of the market, this left only two major manufacturers of portable volume ventilators. I felt that I had many insights and contributions to make to the portable ventilator industry that would benefit the growing population of ventilator-dependent individuals. I met Mr. Jeffery A. Blair, Senior Vice President of Aequitron Medical, Inc., in my office in New York. Mr. Blair had come to New York from Minneapolis where Aequitron Medical, Inc., is headquartered. I presented my credentials and we discussed my potential for becoming a consultant to the portable ventilator division. I was impressed by the Aequitron product and intrigued by Jeff Blair's candid and open manner. In May 1994, I initiated what has become a mutually beneficial relationship with Aequitron. My continued commitment to the new generation of portable volume ventilators and the consequent benefits that are enjoyed by the end-user have been well supported by Jeff Blair's engineers, technical support, and clinical staff. If anything, Aequitron has provided me with an environment that permits me to contribute on a broader scale than was possible with the Puritan-Bennett Corporation. I feel that the intimacy of Aequitron enables it to respond more immediately to the needs of the physicians and patients and to provide an enhanced home care atmosphere.

In a similar way, my work with Paramedical Specialties, Inc., took a new direction when the company was aquired first by Healthdyne, Inc., and subsequently by the Glasrock Home Care Corporation. My work with Glasrock terminated in 1990 when I was offered a more challenging position by a local home care dealer in Westchester County, Respiratory Equipment Supply, Inc. (R.E.S.I.). My role with R.E.S.I. is to assist with the management of their service delivery program, to evaluate quality assurance information, and to recommend appropriate courses of action if a ventilator-dependent client should encounter a problem either in equipment or in service. I am responsible for ensuring client satisfaction by providing a smooth, uninterrupted flow of information between company representatives and the 30 ventilator-dependent R.E.S.I. clients currently living at home.

Most ventilator-dependent patients feel a greater sense of security if they work with someone who is similarly dependent. Ventilator dependency is so complex that many ventilator users feel that the professionals who care for them do not always fully understand their concerns. Following my discharge from Goldwater in 1976, I returned to work with newly disabled ventilator-dependent patients at Goldwater Memorial Hospital. This respiratory rehabilitation center had been my home for more than 20 years. I worked there on a weekly basis to help promote the interface between the rehabilitation and psychology departments and to offer the patients a peer's perspective of ventilator dependency.

The response to these efforts were overwhelmingly positive. The patients needed a role model who would support the premise that they could leave the protective environment of the center. As much as they expressed their dislike of the hospital, to many of them the prospect of living in the world outside was overwhelming when they considered the complexities of community living. Most often, they expressed concern about how the innumerable tasks and the life-sustaining decisions would be accomplished.

Hours turned into weeks and weeks gradually turned into years. The seemingly endless questions and fearful concerns were allayed during our lengthy discussions. The concerns dealt with everything from power failures to future employment, to girlfriends, sexuality, transportation, and the management of personal care attendants.

My work with the newly dependent patients continued for 2 years. Thereafter, I could not continue my weekly visits to the Goldwater patients. I was becoming increasingly involved in my own work, essentially the organization that I had cofounded—Concepts of Independence, Inc.—which was growing at a rate that demanded more of my time and attention.

The satisfaction with employment and the ability to make a significant and meaningful contribution is as important to a ventilator-dependent person as it is to anyone who is not so dependent.

In addition to the satisfaction of employment, meeting new people, establishing relationships, eating out with friends and business associates, attending concerts, getting away on vacation are all a significant aspect of a fulfilled lifestyle—truly, the goal of any of us, whether disabled, ventilator-dependent, or able-bodied.

IV. Personal Assistance Services

Since coming to live independently in my own home, I have hired, and not incidentally fired, a number of personal care assistants. On average, most assistants have remained with me for 2 or 3 years. I have hired only one man in the past 18 years; I prefer working with women although I sometimes wonder why I have any preference. Certainly gender is no assurance of longevity. The hiring of a personal care assistant who is compatible and sensitive to my needs has been one of the most crucial aspects in a successful community-living experience. I feel that the more complex a home care process, the more difficult it will be to remain dependent on family for the provision of personal care. I feel strongly that most families are too emotionally involved to be objective enough to assist with the complexities of daily living. Overall, a good personal care assistant will enable the individual to live independently within the reasonable limits imposed by the disability. While hiring a personal care assistant, it is essential to take into account the necessity for the ventilator-dependent individual to be self-directing.

In 1977, revisions in the New York City Personal Assistance Program raised the prospect of preventing disabled individuals who were receiving home care assistance from hiring their own personal care attendants. The proposed changes were sufficient motivation for me to begin working with colleagues and friends on establishing our own personal assistant service agency. It was our goal to maintain the essential aspects of employing and individually training personal care attendants who can satisfy the unique home care needs of individual employers. Thus was Concepts of Independence, Inc., conceived. It took 2 years and innumerable meetings with state and city officials before Concepts was awarded its first contract in 1980.

Concepts of Independence, Inc., a consumer-directed personal assistance program in New York City, began business with a staff of five, a client census of 20, and an initial contract of $110,000. During the past 15 years, the organization has grown considerably; its staff now consists of 11 members; its client base has exceeded 400; and its current contract is valued at $17 million. As Cofounder and President of Concepts, I am pleased with the day-to-day responsibility of working with the staff, board of directors, and consultants; this interplay has enabled the company to continue operations and to expand its unique program. The program has proved essential to the city's overall strategy for home care services for the hundreds of clients that the company now serves.

From the perspective of a traditional provider of home care services, Concepts is neither their idea or ideal. But from my perspective, Concepts represents home care with a significant difference. This difference centers on the primary objective of Concepts, i.e., to empower each consumer to self-administer his/her own home care service plan. In the Concepts program, the true provider of service is the consumer who has elected the responsibility of self-determination.

When a ventilator-dependent person requires the assistance of a caregiver for every aspect of daily living, it is imperative that he/she clearly understand the responsibilities that are being assumed. Self-directing ventilator-dependent consumers are clearly not in a position to be left alone for any extended period of time. In hiring personal care assistants ensuring appropriate management is imperative. Foresight and good intuition are essential to the success of this undertaking.

Concepts currently has more than 50 ventilator-dependent clients. These individuals, and I include myself among this group, must use appropriate strategies to cover any unforeseen absence of the assistant. As a general rule, most clients, including myself, do not permit the personal care assistant to leave until the next covering assistant has arrived. When interviewing prospective assistants, I discuss the prospect of the individual having to stay with me, on the job, for an extended period should an illness or other unforeseen circumstance interrupt the normal flow in my personal care attendant schedule.

Clear and appropriate planning by the client with friends and reliable assistants is the cornerstone to success in this vital area. In the 19 years that I have lived at home, I have never experienced a single incidence of abandonment; in only one instance have I encountered gross employee irresponsibility. Of course, as mutual fund companies are so fond of saying, "Past performance is no indication of future performance." I am always aware of my vulnerability, and as a result, I tend to overcompensate for any situation that might place me in a compromising situation. I have given my most trusted assistants a beeper, a small monthly expense for the security it affords. I keep at bedside a list of available individuals, and I live close to close friends who are similarly ventilator-dependent. This sort of preparedness is necessary if a ventilator-dependent individual is to be a successful client with Concepts. Indeed, the successful longevity of any individual who is a ventilator-dependent and intends to live successfully in the community is directly related to his/her level of preparedness.

One area in which planning must come into play is in selecting a provider of ventilatory support services. There are a multitude of home care providers who rent ventilators to ventilator-dependent people. Choosing the one that will provide a timely response in the event of equipment failure is crucial for managing an emergency. In selecting the home care provider from whom I receive services and with whom I work, commitment to this concern was a critical element in shaping my decision process. In working with clients who are served by the home care provider that I utilize as well as with clients who are served by other home care providers, I have found that a company's commitment to timely response is a key component to an enduring and satisfying relationship.

Another area where planning is most important is the proper selection of a responsible transportation company. I have had the misfortune of having been left in the city, with my ventilator battery running down, waiting for a van to pick me up after a meeting. Transporters do not always appreciate the importance of timely pickups. Again, careful planning and a thorough explanation of the situation to the dispatcher is essential.

Transportation is only one element in the complex process of planning that will confront the ventilator-dependent person living outside of the institution. When a client is in an institution, the institution anticipates virtually everything that can go wrong and provides coverage for these eventualities. In the home care situation, this responsibility is placed firmly on the shoulders of the client. The foresight and initiative that are essential for a successful adaptation to community living must be inherent in the person who assumes responsibility for these tasks. It must never be assumed that caregivers will "take care of it."

My discharge from Goldwater 19 years ago reminds me of the enormity of the change and growth in me that have occurred. In my independent life-style, I have grown much beyond the institution's definition of "home care"; to accomplish this independent life-style, I require the constant support of properly selected personal care assistants. I live an extremely busy and complex life. My daily activities frequently require that I wake at 4:30 A.M. in order to leave for my office at 9:30 A.M. When at the office, I manage the Concepts home care program with the assistance of a staff of 11 individuals, plus the necessary legal and financial consultants. In addition to managing the home care program, I direct a group of trustees in the management of a $2,000,000 health and pension fund. Another project in which I am actively engaged, with our Program Director, Ed Litcher, and Assistant Director, Jacob Mathieu, is in the selection of new office space to replace the outgrown capacities of our current offices. Negotiations have entailed more than 8 months of interplay with brokers, architects, and telecommunication and computer salespeople. On the days that I do not go to the office, I am in continuous telephone communication with Ed and Jacob and our consultants. The days that are not spent at Concepts provide me with the opportunity to develop my reports and engage in my consultative agenda with Aequitron Medical, Inc.

Living in New York City affords me access to the comprehensive personal assistance services that I require; these services are operative 24 hr/day, 7 days/week. This level of comprehensive coverage permits me to live in a manner that allows me the flexibility and the dignity of executing my own decisions; it also provides me the ability to make appointments with a schedule that allows for my individuality.

The cost-effectiveness of the Concepts program has attracted national attention. The economies by which services are provided offer a compelling reason for the utilization of a Concepts-style program of home care. The Concepts program enjoys a high level of cost-effectiveness because it relies on the consumer to provide much of the case management; this reliance decreases labor intensiveness since Concepts provides all services at the personnel care level. In New York State, participants in consumer-directed home care programs such as Concepts are afforded a waiver from the usual constraint of the Nurse Practice Act. Consumers in the Concept's program are enabled to receive services from a personal care assistant. These required services are generally regarded as skilled, calling for a home health aide if not a licensed practical or registered nurse. When the costs of home care provided by Concepts are compared to those of traditional home care agencies, we estimate that for every 20 "high needs" consumers serviced by Concepts, the savings to the state Medicaid program are on the order of $1 million per year.

As stated in a recent article (1):

> . . . safety and substantial savings can be achieved by maintaining self-directed ventilator assisted individuals at home with personal care [assistants] as necessary rather than institutionalization under the least expensive circumstances. Conversion of ventilator assisted individuals to the use of noninvasive methods of supported ventilation facilitates disposition to be community by simplifying personal care needs and under current laws in most states by avoiding the need for home nursing care for tracheal suctioning.

In this era of budget cuts and shrinking allocations, the advantages of personal assistance services provided to ventilator-assisted individuals make more sense than ever. Obviously, the singular advantage is the achievement of the sensitivity and responsibility inherent in a consumer-directed program. Utilizing this program modality enables the severely disabled individual who is ventilator-compromised to reenter the mainstream of functional productivity and to become a contributing individual.

V. Setting Priorities and Goals

Many years have elapsed since I entered that iron lung in Boston in August 1955. Having lived almost 40 years as a ventilator-dependent quadriplegic, I feel that my need to establish goals and to satisfactorily achieve objectives has been one of the major factors in my successful life.

The accomplishments that can and are being made by ventilator-dependent people in today's world are both startling and real. I am pleased and proud to know many others like myself who are functional, productive people living full and active lives. The possibilities are truly endless. There are problems that I share with those who do not use ventilators and there are problems that I must solve within myself; the process goes on. In reviewing my accomplishments, I am pleased and proud that I have been given the opportunity to direct myself toward the solution of problems that disabled people and those of us who are ventilator-dependent must face at work and in our personal lives. People have asked me to tell them which year I would consider most fulfilling, what period of my life I feel reflects my most extensive accomplishment. I would say that overall, the present is most deeply satisfying.

A ventilator-dependent person should be given every opportunity to access personal assistance and today's technology. If the decision to provide a ventilator to a patient is made, then a commitment to that patient must be part of the offering. The commitment must include the opportunity for the individual to access whether essential services are necessary to ensure that the quality of life will be the foremost objective. To offer community-based services to a ventilator-dependent person who is not capable of managing his/her ventilatory support services is, at best, questionable, but to deny support services to a patient who is aware and who has the potential to be a functional and productive person is a disservice to that individual and to society.

References

1. Bach JR, Intintola P, Alba AS, Holland IE. The ventilator assisted individual. The cost analysis of institutionalization vs rehabilitation and in-home management. Chest 1992; 101(1):26–30.
2. Holland IE. The home care alternative for ventilator-dependent patients. J Respir Care Pract 1993; 5:20–34.

27

Psychological Aspects of Pulmonary Rehabilitation with the Ventilator-Dependent Patient

LISA ISAAC

Mercy Catholic Medical Center
Darby, Pennsylvania

GERARD J. CRINER

Temple University School of Medicine
Philadelphia, Pennsylvania

Routinely, health care providers are faced with patients who challenge the most effective management strategies. Many of these patients have a psychological component to their medical problem that complicates their treatment, rehabilitation, and recovery. The risk for psychological problems is greatly increased in patients with critical (1,2) and chronic (3) illnesses, patients relying on life support technology (4), and patients undergoing open heart surgery (5,6).

Although psychological problems have been reported to adversely affect weaning in patients undergoing mechanical ventilation (7), data concerning psychological function in ventilated patients are extremely limited. This paucity is surprising, since the ventilator-dependent patient is subject to many factors that adversely affect psychological status, such as the intensive care unit (ICU) environment, dependence on machines for life support, and the presence of a chronic illness.

Most ventilator-dependent patients receive all or some portion of their hospital treatment in the ICU; overall, they are likely to be sicker than nonventilated patients and are more likely to have underlying cardiopulmonary diseases that cause chronic hypoxemia or to receive medications that increase their risk for impaired neuropsychological function.

The process of mechanical ventilation further predisposes the patient to the development of psychological problems by rendering the patient immobile, impeding natural communication ability, limiting independent function, and thereby, increasing the patient's apprehension and sense of isolation. Thus, a variety of factors increase the risk for psychological problems in the ventilator-dependent patient; these problems can interfere with their clinical management and rehabilitation.

This chapter integrates information about psychological problems in patients with pulmonary disorders and life-threatening illnesses with the limited data available about the psychological effects of long-term mechanical ventilation. First, psychological disturbances that have been documented in the ICU setting are described and specific environmental aspects of the critical care milieu that contribute to psychological problems are reviewed. Second, special psychological considerations for the ventilator-dependent pulmonary patient are discussed. Finally, a strategy is proposed for the evaluation and treatment of psychological problems that can interfere with weaning and rehabilitation.

I. Psychological Problems in the ICU Patient

A. Incidence and Etiology of Psychological Disturbances

As noted above, most patients who undergo long-term ventilation receive at least a portion of their care in the ICU. Psychological problems have been reported to occur in 14–72% of patients in the ICU whereas the frequency is less than 1% of hospitalized patients not in the ICU (8). Psychological reactions in the ICU can include anxiety, agitation, apathy, depression, fear, and delirium; these disturbances range in severity and can occur either singly or in combination, for patients receiving ICU care for as few as 5–7 days. Kornfeld and colleagues (5) reported that after open heart surgery, 38% of patients in the ICU developed delirium, characterized by progressive disorientation to time, person, and place, which was associated with varying degrees of cognitive impairment. Others confirmed these findings, reporting that delirium or other psychological disturbances occurred during the postoperative period after open heart surgery in 25–57% of their patients (6,9,10).

The psychological disturbances are probably multifactorial in etiology, including such factors as the patient's age, baseline psychological function, medications, and the underlying medical illness. Environmental features of the critical care milieu, and the quantity and quality of the patient's interactions with the medical staff, may also be important in contributing to the psychological disturbance.

B. Sleep Deprivation

The ICU setting is typically designed with the goal of streamlining critical levels of patient care rather than providing a stimulating environment for the patient. The unfortunate result is that the ICU environment can contribute to sleep and sensory disturbances, both of which can promote the development of psychological problems (6,11).

Up to 80% of hospitalized patients who require psychiatric consultation have an underlying sleep disturbance (12). Restless sleep, the development of nightmares, and the total absence of dreaming are common in patients in the ICU who develop delirium or other psychological disturbances.

While critical intermittent treatment and interventions, e.g., suctioning and aerosol delivery, interrupt continuous normal sleep, ongoing noise generated by the ventilator equipment, monitors, and oxygen outlets also contributes to sleep deprivation. Woods and Falk (13) measured mean noise levels at the head of patient beds in the ICU and found that for 90% of the time, the noise levels generated by ventilators, alarms, and oxygen equipment were equivalent to that of a radio playing at full volume.

In addition to ongoing noise, nighttime nursing activities and other interventions are not conducive to restful sleep. Sleep is a cyclical process and the normal adult alternates between non-rapid eye movement (NREM) and rapid eye movement (REM) sleep phases approximately five times in an 8-hr period, with approximately 25% of that time spent in REM sleep. For critically ill patients in the ICU who require multiple interventions, even one full, uninterrupted sleep cycle per night may be unobtainable, and depending on the nature of the underlying illness, this pattern may continue for several consecutive nights. Sleep studies for two to four consecutive nights in hospitalized patients who were not in the ICU showed that all had less than or equal to 2 hr of total sleep and severe reductions in stage 3–4 sleep, and none experienced any REM sleep (13). Medications frequently used in treating the critically ill ICU patient, i.e., narcotic analgesics, barbiturates, catecholamine infusions, and long-acting benzodiazepines, have all been reported to either significantly reduce or delay the onset of REM sleep (14).

Failure of nurses and physicians to recognize the importance of sleep quality and to intervene to ensure adequate sleep can also adversely influence the quality of sleep in the ICU. For example, in one study, nurses in the ICU reported that patients had slept all night, even though concurrent polysomnographic studies showed that no patient had slept for more than 2 hr (15). In another study, hospitalized patients who had significant sleep disorders were found to have no documentation of the quality of their sleep in their records (11).

C. Sensory Deprivation

A variety of abnormal auditory and visual stimuli, as well as sensory deprivation, that are routinely encountered during long-term ventilation in the ICU may predispose susceptible patients to the development of psychological problems. ICUs typically are monochromatic and unadorned. The incidence of delirium in postoperative patients treated in ICUs without windows was threefold greater than in ICUs with windows (1).

Because of the constraints imposed on mobility by the ventilatory support, visual stimuli of patients undergoing long-term ventilation are usually restricted to the overhead white ceiling tiles or plain white walls. Also, because of the need for round-the-clock care in the ICU, lighting is usually extremely bright, so it is never truly nighttime in the ICU.

Except for the unpleasant sounds of the ventilator apparatus, the oxygen outlets, and the monitors, acoustic stimulation is sparse and intermittent. Intermittent auditory stimulation can produce visual and auditory hallucinations even in normal subjects (16). Moreover, after open heart surgery, intermittent clicking, i.e., 1–6 clicks per second for several days, seemed to cause hallucinations and thought disorders (6).

II. Psychological Problems in Chronic Pulmonary Illness and Mechanical Ventilation

Abnormalities in central respiratory drive and gas exchange are common in patients undergoing long-term ventilation and may be associated with hypoxemia and hypercapnia, which, in turn, can elicit a variety of psychological and cognitive disorders, e.g., disturbed judgment, impaired short-term memory, inappropriate behavior, perceptual changes, and indifference or inattention (17).

Medications used to treat pulmonary illnesses can produce psychological and behavioral side effects. For example, excitation and agitation may result from the use of sympathomimetic agents. Aminophylline has been reported to affect patient mood, behavior, and performance on neuropsychological testing, possibly related to an acute reduction in regional cerebral blood flow (18).

Corticosteroids can evoke affective disturbances and inappropriate behavior. Adrenocorticotropic hormone (ACTH) may adversely affect attention span and memory (19). The effects of chronic administration of corticosteroids may be dose-related. In a review of more than 700 hospitalized patients treated with corticosteroids, the incidence of psychiatric disturbances was only 1% in patients receiving less than 40 mg of prednisone per day, 5% in patients receiving 40–80 mg of prednisone per day, and 18% in patients receiving more than 80 mg of prednisone per day (20). Also, in patients receiving more than 20 mg of prednisone per day, the incidence of psychological disturbances approached 2% (21). These data suggest that corticosteroid therapy may have an important effect on attention span and memory in some patients. However, significant psychological impairment can be minimized by corticosteroid doses that are less than, or equal to, 20 mg of prednisone per day.

The sensation of *dyspnea* is important in the patient's tolerance of long-term ventilation and ability to wean successfully from the ventilator. Dyspnea in the mechanically ventilated patient may be multifactorial in etiology and secondary to a variety of causes: the underlying disease, changes in acid-base status, respiratory pump dysfunction, impaired gas exchange, the presence of intrinsic PEEP, or the choice of ventilator modality and underlying ventilatory apparatus, i.e., tracheostomy tube, ventilator circuit, or ventilator settings. The sensation of dyspnea often causes or increases anxiety, which, in turn, increases the sense of breathlessness even though there are no causative physiological changes.

In some patients, the etiology of dyspnea may be unclear and limit their ability to tolerate the ventilator or to wean efficiently. In these patients, dyspnea may be misinterpreted as a lack of cooperation on the part of the patient. Also, fear of dyspnea can lead to decreased expression of any emotion since even positive emotions, such as joy or laughter, can increase the demand for oxygen, thereby increasing dyspnea. The phenomenon of limited expression of emotions and feelings in the pulmonary patient has been described as "living in an emotional straitjacket" (22). In some patients, tolerance for breathlessness decreases over time; these individuals may become anxious in anticipation of any physical activity that they fear will increase their dyspnea and they may attempt to avoid the physical exertion. In patients on long-term ventilator care who have developed anticipatory fears and anxiety related to dyspnea, initiation of trials of weaning or of a physical exercise program can provoke anxiety and fear that is more related to the anticipation of dyspnea rather than to the stress of the activity itself.

A. Effects of Mechanical Ventilation on Psychological Function

Ventilator-dependent patients experience the unique stress of *depending on a machine* for breathing moment to moment, hour to hour, and day to day. The inability to communicate, disorientation, memory loss, pain, and discomfort are all perceived by patients to be extremely important problems (23). A retrospective review of patients' recall of their reactions to mechanical ventilation after hospital discharge disclosed that 47% of patients felt anxious or fearful during mechanical ventilation and that 90% remembered the experience as stressful or unpleasant as long as 4 years after treatment (24).

The *ventilator equipment* can also contribute to psychological stress. The incessant beeping of ventilator alarms can be perceived by the patient as indicating serious developments, i.e., equipment failure, and contribute to feelings of anxiety, apprehension, and even impending death. The noises emitted by the mechanical ventilator are monotonous and unnatural and contribute to aberrant sensory input and sleep disturbances. Endotracheal tubes and nasal intubation can cause tracheal trauma; most patients describe endotracheal suctioning as extremely unpleasant, comparing the experience of suctioning to suffocating or gagging. Patients undergoing mechanical ventilation are usually limited in the distance that they can travel, e.g., typically to the 6 ft length of tubing, further increasing their sense of isolation.

Patients are especially concerned about *fears of death or abandonment* by family and staff; these feelings may predominate and precipitate symptoms of anxiety, depression, or dependent behaviors. Often, adverse psychological problems can be manifested by the patient (and misinterpreted by those caring for the patient) as behavioral problems; in addition to fearfulness, apprehension, and anxiety, the patient may also display demanding, questioning, or withdrawing behaviors or be uncooperative with the staff, the treatment plan, or the rehabilitation effort. Depression is common and can range from poor motivation and despair to hopelessness and frank suicidal ideation. Some patients become inordinately dependent on others for activities relating to self-care, thereby gaining attention and support from family or staff that might otherwise be unavailable.

There are few data concerning the prevalence of *cognitive compromise* in patients receiving long-term mechanical ventilation. In one situation in which 20 patients in the ICU requiring chronic ventilation were compared with 20 nonventilated patients of similar age and severity of illness, cognitive status, memory, and conceptual performance were more impaired in ventilator patients than in ICU controls (25).

Recently, we evaluated the prevalence and distribution of neuropsychological deficits in ventilator-dependent patients admitted to our tertiary care ventilator rehabilitation unit (VRU) (26). A clinical psychologist performed bedside neuropsychological assessment with 28 patients with a variety of underlying disorders requiring mechanical ventilation for a minimum of 21 days. Figure 1 shows that 86% of patients displayed deficits in short-term recall ability, 50% of patients were disoriented or had impaired reasoning, and 36% of patients had impaired long-term memory and language function. Figure 2 shows that the majority of patients had deficits in three or more cognitive areas, and only 7% of patients had no abnormalities on cognitive review. These data suggest that cognitive deficits are common in patients receiving prolonged ventilation and may be an important factor in the development of psychological disturbances.

In summary, the stresses facing mechanically ventilated patients are similar to those encountered by the critically ill, but include the added stresses of continuous dependence on a machine for breathing. The complex relationship between physiological changes due to the underlying lung disease and dependence on technology that limits the ability to communicate and be functionally independent, combined with the potential for undetected cognitive deficits, re-

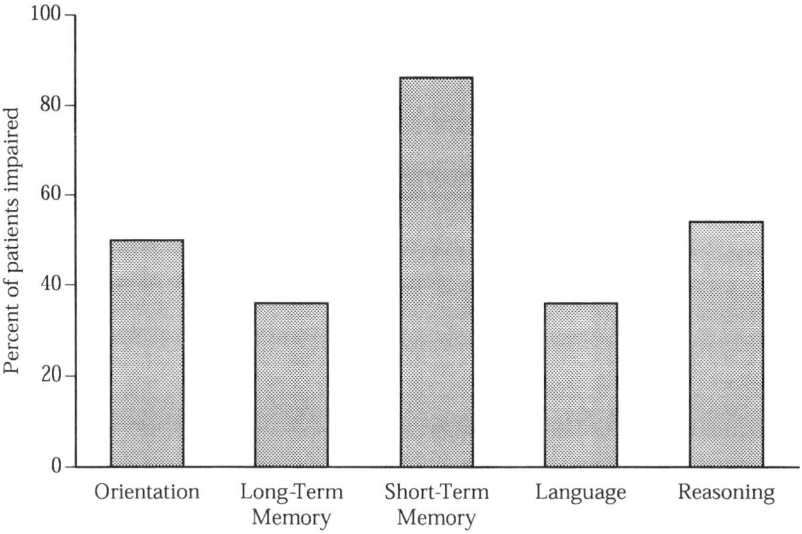

Figure 1 The frequency of cognitive deficits in 28 patients undergoing prolonged mechanical ventilation. Most patients displayed deficits in short-term memory. Disorientation and impaired reasoning were observed in 50% of the patients; in 36% of the patients, long-term memory and language function were impaired.

sults in a number of factors that can precipitate the development of psychological problems specific to the patient requiring mechanical ventilation.

III. Evaluating Psychological Function

A. General Assessment Strategies

The assessment of psychological function, and of the impact of psychological stresses and reactions in the patient receiving long-term ventilation, falls well within the repertoire of evaluation skills of most of the clinical management team. Thus, psychological assessment can be incorporated into the routine assessment strategy of the physicians, nurses, and respiratory and rehabilitation therapists. Although a psychologist or psychiatrist is a welcome addition to the clinical management team, a mental health professional is not a prerequisite for measuring and addressing psychological issues.

The evaluation of psychological function begins with a comprehensive history and physical examination. However, in contrast to the routine medical history and physical examination, the quality of psychological assessment is largely influenced by the affect and communication skills of the interviewer. If the initial encounter with the patient is successful, it will have a positive impact

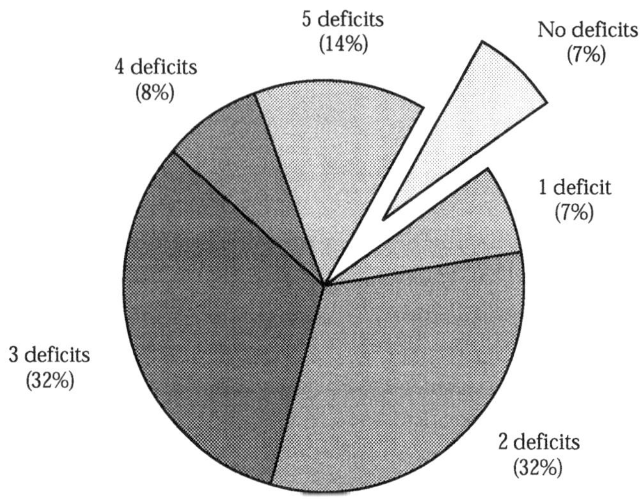

Figure 2 Distribution (in percent) of cognitive deficits in 28 ventilator-dependent patients. Only 7% of patients were normal in all areas of cognitive function evaluated. Most patients showed multiple cognitive deficits.

on establishing good rapport and facilitate the completion of a thorough psychological examination. Throughout the assessment process, the interviewer should be supportive and reassuring, use nonverbal skills such as direct eye contact, sit close to the patient, and reassure by touch. Disclosure of feelings and concerns is facilitated by using open-ended questions, allowing silence while the patient formulates his/her answer, and restating the patient's words to clarify feelings.

The main goal of the psychological examination is to identify those factors that may be contributing to, or exacerbating, the patient's psychological state. Three broad areas should be assessed: features of the underlying disease, aspects of the underlying psychological status and behavioral style, and reactions specific to the medical treatment.

B. Assessing the Psychological Impact of the Disease Process

The course of a patient's disease plays a large role in determining how the patient reacts to the stresses of illness in general and responds to treatment and interventions. Although there is a general similarity in the range of psychological responses across patients with different types of chronic debilitating illnesses, patients with newly diagnosed medical problems tend to show poorer adjustment than do patients who had been living with a chronic illness for a long time (3). There is a marked difference between the reactions of patients receiving mechanical ventilation for the first time, e.g., for acute respiratory failure, and those who have had multiple experiences with mechanical ventilation for chronic obstructive pulmonary disease (27). The newly ventilated patient is usually fearful and bewildered by ventilator treatment, but has a hopeful outlook and high expectations for weaning and independence. The chronically ventilated patient may be more familiar with ventilator treatment, but is usually less hopeful and more discouraged about the outcome.

An additional consideration relating to the individual patient are the limitations that the patient imposed on his/her own levels of activity before the exacerbation of the illness that led to hospitalization and mechanical ventilation. Many patients with chronic respiratory disease severely restrict their daily activities and level of independence as dyspnea and fatigue increase; this limitation decreases their expectations about optimal levels of functioning and, in turn, decreases the family's expectations with respect to physical rehabilitation and education in self-care skills before discharge. In this regard, the goals and expectations of the management team may differ considerably from those of the patient and the family.

C. Assessing Psychological Status and Behavior

A good psychological history should include questions about the patient's education, past learning behavior, marital discord, family support, socioeconomic status, living arrangement, work history, and drug and alcohol use. The interviewer should also inquire about psychological or psychiatric symptoms in the patient and family and their style of coping with physical illnesses and death. Among the more sensitive indicators of affective function, such as anxiety and depression, are not only mood symptoms such as feelings of sadness, tension, and nervousness, but also somatic symptoms such as changes in appetite, sleep disturbance, or fatigue, motivational symptoms such as inertia or difficulty concentrating or reaching decisions, and cognitive symptoms such as low self-esteem, worthlessness, or guilt. It is important to determine the relative impact of emotional concerns versus physiological determinants on complaints of anxiety and depression, because patients frequently misinterpret the physical symptoms of pulmonary disease, e.g., trembling and restlessness, as signs that they are anxious or depressed.

It should also be determined whether the patient is experiencing frank psychiatric symptoms such as visual or auditory hallucinations, paranoid ideations, or delusions. Standardized bedside neuropsychological tests, e.g., the Mini-Mental State Examination (28) or the Mattis Dementia Rating Scale (29), can be used to objectively assess mental status and cognitive function. Areas to be assessed include orientation to person, place, and time, capacity for sustained attention, immediate and delayed memory function, and reasoning ability. Other skills that can be assessed in the interview include visual skills, motor function, long-term memory, receptive and expressive language function, reading ability, and the style of both abstract and logical thinking.

D. Assessing the Psychological Reactions to Treatment

The effects on the patient of the physical environment and the ventilator apparatus have been noted above. Sleep and sensory deprivation can cause delirium. It is important to establish the patient's level of orientation, not only to person, place, and time, but also to the salient aspects of daily management including scheduled treatments, rehabilitation therapies, and members of the treatment team.

Psychological problems related to the weaning process are especially important. An assessment should be made of the patient's perception of the ventilator apparatus, the process of weaning from ventilation, and the goals for weaning. Weaning is often perceived differently by different patients; it is important to ascertain the patient's perspective before implementing a trial of weaning. For example, weaning may be viewed as a significant improvement in some patients by increasing their ability to communicate verbally and to become more mobile. In contrast, other patients may view weaning as uncomfortable and anxiety-provoking. Patients may also misunderstand the weaning process, lack confidence in their ability to breathe without the ventilator, feel unable to regulate their breathing, or feel abandoned by staff. Thus, a detailed assessment of the patient's perception of the weaning process, his/her goals for the outcome of weaning, and the likelihood of weaning success should be established to minimize psychological dysfunction.

IV. Treatment of Psychological Problems

The approach to treating psychological problems in the ventilator-dependent patient consists of two components: (1) the basic strategies used to treat psychological disorders in patients suffering from advanced lung disease and critical illnesses, and (2) a treatment plan directed at the special problems created by the process of mechanical ventilation. Factors contributing to abnormal psychological reactions precipitated by the necessity of mechanical ventilation, e.g., limited mobility, sterile environment, impaired communication and swallowing, should be identified and systematically treated to improve the patient's sense of control and ability to interact with family members and the medical staff.

A. The Environment

An initial goal for psychological intervention is to provide a setting that minimizes patient seclusion and enhances interaction with the family and medical staff. The optimal setting is an environment in which patients are in individual rooms: interventions that disturb sleep are then minimized; monotonous sensory input is reduced by placing unnecessary monitoring equipment outside the patient's room; inside the room are orientation aides such as clocks, calendars, and family artifacts; mobility of the patient can be maximized; and an outside window is visible to the patient. In shared rooms, attempts should be made to approach this ideal.

While one goal of psychological treatment is to minimize conditions that contribute to disorientation and confusion, concomitantly an effort should be made to provide compensatory strategies for cognitive problems. Patients receiving long-term mechanical ventilation are prone to cognitive disturbances, including memory impairment (23–25) and disorientation (23,25), as well as deficits in verbal functioning and abstract reasoning (25). A cognitive evaluation should be performed on all patients to detect subtle cognitive problems that could interfere with active participation in rehabilitation and with the retention of skills taught for self-care. Among the compensatory strategies could be multiple repetitions of information in highly simplified and concrete ways and the delivery of information not only verbally, but also visually, via pictures and gestures. Patients should be encouraged to wear their eyeglasses, hearing aids, and dentures. By systematically providing cues and compensatory strategies for cognitive problems, deficits that could interfere with tolerance of mechanical ventilation or rehabilitation can be minimized.

B. Communication and Swallowing

An important step in minimizing the consequences of cognitive dysfunction is to reestablish the patient's ability to communicate. Improved communication between ventilator-dependent patients, families, and staff decreases stress, improves decision making, and decreases the likelihood of patient isolation. Several modalities are available to facilitate written or verbal communication. Some of these can even be employed while patients are on full ventilatory support, e.g., buccal resonator, talk trach, Electrolarynx. Others can be applied during periods of spontaneous breathing by using devices that allow airflow through the vocal cord and more natural speech, such as fenestrated or bidirectional flow tracheostomy tubes, or Passey-Muir valves. Regardless of the method used, a special effort should be made by the entire staff to encourage the patient to use the device as much as possible in order to improve his/her communication skills and decrease the sense of isolation.

One of the most important processes for the sake of the patient's sense of well-being is restoration of the ability to eat. In addition to its obvious role in providing sustenance, eating, rather than being fed intravenously or enterally, provides a sense of independence, social interaction, and enjoyment that can be psychologically uplifting for patients who have been receiving long-term ventilatory support. An evaluation by an experienced speech pathologist can help to direct the return to oral intake and swallowing. Compensatory mechanisms, including adjusting for head posture, alternating the consistency of food, and making repetitive swallows after a bolus of food, can improve swallowing ability in long-term ventilator-dependent patients who were previously unable to eat (30). Reinstitution of oral intake can be a significant psychological victory and milestone in the recovery of the ventilator-dependent patient.

C. Rehabilitation Goals and Gains

Patients on long-term mechanical ventilation may have decreased tolerance for physical exercise and exertion due to severe deconditioning and fears that exercise will exacerbate their pulmonary condition. Also, patients may have poor appreciation of the need for increased endurance because they had a sedentary life-style even before their pulmonary illness worsened, because they were not routinely encouraged to exercise in the acute phases of their hospitalization in the ICU, or because they are unaware of the relationship between exercise endurance and functional capacity. For these reasons, it is critical to structure the rehabilitation effort to include teaching about exercise and endurance, to include the patient in setting rehabilitation goals, and to provide strong, positive feedback about gains to enhance motivation.

Ventilated patients tend to focus on independent breathing without mechanical assistance as their ultimate goal, and to view increased self-care and changes in functional status as secondary objectives. Likewise, patients may feel disappointed with the slow progress by which rehabilitative gains are achieved, thereby diminishing their motivation and participation. For these reasons, in addition to major goals such as ambulation, patients should receive structured therapies that include modest goals that are achievable daily, e.g., accomplishing increased repetitions of leg and arm lifts. Providing a means by which the patient can appreciate his/her accomplishments visually, e.g., graphs of daily progress, can help to remind the patient of achievements and increase motivation. Encouraging patients to be dressed in their own street clothes, e.g., sweatsuits, not only diminishes self-consciousness about exercising in immodest hospital gowns, but also reinforces the patient's sense of transition from complete care to independence.

D. Comprehensive Multidisciplinary Treatment Teams

Several studies of patients with obstructive lung disease and of patients undergoing long-term ventilatory support have shown that involvement of the patient and family in a comprehensive rehabilitation program can improve the patient's physical and psychological function (31,32). These programs usually include both pulmonary and whole-body rehabilitation and employ a multidisciplinary team comprised of occupational and physical therapists, respiratory therapists, nutritionists, psychologists, speech therapists, social workers, nurses, and physicians to collaborate with patients and families on rehabilitative goals. The impact of multidisciplinary units on the outcome and cost of care in patients receiving long-term ventilation is being measured by the Chronic Ventilator Demonstration Project conducted by the Health Care Financing Administration (33). Preliminary data from this project suggest that a significant improvement in patients' functional and psychological status is obtained when ventilator-dependent patients are enrolled in such treatment programs (34,35).

As a participant in the Chronic Ventilator Demonstration Project, we have studied the effects of a comprehensive multidisciplinary rehabilitation program on affective disorders and cognitive function in patients receiving long-term chronic ventilation in a noninvasive respiratory care unit (VRU) (36). We recently asked a cohort of patients and their families to rate their perceptions about the VRU as compared to the ICU (Fig. 3). Patients and families reported an overall reduction in cognitive impairment and affective problems in the

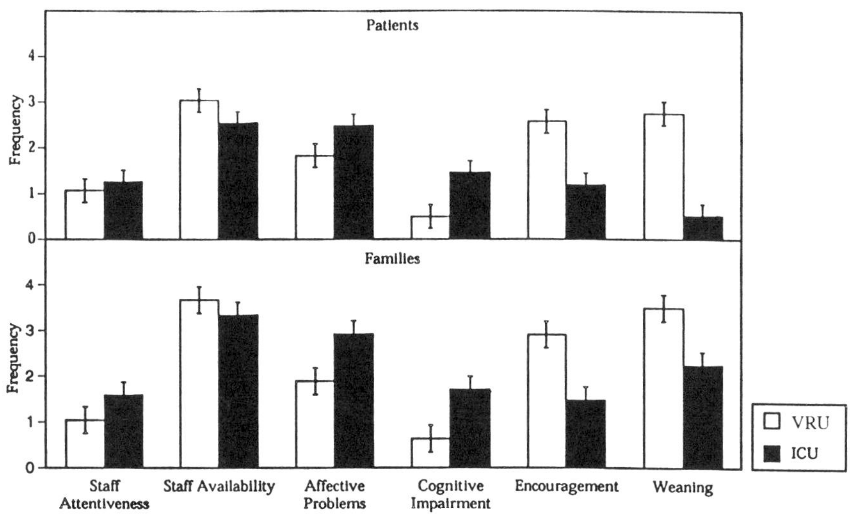

Figure 3 Mean ratings by patients and their families of their perceptions of the VRU as compared to the ICU. A five-point scale was used to rate each item corresponding to how often the patient or family member perceived the feelings listed: 0 = never, 1 = occasionally, 2 = sometimes, 3 = often, 4 = very often. Patients reported a lower incidence of affective and cognitive problems in the VRU than in the ICU; their families concurred. Patients and families noted more encouragement by staff and a greater emphasis on mechanical ventilation and weaning in the VRU.

VRU as compared to the ICU. Patients in our VRU were provided with clocks and calendars to maintain orientation, and specific strategies were used to compensate for particular memory disturbances. Ongoing psychological support was an integral part of the treatment effort, with the goal of minimizing emotional distress and of providing counseling that addressed concerns about coping and adjustment. In the VRU, mechanical ventilation is generally delivered via portable volume ventilators that liberate patients from large stationary ventilators that restrict them to within several feet of a power source, thereby facilitating whole-body reconditioning and patient mobility. Portable ventilators not only improve patient mobility, but also make possible ambulation and out-of-the-hospital activities that enhance the sense of independence, improve functional status, and limit the effects of isolation on psychological function. Patients and families also reported greater impetus to independent functioning and better understanding of the weaning goals in the VRU as compared to the ICU (Fig. 3). Such preliminary data from multidisciplinary treatment programs suggest that functional status and recovery from long-term ventilatory support can be facilitated by treatment in such units.

E. Biofeedback

Respiratory biofeedback has been used recently in patients undergoing mechanical ventilation as a mechanism for reducing anxiety and facilitating weaning. Biofeedback teaches patients to control their physiological responses, e.g., blood pressure, respiratory rate, heart rate, by combining auditory and visual signals with relaxation techniques to achieve certain training goals. This technique has been shown to be useful for the control of dyspnea in asthmatic patients (37). In a prospective, controlled, randomized study, Holliday and Hyers (38) used respiratory biofeedback to improve the weaning outcome of 40 patients who were ventilated for 7 days or longer. Impedance plethysmography was used to provide visual and auditory feedback from the ribcage and abdomen; electromyographic activity of the frontalis muscle was displayed as a strategy for controlling anxiety by muscle relaxation. Patients randomized to the biofeedback group received 30 to 50-min training sessions for 5 days/week until they were extubated. The average number of days on the ventilator was significantly less in the biofeedback group than in the control group, i.e., 20.6 $\pm$ 8.9 versus 32.6 $\pm$ 17.6 days. Also, the decrease in ventilator days was associated with a significant increase in tidal volume (415 $\pm$ 45 versus 295 $\pm$ 41 ml), mean inspiratory flow (560 $\pm$ versus 361 $\pm$ 40 ml), and V_T/diaphragm electromyogram (0.94 $\pm$ 0.21 versus 0.33 $\pm$ 0.09 L/mv). The patients who underwent biofeedback stated that they felt more relaxed and experienced less anxiety.

While such observations on sophisticated respiratory biofeedback are encouraging, widespread use of these techniques with patients receiving long-term mechanical ventilation is limited by the need for special equipment and trained personnel. However, it has recently been shown that less sophisticated strategies may suffice: the digital display of respiratory rate and expired tidal volume on the ventilator was recently used successfully as visual feedback to wean patients who had difficulty in weaning and to decrease their anxiety (39). Although these results are preliminary, they are encouraging.

V. Summary and Conclusions

Ventilator-dependent patients may be at increased risk for psychological problems that can complicate their management, weaning, and rehabilitation. Assessment of psychological issues can be performed by each member of the treatment team as part of the initial and ongoing evaluation of the patient. Evaluation of psychological factors should include reactions specific to the patient's disease course, psychosocial and behavioral problems, cognitive function, and reactions to the environment and the ventilator equipment. Treatment strategies that focus on identifying the etiology of psychological disturbances, minimizing environmental stressors, compensating for cognitive dysfunction, and facilitating independence and communication have the greatest likelihood of improving the patient's functional status and facilitating tolerance of ventilation and rehabilitation. Comprehensive multidisciplinary rehabilitation programs may be an efficient method by which psychological problems in patients receiving long-term ventilation can be addressed. Biofeedback may also provide a treatment option to reduce anxiety and increase the perceived control of breathing in patients whose ventilator course is complicated by psychological problems.

References

1. Wilson M. Intensive care delirium. Arch Intern Med 1972; 130:225–226.
2. Tomlin PJ. Psychological problems in intensive care. Br Med J 1977; 2:441–443.
3. Cassileth BR, Lush EJ, Strouse TB, et al. Psychosocial status in chronic illness: a comparative analysis of six diagnostic groups. N Engl J Med 1984; 311:506–511.
4. Abrams HS. Survival by machine: the psychological stress of chronic hemodialysis. Psychiatric Med 1970; 1:37.
5. Kornfeld DS, Zimbers S, Malm JR. Psychiatric complications of open heart surgery. N Engl J Med 1965; 273:287–292.
6. Egerton N, Kay JH. Psychological disturbances associated with open heart surgery. Br J Psychiatry 1964; 110:439–443.
7. Tobin MJ, Yang K. Weaning from mechanical ventilation. Crit Care Clin 1990; 6:725–747.

8. Wilson VS. Identification of stressors related to patient's psychologic responses to the surgical intensive care unit. Heart Lung 1987; 16:267–273.
9. Blachy PH, Starr A. Post-cardiotomy delirium. Am J Psychiatry 1964; 121:371–375.
10. Rubinstein D, Thomas JK. Psychiatric findings in cardiotomy patients. Am J Psychiatry 1969; 126:60–68.
11. Berlin RM, Litovitz GL, Diaz MA, et al. Sleep disorders on a psychiatric consultation service. Am J Psychiatry 1984; 141:582–584.
12. Sveinnson I. Postoperative psychosis after heart surgery. J Thorac Cardiovasc Surg 1975; 70:717–726.
13. Woods N, Falk S. Noise stimuli in the acute care area. Nurs Res 1974; 23:144–150.
14. Nicholson AN, Bradley CM, Pascoe PA. Medications: effect on sleep and wakefulness. In: Kryger MH, Roth T, Dement WC, eds. Principles and Practice of Sleep Medicine. Philadelphia: WB Saunders, 1989:228–236.
15. Aurell J, Elmguist D. Sleep in the surgical intensive care unit: continuous polygraphic recording of sleep in nine patients receiving post-operative care. Br Med J 1985; 290:1029–1032.
16. Neher A. Auditory driving observed with scalp electrodes in normal subjects. Electroencephal Clin Neurophysiol 1961; 13:449–451.
17. Grant I, Prigatano GP, Heaton RK, et al. Progressive neuropsychological impairment in relation to hypoxemia in chronic obstructive pulmonary disease. Arch Gen Psychiatry 1987; 44:999–1006.
18. Young LD, Bouton D, Alford P, et al. Do medications reduce cerebral blood flow in COPD patients? Psychosomatics 1986; 27:240.
19. Schraa JL, Dirks JF. The influence of corticosteroics and theophylline on cerebral function. Chest 1982; 82:181–185.
20. Boston Collaborative Drug Surveillance Program. Acute adverse reactions to prednisone in relation to dosage. Clin Pharmacol 1972; 13:694–698.
21. Smyllie H, Connolly C. Incidence of serious complications of corticosteroid therapy in respiratory disease. Thorax 1968; 23:571–581.
22. Sandu HS. Psychosocial issues in chronic obstructive pulmonary disease. Clin Chest Med 1986; 7:629–642.
23. Riggio RE, Singer RD, Hartaran K, et al. Psychological issues in the care of critically ill respirator patients: differential preceptions of patients, relatives, and staff. Psychol Rep 1982; 51:363–369.
24. Bergbom-Engberg I, Haljamae H. Assessment of patient's experience of discomforts during respirator therapy. Crit Care Med 1989; 17:1068–1072.
25. Franco KN, McSweeny AJ, Verbosky L, et al. Cognitive and emotional findings in ventilator patients (submitted for publication).
26. Isaac L, Hungerpillar J, Criner G. Neuropsychologic deficits in chronic ventilator-dependent patients. Chest 1989; 96:255S.
27. Gale J, O'Shannick GJ. Psychiatric aspects of respiratory treatment and pulmonary intensive care. Adv Psychosom Med 1985; 14:93–108.
28. Malloy DW, Alemayehu E, Roberts R. A Standardized Mini-Mental State Exami-

nation (SMMSE); its reliability compared to traditional Mini-Mental State Examination (MMSE). Am J Psychiatry 1991; 148:102–105.
29. Mattis S. Mental status examination for organic mental syndrome in the elderly patient. In: Bellack L, Karusu TB, eds. Geriatric Psychiatry. New York: Grune & Stratton, 1976.
30. Hungerpiller J, Leonard C, Criner GJ. Swallowing function in trached patients requiring mechanical ventilation. Chest 1989; 96:296S.
31. Fishman DB, Petty TL. Physical, symptomatic and psychological improvement in patients receiving comprehensive care for chronic airway obstruction. J Chronic Dis 1971; 24:775–785.
32. Make B, Gilmartin M. Rehabilitation and home care for ventilator-assisted individuals. Clin Chest Med 1986; 7:679–681.
33. O'Donohue WJ. Chronic ventilator-dependent units in hospitals: attacking the front end of a long-term problem. Mayo Clin Proc 1992; 67:198–200.
34. Gracey DR, Viggiano RW, Nawssens JM, et al. Outcomes of patients admitted to a chronic ventilator-dependent unit in an acute care hospital. Mayo Clin Proc 1992; 67:131–136.
35. Criner GJ, Kreimer DT, Pidloan L. Outcome of patients receiving prolonged mechanical ventilation. Am Rev Respir Dis 1993; 147:A874.
36. Isaac L, Criner G. Patient and family perceptions on weaning from mechanical ventilation in a specialized rehabilitation unit. Am Rev Respir Dis 1990; 141:A411.
37. Feldman GM. The effect of biofeedback training on respiratory resistance of asthmatic children. Psychosom Med 1976; 38:27–34.
38. Holliday JE, Hyers TM. The reduction of weaning time from mechanical ventilation using tidal volume and relaxation biofeedback. Am Rev Respir Dis 1990; 141:1214–1220.
39. Yarnal J, Herrell D, Sivak E. Routine use of biofeedback in weaning patients from mechanical ventilation. Chest 1981; 79:127–128.

Part Five

SPECIFIC DISORDERS AND INTERVENTIONS

28

Comprehensive Pulmonary Rehabilitation in Chronic Obstructive Pulmonary Disease

BRUCE A. STAATS and PEGGY M. SIMON

Mayo Clinic
Rochester, Minnesota

In this chapter, we will describe a workable model for a pulmonary rehabilitation program. Pulmonary rehabilitation is by design a multidisciplinary effort of many health professionals. We recognize that a successful program takes advantage of the professionals who are available and who are interested in pulmonary rehabilitation. Therefore, a program's design is heterogeneous and not all types of health professionals are available in every program. For instance, breathing exercises may be taught by a physical therapist, respiratory therapist, nurse, physician, or other person. Pharmacotherapy issues may be covered by a pharmacist, physician, nurse, or other respiratory care practitioners. The important point in a successful program is that all of the topics of pulmonary rehabilitation are addressed, not who addresses them.

I. Definition of Rehabilitation in Chronic Obstructive Pulmonary Disease

Rehabilitation medicine staff are committed to improving the functional capabilities and the quality of life of the population it serves. The Council of Rehabilitation reflects this commitment in their original definition of rehabilitation in 1942. In 1974, the ad hoc committee of the American College of Chest Physicians developed the following definition specific to pulmonary rehabilitation (1):

> Pulmonary rehabilitation may be defined as an art of medical practice wherein an individually-tailored, multidisciplinary program is formulated which through accurate diagnosis, therapy, emotional support, and education, stabilizes or reverses both the physio- and psycho-pathology of pulmonary diseases and attempts to return the patient to the highest possible functional capacity allowed by his pulmonary handicap and overall life situation.

The College used this definition (later endorsed by the American Thoracic Society in 1981) (2) to outline essential components of a pulmonary rehabilitation program in an attempt to dictate standards for newly developing programs around the country.

Recently, a new definition for pulmonary rehabilitation has emerged to reflect steps taken to become more invested in science. In April 1993, two components of the National Institutes of Health (the Division of Lung Diseases of the National Heart, Lung, and Blood Institute and the newly formed National Center for Medical Rehabilitation Research) convened a workshop on pulmonary rehabilitation research. The workshop arrived at the consensus that pulmonary rehabilitation's designation as an "art" was inappropriate. To reflect the deliberations of the NIH workshop (3), they offered the following definition:

> Pulmonary rehabilitation is a multidimensional continuum of services directed to persons with pulmonary disease and their families, usually by an interdisciplinary team of specialists, with the goal of achieving and maintaining the individual's maximum level of independence and functioning in the community.

Regardless of the definition used, pulmonary rehabilitation's goal is to restore patients to an independent, productive, and quality life and to prevent further clinical deterioration to the maximal extent congruous with the stage of the disease. Ideally, this would include return to gainful employment; however, this has not been a realistic goal for most patients with chronic obstructive pulmonary disease (COPD) who have been obliged to give up their employment.

II. Patient Selection

Traditionally, the preoccupation of pulmonary rehabilitation has been with COPD, although the effectiveness of a comprehensive program individually tailored to patients with other chronic lung diseases has been shown (4,5). With program success increasingly measured in terms of functional outcome and health-related quality of life rather than physiological outcomes, clinicians' criteria for enrolling patients into pulmonary rehabilitation has also changed.

In general, any patient whose breathlessness from COPD has resulted in functional limitations that affect his or her quality of life should be considered a candidate for pulmonary rehabilitation. The intensity of the exercise program will obviously depend on the severity of the underlying lung disease, but even severely limited patients can better perform the activities of daily living following pulmonary rehabilitation. Furthermore, other objectives, such as understanding and developing methods to cope with the disease, developing a perception of well-being, and decreasing the number of hospitalizations, can be achieved in severely limited patients. Studies have shown that the magnitude of change in both physiological and psychological parameters of patients completing an outpatient pulmonary rehabilitation program is independent of lung function (6,7). These studies support the view that the benefits of rehabilitation can extend to all patients with chronic lung disease, regardless of the severity of preexisting pulmonary dysfunction. This is contrary to earlier studies that suggest that pulmonary rehabilitation is most helpful only in patients who are not severely exercise-limited (8,9).

Clearly the patient's willingness and ability to learn about his or her disease and the motivation to devote the time and effort required to benefit from a comprehensive program are important assets when evaluating potential candidates. Since family members can be strong motivators, family support is also helpful, even if the family members do not wish to participate in the program. A careful assessment of the family status and the geographical area where the patient lives supplies useful information in planning the program.

Patients should be stabilized on standard medical therapy before beginning a program so that assessment and treatment can be based on the patient's optimal baseline function. Resting hypercapnia is not a contraindication to participation in rehabilitation. Foster and colleagues (10) demonstrated similar benefits to patients with COPD independent of whether or not they had hypercapnia. Patients with disabling or unstable conditions that would limit their ability to participate in rehabilitation should be excluded. These include, but are not limited to, unstable heart disease (such as severe coronary artery disease, congestive heart failure, or uncontrolled arrhythmias), major neurological disorders, and organic brain syndrome. Unsuitable rehabilitation candidates also include those with a history of medical noncompliance and those with persistent nicotine addiction who lack the motivation to attempt to quit smoking.

Financial resources cannot be ignored but rather should be resolved before the patient begins the program. Most outpatient programs are reimbursable according to guidelines that vary across the nation. However, controversies about the medical necessity of part of the services or technical errors in drawing up the bill can cause the patient unexpected expenses. An understanding of the patients' financial concerns and the amount of out-of-pocket expenses for the program is key to their participation.

III. Director of the Program

An enthusiastic person is required to lead a pulmonary rehabilitation program. This person could be a respiratory therapist, nurse, physician, or physical therapist. Important qualifications include an interest in patients with COPD and the ability to work with their families and to lead a group of professionals and other support personnel.

Medical input is also important; usually a pulmonologist is director but other physicians also participate. A working relationship should be fostered between the medical director and the patient's primary physician, as the medical director usually does not serve as the primary physician after the patient has left the program. Certain primary medical care issues may need to be addressed while the patient is participating in the program.

IV. Components of a Pulmonary Rehabilitation Program for COPD

Many questions concerning what constitutes an optimal program remain unanswered. Most pulmonary rehabilitation specialists agree on a multidisciplinary team approach and certain key components of a program. However, such questions as type of exercise evaluation, mode and intensity of exercise, the duration of the program, and the setting, i.e., inpatient, outpatient, or home-based, are not clear. The variety of "successful" programs reported in the literature suggests there is more than one answer to these questions.

A. Initial Evaluation

Whether patient referral is self-generated or from a primary physician, an initial evaluation including a history and physical examination should be performed by a physician involved with the program. Tests ordered should include spirometry pre- and postbronchodilator, lung volume study, diffusion capacity, resting arterial blood gas, exercise study (following initial physician evaluation), complete blood count, chemistry profile, theophylline level (if applicable), electrocardiogram (ECG), and chest X-ray (posteroanterior and lateral). These are important to assure clinical stability for exercise and overall ability to participate in the rehabilitation program. Review of medications and recommendations for maximization of pharmacotherapy are also important aspects of the initial evaluation. In most circumstances, direct communication with the referring physician prior to alteration of the medical regimen should be carried out. Alteration of medication or dosage should not necessarily delay entry into the program, unless the patient is undergoing an exacerbation of his or her underlying disease or if alteration of the medical regimen will likely result in a considerable improvement in respiratory symptoms.

Whenever possible, results of pulmonary function tests including spirometry (pre- and postbronchodilator), maximal voluntary ventilation, lung volumes, diffusion capacity for carbon monoxide (DLCO), and a resting room air arterial blood gas (ABG) should be available at the initial evaluation. ABG is mandatory because an oximetry study cannot assess hypercapnia or consistently provide an accurate measurement of oxygenation; the degree of correlation between the oxygen saturation from the ABG with that from an oximeter can also be evaluated. A carbon monoxide level obtained from arterial blood is helpful to assess compliance in smoking cessation for those patients who have recently quit. Furthermore, elevated carbon monoxide levels will result in spurious readings during oximetry monitoring (11). The DLCO provides a rough correlation of the degree of emphysema (12) and of the potential for arterial oxyhemoglobin desaturation with exercise (13). Although lung volume studies from plethysmography are helpful in evaluating degree of hyperinflation, they are not essential.

An exercise evaluation (a 6- or 12-min walk or a formal test on a bicycle or treadmill) is sometimes performed prior to the initial evaluation. However, the exercise evaluation should wait until after the medical director's initial history and physical. Ultimately, it is the medical director's responsibility to assure that the patient is safe for exercise. A formal cardiac evaluation is sometimes necessary prior to an exercise evaluation and entrance into the program. Twelve-lead ECG monitoring during formal exercise testing is strongly recommended, not only because of "occult" coronary disease, but also because of difficulty distinguishing whether symptoms of shortness of breath with activity and "atypical" chest discomfort are pulmonary or cardiac in origin. Other aspects of the exercise program will be dealt with in the subsequent exercise section.

A comprehensive history, physical examination, pulmonary function testing, and exercise evaluation help to assess the physical impairment. This should include an assessment of respiratory symptoms, sleep disturbances, ambulation problems, mobility, and cognitive impairment. However, the functional assessment must also include the emotional and social consequences of the individual's disability that have a major impact on his or her ability to perform the activities of daily living, including personal care, household, and vocational tasks; this will include dependency issues, emotional response to disease impact, perception of functional capabilities, and social limitations. The pulmonary rehabilitation team needs to incorporate methods to evaluate, quantify, and monitor the variables that are important determinants of a patient's quality of life. Functional assessment as it relates to different components of the pulmonary rehabilitation program is outlined in subsequent sections of this chapter. Methods of assessing health-related quality of life in patients with chronic pulmonary disease are detailed in another chapter.

B. Overview of the Program

The essential components of a pulmonary rehabilitation program are outlined in Table 1 and discussed in subsequent sections and other chapters. The organization and structure of a program may vary among facilities, but the essential components of pulmonary rehabilitation are the same. Therefore, pulmonary

Table 1 Essential Components of a Pulmonary Rehabilitation Program

Medical and functional assessment by team
Medical director's initial evaluation
Respiratory care practitioner—nurse and/or respiratory therapist
Physical therapist
Occupational therapist
Registered dietician (nutritionist)
Social worker
Education and patient training
Disease process
Medications, including inhalation technique
Bronchial hygiene and infection control
Proper nutrition
Breathing retraining and energy conservation
Relaxation and control of panic
Activities of daily living
Sexuality
Exercise program
Conditioning and strengthening
Upper-extremity strengthening
Ventilatory muscle training
Home program plan
Psychosocial intervention
Coping skills
Support structure
Dependency issues
Treatment of anxiety and depression
Counseling

rehabilitation is not merely an educational or an exercise program, but rather a carefully integrated program that is individualized to meet the needs of each participant.

Within this general framework, pulmonary rehabilitation programs have been successfully established with different formats (individual or group) and in different settings, e.g., inpatient or outpatient, hospital- or practice-based. Inpatient management may offer some advantage to patients with very severe disease, particularly in the early phases of rehabilitation. Some pulmonary rehabilitation teams become involved with a patient during hospitalization for an acute exacerbation and then outline a program that the patient will continue as an outpatient. However, pulmonary rehabilitation is largely an outpatient activity, in part because third-party payers are unwilling to pay for hospital care for those who are not acutely ill. How a program is structured, e.g., the frequency of weekly visits, program duration, and subsequent follow-up, depends on a number of factors including the location of the facility relative to the population it serves, patient characteristics, costs, available staff and resources, and social considerations. Outpatient programs vary considerably in program length and frequency of follow-up. Traditionally, programs have been composed of 12–24 visits over a 6- to 12-week period. More recently, shorter programs designed to address the needs of rural-based referral populations have been reported to demonstrate results similar to those of the longer-duration programs (14).

It is difficult to compare outcomes among differently structured pulmonary rehabilitation programs for several reasons. Outcomes have been based on a variety of indices whose end-points are usually measured qualitatively. The diversity of the different populations' severity of disease and the broad range of therapeutic interventions makes comparison between programs difficult. Before clinical trials of pulmonary rehabilitation can be undertaken, developing tools to better quantify functional state, clinical outcome, and quality of life is necessary, along with better definition of the spectrum of disease incorporated under the term "COPD."

C. The Exercise Program in Pulmonary Rehabilitation

One of the anticipated outcomes of pulmonary rehabilitation is the performance of physical activities with less dyspnea and fatigue. Realization of this goal depends on many factors including the design of the program, patient motivation, underlying medical and orthopedic conditions, and severity of pulmonary disease. The patient and the staff need to set realistic goals for the degree of improvement in overall physical performance. Initial quantitative assessment of physical performance is important.

Deconditioning is loss of the ability to perform external work; specifically, it is a reduction in cardiac performance, muscle strength, peripheral distribution of blood flow, and mitochondrial mass and number. Deconditioning is prevalent in many patients with chronic illnesses, particularly those who become sedentary. In COPD patients, a downward spiral frequently develops with initial limitations imposed by the disease (that may be both real and perceived) leading to the global effects of deconditioning (15). At a level of work that once was comfortable, the patient now experiences tachycardia, hyperpnea, and, at times, hyperventilation. To avoid these unpleasant sensations, patients may avoid further exertion. Without exercise, further deconditioning results, perpetuating the downward spiral of inactivity. It may be difficult for the markedly deconditioned patient with severe pulmonary disease to achieve substantial improvement in a pulmonary rehabilitation program. However, normal subjects can experience a brisk reconditioning effect after bed rest for several weeks and a subsequent exercise program (16).

Studies have demonstrated that there is a gradation in degree of exercise limitation in COPD patients (17). Patients with mild obstruction have cardiovascular limitation like normal subjects. Patients with moderate disease have exercise limitation caused by both cardiovascular limitation and lowered ventilatory capacity. Patients with severe COPD generally are limited by ventilatory and gas exchange abnormalities, although some patients may have coexisting cardiac limitation or deconditioning (Table 2) (18). Because there may be several reasons for exercise limitation, cardiopulmonary exercise testing is useful

Table 2 Purported Causes of Exercise Limitation in COPD

Ventilatory factors
Airway obstruction
Respiratory muscle weakness or fatigue
Abnormal gas exchange
Hypoxemia
Hypercapnia
Acidosis or alkalosis
Deconditioning
Peripheral muscle weakness
Cardiac dysfunction
Pulmonary hypertension
Left ventricular dysfunction
Dysrhythmias
Psychological factors
Depression
Inordinate fear of dyspnea
Effects of smoking

in determining the cause of exercise intolerance and in directing the exercise component of the rehabilitation program. For programs limited in scope or for severely obstructed patients, a less involved form of exercise testing (such as the 6-min walk) may be more appropriate.

Patients can undertake several types of exercise depending on their coexisting medical and orthopedic conditions. The larger skeletal muscles must be exercised to reverse the effects of generalized deconditioning. Some rehabilitation programs recommend stationary cycling; others utilize various forms of walking. Walking most clearly approximates the lower-extremity exercise patients perform in their homes. Some patients have become devotees of other modes of exercise including ski trainers and stair steppers. The patient should choose a form of exercise that he or she is likely to perform on a continual basis (Table 3), and it should be varied. This approach not only allows the use of more groups of muscles, but also helps to alleviate the boredom that easily occurs when there is only one form of exercise. Some patients may be bedridden or too ill to accomplish any degree of physical training. They should be encouraged to perform range-of-motion and flexibility exercises. If weakness of a specific group of muscles is identified, exercises tailor-made for that group should be performed.

There are two general methods to assist the patient in determining the level of exercise necessary to attain physical conditioning. Target heart rate is advocated by some (19). The patient is taught to measure the pulse by one of several methods. In general, a target level of 100–120 beats/min is chosen, depending on age, medical condition, and current medications. The patient then exercises to a level sufficient to maintain the pulse to that prescribed level. As conditioning improves, the level of exercise will need to be increased for the

Table 3 Physical Training in Pulmonary Rehabilitation

Type	Advantages	Disadvantages
Stationary cycling	Safe Readily available	Boring to some Primarily legs
Treadmill	Fairly safe	Expensive Primarily legs Boring to some
Walking	Readily available Mimics normal activities	Weather No available location
Swimming	Total-body exercise	Requires a pool Need to be able to swim
Ski simulator	Total-body exercise	Expensive Athletic ability

same heart rate to occur. In the normal but deconditioned subject, the temporal effect of the training response is fairly steep with a rapid increase in exercise level in the first few weeks followed by a slower rise or plateau. The heart rate response in mild to moderate COPD patients is close to that of a normal patient (20), but for severe COPD patients the response is somewhat blunted. The other method to gauge exercise intensity is exercising to a specific perceived exertion or Borg scale (21). This method requires that the patient estimate the degree of discomfort associated with a given level of exercise. An exercise level of 10–12 on a 20-point scale is usually recommended. This method is not objective unless some quantitative measurement of external workload or oxygen uptake is performed. It may be easier for the patient to monitor perceived exertion. This methods allows flexibility in the exercise regimen to account for good and bad days so often experienced by COPD patients.

Training is directed to both upper and lower extremities. The upper extremities can be trained and should not be neglected; however, the lower extremities are required for ambulation. Training has been found to be muscle-group-specific in COPD; i.e., training the legs does not condition the arms, and vica versa (22).

The duration and frequency of exercise necessary to obtain a higher level of physical conditioning have not been well established in patients with severe COPD. However, a study in patients with mild to moderate COPD suggests that a high-intensity program is better than a low-intensity program (6). Duration and frequency of the formal exercise program is dependent on many factors, including the patient's cooperation, severity of disease, and design of the program.

There are very few controlled and randomized studies that have evaluated exercise capacity in COPD patients going through a pulmonary rehabilitation program. In an 8-week program of twice-weekly exercise, Toshima et al. (23) documented improvement in treadmill walking from 12.5 to 23 min in the exercise group and no improvement in the control group. The exercise group was encouraged to continue their exercise program and was restudied 6 months later: the improvement persisted. General conditioning exercise improves performance in most COPD patients. This does not mean that all COPD patients must undergo a conditioning type of exercise for a pulmonary rehabilitation program to be successful. It is very important that the patient continue to do some exercise after the formal program is over; otherwise the improvement may be lost.

Initial evaluation should include some assessment of exercise capacity. Either a graded cardiopulmonary exercise test or less formal exercise such as treadmill walking or a 6- or 12-min walk is used in most programs. There are advantages and disadvantages to both (Table 4). A final evaluation should be

Table 4 Exercise Capacity Assessment in COPD

Test	Components	Advantages	Disadvantages
Formal maximal exercise test	Bicycle or treadmill Maximal effort Expired gases Electrocardiogram Oxygen saturation Blood gases	Many measurements Quantitative	Expensive Time Invasive
Submaximal exercise test	Bicycle or treadmill Submaximal effort Electrocardiogram Oxygen saturation	Easier to perform	Fewer measurements
6- or 12-min walk	Stopwatch Measured course	Readily available Reproducible Inexpensive	Limited measurements

performed in similar fashion to demonstrate to the patient, family, and staff the objective degree of improvement in physical performance.

D. Pharmacotherapy

This section provides only a brief overview of pharmacotherapy. In patients with COPD, bronchodilators generally increase airflow, reduce dyspnea, and improve exercise tolerance. Failure of a single trial of a bronchodilator to show a reversible effect in airflow limitation does not necessarily indicate that a bronchodilator should not be prescribed. It is important to remember that a single trial may not identify all patients with reversible disease nor predict the response to long-term bronchodilator therapy. A typical treatment regimen is depicted in Figure 1.

Inhaled anticholinergic agents and beta agonists are the mainstay of treatment for patients with COPD. Ipratropium bromide (Atrovent) has been reported to produce a greater degree of bronchodilation than conventional doses of beta agonists (24), although studies using maximal doses of beta agonists have shown similar degrees of bronchodilation (25). Whether the use of both medications potentiates the action of the other remains controversial (25–27). Unlike sympathomimetics, the dose of ipratropium bromide may be doubled or tripled without noticeable side effects. In contrast to atropine, it does not affect the viscosity of the sputum. However, it is important to teach the patient that ipratropium bromide is slower in onset and therefore should be used on a more regular basis rather than only when symptomatic.

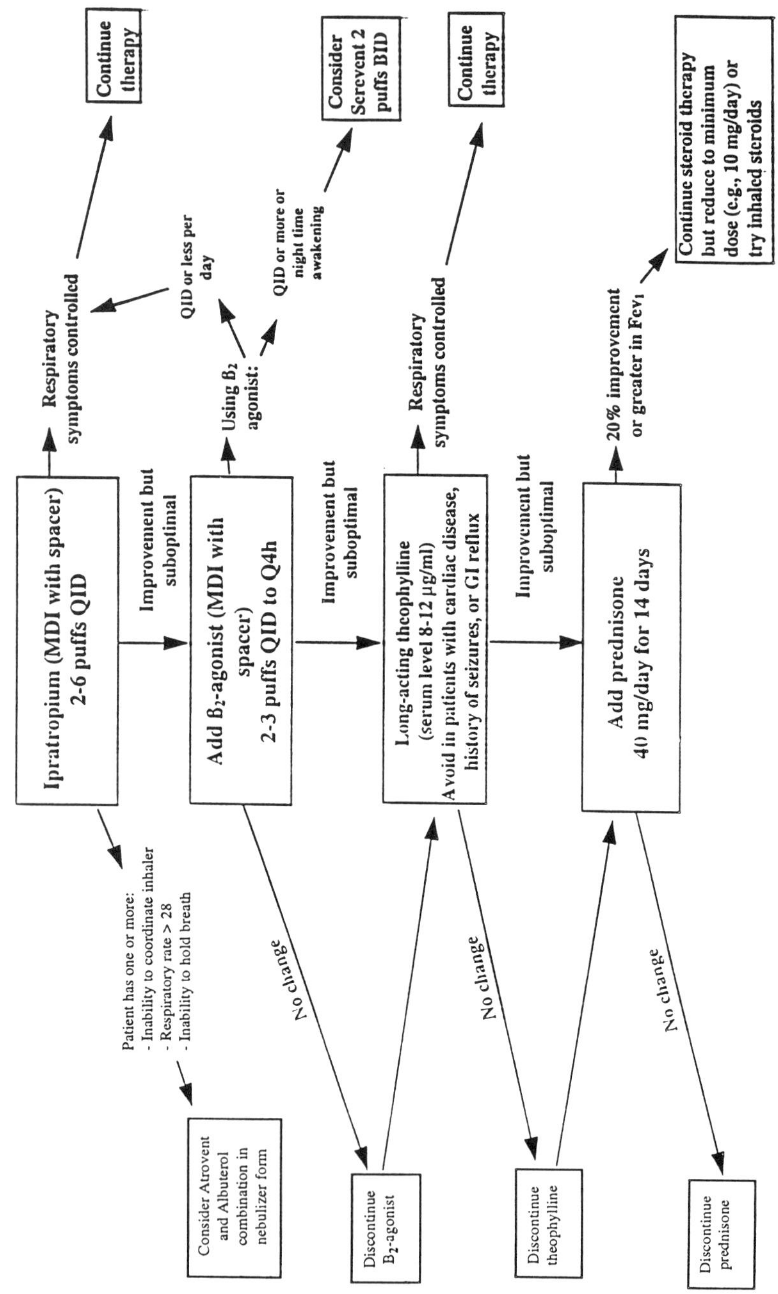

Figure 1 Typical regimen for treating COPD. Medication usage described in detail in the text.

In summary, ipratropium bromide is generally considered to be the first-line bronchodilator in patients with COPD. Adding an inhaled beta agonist to the regimen is reasonable in patients who remain symptomatic or who have episodes of acute shortness of breath and need faster bronchodilation. If patients are using beta agonists routinely four or more times a day, substituting salmeterol (a long-acting beta agonist) can decrease the use of the shorter-acting beta agonists. Salmeterol (Serevent) has been helpful in preventing nocturnal symptoms in asthmatics (28). Common mistakes in medical management of these patients include inadequate teaching about the medications, improper technique for using metered-dose inhalers (MDI), suboptimal dosing, and insufficient monitoring. Using a spacer with a MDI simplifies inhalation therapy, assures better deposition of the drug in the airways, and improves compliance. Bronchodilation is equivalent whether a MDI (optimal dosing and good technique) or a nebulizer is used to deliver medication. Those patients with severe symptoms, e.g., those whose respiratory rate is greater than 28 breaths/min, who have difficulty holding their breath, or who have difficulty coordinating an inhaler, may require a nebulizer.

The role of theophylline in the treatment of COPD is controversial. Its use in the treatment of hospitalized patients with COPD exacerbations has not been shown to give additional benefit beyond that of aerosolized bronchodilators and steroids (29). However, as a maintenance therapy, adding theophylline has been reported to produce small improvements in respiratory function, gas exchange, and dyspnea (30). Theophylline has also been shown to reduce nocturnal decreases in FEV_1 and morning respiratory symptoms (31). Therefore, it is reasonable to consider theophylline in those patients who remain symptomatic despite optimal inhaled bronchodilator therapy. Theophylline at therapeutic serum levels can exacerbate cardiac arrhythmias, potentially lower seizure threshold in patients with seizure disorders, and cause gastrointestinal symptoms, particularly in those with underlying gastroesophageal reflux.

The role of oral corticosteroids in treating COPD is controversial. Many clinicians prescribe steroids if patients have acute, severe exacerbations, although there are few studies to support this practice. It is not possible to predict which patient will benefit from either short- or long-term administration. A closely monitored trial of prednisone therapy, e.g., 40 mg/day for 2 weeks, should be considered in patients who have continuing symptoms despite maximal therapy with other agents. Documentation of objective improvement with spirometry (20% increase in FEV_1) is important, particularly since subjective improvement is not uncommon. The lowest possible effective dose should be prescribed.

As yet, data concerning the use of inhaled steroids in COPD patients are lacking. Some patients with COPD who respond to oral steroids have been shown to benefit from inhaled steroids (32); therefore, it is reasonable to attempt switching from the oral to the inhaled form. Moreover, it seems reasonable to add inhaled steroids to the regimen of patients with a significant element of reversible disease or episodic bronchospasm (frequent cough and wheezing); however, there are no published data to support this practice.

Antibiotic usage in patients undergoing an acute exacerbation of COPD has been shown to decrease the duration of symptoms and the relapse rate (33). A reasonable approach would be to add an antibiotic when patients complain of an increase in two or more of the following symptoms: dyspnea, cough, or phlegm production.

E. Physical Therapy Issues in Pulmonary Rehabilitation

Assessment of physical therapy needs is an important aspect of a comprehensive pulmonary rehabilitation program. Typical activities of a physical therapist include: (1) assessing overall strength and flexibility; (2) assessing stability and gait; (3) designing and assisting the patient in carrying out an exercise program (including upper-extremity, back, and lower-extremity exercises); and (4) teaching breathing exercises.

Several of the breathing techniques currently used in pulmonary rehabilitation are particularly useful (Table 5). Patients learn by observing and practicing the various breathing techniques. Repetition and reinforcement are important in adopting new methods.

In pursed-lip breathing, the patient exhales slowly through pursed lips keeping the nasal passages occluded by the soft palate. Exercise tolerance and gas exchange improve when the patient breathes through pursed lips (34). Many patients had taught themselves pursed-lip breathing long before the technique was shown to them. The key is to unconsciously utilize pursed-lip breathing in all situations associated with dyspnea.

Another technique is diaphragmatic breathing (35), which is taught by having the patient place one hand on the epigastrium; on inspiration, the abdomen should push out as monitored by motion of the hand; the reverse should

Table 5 Breathing Maneuvers Utilized in Pulmonary Rehabilitation

Pursed-lip breathing
Diaphragmatic breathing
Controlled-rate breathing
Specific bronchopulmonary segment breathing
Postural drainage techniques
Cough-assist techniques

occur on expiration. This technique should also become "automatic" for the dyspneic COPD patient.

Other techniques can be helpful. For example, controlling the respiratory rate is perhaps the simplest technique; the patient should consciously slow the breathing frequency and thereby increase tidal volume. Postural drainage, coupled with cough, vibration, percussion, and gravity, allows various bronchopulmonary segments to "drain" their secretions (36).

F. Occupational Therapy Issues in Pulmonary Rehabilitation

The occupational therapist interviews the patient and assesses how COPD affects the patient's ability to engage in activities both inside and outside the home (37). Evaluation of the home situation includes a number of key elements such as accessibility, location of the home in relation to shopping or other activities, and transportation.

Activities of daily living (ADL) are an important part of patient assessment prior to entering the program: dressing, undressing, cooking, cleaning, and other activities are evaluated. The occupational therapist can provide guidance in performing ADL in a more energy-efficient manner. For instance, grooming with the arms placed above the head may increase dyspnea in COPD patients. Leisure time activities and ability to drive safely are also considered. A visit to the patient's home and observation during the performance of ADL can be quite helpful.

G. Nutrition Issues in Pulmonary Rehabilitation

An important aspect of pulmonary rehabilitation is identifying the patient's nutritional needs and determining whether they are being met. Weight loss is a common finding in severe COPD. The causes are multifactorial, including increased metabolic needs of the ventilatory muscles and inadequate dietary intake, due to depression, poor selection of foods, side effects of medications, and gastrointestinal disorders (38).

In some patients, a dietary consultation is necessary. Ideally, a family member should be present during the interview to confirm the details of the dietary history and to listen to the dietitian's recommendations. The Harris-Benedict equation is often utilized to calculate the predicted caloric requirement. The adjustment necessary for the increased metabolic needs of COPD patients has not been well characterized. One method is to use the basal caloric requirement plus 50%. Depending on the patient's goal weight, an adjustment can then be made in the patient's current caloric intake. The dietary intake relative to the proportion of recommended food groups should also be considered and changes in the diet should be made when appropriate. In general, patients should be cautioned to eat small and frequent meals, rather than large ones. Some foods cause excess abdominal gas and should be avoided.

In malnourished patients, a nutritional assessment that includes biochemical markers such as albumin and nitrogen balance measurements can be helpful. To document improvement, these measurements are then followed during the rehabilitation program, provided the program is long enough to induce changes.

Obesity is also detrimental to the outcome of a successful rehabilitation program. The increased metabolic requirements to move the body mass and the mechanical disadvantage at which the diaphragm and chest wall operate can interact to increase dyspnea. Most obese patients should visit a dietitian during a rehabilitation program to discuss methods of weight reduction.

H. Psychological Issues in Pulmonary Rehabilitation

Most chronic illnesses are accompanied by varying degrees of anxiety and depression, and in COPD these feelings are particularly common (39). These feelings can be detrimental to patients with COPD because anxiety may lead to dyspnea and the preoccupation that some patients develop with breathing may precipitate further anxiety, even causing panic episodes. Fear of dyspnea may lead to a sedentary life-style, which promotes deconditioning. Medications prescribed to alleviate anxiety, such as the benzodiazepams, may have deleterious effects on mental functioning and ventilatory control and may worsen gas exchange. These side effects have led to interest in nonpharmacological means to reduce anxiety (see Table 6). These therapies require the patient's cooperation and are addressed in comprehensive pulmonary rehabilitation.

Most studies have found depression to be very common in COPD patients (40). A reasonable goal of rehabilitation is to reduce the degree of depression; however, this may be difficult to prove. The Beck Depression Inventory has been used to detect and quantify the degree of depression in patients with

Table 6 Nonpsychopharmacological Methods to Reduce Anxiety

Desensitization to dyspnea
Adoption of breathing maneuvers (pursed-lip breathing)
General relaxation techniques
Review of medications that may cause anxiety
Discussion within a peer group
Increased knowledge regarding pathophysiology of COPD
Reassuring attitude of family and friends
Improved continuity of care (physician, nurse, health aide, etc.)

COPD. An overall assessment of psychological status, such as the Minnesota Multiphasic Personality Inventory (MMPI), may prove beneficial in selected patients. In addition to quantifying anxiety and depression, the MMPI may help identify personality factors that may adversely affect rehabilitation. Formal psychiatric consultation is beneficial in some patients, especially in those who may need psychiatric medication intervention.

The others patients in the pulmonary rehabilitation program group are an important component. The support offered by others with a similar illness can be invaluable. Many patients are initially skeptical about group interaction but, with time, most become receptive. The "group" may stay together long after the formal rehabilitation program ends and serves as a means of continuing encouragement. If possible, the pulmonary rehabilitation program should foster the development of a cohesive patient group.

I. Management of Dyspnea

Dyspnea is the most disabling symptom experienced by patients with COPD and frequently the most frustrating symptom to relieve, particularly in those already on optimal pharmacological therapy. Frequently, patients are seen with similar levels of pulmonary function whose magnitude of breathlessness is quite different. It is important to recognize that dyspnea is a perceived sensation rather than a measurable physical parameter. The intensity of breathlessness can be influenced not only by physiological derangements, but also by the psychological state.

In the management of dyspnea, it is important to rule out other medical disorders in patients with COPD, such as concomitant cardiac dysfunction, anemia, pneumonia, lung carcinoma, upper airway problems, pneumothorax, or pleural effusion, that may exacerbate their breathlessness.

Use of a measurement tool to assess dyspnea is helpful in quantifying both the baseline dyspnea and the effect on dyspnea of the various therapeutic modalities to which the patient is exposed in a pulmonary rehabilitation program. Exercise testing is helpful in determining the degree to which dyspnea limits function; later, exercise testing can estimate the effect of treatment in patients who are limited by dyspnea.

A graded exercise protocol or a 6- to 12-min walk test along with a category scale can provide a measure of both the level of dyspnea at any given workload and the total work achieved. A popular scale is the original, or modified, Borg scale. Clinical methods of assessing dyspnea, e.g., the British Medical Research Council (MRC) scale, have depended primarily on the estimation of the magnitude of the exertional task with respect to the ADL that produce dyspnea. However, these techniques that focus only on the magnitude of the task without directly addressing functional status can be somewhat imprecise and insensitive to small changes. Other indices of dyspnea, such as the baseline and transitional dyspnea index of Mahler et al. (41), appear to be more useful in measuring overall impairment and in providing a more sensitive tool to detect small changes.

There are a number of approaches to managing dyspnea in patients with COPD (Table 7). For example, bronchodilator therapy to decrease airflow obstruction, or diuresis in the patient with concomitant congestive heart failure to increase lung compliance, may help to decrease the work of breathing. Several studies of the use of theophylline in patients with COPD have demonstrated a decrease in dyspnea (42).

Supplemental oxygen should be given to all patients with resting arterial hypoxemia and should be considered in those who develop arterial hypoxemia during exercise. Although the degree of improvement is somewhat unpredictable, some patients will experience significant relief from exertional dyspnea while breathing oxygen-enriched air; however, a placebo effect can be difficult to exclude.

Although inspiratory muscle training can result in increased respiratory muscle strength and endurance, whether patients achieve any significant improvement in exercise performance is still controversial. Breathing techniques or breathing retraining (see Section IV. E) teaches patients to modify their breathing patterns, which, in turn, can improve gas exchange, decrease the work of breathing, and reduce dyspnea. Furthermore, breathing retraining builds self-control and self-confidence that can prevent the panic that can lead to worsening dyspnea and respiratory failure. A regular program of exercise training has been shown to improve exercise tolerance in patients with COPD;

Table 7 Management of Dyspnea

Optimization of bronchodilators and oxygen therapy
Breathing retraining (breathing maneuvers)
Desensitization to dyspnea through exercise program
Treatment of psychological component
Relaxation techniques
Biofeedback
Pharmacotherapy when warranted for anxiety and/or depression
Surgical intervention
Bullectomy
Lung volume reduction surgery
Lung transplantation
Medications to relieve dyspnea
Dihydrocodeine
Morphine

desensitization to dyspnea is probably the key factor. Both an exercise program and breathing retraining are probably the most effective methods to alleviate breathless and improve functional capacity.

As alluded to earlier, it is important to recognize and treat major psychological components, e.g., anxiety or depression, that are prevalent in this group of patients. In some patients, appropriate management of these disorders can successfully reduce dyspnea.

Surgical intervention may be an option for some patients with COPD whose dyspnea has resulted in severe functional limitation. Surgical procedures available include bullectomy (43), lung volume reduction (44), and lung transplantation (45).

Another approach to reducing dyspnea is directed at pharmacologically blunting the respiratory drive. However, the effects of diazepam and aprazolam have been inconsistent (46,47). On a short-term basis, dihydrocodeine and morphine have improved exercise tolerance and reduced breathlessness at rest (48,49). These medications can cause many side effects including drug addiction. Furthermore, any intervention that depresses respiratory drive will cause hypoventilation and may aggravate blood gas abnormalities. Therefore, these drugs cannot be recommended except perhaps in end-stage lung disease to improve quality of life.

J. Chemical and Tobacco Abuse Issues in Pulmonary Rehabilitation

Alcoholism and COPD appear to be responsible for the greatest comparative mortality when normalized for socioeconomic status (50). Alcoholism is not common in patients with severe COPD: Yellowlees et al. (51) noted that only 4% of a group of severe COPD patients admitted to the hospital were definitely alcoholic; however, half drank regularly. Alcohol may lessen the sensation of dyspnea and it has a generalized sedative effect in anxious patients. A history of alcohol intake should be obtained in all patients, with special attention to general questions such as: (1) Have you ever needed a drink the first thing in the morning? (2) Have you ever felt guilty about your drinking? (3) Have relatives or friends ever criticized you about your drinking? (4) Have you ever felt you should drink less?

The daily use of alcohol has been associated with chronic bronchitis but not with progressive airway obstruction. Alcohol use can lead to blunting of the hypercapnic ventilatory response (52) and exacerbation of snoring and obstructive sleep apnea (53). In years past, sedatives (particularly the benzodiazepams) were commonly given to COPD patients; some of those patients developed sedative dependence. In recent years, this practice has become less common. A thorough drug history obtained at the beginning of the program and confirmed by a family member is important to detect the occasional patient who may be abusing drugs. Alcohol or sedative abuse can interfere with a pulmonary rehabilitation program. When addiction is suspected, the patient should be referred to a counselor; if the patient is found to be chemically dependent, this should be treated prior to commencing the rehabilitation program.

Although one would like all patients who smoke to quit prior to entering a pulmonary rehabilitation program, this cannot always be accomplished (54). There is a philosophical debate about whether patients should be required to stop smoking before beginning rehabilitation. Few would challenge this requirement for patients waiting for lung transplantation. A realistic approach would be to consider smoking cessation as a goal of rehabilitation rather than a requirement. Kass et al. reported the 1-year success rate of smoking cessation once in rehabilitation to be 23% (55). This is approximately the quit rate of a community-based pulmonary function screening program in which 21% of smokers with abnormal function quit and only 12% of smokers with normal function quit (56). The current smoker entering rehabilitation should be referred to the smoking cessation counselors if a defined program exists. In this way, those involved in the rehabilitation program do not dilute their efforts by the time required for smoking cessation counseling. For patients who do quit, some form of abstinence monitoring (such as CO monitoring or cotinine measurements) at follow-up may prove beneficial. After the formal rehabilitation program has ended, follow-up should include continuing encouragement not to smoke.

K. Oxygen Therapy Issues in Pulmonary Rehabilitation

Supplemental oxygen is the only therapy found to prolong life in hypoxic COPD patients (57). Proposed mechanisms include reduction in pulmonary hypertension, reduction in airways resistance, and reduction in hematocrit (58,59).

An initial goal of a pulmonary rehabilitation program should be to determine which patients need oxygen. At first glance, this would appear reasonably straightforward. The criteria specified in the British Medical Research Council Study (57) and the Nocturnal Oxygen Therapy Trial (60) have been adopted and later modified by Medicare and third-party payers. These criteria are detailed in Table 8. However, not all patients who could benefit from oxygen are included within these guidelines. Fletcher et al. (61) reported a group of patients who had nonapneic arterial hypoxemia during REM sleep even though the arterial Po_2 during wakefulness exceeded 60 mmHg. This study compared oxygen-treated to placebo groups and found that oxygen prevented bouts of arterial hypoxemia and increases in pulmonary artery pressure; however, there was no difference in 3-year mortality in the oxygen versus control groups. The clinical use of overnight oximetry can identify patients with episodic arterial

Table 8 Certification of Supplemental Oxygen in the United States

Initial certification[a] includes
Pa_{O_2} of 55 mmHg or less or Sp_{O_2} of 88% or less breathing room air or
Pa_{O_2} of 59 mmHg or less or Sp_{O_2} of 89% or less if
cor pulmonale or
erythrocytosis (hematocrit 57% or greater)
Blood analysis in a "Medicare qualified" laboratory
Recertification[a] of the above criteria within 90 days if the patient was not previously on supplemental oxygen
Renewal[a] yearly; blood gas or Sp_{O_2} determination is not necessary but recommended

[a]Certificate of Medical Necessity Form (HCFA-484) must be filled out and signed by the physician.

desaturation. Until there are long-term confirmatory studies, some uncertainty will continue about which patients deserve a trial of supplemental oxygen.

Another problem arises in patients initially discharged from the hospital on oxygen therapy but who, when restudied within 90 days, no longer qualify on the basis of P_{O_2} or Sp_{O_2} levels. It is estimated that 30–45% of all patients begun on supplemental oxygen while in the hospital improve sufficiently to no longer qualify for supplemental oxygen (62). The prospect that improved oxygenation may be a direct beneficial effect of oxygen therapy raises the possibility that, in these patients, supplemental oxygen should be continued.

Oximetry is useful in identifying patients who develop arterial hypoxemia during exercise. Supplemental oxygen is usually prescribed for symptomatic relief when desaturation does occur. However, there is no proof that the administration of supplemental oxygen during exercise reduces morbidity or mortality. Furthermore, some patients who become hypoxemic during exercise do not become less dyspneic when given supplemental oxygen. Adding to the confusion of which patients to place on oxygen, the study by Woodcock et al. (63) demonstrated that some patients who do not become hypoxemic are able to exercise for longer periods on oxygen. A common problem for some patients who do not quality for oxygen at rest but do need it while ambulating is difficulty in finding a provider. If oxygen is prescribed for use during ambulation but not for continuous or nocturnal use, current Medicare reimbursement is so low that suppliers may not be willing to provide it. In some instances, this has led to "pressure" on the physician to consider the use of continuous oxygen in patients who do not technically meet the guidelines.

Difficult questions regarding oxygen therapy commonly arise during pulmonary rehabilitation. Decisions regarding oxygen must be individualized; some patients clearly should remain on oxygen and others should be given a trial of oxygen. In situations where denial is anticipated, we have found that advocate letters written to the local Medicare insurance carrier may prove beneficial. The solution to this conundrum is further research into the utility of supplemental oxygen during sleep and exercise.

Most patients utilize an oxygen concentrator as their home oxygen source and compressed gas cylinders for ambulatory oxygen. Liquid oxygen is available in some areas of the country; portable oxygen is then obtained from a small liquid oxygen tank, which is filled from the reservoir container in the patient's home. The latter is the best system for the patient who is fully ambulatory. Patients should be encouraged to "shop around" to obtain a liquid oxygen system. Unfortunately, the type of oxygen used is often decided by economic factors rather than by patient wishes.

A great deal has been written about saving oxygen in patients on continuous oxygen. Perhaps the greatest savings can be obtained by carefully titrating the patient's arterial O_2 saturation to 90–92%, at rest and during exercise. In this way, the flow can often be decreased by up to 50%.

In patients who are ambulatory and likely to be away from home for extended periods, some of the oxygen conservation devices may prove useful. Broadly classified, there are three types of oxygen-conserving devices: (1) *Demand valve systems* are attached to the portable oxygen container and sense inspiration. A "puff" of oxygen is administered at the onset of inspiration, saving the oxygen from being vented on expiration. (2) *Reservoir devices* include those that have a small bladder in the oxygen tubing that fills during expiration and is emptied during inspiration. (3) *Transtracheal oxygen* is administered directly into the trachea through a small-diameter catheter; the oxygen tubing is connected directly to the catheter. Transtracheal oxygen delivery has some side effects and the catheters may not be reimbursed by Medicare. This means of delivery is particularly useful in patients requiring oxygen in excess of 5 L/min.

Many modifications can be made in oxygen therapy, including the source, rates of flow, duration, and use of oxygen-saving devices. The pulmonary rehabilitation program is an excellent time to introduce the patients to alternative means of oxygen therapy and to "fine tune" their program.

L. Role of Sleep Evaluation in Pulmonary Rehabilitation

Patients with severe COPD often complain of poor nocturnal sleep. In general, patients with COPD sleep poorly, with an increase in stage 1 sleep, reduction in stage 2 sleep, and an increased number of arousals and shifts in the stages of sleep (64). In spite of disturbed nocturnal sleep, there is no evidence of daytime sleepiness as measured by the multiple sleep latency test (65). Initial evaluation of patients for pulmonary rehabilitation should include questions regarding their sleep habits, subjective sleep quality, and an observer's report of the patient's sleep. Sleep disorders and disruptions that we have found prevalent in patients with COPD are shown in Table 9. The relative frequency of these conditions is unknown and, in part, dependent on the severity of COPD and the resulting arterial hypoxemia.

Assessment of gas exchange is an important aspect of pulmonary rehabilitation. Most patients undergo a determination of arterial blood gas composition. If hypoxemia is present while the patient is awake, or if there is suspicion of disordered nocturnal breathing (such as cor pulmonale, nocturnal arousals associated with dyspnea, snoring, witness breathing pauses), then overnight trend oximetry may be useful. This test can be performed in the home or hotel (as opposed to the hospital or sleep laboratory) by using the storage capabilities of the pulse oximeter and a computer program that assists in analysis of the nocturnal saturation data (66). Trend oximetry is usually performed while the patient breathes room air unless the patient is already on supplemental oxygen and there is a question of adequacy of nocturnal saturation. Desaturation during REM sleep is quite common in patients with COPD (67), particularly in those who are obese and in those who have chronic bronchitis with impaired gas exchange. A typical overnight oximetry pattern is shown in Figure 2.

If overnight oximetry reveals repetitive "dips" in oxygen saturation or if there is a history of serious daytime sleepiness, apnea, or snoring-related arousals, then formal sleep consultation is indicated. Sleep-disordered breathing is best evaluated with formal nocturnal polysomnography. Without documentation of sleep stage, breathing pattern, body position, and arterial O_2 saturation, it is difficult to sort out the contributing effects of hypoventilation and upper airway obstruction.

Significant obstructive apnea or hypopnea is often treated with nasal con-

Table 9 Sleep Disorders of Patients with Severe COPD

Poor quality of nocturnal sleep (may lead to hypersomnia)
Generally poor sleep, associated with COPD
Arousals related to airways obstruction or coughing
REM-sleep-related arousals due to desaturation
Obstructive sleep apnea/hypopnea or snoring arousals
Alveolar hypoventilation
Arousals related to effect of nicotine or caffeine
Medication-induced, such as theophylline
Related to devices (ventilators, oxygen delivery, etc.)
Other sleep disorders (such as nocturnal myoclonus)
Insomnia (may lead to increased daytime fatigue)
Psychophysiological (learned or behavioral insomnia)
Psychiatric disorders (such as anxiety or depression)
Due to adverse effects of poor sleep hygiene (such as excesive napping and variable sleep schedule)

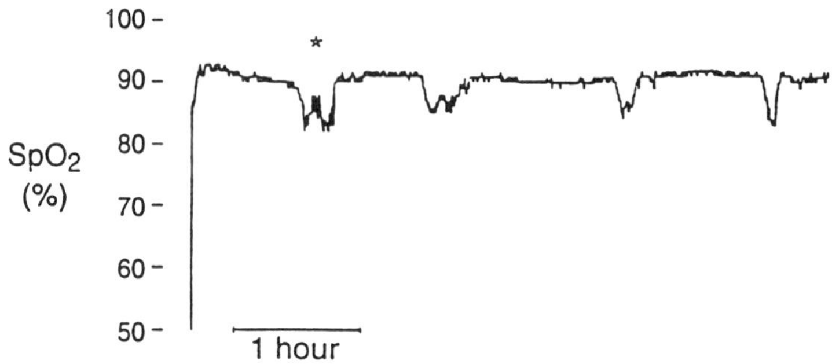

Figure 2 Trend oximetry tracing obtained in the home of a patient with severe COPD. The study was performed on room air. Spo_2 is the pulse oximeter oxygen saturation value. The baseline oxygen saturation was 93%. The asterisk (*) denotes a "broad-based" dip in oxygen saturation compatible with a REM-sleep-related fall in oxygen saturation. There were four "dips" in all. The awake oxygen saturation was above 88%; therefore, by standard guidelines the patient would not qualify for nocturnal oxygen therapy.

tinuous positive airway pressure. Alveolar hypoventilation generally becomes worse in REM sleep and as the night progresses. Patients who hypoventilate severely may have nighttime awakenings with severe dyspnea, and they may wake up in the morning with a headache and confusion. In this type of patient, overnight oximetry and arterial blood gases at the beginning of the night and on awakening may demonstrate progressive arterial O_2 desaturation and carbon dioxide retention. These patients should be considered candidates for intermittent nocturnal noninvasive ventilation, with either a volume ventilator or bilevel positive airway pressure support.

Caffeine, nicotine, theophylline, and inhaled or oral beta agonists (68–70) can adversely affect sleep. If there is a complaint of poor nocturnal sleep with frequent awakenings or the feeling of nonrestoration in the morning, then the above drugs should be considered as potential causes and therapy should be modified accordingly.

Insomnia is not uncommon in COPD. Because of nocturnal awakenings, dyspnea, and perhaps a fear of death, some patients "dread the night." Negative connotations about sleep inhibit the patient from falling asleep and thus become self-perpetuating. This condition is called "psychophysiological" or "learned" insomnia (71). Chronic anxiety and depression may also be expressed by poor nocturnal sleep. Poor sleep hygiene (72) may be brought out by a detailed sleep history. The history should include questions regarding habits of napping, variability of sleep times, poor sleep environment, and the use of sleep aids (including an alcoholic "nightcap").

If insomnia is severe, referral to a sleep disorders center can be beneficial. Formal evaluation and treatment is preferable to prescribing hypnotics; these medications are effective only for short periods of time and may depress respiration. It is much better to approach insomnia from a behavioral approach than a pharmacological one.

M. Interval Conferences with the Patient and the Family

After the individual goals of the rehabilitation program have been decided upon and the program is underway, it is important for the patient to have feedback about how he or she is progressing. In some instances, goals may have been too optimistic and need to be modified. More often, the patient learns that he/she can do more than was initially thought. Goals can then be "renegotiated" so that the patient remains challenged during the program. For example, treadmill speed or minute walk distance can be increased or ADL modified once the patient becomes reconditioned.

N. Final Outcomes of Pulmonary Rehabilitation

It is important to assess the patient's improvement in all spheres at the end of the rehabilitation program. Outcome assessment is beneficial to both the program and the patient. With a "report card," the patient can see objective improvements and note specific areas where further progress can be made. This assessment can also serve as a level to maintain after the program is over. Review of the results with family members or caregivers may help clarify misunderstandings about expected activities at home.

If an initial exercise test (treadmill, 6-min walk, or other) was performed, repeating this test at the end of the program will be informative to the patient. The patient can note objective changes, and the level of improvement may assist the person directing the exercise program in setting goals for future patients. Unless the patient was markedly deconditioned or exhibited an initial fear of developing dyspnea, large improvements in exercise tolerance are uncommon in pulmonary rehabilitation. Nevertheless, even small improvements are usually accompanied by a reduced sensation of dyspnea at a given activity level. Reducing the level of dyspnea in a patient with severe obstructive disease of the airways is perhaps a more important outcome than a longer exercise time. Unless there are special circumstances, e.g., optimization of pharmacological management, it is probably not worthwhile to assess pulmonary function since most studies have shown little change.

Tools to assess quality of life, dyspnea, and exercise tolerance upon entry and completion of the pulmonary rehabilitation program are also helpful in assessing the program; such an assessment may be required in the future to justify the program's existence and for reimbursement purposes.

A typed summary of the program including medications, recommendations regarding exercise, oxygen therapy, and ADL should be given to the patient. In this way the patient can refer back to the summary as a reminder to continue all aspects of the program. It is helpful to provide a telephone number for the patient to call if there are further questions. Finally, it is important to communicate to the primary physician the results of the pulmonary rehabilitation program, the recommendations given to the patient, and an outline for follow-up. The primary physician will most likely be responsible for monitoring the medication program and for encouraging the patient to continue the recommendations.

O. Follow-Up Evaluation

The ideal frequency for follow-up and the duration between visits is unknown, nor will it likely be determined in the future because of the variability between pulmonary rehabilitation programs and the heterogeneity of the population each program serves. Patients should be encouraged to have periodic follow-up on a long-term basis after completing a pulmonary rehabilitation program. This is particularly helpful to patients with COPD, who, as their disease progresses and their dyspnea worsens, may need their medical regimens altered, other coping skills taught, previous goals modified, and support and encouragement provided.

Existing pulmonary rehabilitation programs vary tremendously with respect to the frequency of follow-up after the program is completed and the intervals between visits. This may be inherent in the structure of the program or related to the geographical area of the population it serves, i.e., travel distance to the facility. In part, follow-up should be individualized for each patient, taking into consideration whether close supervision and follow-up can be achieved at a facility closer to home.

Periodically, e.g., every 6–12 months, patients should return to have components of their initial evaluation repeated. Pulmonary function testing, an arterial blood gas at rest, and an exercise evaluation including oximetry monitoring should be performed, in addition to an overall functional assessment, including psychosocial factors. This is particularly helpful to the pulmonary rehabilitation team in determining if the patient has old needs that have not been met or new needs that should be addressed. Previous recommendations given to each patient will likely require modification over time.

References

1. Petty TL. Pulmonary Rehabilitation. Basics of RD. New York: American Thoracic Society, 1975.

2. American Thoracic Society. Pulmonary rehabilitation. Medical Section of the American Lung Association. Am Rev Respir Dis 1981; 124:663–666.
3. NIH Workshop Summary, Fishman AP (chair). Pulmonary rehabilitation research. Am J Respir Crit Care Med 1994; 149:825–833.
4. Foster S, Thomas HM III. Pulmonary rehab in lung disease other than chronic obstructive pulmonary disease. Am Rev Respir Dis 1990; 141:601–604.
5. Goldstein RS, McCullough C, Contreras MA. Approaches to rehabilitation of patients with ventilatory insufficiency. Eur Respir J 1989; 2:655s–660s.
6. Niederman MS, Henderson Clemente P, Fein AM, et al. Benefits of a multidisciplinary pulmonary rehabilitation program: improvements are independent of lung function. Chest 1991; 99:798–804.
7. ZuWallack RL, Patel K, Reardon JZ, Clark BA, Normandin EA. Predictors of improvement in the 12-minute walking distance following a six-week outpatient pulmonary rehabilitation program. Chest 1991; 99:805–808.
8. Mungall IPF, Hainsworth R. An objective assessment of the value of exercise training in patients with chronic obstructive airways disease. Q J Med 1980; 193:77–85.
9. Moser KM, Bokinsky GE, Savage RT, Archibald CJ, Hansen PR. Results of a comprehensive rehabilitation program: physiologic and functional effects on patients with chronic obstructive pulmonary disease. Arch Intern Med 1980; 140:1596–1601.
10. Foster S, Lopez D, Thomas HM III. Pulmonary rehabilitation in COPD patients with elevated P_{CO_2}. Am Rev Respir Dis 1988; 138:1519–1523.
11. Schnapp LM, Cohen NH. Pulse oximetry: Uses and abuses. Chest 1990; 98:1244–1250.
12. Magnussen H, Holle JP, Hartmann V, Schoenen JD. D_{CO} at various breath-holding times: comparison in patients with chronic bronchial asthma and emphysema. Respiration 1979; 37:177–184.
13. Owens GR, Rogers RM, Pennock BE, Levin D. The diffusing capacity as a predictor of arterial oxygen desaturation during exercise in patients with chronic obstructive pulmonary disease. N Engl J Med 1984; 310:1218–1221.
14. Statz E, Will L, Papcke-Benson K, Simon P. Unique pulmonary rehabilitation program with traditional outcomes. Chest 1992; 102:180S.
15. Casaburi R. Exercise training in chronic obstructive lung disease. In: Casaburi R, Petty TL, eds. Principles and Practice of Pulmonary Rehabilitation. Philadelphia: WB Saunders 1993:204–224.
16. Saltin B, Blomquist G, Mitchell JH, et al. Response to exercise after bed rest and training. Circulation 1968; 38:1–78.
17. Babb TG, Viggiano R, Hurley B, Staats B, Rodarte JR. Effects of mild-to-moderate airflow limitation on exercise capacity. J Appl Physiol 1991; 70:223–300.
18. Bye PTP, Farkas GA, Roussos CH. Respiratory factors limiting exercise. Am Rev Physiol 1983; 45:439–451.
19. American College of Sports Medicine Position Stand. The recommended quantity and quality of exercise for developing and maintaining cardiorespiratory and muscular fitness in healthy adults. Med Sci Sports Exerc 1990; 22:265–274.

20. Casaburi R, Patessio A, Ioli F, Zanabouri S, Donner S, Wasserman K. Reductions in exercise lactic acidosis and ventilation as a result of exercise training in patients with obstructive lung disease. Am Rev Respir Dis 1991; 143:9–18.
21. Borg G. Perceived exertion as an indicator of somatic stress. Scand J Rehabil Med 1970; 2:92–98.
22. Belman MJ, Kendregan BA. Exercise training fails to increase skeletal muscle enzymes in patients with chronic obstructive pulmonary disease. Am Rev Respir Dis 1981; 123:256–261.
23. Toshima MT, Kaplan RM, Ries AL. Experimental evaluation of rehabilitation in chronic obstructive pulmonary disease: short-term effects on exercise endurance and health status. Health Psychol 1990; 9:237–252.
24. Tashkin DP, Ashutosh K, Bleecker ER, et al. Comparison of the anticholinergic bronchodilator ipratropium bromide with metaproterenol in chronic obstructive pulmonary disease: A 90-day multi-center study. Am J Med 1986; 81:81–90.
25. Easton PA, Jadue C, Dhingra S, et al. A comparison of the bronchodilating effects of a beta-2 adrenergic agent (albuterol) and an anticholinergic agent (ipratropium bromide) given by aerosol alone or in sequence. N Engl J Med 1986; 315:735–739.
26. LeDoux EJ, Morris JF, Temple WP, et al. Standard and double dose ipratropium bromide and inhaled metaproterenol in COPD. Chest 1989; 95:1013–1016.
27. COMBIVENT Inhalation Aerosol Study Group. In chronic obstructive pulmonary disease, a combination of ipratropium and albuterol is more effective than either agent alone: An 85-day multicenter trial. Chest 1994; 105:1411–1419.
28. Pearlman DS, Chervinsky P, LaForce C, et al. A comparison of salmeterol with albuterol in the treatment of mild-to-moderate asthma. N Engl J Med 1992; 327:1420.
29. Rice KL, Leatherman JW, Duane PG, et al. Aminophylline for acute exacerbations of chronic obstructive pulmonary disease: A controlled trial. Ann Intern Med 1987; 107:305–309.
30. Murciano D, Auclair MH, Pariente R, et al. A randomized, controlled trial of theophylline in patients with severe chronic obstructive pulmonary disease. N Engl J Med 1989; 320:1521–1525.
31. Martin RJ, Pak J. Overnight theophylline concentrations and effects on sleep and lung function in chronic obstructive pulmonary disease. Am Rev Respir Dis 1991; 145:540–544.
32. Weir DC, Gove RI, Robertson AS, et al. Corticosteroid trials in non-asthmatic chronic airflow obstruction: a comparison of oral prednisolone and inhaled beclomethasone dipropionate. Thorax 1990; 45:112–117.
33. Anthonisen NR, Manfreda J, Warren CP, et al. Antibiotic therapy in exacerbations of chronic obstructive pulmonary disease. Ann Intern Med 1989; 106:196–204.
34. Rodenstein DO, Stanescu DC. Absence of nasal air flow during pursed lips breathing. Am Rev Respir Dis 1983; 128:716–718.
35. Miller WF. A physiologic evaluation of the effects of diaphragmatic breathing training in patients with chronic pulmonary emphysema. Am J Med 1954; 17:471–477.

36. March H. Appraisal of postural drainage for chronic obstructive pulmonary disease. Arch Phys Med Rehabil 1971; 52:528–530.
37. Spencer EA. Neurologic, arthritic, orthopedic, cardiac, and pulmonary conditions. In: Hopkins HL, Smith HD, eds. Occupational Therapy. Philadelphia: JB Lippincott, 1993:621–656.
38. Edelman NH, Rucker RB, Peavy HH. NIH workshop summary: nutrition and the respiratory system: chronic obstructive pulmonary disease (COPD). Am Rev Respir Dis 1986; 134:347–352.
39. Dudley DL, Verhey JW, Masuda M, Martin CJ, Holmes TH. Long-term adjustment, prognosis, and death in irreversible diffuse obstructive pulmonary syndromes. Psychosom Med 1969; 31:310–325.
40. McSweeny AJ, Grant I, Heaton RK, Adams KM, Timms RM. Life quality of patients with chronic obstructive pulmonary disease. Arch Intern Med 1982; 142:473–478.
41. Mahler DA, Weinberg DH, Wells CK, Feinstein AR. The measurement of dyspnea: contents, interobserver agreement, and physiologic correlates of two new clinical indexes. Chest 1984; 85:751–758.
42. Mahler DA, Matthay RA, Snyder PE, Wells CK, Loke J. Sustained-release theophylline reduces dyspnea in nonreversible obstructive airway disease. Am Rev Respir Dis 1985; 131:22–25.
43. Nickoladze GD. Functional results of surgery for bullous emphysema. Chest 1992; 101:119–122.
44. Cooper JD, Trulock EP, Triantafillou AN, et al. Bilateral pneumectomy (volume reduction) for chronic obstructive pulmonary disease. J Thorac Cardiovasc Surg 1995; 109:106–119.
45. Mal H, Andreassian B, Pamela F, et al. Unilateral lung transplantation in endstage pulmonary emphysema. Am Rev Respir Dis 1989; 140:797–802.
46. Woodcock AA, Gross ER, Geddes DM. Drug treatment of breathlessness: contrasting effects of diazepam and promethazine in pink puffers. Br Med J 1981; 283:343–346.
47. Man GCW, Hsu K, Sproule BJ. Effect of alprazolam on exercise and dyspnea in patients with chronic obstructive pulmonary disease. Chest 1986; 90:832–836.
48. Woodcock AA, Gross ER, Gellert A, Shah S, Johnson M, Geddes DM. Effects of dihydrocodeine, alcohol, and caffeine on breathlessness and exercise tolerance in patients with chronic obstructive lung disease and normal blood gases. N Engl J Med 1981; 305:1611–1616.
49. Light RW, Mura JR, Sato RI, Stansbury DW, Fischer CE, Brown SE. Effects of oral morphine on breathlessness and exercise tolerance in patients with chronic obstructive pulmonary disease. Am Rev Respir Dis 1989; 139:126–133.
50. MMWR—Morbid Mortal Weekly Rep 1988; 37:155–157.
51. Yellowlees PM, Alpers JH, Bowden JJ, Bryant GD, Ruffin RE. Psychiatric morbidity in patients with chronic airflow obstruction. Med J Aust 1987; 146:305–307.
52. Sahn, SA, Lakshminarayan S, Pierson D, et al. Effect of ethanol on the ventilatory responses to oxygen and carbon dioxide in men. Clin Sci Mol Med 1975; 49:33–38.

53. Issa FG, Sullivan CE. Alcohol, snoring and sleep apnea. J Neurol Neurosurg Psychiatry 1982; 45:353–359.
54. Daughton DM, Fix AJ, Kass I, Patil KD. Smoking cessation among patients with chronic obstructive pulmonary disease (COPD). Addict Behav 1980; 5:125–128.
55. Kass I, Daughton DM, Fix AJ, Bell CW, Patil KD. The Nebraska COPD Rehabilitation Project II: a program to identify the predictive criteria involved in the rehabilitation of patients with chronic pulmonary disease. Final report. Spec Educ Rehabil Serv 1982; 20–23.
56. Hepper NGG, Drage CW, Davies SF, et al. Chronic obstructive pulmonary disease: a community-oriented program including professional education and screening by a voluntary health agency. Am Rev Respir Dis 1980; 121:97–104.
57. Report of the Medical Research Council Working Party. Long-term domiciliary oxygen therapy in chronic cor pulmonale complicating chronic bronchitis and emphysema. Lancet 1981; 1:681–686.
58. Kitchin AH, Lowther CP, Matthews MB. The effects of exercise and of breathing oxygen-enriched air on the pulmonary circulation in emphysema. Clin Sci 1961; 21:93–106.
59. Cotes JE, Pisa Z, Thomas AJ. Effect of breathing oxygen upon cardiac output, heart rate, ventilation, systemic and pulmonary blood pressure in patients with chronic lung disease. Clin Sci 1963; 25:305–321.
60. Nocturnal Oxygen Therapy Trial Group. Continuous or nocturnal oxygen therapy in hypoxemic chronic obstructive lung disease. Ann Intern Med 1980; 93:391–398.
61. Fletcher EC, Luckett RA, Goodnight-White S, et al. A double-blind trial of nocturnal supplemental oxygen for sleep desaturation in patients with chronic obstructive pulmonary disease and a daytime Pao_2 about 60 mm Hg. Am Rev Respir Dis 1992; 145:1070–1076.
62. Timms RM, Kvale PA, Anthonisen NR, et al. Selection of patients with chronic obstructive pulmonary disease for long-term oxygen therapy. JAMA 1981; 245:2514–2516.
63. Woodcock AA, Gross ER, Geddes DM. Oxygen relieves breathlessness in "pink puffers." Lancet 1981; 1:907–909.
64. Fleetham J, West P, Mezon B, et al. Sleep, arousals and oxygen desaturation in chronic obstructive pulmonary disease. Am Rev Respir Dis 1982; 126:429–433.
65. Orr WC, Shamma-Othman Z, Levin D, et al. Persistent hypoxemia and excessive daytime sleepiness in chronic obstructive pulmonary disease. Chest 1990; 97:583–585.
66. Series F, Marc I, Cormier Y, La Forge J. Utility of nocturnal home oximetry for case finding in patients with suspected sleep apnea hypopnea syndrome. Ann Intern Med 1993; 89:533–539.
67. Catterall JR, Calverley PMA, MacNee W, et al. Mechanism of transient nocturnal hypoxemia in hypoxic chronic bronchitis and emphysema. J Appl Physiol 1985; 59:1698–1703.
68. Curatolo PW, Robertson D. The health consequences of caffeine. Ann Intern Med 1983; 98:641–653.

69. Soldatos CR, Kales JD, Scharf MB, et al. Cigarette smoking associated with sleep difficulty. Science 1980; 207:551–552.
70. Kaplan J, Frederickson PA, Renaux SA, O'Brien PC. Theophylline's effect on sleep in normal subjects. Chest 1993; 103:5–6.
71. Hauri P, Fisher J. Persistent psychophysiologic (learned) insomnia. Sleep 1986; 9:38–53.
72. Zarcone VP Jr. Sleep hygiene. In: Kryger MH, Roth T, Dement WE, eds. Principles and Practice of Sleep Medicine. Philadelphia: WB Saunders 1994:542–546.

29

Pulmonary Rehabilitation in Chronic Pulmonary Interstitial Disease

RICHARD S. NOVITCH and HENRY M. THOMAS III

Cornell University Medical College
New York, New York
and Burke Rehabilitation Hospital
White Plains, New York

Pulmonary rehabilitation for interstitial lung diseases (ILD) (1) and for other nonobstructive lung diseases has been reported to be beneficial (2,3), but has received little attention in the literature. To a large extent, this lack of attention is due to the low frequency of nonobstructive diseases relative to chronic obstructive pulmonary disease (COPD). In the United States, the prevalence of COPD is 53.5 cases per 1000 men and 63.5 cases per 1000 women (4). In contrast, Coultas and associates (5), gathering epidemiological data from Bernalillo County, New Mexico, found that the combined prevalence of ILD was only 0.8 cases per 1000 men and 0.67 cases per 1000 women (Table 1). Thus, it is no surprise that the most common diagnosis in any pulmonary rehabilitation program is COPD. This emphasis on COPD can also be seen in the scientific publications, patient educational materials, and promotional literature concerning pulmonary rehabilitation. Furthermore, it is our impression that the rate of referral for rehabilitation may be relatively higher for patients with COPD than with ILD because of pessimism among physicians about ILD patients, once their respiratory status becomes disabling. The long-term prognosis for ILD patients, especially those with idiopathic pulmonary fibrosis, is poor.

Once a pulmonary rehabilitation program is established with strong referral patterns, it becomes apparent to patients and families, as well as to referring

Table 1 Prevalence and Incidence of Interstitial Lung Diseases

	Prevalence/100,000		Incidence/100,000/yr	
	Male (*n*)	Female (*n*)	Male (*n*)	Female (*n*)
Idiopathic pulmonary fibrosis	20.2	13.2	10.7	7.4
Interstitial pneumonitis	1.8	2.8	1.8	1.4
Pulmonary fibrosis	10.1	14.3	3.9	4.1
Connective tissue diseases	7.1	11.6	2.1	3.0
Occupational and environmental fibrosis	20.8	0.6	6.2	0.8
Drug and radiation firosis	1.2	2.2	1.8	1.1
Sarcoidosis	8.3	8.8	0.9	3.6
Pulmonary hemorrhage syndromes	0.6	2.2	1.5	0.8
Other	10.7	11.6	2.7	3.9
Total	81 (*n*=136)	67 (*n*=122)	31 (*n*=106)	26 (*n*=96)

Prevalence and incidence of interstitial lung diseases by sex in Bernalillo, New Mexico, from October 1, 1988, through September 30, 1990. There is apparent overlap between the categories idiopathic pulmonary fibrosis, interstitial pneumonia, and pulmonary fibrosis.
Source: Ref. 5.

and rehabilitation physicians, that pulmonary rehabilitation is useful in a wide spectrum of pulmonary diseases. Regardless of etiology, severe ventilatory limitation has physical consequences that are designated as "disabilities." Both the physician's review of symptoms and the therapist's activity of daily living (ADL) score reveal patterns of impairment that are similar in patients with diverse pathophysiological mechanisms of ventilatory limitation.

Patients with a variety of restrictive pulmonary disorders, including the interstitial lung diseases, represent a small but significant subset of all the patients who present for pulmonary rehabilitation. Foster and Thomas (2) reported that approximately 10% (37/354) of the patients admitted to their institution for inpatient pulmonary rehabilitation in the mid-1980s had pathophysiological mechanisms other than airway obstruction as the cause of ventilatory limitation. These patients improved with rehabilitation to a degree similar to that of patients with COPD (Table 2). However, of the 37 patients, only seven had ILD, and Foster and Thomas felt that patients with ILD fared less well in rehabilitation than did the other patients.

The purpose of this chapter is to focus on pulmonary rehabilitation in patients with ILD and to describe the team approach used at this institution. Patients disabled with ILD are a challenge for the pulmonary rehabilitation team accustomed to treating patients with COPD. Issues that are addressed

Table 2 Effect of Rehabilitation on 6-Min Ambulation Distance in 37 Patients with "Restrictive" Lung Diseases

	n	Admission ambulation	Discharge ambulation	Increase in ambulation
Pulmonary fibrosis	7	231 ± 217	506 ± 422	275 ± 368
Fibrothorax	3	240 ± 104	967 ± 189	727 ± 270
Bronchiectasis	7	284 ± 204	583 ± 330	299 ± 196
Scoliosis	4	441 ± 372	520 ± 464	79 ± 135
Neuromuscular disease	4	179 ± 178	439 ± 268	260 ± 127
Other	7	289 ± 206	573 ± 396	284 ± 307

Values are mean ± SD. All distances measured in feet.
Source: Ref. 2.

include training of the staff in the pathophysiological mechanisms of restrictive ventilatory limitation, revising the treatment program to deal with the different problems found in ILD, and modifying the educational program. We report our experience with 26 patients with ILD admitted to our inpatient pulmonary rehabilitation program from January 1990 through September 1994.

I. Trends in the Rehabilitation of Patients with Pulmonary Diseases

Despite the paucity of data in the current literature regarding pulmonary rehabilitation in ILD, pulmonary rehabilitation has been applied to patients with a variety of restrictive lung diseases for the last 100 years. Probably the earliest roots of pulmonary rehabilitation can be traced to the tuberculosis (TB) sanatorium, which immersed patients with chronic respiratory ailments that were not amenable to pharmacological therapy in a milieu designed to foster rest and rehabilitation. Although the TB sanatorium was not designed for rehabilitation as we know it today, many of the aims and methods were similar.

The second wave of pulmonary rehabilitation followed the polio epidemics after World War II. Pulmonary specialists devised new devices and techniques, including assisted mechanical ventilation, to establish life support during acute poliomyelitis. Afterward, those patients who survived received physical therapy and convalescent care, as well as continued mechanical ventilatory assistance when necessary.

Thus, until relatively recently, pulmonary rehabilitation was not directed at the largest group of patients we treat today, i.e., those with obstructive lung disease. The application of restorative therapy to this group is mostly a phenomenon of the last 25–30 years.

As a reminder of our predecessors' efforts, from time to time patients are seen surviving from earlier therapeutic eras in our current pulmonary rehabilitation practice. For instance, patients who have developed respiratory insufficiency as a result of old TB and old TB treatments are still being seen in chest clinics. The pathophysiological problems include parenchymal damage from volume loss and bronchiectasis, thoracic cage deformity from thoracoplasty, and extrapulmonary fibrosis from therapeutic pneumothorax. After 45–50 years, lung capacity in these patients has diminished to the extent that they can no longer sustain their usual activities. Less frequent are patients with scoliosis and progressive respiratory insufficiency due to old poliomyelitis. As these patients age, they present with hypercapnic respiratory failure due to fatigue of the respiratory muscles, which were originally weakened by poliomyelitis. Decades after having had acute poliomyelitis, they may require supplemental mechanical ventilation and/or pulmonary rehabilitation.

At present, there is an increasing number of patients who, due to effective modern subspecialty care, survive very severe acute respiratory illnesses that previously would have been fatal; these patients now require rehabilitation. These survivors of the intensive care unit (ICU) may be left with permanently damaged lungs that prevent them from returning to their previous active lives. Finally, the availability of a rehabilitation setting capable of caring for complex patients recovering from respiratory insufficiency, has created a bypass leading directly from the ICU to the inpatient pulmonary rehabilitation unit. The bypass of the general medical-surgical ward has the advantage of quicker mobilization of patients at a reduced cost. In addition, the bypass has increased the acuity of patients referred for rehabilitation as well as the pulmonary rehabilitation program itself.

Thus, changing times have led to a broader spectrum of patients needing pulmonary rehabilitation. It is in this setting that this chapter considers the rehabilitation of patients with ILD.

II. Overview of Pulmonary Rehabilitation: ILD Versus COPD

A. General Approach

In chronic diseases, the goal of rehabilitation is to restore function. The origin of disability should be of less importance than the disability itself. That is to say, the inability to ambulate, for instance, is of equivalent distress to the patient, no matter what the etiology. Similarly, impairment of a particular organ system from diverse etiologies may have similar impact on the individual affected. This realization is important for those called on to treat disability as a result of chronic ventilatory limitation.

The general principles of rehabilitation are applied to the specific functional problems presented by the patient. The understanding of lung disease and pathophysiological mechanisms enables the multidisciplinary team to design a program consisting of physical, functional, and educational modalities that will not only recondition the patient, but give him/her "tools" to use after discharge to enhance confidence, coping skills, and motivation.

The American Thoracic Society has made its position clear on the role of pulmonary rehabilitation in the treatment of patients with chronic lung disease. The two principle objectives are: (1) control and alleviate, as much as possible, the symptoms and pathophysiological complications of respiratory impairment, and (2) teach the patient how to achieve optimal capability for carrying out his/her activities of daily living (6,7). (Note that "pulmonary rehabilitation" is a misnomer in that it is the patient, not the pulmonary airways or parenchyma, that is being rehabilitated.)

B. The Team Concept

The goals of pulmonary rehabilitation have been best met using a programmed approach by an interdisciplinary team. The team breaks down comprehensive care of the respiratory patient into its component parts: general conditioning, upper-body exercise (8), lower-body exercise, reduction of dyspnea (9), educational needs, psychosocial needs (10), and medical needs. In general, the worse the overall severity of ventilatory limitation, the less likely the physician alone will be able to handle the broad spectrum of care issues that arise. Physicians may have neither the inclination nor the training to provide comprehensive care once the needs of the patient approach this level. The team approach, therefore, fills the gaps as the severity of disease increases. The team approach, with the physician as team leader, is both less costly and more effective than the physician alone (11).

C. Levels of Care

Patients who present for pulmonary rehabilitation typically fall into one of several categories: (1) too impaired to live at home; (2) able to live at home but too impaired to attend outpatient rehabilitation programs; and (3) able to live at home and participate in outpatient rehabilitation. Inpatient rehabilitation focuses on the most severely ill, those in the first two categories.

Patients in the first category are transferred directly from the acute care setting after having suffered exacerbations with or without respiratory insufficiency. The patients are deconditioned and may be malnourished enough to hinder reconditioning (12,13). Without rehabilitation, the prospect of living outside of an institutional setting is untenable for some of these patients. They have complex needs requiring specialized respiratory care that is not available in nursing homes or subacute facilities. Yet these patients need to be liberated from the constraints of a monitored bed in acute care.

Patients failing at home are a second group suitable for inpatient rehabilitation. They may have been hospitalized numerous times, and all concerned agree that a definitive intervention of intense physical rehabilitation, in addition to close medical scrutiny, should be undertaken.

D. The Trigger for Referral

Patients with chronic pulmonary diseases progress gradually to the stage at which rehabilitation is needed. COPD is a disease of aging (14,15), and the progressive expiratory airflow obstruction of COPD is an exaggeration of the normal trend of airflow obstruction with aging. The disease progresses insidiously to a level of impairment that the patient can sense. Similarly, ILD can worsen gradually, although the overall course is much shorter (16). Patients with COPD or ILD may not present for medical attention until the physiological impairment is severe. In either disease, a variety of physical limitations begin to constrain the patient. The changes are subtle at first and are easy to explain away by invoking age and sedentary life-style. Eventually, the symptoms become obvious and ever-present, as pulmonary function falls below seemingly critical thresholds for patients to be comfortably active. Often, patients are perplexed that they have a seemingly chronic disease that presents in such an acute manner. What they are experiencing, however, is not the rapid onset of disease, but the rapid onset of disability. In time, the patient (and family) struggle to find solutions to the multitude of difficulties that complicate everyday living. The clinical course may culminate in a decompensation brought about by an exacerbation or other comorbidity. The physician and patient see an alternative, which is pulmonary rehabilitation.

At this point, the goal of rehabilitation is to regain the functional capacity that has been gradually or abruptly lost. Most often, however, improvement to a level below the previous plateau is the most that can be achieved.

Physical performance in COPD is only partially correlated with physiological variables of pulmonary function (17,18). The same is true in ILD. In both conditions, impairment of pulmonary function sets an upper limit on exercise capacity, but many patients' exercise capacity is substantially below that predicted from their pulmonary function tests. Occasionally, a patient with either COPD or ILD exhibits tremendous gains in functional capacity early in the rehabilitation program. The likely scenario in this case is that the patient was underachieving relative to the ceiling set by his/her pulmonary limitation. Other factors, such as deconditioning, intercurrent illness, or depression, may have had a dramatic detrimental effect on physical performance and may be reversible during rehabilitation.

E. The Program

The program uses a multidisciplinary approach (19) involving multiple daily therapy sessions to achieve its goals. It involves patients attending multiple daily episodes of didactic and interactive encounters of directed physical activity and communication with staff. Physical, occupational, and respiratory therapists are responsible for moving the patients toward their goals. Therapy can be divided into two components. The first component is exercise reconditioning, which, in our program, is generally of low intensity. The second component consists of the repetition of focused movements that mimic daily life activities. This component reduces the difficulty of dressing, bathing, and grooming and increases the safety and ease of movement in the home. Other members of the rehabilitation team direct their efforts to general education of the patient as well as the formulation of a coherent, supportive discharge plan.

As a general rule, the patients with non-COPD lung diseases participate in the same multidisciplinary rehabilitation program as their counterparts with COPD. They undergo an intensive inpatient program with an average length of stay of 4 weeks. Those patients with hypoxemia are given supplemental oxygen according to ACCP-NHLBI guidelines (20). Exercise desaturation is a prominent component of many patients with ILD, especially idiopathic pulmonary fibrosis. Patients with ILD may therefore require augmented levels of inspired oxygen during physical activity. (Modification of the standard COPD program for patients with ILD is discussed below.)

Physical therapy produces substantial improvement in general conditioning. The patients start with one daily session of individual physical therapy, which is extended after 1 week to a second session of group therapy. The 45-min physical therapy sessions emphasize strength and conditioning through repetitive work against resistance. Included are floor walking, treadmill walking, stationary bicycle riding, and work on an upper-body cycle ergometer; each of these is performed repetitively to the patient's tolerance. Breathing retraining attempts to develop a slow, deep diaphragmatic (abdominal) respiratory pattern and desensitization toward dyspnea.

A 45-min occupational therapy session each day emphasizes upper-extremity resistive exercise to tolerance, improvement in the performance of activities of daily living, and incorporation of breathing techniques into the activities of daily living. There is also training in surface-to-surface transfers, labor-saving techniques, and safety.

Patients participate in either an education or relaxation class for 1 hr daily. Respiratory therapy provides the patient with chest physiotherapy and education in the use of nebulizers and inhalers. Patients are seen at least four times a week by the physician for medical management. Instruction given in the classroom and gym is reinforced in the patient unit by the nursing staff. Progress is assessed at a weekly multidisciplinary conference. The 6-min walk test is performed at both admission and discharge (21).

III. Results of Pulmonary Rehabilitation in Interstitial Lung Diseases

A. Data Summary

A retrospective analysis of patients admitted between January 1, 1990, and September 30, 1994 (22), revealed that ILD was the primary admitting diagnosis in 26 of 751 (3.5%) patients (Table 3). (Seventy-two of these patients, including one patient with ILD, had a total of 84 subsequent admissions for further rehabilitation during that period.) The percentage of pulmonary patients admitted with ILD (3.5%) appears to be increased above our earlier experience (2.0%) (2). A summary of the admitting diagnoses in the 26 patients categorized as having ILD is shown in Table 4. The patients ranged in age from 45 to 86 years old (66 ± 10 SD years). On average, the patients were not significantly underweight. Three patients with idiopathic pulmonary fibrosis did not complete the program; two expired and one was retransferred to an acute care hospital.

Table 3 Diagnosis of Patients Admitted for Pulmonary Rehabilitation Between January 1, 1990, and September 30, 1994

Diagnosis	No. of patients
COPD	628
Pulmonary fibrosis	26
S/P respiratory failure	15
Asthma	12
Diaphragmatic paralysis	11
S/P thoracoplasty	10
Scoliosis	10
Obesity-hypoventilation	4
Neuromuscular disease	4
Bronchiectasis	4
Miscellaneous	27
Total	751

Table 4 Diagnoses of Pulmonary Rehabilitation Patients with Interstitial Lung Disease

Diagnosis	Number
Idiopathic pulmonary fibrosis	17
Scleroderma	2
Sarcoidosis	4
Radiation fibrosis	1
Desquamative interstitial pneumonitis	2
Total	26

Pulmonary function tests for the 23 patients who completed the program are shown in Table 5. The mean forced vital capacity was moderately to severely reduced (50% of the predicted value), and the maximum voluntary ventilation was slightly better preserved (64% of the predicted value). The average Po_2 of the group was 62.6 mmHg while breathing room air.

B. Outcomes

Patients with ILD improved during the rehabilitation program in a number of parameters related to exercise (Table 6). The improvements in 6-min walk distance are comparable to values that we have published for groups of patients with COPD, with COPD and hypercapnia, and with nonobstructive lung diseases participating in our program (2,23). Patients began the program with a

Table 5 Pulmonary Function Values in 23 Patients with ILD

		% of predicted value
FVC, L	1.67 ± 0.78	50 ± 21
FEV_1, L	1.39 ± 0.56	53 ± 20
FEV_1/FVC, %	81 ± 14	
MVV	66 ± 32	64 ± 25
PEmax	77 ± 33	51 ± 18
PImax	56 ± 22	65 ± 20
DLCO, ml/mmHg/min	7.7 ± 3.0	37 ± 16 ($n = 7$)
pH	7.44 ± 0.04	
Pco_2, torr	40 ± 6	
Po_2, torr	63 ± 19	

Mean values ± SD. Except where indicated, values are the means of the 23 patients who completed the rehabilitation program.

Table 6 Results of Pulmonary Rehabilitation in Patients with ILD

Activity	Admission	Discharge	p
6-min ambulation, ft	315±348	719±537	.0001
No. of stairs climbed	12±11	24±19	.0004
Bicycle ergometry, min	8.3±4.7	12.2±4.7	.025
Arm ergometry, min	5.9±3.3	22.2±34.3	.038

Values are the means ± SD for the 23 patients who completed the rehabilitation program.

wide range of functional impairment as measured by the 6-min ambulation test. The average initial ambulation distance was 315 ft, with a range of 0–1150 ft. At the time of completion of the program, there was approximately a doubling of the mean 6-min ambulation distance, with a mean distance of 719 ft traversed in 6 min. Stair climbing, upper-extremity ergometry, and lower-extremity (bicycle) ergometry also improved significantly.

These data demonstrate that a standard program of multidisciplinary inpatient pulmonary rehabilitation is effective in patients with ILD. This is interesting in that the pathophysiology of ILD is very different from that of COPD. We see that similar gains in timed ambulation distance can be achieved across diagnostic categories. We also conclude from these results that the aim of pulmonary rehabilitation is to improve functional capacity and treat disability rather than to increase maximal oxygen uptake. This conclusion is compatible with published results that show poor correlation between the performance in a pulmonary rehabilitation program and measured pulmonary function and the inability of pulmonary rehabilitation to alter any parameter other than measures of functional impairment or the ventilatory equivalent of exercise.

IV. Principles of Rehabilitation in Patients with ILD

A. Level of Exercise Required for Pulmonary Rehabilitation

Wasserman et al. (24) and Casaburi and co-workers (25) have emphasized the importance of exercising above the anaerobic threshold to obtain the well-known training effect on the heart. Although most of the patients in our inpatient program were unable to exercise at levels that would raise lactic acid concentration above the anaerobic threshold, repeated exercise at the rather low levels that the patients could tolerate definitely improved their ability to exercise. Further, Casaburi and colleagues (26) have demonstrated that increases in maximal oxygen consumption were achieved by patients with severe COPD whose mean lactic acid level during the exercise program was only 2.0 mEq/L.

Thus, it seems that there are multiple benefits from pulmonary rehabilitation. First, in the less impaired patients, the well-known training effect noted above can be obtained from intense exercise. Second, in the more severely impaired, other factors that are less well understood come into play. For example, many of these patients are more deconditioned than others with the same degree of impairment of lung function. Thus, the second major benefit of rehabilitation may be the regaining of function the loss of which is attributable to inactivity and deconditioning rather than to the pulmonary limitation. Third, exercise capacity of patients with all degrees of exercise limitation seems to improve more than can be explained by either of the two factors above. Part of this improvement may be due to desensitization to dyspnea and to encouragement rather than to physiological improvement.

B. Selection of ILD Patients for Rehabilitation

It may be helpful to stratify patients with ILD when considering patient selection for pulmonary rehabilitation. Schulman has noted that patients with idiopathic pulmonary fibrosis (IPF) who are awaiting lung transplant are less likely to survive the wait before surgery than patients with other diseases (Schulman LL, personal communication). This corroborates our impression that patients with ILD (IPF) who are in rapid decline in the end-stage cannot be helped by rehabilitation. Some patients have a rapid downhill course while others may be relatively stable and others may be responding to treatment (27,28). Panos and colleagues (29) found that the most common reason for clinical deterioration of patients with IPF was not complications, but rather worsening of the underlying disease. Watters et al. (30) explored a strategy for assessing the clinical status of patients with IPF. A composite clinical-radiographic-physiological (CRP) scoring system was devised using seven variables: dyspnea, chest radiograph, spirometry, lung volume, diffusion capacity, resting alveolar-arterial Po_2, and exercise O_2 saturation. Watters et al. found that the initial CRP score determined at the time of open lung biopsy correlated significantly with the pathology score. The change in CRP score after 6 months of corticosteroid therapy tended to reflect the cellular histopathological component of the open lung biopsy.

Some patients may be too ill to undertake rehabilitation. Reviewing the three patients who did not complete the rehabilitation program, it is evident that they failed to improve because they were very ill. Two of the patients died in the rehabilitation hospital. One of them was initially able to walk 180 ft in 6 min, but was the only one of the 26 patients with ILD who presented with an S3 gallop, indicating severe right ventricular decompensation. The second patient who died had never left the acute hospital after his open lung biopsy and was far under ideal body weight. The third patient, a woman who had to be transferred back to acute care, had been hospitalized for months prior to rehabilitation. Neither of these latter patients could walk 10 ft upon admission to rehabilitation.

However, a number of patients with very severe ventilatory limitation (FVC less than 30% of predicted), very severe limitation of exercise capability (6-min walk distance less than 100 ft), or both had satisfactory improvement with rehabilitation. We believe it is reasonable to try rehabilitation in all but the moribund, realizing that occasional patients will have a downhill course during rehabilitation. Complications during the rehabilitation process are not unexpected (31).

In summary, pulmonary rehabilitation in patients with IPF may be reserved for those patients who are clinically stable, or who respond to pharmacological treatment, or whose recent loss in overall function exceeds that attributable to loss of pulmonary function. Patients with rapidly progressing ILD may not be as suited for rehabilitation.

C. Unique Characteristics of Rehabilitation in Patients with ILD

The major goals of the rehabilitation staff for patients with ILD are exactly the same as those for all other patients with chronic ventilatory limitation. Specific goals for the rehabilitation staff dealing with ILD patients are listed in Table 7. Ideally, all members of the team should be aware of the diagnosis of each patient. In-service education should be undertaken to familiarize all concerned with the nature of ILD. Reassurance should be given to the patient that the same rehabilitation program is effective in both obstructive and restrictive lung diseases. Patients and staff should be taught that the patterns of disability in ILD are the same as in COPD, and that patients with COPD and ILD both have difficulty with any activity requiring increased ventilation. Dyspnea is a

Table 7 Staff Goals for Treatment of Patients with Interstitial Lung Diseases

1. Identification of a patient with interstitial diagnosis to nursing and therapy staff
2. Staff education in physiology of interstitial lung disease in general and explanation of pathophysiology of the specific presenting interstitial disorder
3. Modification of education materials for diagnosis
4. Education of patient regarding particular restrictive diagnosis
5. Physician responsibilities
   a. Assure patient that the staff is aware of the "unusual" diagnosis
   b. Assure patient that the rehabilitation program is applicable equally to all pulmonary disorders and any special needs of the patient will be met
   c. Do not refer to COPD as the "problem"
   d. Encourage patient to attend all education and relaxation programs, apply what pertains to the condition, and disregard the remainder

prominent feature, and severe cough may be extraordinarily limiting in and of itself. The patient has difficulty with self-care activities, including both dressing and grooming. Showers are a singularly difficult undertaking. These difficulties may be partly due to interference with ventilation by unsupported arm exercise (8).

Although breathing retraining may be an appropriate rehabilitation modality for COPD, it may not be so for ILD. Although Gallagher and Younes (32) found that the breathing pattern during exercise and recovery were similar in COPD and ILD and that both differed from the recovery pattern in cardiac disease, we suspect that breathing techniques, as practiced by most patients, are primarily an effective psychophysiological tool.

D. Physiology of Exercise Limitation in ILD

Ventilation

In the presence of moderate to severe ILD, the impairment in lung mechanics and in gas exchange is severe enough to cause increased ventilation and energy expenditure, even in the basal state (33,34). The ability of patients with restrictive lung diseases to maintain a high level of ventilation in the presence of an increased elastic load was noted by Austrian and colleagues (35). The strategy employed to minimize the work of breathing in these patients during exercise is to increase minute ventilation solely by increasing respiratory frequency while maintaining a constant tidal volume (36). However, the maximal exercise capacity is limited and correlates with the decline in vital capacity (37).

In cardiopulmonary exercise testing, exercise limitation deemed to be ventilatory in origin is characterized by $\dot{V}_E$max that is greater than 70% of the maximum voluntary ventilation (MVV) (38). MVV is correlated with respiratory muscle strength in normals (39,40) and in patients with restrictive lung disease (41) whereas it is correlated with airway resistance in COPD (42,43). Therefore, reduction in both the vital capacity and respiratory muscle strength contributes to reductions in the maximum sustainable exercise ventilation in patients with restrictive lung disease.

Gallagher et al. (44) found that maximal levels of sustained exercise ventilation were 71, 76, and 111% of MVV in normals, subjects with ILD, and patients with COPD, respectively. The tendency of patients with restrictive lung disease to exercise at a lower percentage of MVV than those with COPD may postpone the onset of respiratory muscle fatigue. This scenario is different from that of COPD in which hyperinflation places the respiratory muscles on a disadvantageous portion of their length-tension curve. In restrictive lung diseases, volume reduction tends to maximize inspiratory muscle strength in accord with the Laplace relationships (45). In patients with COPD, the activation of the inspiratory muscles throughout the respiratory cycle may predispose to early respiratory muscle fatigue (46). On the other hand, increases in static recoil pressure in ILD facilitate the return of the lung to resting end-expiratory lung volume passively.

Gas Exchange

Abnormal gas exchange is a prominent feature in ILD. This can be overtly apparent in the rehabilitation program during exercise in the form of central cyanosis, systemic hypertension, and a drop in arterial blood oxygen saturation as measured by pulse oximetry. However, several studies have shown that impairment in gas exchange can vary in interstitial lung disease according to the underlying diagnosis (47). Thus, Agusti and co-workers (48) demonstrated that arterial hypoxemia during exercise in IPF was a result of substantial diffusion limitation as well as ventilation-perfusion abnormality. Hypoxic pulmonary vasoconstriction, which helps to minimize ventilation-perfusion abnormalities in mild to moderate ILD, appears to be lost as pulmonary hypertension caused by the pathological process supervenes in severe ILD (48). Harris-Eze and co-workers (49) found that by augmenting the concentration of oxygen in inspired gas ($Fio_2 = 0.6$), diffusion impairment during exercise could be overcome, with the result that peak $\dot{V}o_2$ exercise duration and maximal workload increased. At equivalent levels of exercise, supplemental O_2 reduced tidal volume and increased the frequency of breathing, indicating that factors other than arterial oxygen desaturation are primarily responsible for the rapid shallow breathing pattern found in ILD. In a group of patients with mild sarcoidosis studied by cardiopulmonary exercise testing, Sietsema et al. (50) found an abnormal response of $\dot{V}o_2$ during exercise in nine of 20 subjects, suggesting a defect in cardiocirculatory function.

Exercise Limitation

Exercise limitation in ILD is a result of several factors. The symptom that limits activity in lung disease is usually dyspnea or leg fatigue (51–53). The increase in the work of breathing during exercise produces disabling dyspnea. Abnormalities of gas exchange, especially diffusion limitation of oxygen with desaturation of arterial blood during exercise, pose a substantial pathophysiological obstacle. In severe ILD, destruction of the alveolar vasculature leads to pulmonary hypertension (54), which can impair right ventricular function and exercise capacity. Idiopathic pulmonary fibrosis, among all the interstitial lung diseases, may cause the greatest exercise limitation and functional impairment due to its profound effect on the pulmonary vasculature. Finally, an intact respiratory musculature is crucial in maintaining maximum sustainable exercise ventilation—the primary compensatory mechanism for diffusion limitation in ILD.

V. Conclusion

Patients with ILD pose an important challenge to those interested in pulmonary rehabilitation. Our experience is that this group of patients has as much to gain as those with COPD traditionally treated in rehabilitation programs. Certainly, the health benefits of an exercise program have no reason to be less important in ILD than COPD. It is also noteworthy that the favorable results of ILD rehabilitation validate its utility in the preoperative preparation of potential lung transplant recipients.

References

1. Schwarz MI, King TE Jr, Cherniack RM. General principles and diagnostic approach to the interstitial lung diseases. In: Murray JF, Nadel JA, eds. Textbook of Respiratory Medicine. Vol 2. Philadelphia: WB Saunders, 1994:1803–1826.
2. Foster S, Thomas HM III. Pulmonary rehabilitation in lung disease other than chronic obstructive pulmonary disease. Am Rev Respir Dis 1990; 141:601–604.
3. Novitch RS, Thomas HM III. Rehabilitation of patients with chronic ventilatory limitation from nonobstructive lung diseases. In: Casaburi R, Petty TL, eds. Principles and Practice of Pulmonary Rehabilitation. Philadelphia: WB Saunders, 1993:416–423.
4. Higgins M. Epidemiology of obstructive pulmonary disease. In: Casaburi R, Petty TL, eds. Principles and Practice of Pulmonary Rehabilitation. Philadelphia: WB Saunders, 1993:10–17.
5. Coultas DB, Zumwalt RE, Black WC, Sobonya RE. The epidemiology of interstitial lung diseases. Am J Respir Crit Care Med 1994; 150:967–972.
6. American Thoracic Society. Medical Section of the American Lung Association. Pulmonary rehabilitation. Official ATS statement adopted by the ATS Executive Committee, March 1981.
7. American Thoracic Society. Medical Section of the American Lung Association. Standards for the diagnosis and care of patients with chronic obstructive pulmonary disease (COPD) and asthma. Official statement of the American Thoracic Society adopted by the ATS Board of Directors, November 1986.
8. Martinez FJ, Couser JI, Celli BR. Respiratory response to arm elevation in patients with chronic airflow obstruction. Am Rev Respir Dis 1991; 143:476–480.
9. Reardon J. Awad E, Normandin E, Vale F, Clark B, ZuWallack RL. The effect of comprehensive outpatient rehabilitation on dyspnea. Chest 1994; 105:1046–1052.
10. Emery CF, Leatherman NE, Burker EJ, MacIntyre NR. Psychological outcomes of a pulmonary rehabilitation program. Chest 1991; 100:613–617.
11. Haggerty MC, Stockdate-Wooley R, Nair S. Respi-Care. An innovative home care program for the patient with chronic obstructive pulmonary disease. Chest 1991; 100:607–612.
12. Donahoe M, Rogers RM, Wilson DO, Pennock BE. Oxygen consumption of the

respiratory muscles in normal and in malnourished patients with chronic obstructive pulmonary disease. Am Rev Respir Dis 1989; 140:385–391.
13. Wilson DO, Rogers RM, Wright EC, Anthonisen NR. Body weight in chronic obstructive pulmonary disease. Am Rev Respir Dis 1989; 139:1435–1438.
14. Sorlie PD, Kannel WB, O'Connor G. Mortality associated with respiratory function and symptoms in advanced age. Am Rev Respir Dis 1989; 140:379–384.
15. Tager IB, Segal MR, Speizer FE, Weiss ST. The natural history of forced expiratory volumes. Effect of cigarette smoking and respiratory symptoms. Am Rev Respir Dis 1988; 138:837–849.
16. Crystal RG, Gadek JE, Ferrans VJ, Fulmer JD, Line BR, Hunninghake GW. Interstitial lung disease: current concepts of pathogenesis, staging and therapy. Am J Med 1981; 70:542–568.
17. Neiderman MS, Clemente PH, Fein AM, et al. Benefits of a multidisciplinary pulmonary rehabilitation program. Improvements are independent of lung function. Chest 1991; 99:798–804.
18. Novitch RS, Fried ED, Carson R, Thomas HM III. Relative improvement during rehabilitation is inversely correlated to admission function in severe COPD. Am Rev Respir Dis 1991; 143:A77.
19. Fishman DB, Petty TL. Physical, symptomatic and psychological improvement in patients receiving comprehensive care for chronic airways obstruction. J Chronic Dis 1971; 24:775–785.
20. Fulmer JD, Snider GL. American College of Chest Physicians (ACCP). National Heart, Lung and Blood Institute (NLHBI) Conference on Oxygen Therapy. Arch Intern Med 1984; 144:1645–1655.
21. Butland RJA, Pang J, Gross ER, et al: Two, six and 12 minute walking tests in respiratory disease. Br Med J 1982; 284:1607–1608.
22. Novitch RS, Thomas HM III. Pulmonary rehabilitation in patients with interstitial lung disease. Am Rev Respair Dis 1995; A684.
23. Foster S, Lopez D, Thomas HM III. Pulmonary rehabilitation in COPD patients with elevated Pco_2. Am Rev Respir Dis 1988; 138:1519–1523.
24. Wasserman K, Sue DY, Casaburi R, et al. Selection criteria for exercise training in pulmonary rehabilitation. Eur Respir J 1989; 2 (Suppl 7):604S–610S.
25. Casaburi R, Wasserman K, Patessio A, et al. A new perspective in pulmonary rehabilitation: anaerobic threshold as a discriminant in training. Eur Respir J 1989; 2 (Suppl 7):618S–623S.
26. Casaburi R, Burns M, Cooper C, Singer E, Chang R, Porszasz J. Physiological benefits of exercise training in severe COPD. Am J Respir Crit Care Med 1994; 149:A598.
27. Crystal RG, Ferrans VJ, Basset F. Biologic basis of pulmonary fibrosis. In: Crystal RG, West JB, eds. The Lung Scientific Foundations. New York: Raven Press, 1991:2031–2046.
28. King Jr TE, Cherniack RM, Schwarz MI. Idiopathic pulmonary fibrosis and other interstitial lung diseases of unknown etiology. In: Murray JF, Nadel JA, eds. Textbook of Respiratory Medicine. Vol. 2, Philadelphia: WB Saunders, 1994:1827–1849.

29. Panos RJ, Mortenson RL, Niccoli SR, King TE Jr. Clinical deterioration in patients with idiopathic pulmonary fibrosis: causes and assessment. Am J Med 1990; 88:396–404.
30. Watters LC, King TE, Schwarz MI, Waldron JA, Stanford RE, Cherniak RM. A clinical, radiographic, and physiologic scoring system for the longitudinal assessment of patients with idiopathic pulmonary fibrosis. Am Rev Respir Dis 1986; 133:97–103.
31. Siegler EL, Stineman MG, Maislin G. Development of complications during rehabilitation. Arch Intern Med 1994; 154:2185–2190.
32. Gallagher CG, Younes M. Breathing pattern during and after maximal exercise in patients with chronic obstructive lung disease, interstitial lung disease, and cardiac disease, and in normal subjects. Am Rev Respir Dis 1986; 133:581–586.
33. Lourenço RV, Turino GM, Davidson LAG, et al. The regulation of ventilation in diffuse pulmonary fibrosis. Am J Med 1965; 38:199–216.
34. Fitting JW, Frascarolo P, Jequier E, et al. Resting energy expenditure in interstitial lung disease. Am Rev Respir Dis 1990; 142:631–635.
35. Austrian R, McClement JH, Renzetti AD, et al. Clinical and physiologic features of some types of pulmonary diseases with impairment of alveolar-capillary diffusion. Am J Med 1951; 11:667–684.
36. Bradley GW, Crawford R. Regulation of breathing during exercise in normal subjects and in chronic lung disease. Clin Sci Mol Med 1976; 51:575–582.
37. Burdon JGW, Killian KJ, Jones NL. Pattern of breathing during exercise in patients with interstitial lung disease. Thorax 1983; 38:778–784.
38. Wasserman K, Hansen JE, Sue DY, et al. Principles of Exercise and Interpretation. Philadelphia: Lea & Febiger, 1987.
39. Ringqvist T. Ventilatory capacity in normal subjects: analysis of causal factors with special reference to the respiratory forces. Scand J Clin Lab Invest 1966; 88 (Suppl):1–179).
40. Lavietes MH, Clifford E, Silverstein D, et al. Relationship of static respiratory muscle pressure and maximum voluntary ventilation in normal subjects. Respiration 1979; 38:121–126.
41. De Troyer A, Yernault J-C. Inspiratory muscle force in normal subjects and patients with interstitial lung disease. Thorax 1980; 35:92–100.
42. Rochester DF, Arora NS, Braun NMT, et al. The respiratory muscles in chronic obstructive pulmonary disease (COPD). Bull Eur Physiopathol Respir 1979; 15:951–975.
43. Aldrich TK, Arora NS, Rochester DF. The influence of airway obstruction in respiratory muscle strength on maximal voluntary ventilation in lung disease. Am Rev Respir Dis 1982; 126:195–199.
44. Gallagher CG, Im Hof V, Younes M. Effect of inspiratory muscle fatigue on breathing pattern. J Appl Physiol 1985; 59:1152–1158.
45. Gibson GJ, Pride NB. Pulmonary mechanics in fibrosing alveolitis. The effects of lung shrinkage. Am Rev Respir Dis 1977; 116:637–647.
46. Campbell EJM, Agostoni E, Davis JN. The Respiratory Muscles. Mechanics and Neural Control. Philadelphia: WB Saunders, 1970.

47. Risk C, Epler GR, Gaensler EA. Exercise alveolar-arterial oxygen pressure difference in interstitial lung disease. Chest 1985; 85:69–74.
48. Agusti AGN, Roca J, Gea J, Wagner PD, Xaubet A, Rodgriguez-Roisin R. Mechanisms of gas-exchange impairment in idiopathic pulmonary fibrosis. Am Rev Respir Dis 1991; 143:219–225.
49. Harris-Eze AO, Dridhar G, Clemens RE, Gallagher CG, Marciniuk DD. Oxygen improves maximal exercise performance in interstitial lung disease. Am J Respir Crit Care Med 1994; 150:1616–1622.
50. Sietsema KE, Kraft M, Ginzton L, Sharma OP. Abnormal oxygen uptake responses to exercise in patients with mild pulmonary sarcoidosis. Chest 1992; 102:838–845.
51. Killian KJ, Summers E, Jones NL, Campbell EJ. Dyspnea and leg effort during incremental cycle ergometry. Am Rev Respir Dis 1992; 145:1339–1345.
52. Killian KJ, Jones NL. Mechanisms of exertional dyspnea. In: Clinics in Chest Medicine. Clinical Exercise Testing. Philadelphia: WB Saunders, 1994:247–257.
53. Marciniuk, DD, Gallagher CG. Clinical exercise testing in interstitial lung disease. In: Clinics in Chest Medicine. Clinical Exercise Testing. Philadelphia: WB Saunders, 1994:287–303.
54. Enson Y, Thomas HM III, Bosken CH, Wood JA, Wigger HJ, Harvey RM. Pulmonary hypertension in interstitial disease: relation of vascular resistance to abnormal lung structure. Trans Assoc Am Physicians 1975; 88:248–255.

30

Pulmonary Rehabilitation in Musculoskeletal Disorders

JOHN R. BACH

University of Medicine and Dentistry–New Jersey Medical School
Newark, New Jersey

The precepts of pulmonary rehabilitation that have traditionally been applied to patients with chronic obstructive pulmonary disease (COPD) apply equally well to patients with neuromuscular or paralytic/restrictive conditions. Many of these patients spend a considerable part of their lives using ventilatory assistance. Even when patients with neuromuscular disease can breathe autonomously, restrictive pulmonary syndromes and impaired cough mechanisms greatly increase the risk and incidence of pulmonary complications and contribute to mortality. For example, although most spinal cord–injured (SCI) individuals do not require long-term ventilatory support, because of weakened inspiratory and especially expiratory muscles, their risk of death from pneumonia is at least 10 times higher than that of the general population (1).

Noninvasive physical medicine interventions can prevent pneumonia and eliminate the need for hospitalization, endotracheal intubation, and indwelling tracheostomy tubes. The interventions do so by reversing ventilatory insufficiency and airway encumberment. Unfortunately, the great majority of physicians who care for patients with paralytic/restrictive pulmonary syndromes have no experience in the use of noninvasive respiratory muscle aids as alternatives to tracheostomy. Also, influenced by their negative bias toward ventilatory support via tracheostomy, they discourage ventilator use in general (2).

Individuals with paralytic/restrictive pulmonary syndromes usually have nonpulmonary impairments that must also be addressed. These include a tendency for articular degeneration and loss of range of motion, muscle weakness, decreased endurance, dysphagia, impaired communication, mobility, transfers, personal hygiene and dressing skills, and bowel and bladder dysfunction. Psychosocial and vocational impairments are also common. In addition, many of these individuals are candidates for developing pressure ulcers, thrombophlebitis, reactive depression, and dependency on others for financial support, transportation, and most activities of daily living (ADL). Throughout the rehabilitation process, these issues must be addressed. The self-directed patient should be prepared to assume responsibility for his/her management decisions and for the instruction and direction of those who provide rehabilitative care.

Respiratory muscle disability that necessitates the use of physical medicine interventions results from conditions in which: (1) the dysfunction of both the skeletal and respiratory muscles is progressive; (2) the skeletal and respiratory muscle dysfunction is sudden in onset and permanent; (3) the dysfunction of both the skeletal and respiratory muscles either remits or undergoes intermittent exacerbations and remissions.

I. The Progressive Neuromuscular Conditions

To cite the Honourable Justice Sam Filer, who uses a computer-assisted communication system for communication, "Throughout the ALS [amyotrophic lateral sclerosis] process, I have learned many things. I have learned that having ALS does not necessarily mean a death sentence, that I am not living with a life threatening disease, but rather with a life enhancing condition." For seven years, Justice Filer, who has no measurable vital capacity (VC) because of amyotrophic lateral sclerosis (ALS), has served as a municipal court judge despite lack of motor function of his extremities and his ventilator dependence (3).

A. Characterization

The progressive neuromuscular conditions include the muscular dystrophies and certain other generalized myopathies and myotonias, the spinal muscular atrophies, and progressive motor neuron diseases. Respiratory failure is the most common cause of morbidity and mortality for individuals with these conditions (3–5). In addition, individuals who are postpoliomyelitis (6) and others with certain congenital myopathies, or conditions that are considered to be stable, such as chronic spinal cord injury (7), can also undergo insidious deterioration that leads to late-onset ventilatory failure.

In some severe, infantile-onset, neuromuscular conditions, particularly spinal muscular atrophy type I (8), the normal motor milestones are never achieved and patients may require ventilatory support to survive the neonatal period. However, in most neuromuscular conditions, the motor milestones are achieved and then eventually lost as the patients develop increasingly generalized weakness and musculotendinous contractures. The most common of these disorders is Duchenne muscular dystrophy (DMD). This disorder almost invariably presents three clinical stages (Table 1). The management options in each stage of DMD can be applied to individuals with other neuromuscular conditions. With proper treatment and support in each stage, patients can remain active in the community even though many eventually need to use respiratory muscle aids for up to 24 hr a day.

Of the postpoliomyelitis patients who had been weaned from ventilators during the acute period, many have developed late-onset ventilatory failure and have become long-term ventilator users. Although the first report of postpolio late-onset ventilatory failure was only 25 years ago (9), most of the current ventilator users are late-onset (6,10); this includes some postpolio individuals who did not require ventilatory assistance during the acute poliomyelitis period (6,10,11). In a recent national survey of the late effects of poliomyelitis, 42% of the respondents reported new breathing problems (12).

Table 1 Management Principles for Neuromuscular Disease Stages

Ambulatory stage

1. Early establishment of the diagnosis and genetic counseling
2. Early and informed counseling and psychological support to prevent counterproductive family psychodynamics, to encourage goal-oriented activities, and to prepare the patient and family for current and future therapeutic interventions
3. Early management of musculotendinous skeletal and chest wall contractures and orthopedic interventions in some situations
4. Appropriate use of supportive physical and occupational therapy and possibly splinting and therapeutic exercise
5. Monitoring for prevention of cardiac complications

Wheelchair-dependent stage

1. Facilitation of ADL independence with assistive devices
2. Early prevention or correction of spinal deformity
3. Ongoing monitoring for and management of cardiac insufficiency
4. Maintenance of pulmonary compliance and alveolar ventilation

The stage of prolonged survival

1. Patient instruction and encouragement for taking responsibility for management decisions and directing caregivers
2. Facilitation of ADL independence with assistive devices
3. Timely introduction of appropriate noninvasive respiratory muscle aids to assist alveolar ventilation and clear airway secretions as needed

For kyphoscoliotic individuals, for those who have the obesity hypoventilation syndrome, or for anyone with severe sleep-disordered breathing and chronic alveolar hypoventilation, ventilatory dysfunction can be progressive despite the absence of progressive neuromuscular disease.

B. General Interventions

Individuals with progressive neuromuscular conditions require some of the same general medical interventions as do patients with primary lung disease (13). Counseling is needed to define and explain the various impairments as well as the therapeutic options. In addition, the patient is cautioned to avoid obesity, heavy meals, extremes of temperature, humidity, excessive fatigue, crowded areas or exposure to respiratory tract pathogens, sedatives, and narcotics. The need for early and appropriate attention during respiratory tract infections (RTIs) should also be reinforced as well as the need for vaccinations against viral (influenza) and bacterial (*Pneumococcus*) infections. Since treated patients with progressive neuromuscular diseases can have much greater life expectancies than previously thought possible, they should also be encouraged to undertake goal-oriented activities and plan for their futures.

Nutrition

Heavy meals and obesity should be avoided. Although some clinicians suggest high caloric and protein intake for certain muscular dystrophy patients (14), most feel that wheelchair-dependent adolescents should be limited to about 1200 calories, i.e., about one-half of normal levels. Malnutrition is more likely to be a problem in the advanced stages of the disease; serum albumin and protein levels should then be monitored. In one study, the average weight of 40 neuromuscular patients at the initiation of assisted ventilation was 70 lb (15). Dysphagia and fear of choking can limit oral intake to thick liquids and high-calorie dietary supplements; placement of a gastrostomy tube may become necessary. Eating difficulties can also be due to shortness of breath and fatigue associated with chronic alveolar hypoventilation (16). These difficulties often resolve and patients gain weight when inspiratory muscle aids are used (16,17).

Orthopedic Intervention

Extremity contractures can decrease function, cause discomfort, detract from appearance, and hamper efforts at maintaining good personal hygiene. Lower-extremity contractures can prematurely preclude ambulation. Although most neuromuscular patients who require pulmonary intervention are wheelchair-dependent, some who require up to 24-hr ventilatory support can ambulate (18). Although musculotendinous releases and tibialis posterior transfers can be done after, or at the time of, wheelchair dependence (19,20), earlier interventions may prolong ambulation without bracing or extensive physical therapy (21,22).

Kyphoscoliosis, common in these individuals, disturbs the normal length-contraction relationships that enable optimal contraction of the diaphragm. Although it is debatable if surgical correction of spinal deformity is helpful in slowing the rate of decrease in VC, it is clear that patients with severe scoliosis do develop cardiopulmonary compromise even in the absence of intrinsic disease of the respiratory muscles. Moreover, prevention or correction of scoliosis permits the use of a wider variety of noninvasive inspiratory aids such as the intermittent abdominal pressure ventilator (IAPV) and the chest shell ventilator. Severe scoliosis may eventually prevent assumption of the upright position because of impingement on the abdomen by the ribcage. Lumbar radiculopathy and back and ischial pain are also caused by spinal deformity. Since only surgical intervention can prevent or impede the development of scoliosis in these individuals, it should be performed in a timely manner for all pediatric patients with neuromuscular disease who develop it (23). However, adult scoliotic patients have more rigid, less reversible, curves and are more prone to surgical complications.

Exercise Therapy

There is evidence that increased functional demand can damage weakened muscles (24). Creatinine kinase levels increase more following exercise in dystrophic patients than in normals. Comparisons of the strength of the preferred upper (25) and lower (26) extremities of dystrophic individuals with that of the opposite extremities have shown that the preferred extremities are weaker; i.e., greater use of the preferred limb muscles appears to lead to overuse weakness. For patients with severe disease who use ventilatory assistance, the routine ADL may cause overuse atrophy. Resistance exercises have been shown to benefit patients only when the initial muscle strength is greater than 15–20% of normal (27). Exercise training with the use of weights may be used if: the degree of weakness is not severe, the rate of clinical progression is relatively slow, the rate of increasing the intensity of the exercise program is relatively slow, and the period of daily exercise is limited and takes into account the individual's level of daily physical activity (28). Thus, exercise programs cannot benefit individuals who are most in need of help. However, all patients should, be encouraged to remain as active as possible with activities they enjoy while avoiding muscle strain. Patients who are bedridden because of acute illness or surgical procedures should receive daily physical therapy with active exercises until they recover their strength. With the fact that in normals only 50% of motor units remain by the 6th decade, it becomes clear how difficult muscle strengthening can be for aging neuromuscular patients, particularly those with anterior horn cell diseases whose remaining motor neurons have the burden of innervating many additional muscle fibers.

Activities of Daily Living

ADL can be greatly facilitated by the use of a wheelchair, adaptive equipment, and energy conservation. A multitude of orthoses and other assistive devices are at the disposal of occupational and physical therapists, that can assist paretic individuals in dressing, grooming, personal hygiene, transfers, wheelchair mobility, and, possibly, ambulation (29,30). Environmental control systems can permit access of the severely disabled individual to the telephone and electrical appliances. One especially helpful assistive device is the wheelchair-mountable robotic arm (31). This can permit wheelchair-bound neuromuscular ventilator users with several inches of finger excursion to feed themselves, open doors, perform some personal hygiene, and manipulate objects. This option is potentially widely applicable since, with the exception of patients with severe motor neuron disease, the great majority of these individuals do not lose finger excursion. Also, since 95% of these patients often retain eyelid and extraocular movements, they can communicate with the use of computerized voice synthesizers (3).

For many, an efficient bowel and bladder management program is one of the greatest facilitators of the ADL. Constipation associated with an increase in gastrointestinal transit time is common. High fluid and fiber intake should be encouraged, hypokalemia avoided, and prudent dietary habits, including a high intake of fruit and vegetables, should be developed (32). A regular daily or every-other-day bowel program involving the use of cathartics, such as aloes, suppositories, and occasionally enemas, may be necessary. The most useful single technique for facilitating a bowel movement is having it from a lift in which the hips are flexed and the buttocks are in dependent position over a commode chair. This can decrease the waiting time for postsuppository evacuation from hours to minutes. An effective bowel program can also decrease the incidence of "bowel accidents," which would otherwise interfere with the ADL. Although there are few progressive neuromuscular or postpoliomyelitis patients with neurogenic bladders, wheelchair dependence and impaired upper-extremity function can also make bladder evacuation an ordeal that can interfere with social reintegration and ADL. In this case, a condom-catheter drainage system will permit the individual to urinate without interrupting ADL.

Bed mobility in these severely impaired ventilator users necessitates frequent assistance in turning during the night. Patients are often awakened by discomfort from skin pressure. To ease the burden on caregivers and to improve the quality of the patient's sleep, alternating pressure pad mattresses can be helpful. Even more effective, but more expensive, are motorized beds that rotate patients slowly from side to side (Motion Bed, J. H. Emerson Company, Cambridge, MA). These can completely eliminate the need for assisted turning, but can inadvertently loosen the nasal interfaces used for intermittent positive-pressure ventilation (IPPV) and cause the patient to seek help.

Psychological Concerns

The great majority of severely involved neuromuscular and poliomyelitis ventilator users have the same positive satisfaction with life as does the general population (33,34). They also consider their lives to be interesting, enjoyable, worthwhile, friendly, full, hopeful, and rewarding. Health care professionals, on the other hand, incorrectly judge that these patients consider their lives to be boring, miserable, useless, lonely, empty, and discouraging. The ventilator users are generally dissatisfied only with their general health and their sex lives (33,34). The latter is in part true because of the restrictive and overprotective attitudes of relatives and of society in general (35). Unfortunately, physicians rarely discuss sexual concerns with neuromuscular patients who are ventilator users. Indeed, as noted above, most physicians not only fail to advise about these concerns, but are also biased against ventilator use in general and misinformed about options for ventilator use (2). Purtilo has called attention to popular misconceptions of physicians about the undesirability of "going on a respirator (and the quality of life of ventilator users)." She has also noted that these misconceptions have "far-reaching negative effects for chronically-impaired individuals who could be happily supported on a respirator" (36).

C. Respiratory Interventions

Respiratory Muscle Exercise

Rest for the respiratory muscles and training of the inspiratory muscles has been reported to improve the strength and endurance of the respiratory muscles in neuromuscular patients during weaning from the ventilator (37). However, in individuals with stable or slowly progressive conditions, short daily sessions of exercise training with increased inspiratory resistance have not been shown to affect lung volumes or maximum inspiratory or expiratory pressures (38–40), but they can improve the endurance of the respiratory muscles (38,40). Unfortunately, the degree of improvement in endurance correlated directly with the VC and maximum inspiratory pressure at the outset of the training: no patient with a VC less than 30% of predicted normal showed improvement in endurance (38). However, such patients often require nocturnal ventilatory aid and develop respiratory failure during RTIs (16). Despite suggestions to the contrary, there is no evidence that beginning an exercise program earlier can prevent or delay ventilatory failure (38). On the contrary, mildly affected ALS patients appear to respond to an exercise program entailing increased inspiratory resistance with a decrease in VC and inspiratory pressures (41).

Prevention of Chest Tightness

A basic intervention in physical medicine is to increase the range of motion of hypomobile tissues by the use of appropriate exercises. This principle should also be applied to the lungs and chest walls of neuromuscular patients. To this end, a program designed to provide increasingly greater insufflations should be instituted; the goal of such a program is to attain the predicted inspiratory capacity of the patient. Incentive spirometry is useless for this purpose. By applying range of motion to musculoskeletal articulations of the chest wall, short periods of mild mechanical hyperinflation can transiently increase dynamic pulmonary compliance (42). However, such limited treatments applied late in the course of the disease do not improve static compliance (43). Therefore, it may be beneficial to use maximum insufflations on a daily basis long before the VC drops to 50% of predicted normal. Deep insufflation methods include glossopharyngeal breathing (GPB) (44), maximal intermittent positive-pressure breathing (IPPB) via an IPPB machine, a blower (Zephyr, Lifecare Inc., Lafayette, CO), or, a ventilator. If the lips are too weak to grasp a mouthpiece, deep insufflations may be delivered via a nasal interface. The delivered volumes should be increased gradually, as tolerated, to approach the predicted normal inspiratory capacity (45,46). It has been suggested that regular lung hyperinflation can improve the VC (47,48). We, too, have seen many instances where the initiation of hyperinsufflation exercises or regular periods of noninvasive IPPV has resulted in increases in VC.

Glossopharyngeal Breathing

Glossopharyngeal breathing or "frog breathing" is a technique used by some patients with neuromuscular disease who are dependent on ventilators to increase maximal inspirations to assist coughing, to increase the volume of the voice, and to increase breathing time while off the ventilator (44). Many patients learn this technique on their own although video instruction tapes, and training manuals are available (49,50). With this technique the tongue and pharyngeal muscles "gulp" boluses of air past the vocal chords. Six to eight gulps of 60–100 ml constitute one breath. A normal minute ventilation can be maintained for hours by individuals who otherwise have no measurable VC. Glossopharyngeal breathing is ineffective when bulbar muscle dysfunction is severe.

Normalization of Alveolar Ventilation and Oximetry Biofeedback

Hypoventilation increases the risk of developing pneumonia and acute respiratory failure (4). As restriction of lung motion, hypoventilation, and hypoxemia progress, the hypoxemic stimulus to breathing becomes increasingly blunted and pulmonary hypertension develops. Nocturnal use of noninvasive IPPV becomes less effective in maintaining normal oxyhemoglobin saturation (Sa_{O_2}) and P_{CO_2} during sleep if the patient hypoventilates during the day (16). The goal, therefore, is to maintain normal Sa_{O_2} day and night and, using the oximeter as biofeedback, to facilitate achievement of this goal.

An oximeter can be used to estimate alveolar ventilation during ambient-air breathing. Patients who hypoventilate usually have prolonged periods of Sa_{O_2} less than 95%. By increasing breathing rate, depth, or both, the patient can observe normalization of his/her Sa_{O_2} and, therefore, improvement in alveolar ventilation. However, the patient learns that he/she cannot sustain the effort required to accomplish this all day without the use of inspiratory muscle aids. Once introduced to noninvasive intermittent positive-pressure ventilation (IPPV) and chronic fatigue and dyspnea are relieved, many go on to use these techniques for increasingly longer periods as the need arises. They soon learn that occasional deep insufflations can cause Sa_{O_2} to exceed, and to remain, greater than 94%. During the training period, an alarm can be set to sound when the Sa_{O_2} decreases below an unacceptable level, e.g., 93%, to remind the patient to take a few assisted breaths using a mouthpiece.

Overnight ventilatory assistance is usually needed when the supine VC diminishes to about 30% of predicted (16). However, these individuals often remain free of ventilator use, albeit at the expense of hypercapnia and fatigue, until an intercurrent respiratory tract infection causes acute respiratory failure. During these episodes, bronchial mucus plugging, fatigue, and exacerbated respiratory muscle weakness (51) can necessitate the use of inspiratory muscle aids (noninvasive IPPV) for up to 24 hr a day (17). The use of expiratory muscle aids (52) (manually and mechanically assisted coughing) is also critical if hospitalization, intubation, bronchoscopy, and tracheostomy are to be avoided (53). While using respiratory aids, changes in Sa_{O_2} signal the presence and then the clearance of mucus plugs and the resultant atelectasis; changing values for Sa_{O_2} can also be useful in screening for the onset of clinically significant intrinsic lung disease (53). Finally, nocturnal oximetry is also useful in documenting the effectiveness of nocturnal ventilatory support (16,53,54).

The Inspiratory Muscle Aids

Inspiratory muscle aids are used to provide ventilatory support for up to 24 hr a day as an alternative to endotracheal methods; they also provide deep breaths that facilitate coughing and increase the volume of the voice as well as expand the lungs. Although the rocking bed and negative-pressure body ventilators are noninvasive aids and were the first widely used ventilatory support methods (55), they are now infrequently used for patients with alveolar hypoventilation, except possibly during tracheal extubation and switching to noninvasive IPPV (56). Since noninvasive IPPV methods are better tolerated, more effective, and more convenient, the following discussion will be limited to them.

IPPV delivered via a mouthpiece has been used for many years by many individuals with progressive neuromuscular disorders for ventilatory support (54). The mouthpiece is fixed onto motorized wheelchair chin, tongue, or sip-and-pull controls. For wheelchairs not having these controls, it is positioned adjacent to the mouth, held in place by a gooseneck clamp attachment to the wheelchair frame (Fig. 1). As weakness increases, sometimes guided by oximetry biofeedback (53), many patients require one or more additional hours per day of mouthpiece IPPV use each year to maintain adequate ventilation during daytime hours (57).

Patients usually prefer to use nasal IPPV for nocturnal ventilatory support (58). Nocturnal IPPV is delivered via a comfortable nasal interface. The patient

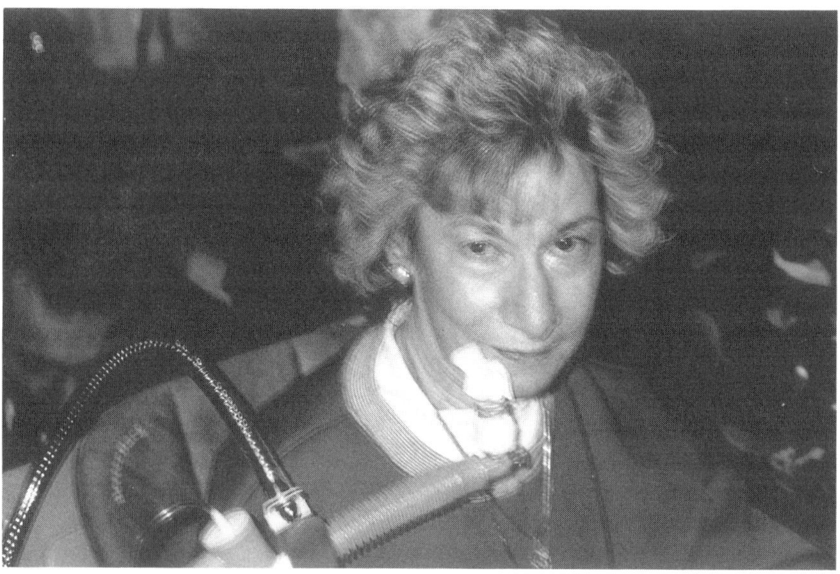

Figure 1 Amyotrophic lateral sclerosis patient with functional bulbar musculature but a vital capacity of 220 ml and no ventilator-free breathing time. She is using mouthpiece IPPV during daytime hours, seen here, and nasal IPPV overnight.

is given the opportunity to try at least three or four varieties of "CPAP masks" in order to find the ones with which he/she is most comfortable (53). A large number of nasal interfaces are now commercially available (Respironics, Monroeville, PA; Puritan-Bennett Inc., Pickering, Ontario; Lifecare International Inc., Westminster, CO; and others). When these interfaces are not well tolerated, custom-molded varieties have to be fabricated (Figs 2. and 3) (58,59). Although usually only preferred for nocturnal use or when the patient is in bed, nasal IPPV has been used up to 24 hr a day by ventilator users whose lips or neck are too weak to accommodate mouthpiece IPPV during the daytime.

Some ventilator users prefer mouthpiece IPPV for use overnight with lipseal retention (Fig. 4) (Puritan-Bennett, Pickering, Ontario) (54). The lipseal can completely seal off the mouth to prevent oral leakage of air delivered by the ventilator (insufflation leakage). In our experience, this technique provides excellent alveolar ventilation during sleep with fewer instances of oxyhe-

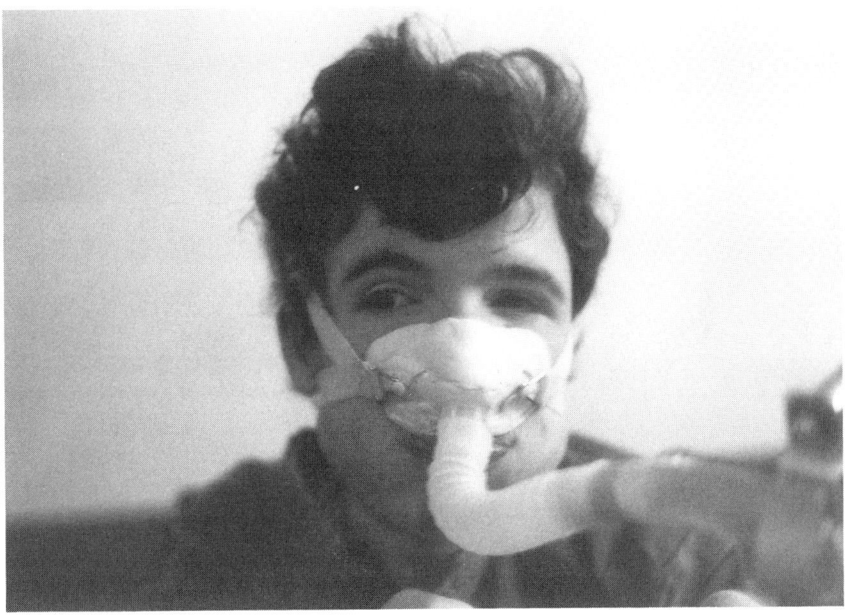

Figure 2 Duchenne muscular dystrophy patient who has required 24-hr ventilatory support for 7 years and currently has less than 2 min of ventilator-free breathing time. Since his lips are too weak to grab a simple mouthpiece, he uses 24-hr nasal IPPV alternating use of various nasal interfaces. Here he is using one of three nasal interface styles custom-molded to his nose (available from Lifecare International Inc., Westminster, CO). He also has a custom-made, molded mouthpiece, which he uses about 2 hr each morning.

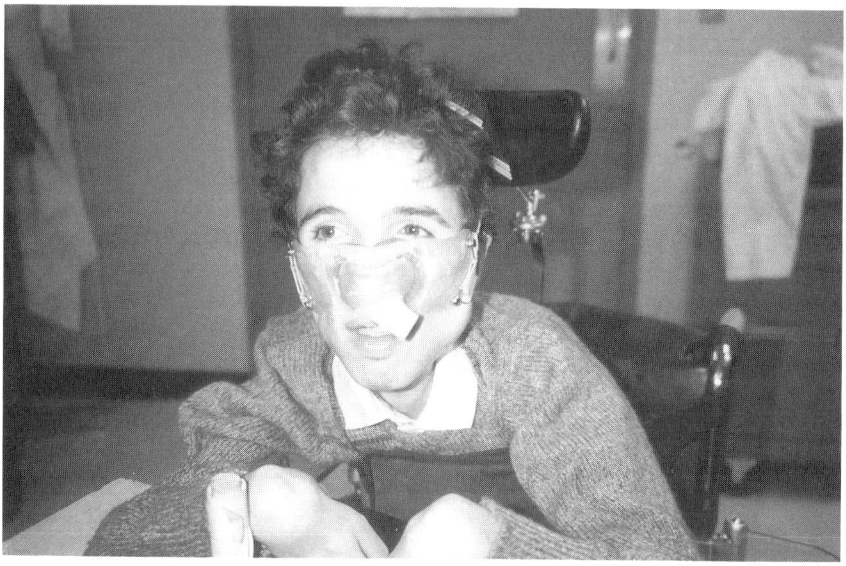

Figure 3 The same patient as in Figure 2 wearing a firm custom, acrylic nasal interface made from a plaster moulage (59).

moglobin desaturation (54); it also improves the quality of sleep. In a few patients, sealing of the nostrils with cotton pledgets has been used to create a closed system of ventilatory support, similar to that of tracheostomy IPPV with an inflated cuff.

In addition to the possibility of offering mouthpiece and nasal IPPV alternatives to intubation and tracheostomy, custom-molded strapless acrylic interfaces, which cover both the nose and mouth, have been used for nocturnal support (59,60). These interfaces are retained by a biteplate that is attached to an outer shell, i.e., essentially an acrylic lip and nose seal; the biteplate can be thrust out of the mouth by a movement of the tongue. This interface is indicated for ventilator users who live alone and who have some upper-extremity function, but insufficient function to don the straps of strap-retained interfaces. The disadvantages of this device are expense and the need for stable dentition.

Noninvasive IPPV can be provided by using pressure-triggered or volume-triggered ventilators. The former include bilevel positive airway pressure (BiPAP) devices. When BiPAP is used, the greater the differential between inspiratory positive airway pressure (IPAP) and the expiratory positive airway pressure (EPAP), the greater the inspiratory muscle support. BiPAP devices have the advantages of being lighter and less expensive than volume-triggered ventilators and lack the annoying, and usually useless, alarm systems of the latter. However, it can be difficult to assess the extent of inspiratory muscle aid by BiPAP since the pressure gauges on the machine indicate the same pressures regardless of whether the patient is receiving adequate tidal volumes. BiPAP is also usually mistakenly used at inadequate IPAP pressures. Moreover, an adapter is needed for the BiPAP machine to be powered by direct current. In general, clinicians with little experience in the use of noninvasive aids should use portable volume ventilators and reserve BiPAP for patients with obstructive apneas or obstructive pulmonary disease for whom the expiratory positive airway pressure may be helpful.

The IAPV or "exsufflation belt" is a respiratory muscle aid that can provide normal alveolar ventilation for some individuals with little or no measurable VC. The IAPV optimizes the appearance, function, and mobility of the patient. It can only be used in the sitting position and in individuals without severe spinal deformity or obesity. It has the advantage of freeing the mouth from mouthpiece IPPV for the performance of ADL by maneuvering objects with a stick on one end in the mouth (mouth stick activities). Tidal volumes up to 1200 ml can be provided by this method (61).

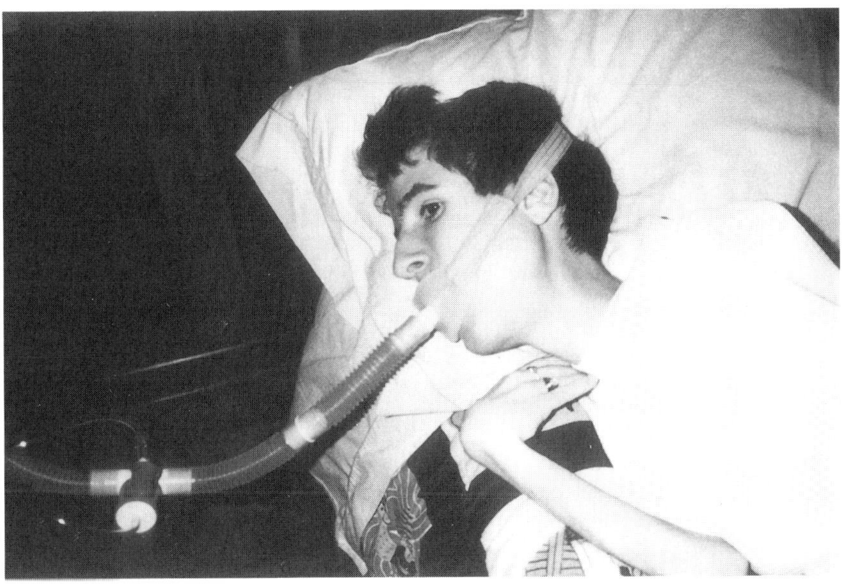

Figure 4 Duchenne muscular dystrophy patient using lipseal (Puritan-Bennett Inc., Pickering, Ontario) IPPV for nocturnal ventilatory support prior to switching to nocturnal nasal IPPV.

The Expiratory Muscle Aids

At least 3 L/sec of peak cough expiratory flow (PCEF) are necessary to eliminate airway secretions effectively (62). PCEF can be increased by delivering precough insufflation volumes that approach the normal precough volumes of 2.3–2.5 L (62,63). Precough insufflation should be provided for individuals in whom the VC is less than 1.5 L (52). After an optimal insufflation and closure of the glottis, cough is manually assisted by an abdominal thrust that is timed to the opening of the glottis. This maneuver can often triple PCEF to levels about 5 L/sec (62). The use of assisted cough is vital during intercurrent respiratory infections and after general anesthesia; it can be necessary long before a patient develops the need for ongoing ventilatory support (3). Assisted coughing techniques are good alternatives to endotracheal suctioning, which can increase secretions and damage the airways. Assisted coughing is less effective in individuals with severe scoliosis or fixed airway obstruction.

Mechanical insufflation-exsufflation (In-Exsufflator, J. H. Emerson Company, Cambridge, MA) involves the use of a device that delivers a deep insufflation (Fig. 5) followed by a rapid exsufflation. Typical pressure drops are

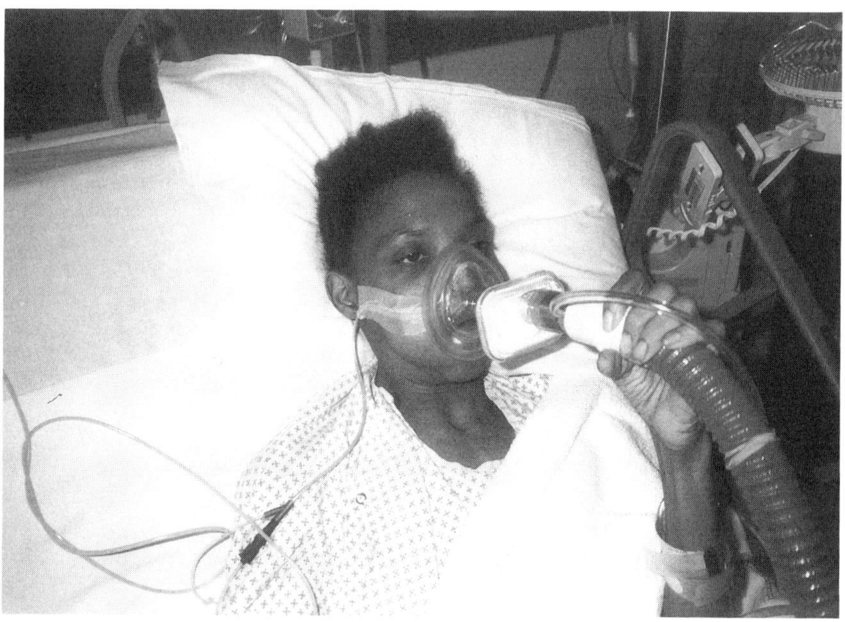

Figure 5 Myasthenia gravis patient self-administering mechanical insufflation-exsufflation. Oxyhemoglobin saturations returned to baseline and vital capacity increased immediately following removal of mucus in this manner.

from 60 to 90 cmH_2O. The resulting 6–10 L/sec of expiratory flow mobilizes airway debris and secretions (62,64–67). The decreases in VC and Sao_2 due to airway mucus plugging are reversed. For most patients an abdominal thrust should also be delivered, timed to the exsufflation phase (52). The insufflation-exsufflation can be delivered via a mask or an endotracheal tube. In the latter case, since routine endotracheal suctioning usually misses the left mainstem bronchus (68), mechanical insufflation-exsufflation can eliminate secretions not accessible to the suction catheter and, thereby, increase postsuctioning pulmonary volumes and Sao_2.

Indications for Tracheostomy

Since noninvasive IPPV is greatly preferred by patients and caregivers with respect to safety, convenience, appearance, comfort, facilitation of speech, sleep, swallowing, and general acceptability, it is always preferable to invasive IPPV (69). Indications for tracheostomy are listed in Table 2.

II. Sudden-Onset Physical and Ventilatory Disability

A. Characterization

The most common causes of sudden-onset, permanent, and severe generalized and pulmonary disability are myelopathies, acute poliomyelitis, and the Guillain-Barré syndrome. Respiratory complications are the most common causes of death in the acute post–spinal cord injury period and account for 14% of overall mortality for SCI individuals (70). The frequency of ventilatory failure in SCI patients, regardless of the level of injury, is 22.6%; ventilatory failure develops, on the average, 4.5 days after admission (72) and lasts for 5 weeks. About 4% of ventilator-supported patients cannot be weaned (56). For SCI tracheostomy IPPV users, mortality by 5 years postdischarge has been reported to be 67% (71).

Of the more than 500,000 people afflicted with paralytic poliomyelitis in the United States from 1928 through 1962 (73), about 15% developed ventila-

Table 2 Contraindications for Long-Term Noninvasive Ventilatory Support

1. Inadequate oropharyngeal muscle function for swallowing or controlling saliva without significant aspiration
2. Significant risk of substance abuse or uncontrolled seizures
3. Inability to cooperate
4. Intrinsic lung disease necessitating supplemental oxygen therapy
5. Orthopedic impediments to IPPV interface use
6. Assisted or unassisted peak cough expiratory flows that fail to exceed 3 L/sec

tory failure, severe impairment of swallowing, or both (74). About 12.5% of these remained ventilator-assisted (74). Late-onset ventilatory failure has been considered in Section I.

B. The Physical Medicine Interventions

The same general medical considerations as those noted in Section I apply to patients who have experienced the sudden onset of physical and ventilatory disability discussed in the preceding paragraphs. Patients with high-level SCI and postpoliomyelitis may also require nutritional intervention because of dysphagia due to bulbar muscle dysfunction.

SCI individuals usually have neurogenic bowels and bladders. A neurogenic bladder can be managed by using an indwelling catheter or intermittent catheterizations. The use of indwelling catheters is associated with a higher incidence of infections; the use of intermittent catheterizations requires much more of the caregivers. Use of a condom catheter drainage system is useful for patients who are incontinent between intermittent catheterizations as well as for severely disabled individuals who are not incontinent. Postvoiding residual volumes are used to establish an appropriate schedule for intermittent catheterizations.

Skin pressure ulcers are the most prevalent postinjury complication in these individuals and interfere the most with ADL. These patients also have a high incidence of cardiac, infectious, circulatory, and gastrointestinal complications. Heterotopic ossification occurs in up to 53% of patients (75). Neuropathic pain, lower-extremity fractures, autonomic dysreflexia, contractures, spasticity, and, less frequently, posttraumatic syringomyelia are other potential problems that require intervention. Rehabilitation efforts are directed at optimizing mobility, environmental control, and ADL, adaptive equipment utilization, bladder and bowel management, coping skills, and community reintegration, and minimizing contractures, spasticity, and other impediments to rehabilitation. For discussion of the many potential rehabilitation interventions for these patients, the reader is referred to more comprehensive sources (76).

C. The Respiratory Interventions

Since most SCI patients who experience ventilatory failure do so 12 hr or more following admission to intensive care units, intubation can be avoided provided there are no contraindications for noninvasive ventilatory support (Table 2). Unless there is a history of recent pneumothorax, patients with decreasing VC are placed on regular maximum tolerated insufflations via a mouthpiece for lung expansion; with decreasing VC, spirometry is performed 3 times a day and oximetry is monitored continuously. If dyspnea and hypercapnia supervene, the patient is supported by mouthpiece or nasal IPPV with frequent sighs as reported in Section I. The administration of O_2-enriched air is avoided unless the mean Sao_2 drops below 90%, the Po_2 is below 60 mmHg, or hypoxia-associated bradycardias occur; intubation may then be indicated. Continuous Sao_2 monitoring can be an adequate gauge of the effectiveness of assisted or unassisted alveolar ventilation if no supplemental oxygen is being administered; when supplemental oxygen is being given, continuous end-tidal CO_2 monitoring or transcutaneous P_{CO_2} monitoring is useful. In general, hypercapnia should be reversed by assisting inspiratory muscles, before oxygen administration is considered. For nocturnal ventilatory support, nasal IPPV or mouthpiece IPPV with lipseal retention is used as previously described. The lipseal straps can be conveniently attached to the posterior posters of a halo or four-poster cervical stabilization brace (56). Airway secretions must be aggressively eliminated by manually assisted coughing, mechanically assisted coughing, or both as described above.

Transorally or transnasally intubated ventilator-supported SCI patients may be candidates for transition to noninvasive aids irrespective of the degree of ventilatory failure. For patients with little or no ventilator free breathing time, the use of a negative-pressure body ventilator may facilitate the transition. The chest shell ventilator is most convenient for this purpose, especially for SCI patients who have no bowel control and for whom a wrap ventilator would be inconvenient. The Porta-lung and iron lung are more effective alternatives to the chest shell ventilator. The effectiveness of the assisted ventilation should be documented by monitoring the blood gases noninvasively. Contraindications to switching to noninvasive IPPV are the same as those noted in Table 2. In addition, placement of a nasogastric tube must be avoided. This tube would hamper the effectiveness of noninvasive IPPV by interfering with closure of the pharynx by the soft palate, with the seal at the nose, with the placement of nasal interfaces, and would increase the risk of abdominal distension.

For the tracheostomized patient, a fenestrated tracheostomy tube is placed. During trials of noninvasive ventilatory aids with the tube capped, the fenestration decreases obstruction to airflow in the upper airways. The use of a negative-pressure body ventilator during extubation can provide adequate alveolar ventilation while the patient is learning noninvasive IPPV techniques and expedite closure of the tracheostomy site. Airway suctioning is minimized or avoided for intubated or tracheostomized patients in favor of manually and mechanically assisted coughing, including exsufflation via the tracheostomy tube.

Some ventilator-free breathing time is helpful for transferring tracheostomized IPPV users directly to noninvasive IPPV without the temporary use of body ventilators (77,78). The effectiveness of noninvasive IPPV is documented by both daytime and nocturnal monitoring of the Sao_2. Once the noninvasive

IPPV has proved to be effective, the tube is removed and a tracheostomy button (Olympic Medical, Seattle, WA) placed. Immediately following button placement, PCEF should be evaluated; after it has been shown to exceed 3 L/sec and noninvasive IPPV has been well tolerated for 24 hr, the button is removed and the site is permitted to close. Once it is closed, the patient is trained in the use of glossopharyngeal breathing (GPB).

The use of noninvasive IPPV methods and mechanically assisted coughing can also facilitate weaning from the ventilator for those who can be weaned (56). In addition, an abdominal binder may be useful to increase diaphragmatic excursion and the VC in seated patients with spinal cord injury.

III. The Remitting or Recurring Conditions

The most common remitting or recurring conditions that lend themselves to the interventions of physical medicine are multiple sclerosis, myasthenia gravis, polymyositis, and Guillain-Barré syndrome.

The characterization of these varied conditions and the possible physical medicine interventions are beyond the scope of this chapter (29). The respiratory interventions are similar to those discussed in the previous sections.

IV. Conclusion

In summary, tracheostomy and intubation are rarely necessary unless PCEF cannot exceed 3 L/sec whether by unassisted or assisted coughing. Noninvasive IPPV methods are the preferred methods of ventilatory support by patients and caregivers and can greatly reduce the cost of mechanical ventilation in the home (79). Adaptive equipment and other assistive devices can improve the ADL for even the most severely affected individuals. The great majority of ventilator users with paralytic/restrictive pulmonary conditions experience considerable satisfaction from life, much of which derives from interpersonal relationships but some of which derives from the attainment of personal goals. Clinicians should recognize their inability to gauge the satisfaction with life that can be achieved by disabled individuals who require ventilator assistance and refrain from letting inaccurate judgment of achievable quality of life misdirect their decisions about how such patients should be managed.

References

1. DeVivo MJ, Black EJ, Stover SL. Causes of death during the first 12 years after spinal cord injury. Arch Phys Med Rehabil 1993; 74:248–254.

2. Bach JR. Ventilator use by muscular dystrophy association patients: an update. Arch Phys Med Rehabil 1992; 73:179–183.
3. Bach JR. Amyotrophic lateral sclerosis: communication status and survival with ventilatory support. Am J Phys Med Rehabil 1993; 72:343–349.
4. Brooke MH, Fenichel GM, Griggs RC, et al. Duchenne muscular dystrophy: patterns of clinical progression and effects of supportive therapy. Neurology 1989; 39:475–481.
5. Rideau Y, Gatin G, Bach J, Gines G. Prolongation of life in Duchenne muscular dystrophy. Acta Neurol 1983; 5:118–124.
6. Bach JR, Alba AS. Pulmonary dysfunction and sleep disordered breathing as post-polio sequelae: evaluation and management. Orthopedics 1991; 14:1329–1337.
7. Bach JR. Inappropriate weaning and late-onset ventilatory failure of individuals with traumatic quadriplegia. Paraplegia 1993; 31:430–438.
8. Wang TG, Bach JR, Avilez C, Alba AS, Yang, GF. Survival of individuals with spinal muscular atrophy on ventilatory support. Am J Phys Med Rehabil 1994; 73:207–211.
9. Hamilton EA, Nichols PJR, Tait GBW. Late-onset of respiratory insufficiency after poliomyelitis. Ann Phys Med 1970; 10:223–229.
10. Fischer DA. Poliomyelitis: late respiratory complications and management. Orthopedics 1985; 8:891–894.
11. Howard RS, Wiles CM, Spencer GT. The late sequelae of poliomyelitis. Q J Med 1988; 66:219–232.
12. Halstead LS, Wiechers DO, Rossi CD. Late effects of poliomyelitis: a national survey: In: Halstead LS, Wiechers DO, eds. Late Effects of Poliomyelitis. Miami: Symposia Foundation, 1985:11–31.
13. Bach JR. Pulmonary rehabilitation. In: Delisa JD, ed. Rehabilitation Medicine: Principles and Practice. Philadelphia: JB Lippincott, 1993:952–972.
14. Goldstein M, Meyer S, Freund HR. Effects of overfeeding in children with muscle dystrophies. J Parenter Enter Nutr 1989; 13:603–607.
15. Bach JR. Pulmonary rehabilitation in neuromuscular disorders. Semin Respir Med 1993; 14:515–529.
16. Bach JR, Alba AS. Management of chronic alveolar hypoventilation by nasal ventilation. Chest 1990; 97:52–57.
17. Bach JR. Update and perspectives on noninvasive respiratory muscle aids. Part 1. The inspiratory muscle aids. Chest 1994; 105:1230–1240.
18. Kirshblum SC, Bach JR. Walker modification for ventilator assisted individuals. Am J Phys Med Rehabil 1992; 71:304–306.
19. Spencer GE. Orthopaedic care of progressive muscular dystrophy. J Bone Joint Surg-A 1967; 49:1201–1204.
20. Roy L, Gibson DA. Pseudohypertrophic muscular dystrophy and its surgical management: review of 30 patients. Can J Surg 1970; 13:13–20.
21. Bach JR, McKeon J. Orthopedic surgery and rehabilitation for the prolongation of brace-free ambulation of patients with Duchenne muscular dystrophy. Am J Phys Med Rehabil 1991; 70:323–331.
22. Rideau Y, Delaubier A, Guillou C. Duport G. Prolongation d'une stade de vie

proche de la normale: premiers reculs de l'évolution de la dystrophie musculaire de Duchenne. Cah Kinésithér 1988; 133:22–29.
23. Rideau Y, Glorion B, Delaubier A, Tarle O, Bach J. Treatment of scoliosis in Duchenne muscular dystrophy. Muscle Nerve 1984; 7:281–286.
24. Dangain J, Vrbova G. Response of normal and dystrophic muscles to increased function demand. Exp Neurol 1986; 94:796–801.
25. Johnson EW, Braddom R. Over-work weakness in facioscapulohumeral muscular dystrophy. Arch Phys Med Rehabil 1971; 52:333–336.
26. Bélanger AY, Noël G, Côté C. A comparison of contractile properties in the preferred and non-preferred leg in a mixed sample of dystrophic patients. Am J Phys Med Rehabil (in press).
27. Milner-Brown HS, Miller RG. Muscle strengthening through high-resistance weight training in patients with neuromuscular disorders. Arch Phys Med Rehabil 1988; 69:14–19.
28. Fowler WM Jr. Management of musculoskeletal complications in neuromuscular diseases: weaknesses and the role of exercise. Phys Med Rehabil S-T-A-Rs 1988; 2:489–507.
29. Smith MB. Physical therapy and management of neuromuscular disease. In: Maloney FP, Burks JS, Ringel SP, eds. Interdisciplinary Rehabilitation of Multiple Sclerosis and Neuromuscular Disorders. Philadelphia: JB Lippincott, 1985:239–258.
30. Brammell CA. Assistive devices for patients with neuromuscular diseases: the role of occupational therapy. In: Maloney FP, Burks JS, Ringel SP, eds. Interdisciplinary Rehabilitation of Multiple Sclerosis and Neuromuscular Disorders. Philadelphia: JB Lippincott, 1985:259–276.
31. Bach JR, Zeelenberg A, Winter C. Wheelchair mounted robot manipulators: long-term use by patients with Duchenne muscular dystrophy. Am J Phys Med Rehabil 1990; 69:59–69.
32. Siegel IM. Update on Duchenne muscular dystrophy. Comprehens Ther 1989; 15:45–54.
33. Bach JR, Campagnolo DI, Hoeman S. Life satisfaction of individuals with Duchenne muscular dystrophy using long-term mechanical ventilatory support. Am J Phys Med Rehabil 1991; 70:129–135.
34. Bach JR, Campagnolo D. Psychosocial adjustment of postpoliomyelitis ventilator assisted individuals. Arch Phys Med Rehabil 1992; 73:934–939.
35. Anderson F, Bardach J, Goodgold J. Sexuality and neuromuscular disease. In: Rehabilitation Monograph No 56. New York: Institute of Rehabilitation Medicine, 1979.
36. Purtilo R. Ethical issues in the treatment of chronic ventilator-dependent patients. Arch Phys Med Rehabil 1986; 67:718–721.
37. Aldrich JK, Karpel JP, Uhrlass RM, Sparapani MA, Eramo D, Ferranti R. Weaning from mechanical ventilation: adjunctive use of inspiratory muscle resistive training. Crit Care Med 1989; 17:143–147.
38. DiMarco AF, Kelling JS, DiMarco MS, Jacobs I, Shields R, Altose MD. The effects of inspiratory resistive training on respiratory muscle function in patients with muscular dystrophy. Muscle Nerve 1985; 8:284–290.

39. Rodillo E, Noble-Jamieson CM, Aber V, Heckmatt JZ, Muntoni F, Dubowitz. Respiratory muscle training in Duchenne muscular dystrophy. Arch Dis Child 1989; 64:736–738.
40. Martin AJ, Stern L, Yeates J, Lepp D, Little J. Respiratory muscle training in Duchenne muscular dystrophy. Dev Med Child Neurol 1986; 28:314–318.
41. Schiffman PL, Belsh JM. Effect of inspiratory resistance and theophylline on respiratory muscle strength in patients with amyotrophic lateral sclerosis. Am Rev Respir Dis 1989; 139:1418–1423.
42. Sinha R, Bergofsky EH. Prolonged alteration of lung mechanics in kyphoscoliosis by positive pressure hyperinflation. Am Rev Respir Dis 1972; 106:47–57.
43. DeTroyer A, Deisser P. The effects of intermittent positive pressure breathing on patients with respiratory muscle weakness. Am Rev Respir Dis 1981; 124:132–137.
44. Bach JR, Alba AS, Bodofsky E, Curran FJ, Schultheiss M. Glossopharyngeal breathing and noninvasive aids in the management of postpolio respiratory insufficiency. Birth Defects 1987; 23:99–113.
45. O'Donohue W. Maximum volume IPPB for the management of pulmonary atelectasis. Chest 1976; 76:683–687.
46. Huldtgren AC, Fugl-Meyer AR, Jonasson E, Bake B. Ventilatory dysfunction and respiratory rehabilitation in post-traumatic quadriplegia. Eur J Respir Dis 1980; 61:347–356.
47. Houser CR, Johnson DM. Breathing exercises for children with pseudohypertrophic muscular dystrophy. Phys Ther 1971; 51:751–759.
48. Adams MA, Chandler LS. Effects of physical therapy program on vital capacity of patients with muscular dystrophy. Phys Ther 1974; 54:494–496.
49. Dail CW, Affeldt JE. Glossopharyngeal Breathing (video). Los Angeles: Los Angeles Department of Visual Education, College of Medical Evangelists, 1954.
50. Dail C, Rogers M, Guess V, Atkins HV. Glossopharyngeal Breathing Manual. Downey, CA: Professional Staff Association of Rancho Los Amigos Hospital, 1979.
51. Mier-Jedrzejowicz A, Brophy C, Green M. Respiratory muscle weakness during upper respiratory tract infections. Am Rev Respir Dis 1988; 138:5–7.
52. Bach JR. Update and perspectives on noninvasive respiratory muscle aids. Part 2. The expiratory muscle aids. Chest 1994; 105:1538–1544.
53. Bach JR. Pulmonary rehabilitation considerations for Duchenne muscular dystrophy: the prolongation of life by respiratory muscle aids. Crit Rev Phys Rehabil Med 1992; 3:239–269.
54. Bach JR, Alba AS, Saporito LR. Intermittent positive pressure ventilation via the mouth as an alternative to tracheostomy for 257 ventilator users. Chest 1993; 103:174–182.
55. Bach JR. Prevention of morbidity and mortality with the use of physical medicine aids. In: Bach JR, ed. Pulmonary Rehabilitation: The Obstructive and Paralytic/Restrictive Syndromes. Philadelphia: Hanley & Belfus (in press).
56. Bach JR. Alternative methods of ventilatory support for the patient with ventilatory failure due to spinal cord injury. J Am Parapleg Soc 1991; 14:158–174.
57. Curran FJ, Colbert AP. Ventilator management in Duchenne muscular dystrophy

and postpoliomyelitis syndrome; twelve years' experience. Arch Phys Med Rehabil 1989; 70:180–185.
58. Bach JR, Sortor S, Saporito LR. Interfaces for noninvasive intermittent positive pressure ventilatory support in North America. Eur Respir Rev 1993; 3:254–259.
59. McDermott I, Bach JR, Parker C, Sortor S. Custom fabricated interfaces for intermittent positive pressure ventilation. Int J Prosthodont 1989; 2:224–233.
60. Bach JR, McDermott I. Strapless oral nasal interfaces for positive pressure ventilation. Arch Phys Med Rehabil 1990; 71:908–911.
61. Bach JR, Alba AS. Total ventilatory support by the intermittent abdominal pressure ventilator. Chest 1991; 99:630–636.
62. Bach JR. Mechanical insufflation-exsufflation: comparison of peak expiratory flows with manually assisted and unassisted coughing techniques. Chest 1993; 104:1553–1562.
63. Leith DE. Cough. In: Brain JD, Proctor D, Reid L, eds. Lung Biology in Health and Disease: Respiratory Defense Mechanisms. Part 2. New York: Marcel Dekker, 1977:545–592.
64. Barach AL, Beck GJ, Bickerman HA, Seanor HE. Physical methods simulating cough mechanisms. JAMA 1952; 150:1380–1385.
65. Sortor S, McKenzie M. Toward Independence: Assisted Cough (video). Dallas: Bioscience Communications of Dallas, 1986.
66. Barach AL, Beck GJ, Smith RH. Mechanical production of expiratory flow rates surpassing the capacity of human coughing. J Med Sci 1953; 226:241–248.
67. Bach JR. Mechanical exsufflation, noninvasive ventilation, and new strategies for pulmonary rehabilitation and sleep disordered breathing. Bull NY Acad Med 1992; 68:321–340.
68. Fishburn MJ, Marino RJ, Ditunno JF Jr. Atelectasis and pneumonia in acute spinal cord injury. Arch Phys Med Rehabil 90; 71:197–200.
69. Bach JR. A comparison of long-term ventilatory support alternatives from the perspective of the patient and care giver. Chest 1993; 104:1702–1706.
70. Higgins ITT. Epidemiology of bronchitis and emphysema. In: Fishman AP, ed. Pulmonary Diseases and Disorders, 2nd ed. New York: McGraw-Hill, 1988:70–90.
71. Wicks AB, Menter RR. Long-term outlook in quadriplegic patients with initial ventilator dependency. Chest 1986; 90:406–410.
72. Jackson AB, Groomes TE. Incidence of respiratory complications following spinal cord injury. Arch Phys Med Rehabil 1994; 75:270–275.
73. Historical Statistics of the United States: Colonial Times to 1970, Bicentennial Edition, Part 1. Washington, DC: U.S. Department of Commerce, Bureau of the Census. 1975:8,77.
74. Lassen HCA. The epidemic of poliomyelitis in Copenhagen, 1952. Proc R Soc Med 1953; 47:67–71.
75. Venier LH, Ditunno JF Jr. Heterotopic ossification in the paraplegic patient. Arch Phys Med Rehabil 1971; 52:475–479.
76. Staas WE, Formal CS, Gershkoff AM, et al. Rehabilitation of the spinal cord injured patient. In: DeLisa JA, ed. Rehabilitation Medicine: Principles and Practice, 2nd ed. Philadelphia: JB Lippincott, 1993:886–915.

77. Bach JR, Alba AS. Noninvasive options for ventilatory support of the traumatic high level quadriplegic. Chest 1990; 98:613–619.
78. Bach JR. New approaches in the rehabilitation of the traumatic high level quadriplegic. Am J Phys Med Rehabil 1991; 70:13–20.
79. Bach JR, Intintola P, Alba AS, Holland I. The ventilator-assisted individual: cost analysis of institutionalization versus rehabilitation and in-home management. Chest 1992; 101:26–30.

31

Pulmonary Rehabilitation in the Intensive Care Unit

KATHY LEE BISHOP

University of Pennsylvania Medical Center
Philadelphia, Pennsylvania

Traditional pulmonary rehabilitation was developed to meet the needs of the individual with chronic obstructive pulmonary disease (1,2). Originally, pulmonary rehabilitation programs were designed for outpatients. But, in time, pulmonary rehabilitation programs were tailored to accommodate the needs of a small subset of patients with neuromuscular diseases and of patients with restrictive pulmonary diseases (3,4). The early rehabilitative literature dealing with the poliomyelitis epidemic describes physiotherapists, physicians, and nurses working to help patients regain pulmonary function (5–8). The poliomyelitis epidemic provided a wealth of understanding about the capability of critically ill patients to achieve a higher level of function and may have been the foundation for all types of pulmonary rehabilitation.

This chapter deals with the pulmonary rehabilitation of the critically ill patient in the current intensive care and step-down units. Pulmonary rehabilitation is envisioned as beginning as early as the first week of admission to the intensive care unit and continued through the step-down unit into the outpatient setting.

I. The Intensive Care Unit

The intensive care unit is a unique environment for pulmonary rehabilitation. The setting is a far cry from the traditional outpatient setting for pulmonary rehabilitation. Moreover, the patients are usually desperately ill with either cardiac or pulmonary diseases and disorders that are life-threatening.

One common disorder found in the intensive care unit is exacerbation of chronic obstructive lung disease that requires intubation for management. Adult respiratory distress syndrome represents another type of pulmonary disorder in the intensive care unit. The underlying disease in patients with the adult respiratory distress syndrome can vary from surgical to medical or be the result of complications following trauma. In addition, cardiac patients admitted to the intensive care unit are likely to be in severe congestive heart failure, frequently complicated by severe arrhythmias. As a rule, with the exception of patients in severe chronic congestive heart failure, cardiac patients are more intact functionally than are those with pulmonary diseases. In pulmonary patients, shortness of breath and physical inactivity have generally led to severe curtailment of the activities of daily life, often complicated by a progressive decline in functional state due to drugs, e.g., corticosteroids, and malnutrition. In contrast, the patient who has recently suffered a myocardial infarction complicated by an episode of congestive heart failure has usually led an active life before the acute episode.

II. Early Mobilization

A major goal of the rehabilitation process is early mobilization. The initial step en route to ambulation is sitting up in bed, followed by sitting in a chair. In addition to avoiding the ill effects of prolonged inactivity, there are several advantages to early out of bed to chair activity, e.g., fewer difficulties with fluid shifts from the periphery to the lungs, and improvements in ventilation, mobilization of secretions, and well-being (9–12). Although the vigor of early ambulation depends on the individual's hemodynamic status, early, not late, mobilization is the mainstay of rehabilitation (9). Unstable arrhythmias, especially those that are symptomatic, or inadequate responses of the blood pressure or heart rate to an orthostatic challenge signal that early ambulation may not always be as feasible as would be desired.

The benefits of early mobilization in patients following coronary bypass graft surgery were shown in a study by Chulay et al. (13). Particular attention was paid to postoperative complications such as atelectasis. The study demonstrated an increase in the frequency of postoperative fever in patients who were not turned as frequently as those in the study. Also, the patients in the study spent less time in the surgical intensive care unit.

III. The Patient with Respiratory Failure

Early mobilization and ambulation have important roles in the care of patients with respiratory failure. Early ambulation of patients in respiratory failure who require prolonged ventilation helps to prevent muscle wasting, thromboembolism, and decubitus ulcers (14). "Aggressive mobilization and frequent position changes" have been suggested in the management of atelectasis and pneumonia (11). Specific exercises have been proposed as a primary tool in the care of patients with pneumonia (15). The effectiveness of these exercises was shown by increases in vital capacity, improvement in ventilation and oxygenation, and improved function of the cardiovascular system, i.e., lower heart rates and greater normalization of blood pressure. As these studies show, early mobilization, in the form of either repositioning in the bed, out of bed activity, or early ambulation, appears to be the key in improving health status and in preventing certain complications.

IV. The Patient with Difficulty in Weaning

The patient in the intensive care unit most likely to benefit from rehabilitation is one who has resisted weaning from the ventilator after prolonged ventilation. The pulmonary patient who is refractory to weaning often has one or more major problems: chronic airway obstruction, pneumonia, pneumonitis related to aspiration, pulmonary collapse related to complications of a neuromuscular disease, or some combination of the above. Not infrequently, the medical problem(s) is complicated by the side effects of corticosteroids, i.e., steroid myopathy, poor skin integrity, and osteoporosis, and the untoward consequences of prolonged bed rest, i.e., muscle wasting. Because of their multisystem involvement, these patients are a challenge to wean because of the balance that must be struck between the demands imposed by each abnormal system and the limited ability of the respiratory pump to meet these demands. Respiratory muscle fatigue during weaning is often the first sign of this imbalance, generally preceding abnormalities in the arterial blood gases or hemodynamics. Many of these individuals can be categorized as "older, debilitated, and/or sicker patients" with underlying disorders, such as chronic obstructive pulmonary disease, obesity, complications of cardiac surgery, or chronic congestive heart failure (16).

The cardiac patient who is resistant to weaning poses distinctive problems. One type of problem is exemplified by the patient who has undergone surgery for coronary artery disease and has developed multiple postoperative complications, i.e., a pseudoaneurysm after removal of the intra-aortic balloon pump, cryogenic damage to the phrenic nerve intraoperatively, or a poorly healing sternum due to infection. A patient with cardiac disease may have persistent arrhythmias that make it difficult to achieve the stable hemodynamic status required for mobilization. In addition, this patient often manifests limited mobility of the chest wall and limited use of the upper extremities because of the weight-bearing restrictions necessary to protect a poorly healing sternum. Such complications after surgery may prolong the need for mechanical ventilation and, because of orthostatic difficulties, inadequate hemodynamic responses to exercise, and overall weak muscles, hinder the progression of activities.

A final example of patients who require prolonged mechanical ventilation and benefit from pulmonary rehabilitation is a small subset of patients previously treated with corticosteroids. Isolated patients will develop quadriparesis following administration of sedatives and paralytics. The muscle abnormalities range from minor weakness to gross absence of muscle contraction. These deficits affect weaning, prolong stays in the intensive care unit or step-down unit, and directly influence the patient's psychological and functional levels. The primary diseases vary considerably in this subset of patients, influencing both functional recovery and the weaning process.

The patients who require prolonged ventilation and have difficulty weaning are likely to benefit from the team approach that characterizes rehabilitation medicine. This approach includes setting goals, outlining a plan, and coordinating the therapeutic program to take into account the needs of the patient with respect to weaning, nutrition, bowel and bladder functions, activities of daily living (bathing, shaving, eating), and functional activities (transfers out of bed to the commode, sitting time in a chair, ambulation in the hall).

V. Comparison Studies on the Intensive Care Unit

Two studies are relevant in reporting the outcomes of pulmonary rehabilitation in the intensive care unit. The first study, by Spicher and White, found that age and functional level prior to development of respiratory failure had the greatest impact on survival. Prolonged mechanical ventilation (longer than 10 days) was associated with poor functional outcome and limited survival (17). The patients with chronic obstructive pulmonary disease had the worst prognosis. The second study, by Gracey et al., found that the total number of days supported by mechanical ventilation did not influence survival in patients over 16 years of age, after the patients had survived greater than 7 days (18). The major difference between the two studies is the patient population. The Spicher and White study had a predominance of patients with respiratory failure secondary to chronic obstructive pulmonary disease, while Gracey et al. reported on postsurgical patients with respiratory failure.

The differences between the results of the two studies underscore the importance of defining the patient population that would benefit from a pulmonary rehabilitation program in the intensive care unit. The age of the patient, the length of time on mechanical ventilation, and the functional status of the patient before hospitalization may influence the outcome of a rehabilitation program.

VI. The Team Approach to Rehabilitation in the Intensive Care Unit

An essential ingredient of the rehabilitation process is that the management of each patient be individualized. In principle, the rehabilitation team consists of the patient, the patient's family or support system, the chest physician or intensivist, the primary care nurse, the respiratory therapist, the physical therapist, the occupational therapist, the speech-language pathologist, the pharmacist, the psychiatrist, the social worker, and the dietitian. The orthotist and physiatrist may also play a role depending on patient need and facility staffing. Not all patients require intervention of the full team. Indeed, in many instances, the "team" consists of the physician, the patient, the family, the nurse, a respiratory therapist, and/or a physical therapist. The nature and vigor of the intervention are determined, in large measure, by the state of the patient, i.e., hemodynamic stability, the extent of functional recovery, and the patient's alertness and ability to participate in the program.

VII. Goals

For the patient who is difficult to wean, the rehabilitation team participates in the weaning process by helping to formulate the plan of care for the day or week. The plan for the day may consist of functional activities early in the morning, followed by a rest period before initiation of the weaning process in the optimal postural position, i.e., sitting upright in bed or sitting upright in the chair. Another rest period is interposed before functional activities are resumed in the afternoon. This program enables the team to evaluate the level of stress that the plan will impose on the patient. Potential sources of stress include the weaning schedule, activities of daily living (eating, washing, shaving, toilet training), functional activities (bed mobility, transfers out of bed to chair, and ambulation), sleep pattern, the effects of medications, and nutritional influences (feeding by mouth or via a tube). The rehabilitation team evaluates the energy cost of each activity and assesses the demand of each activity on the patient. As noted previously, a proper balance of supply and demand on the respiratory pump helps the patient to wean. Conversely, an overzealous activity program places too much demand on the patient and slows the weaning process.

The plan for rehabilitation also addresses prevention and amelioration of the deleterious effects of bed rest, communication, emotional support, psychological well-being, and function. The team plan and goals are helpful to the patient and the patient's support system by tailoring the discharge plan of the patient to the needs of the patient and family. The patient is expected to play an active role in establishing the specific goals and plan.

Examples of specific goals that are addressed by the physical therapist are the promotion of skin integrity and the prevention of a decrease in range of motion. These goals can be achieved by educating staff and family members to assist with positioning and by the use of techniques to prevent, or slow, the progression of muscle atrophy and loss of range. Proper positioning also helps to improve ventilation and oxygenation by improving chest wall excursion, mobilization of secretions, cough effectiveness, and clearance of secretions (11,19–21). The physical therapist also plays a prominent role in setting goals for the rate of improvement in function and in the selection of assistive devices.

Figure 1a–d illustrates the activity and ventilatory progress of patients who were categorized as difficult to wean. Figure 1a represents an initial phase in the process of weaning, i.e., when the patient is off the ventilator during activity. Before this stage, the patient had exercised on the ventilator in the room and had shown no need to increase ventilator settings; she had also demonstrated an appropriate ventilatory and hemodynamic response, i.e., an increase of less than 4–5 breaths/min; no increase in the use of accessory muscles or nasal flaring; no paradoxical breathing pattern; an increase in heart rate of less than 10 beats/min; stable or slightly increased systolic blood pressure. These criteria indicate that the patient is ready for intensification of activity during the weaning process.

The use of assistive devices during graded increase in activity is patient-specific. For example, the rolling platform walker shown in Figure 1b allows the patient to lean forward and to take some body weight off weakened lower extremities. In some cases, it enables the patient to adopt a more comfortable breathing pattern. The rolling walker also allows a more normal gait pattern than does the standard walker, which requires that the patient use the upper extremities to lift and place the walker forward. Steps with a standard walker are stop-and-go and may add to the work done by the patient in lifting the walker. As seen in Figure 1b, the patient may need an orthosis for footdrop secondary to muscle wasting in order to ambulate. A manual respirator that increases the fraction of oxygen inspired can be useful in decreasing the work of breathing for the patient not only during the initial sessions off the ventilator, but also during more demanding functional activities, such as walking in the hallway.

Figure 1c and 1d demonstrate continued progress in the ventilatory and functional levels. In figure 1c the patient no longer requires the orthosis, showing that musculoskeletal strength has improved, and the patient is able to tolerate the physical and respiratory demands of a standard walker. Ventilatory support has been progressively decreased, so the patient now uses a tracheostomy mask that delivers lower concentrations of inspired oxygen. Prior to discharge, the patient had progressed to the use of a cane, as shown in figure 1d. The tracheostomy has been closed and the patient is stair climbing in preparation for discharge from the hospital.

VIII. Obstacles for the Rehabilitation Team in the Intensive Care Unit

The rehabilitation team, including the physical therapist, may have to overcome a variety of obstacles in order to deal appropriately with a particular patient in the intensive care unit. For example, because of isolation procedures, nosocomial pneumonia and hospital-borne infections may confine the patient to activities in the room (22,23). Aspiration and its complications may also slow or delay the rehabilitation process. Therefore, the proper positioning of the patient who has poor trunk and neck support or poor oral motor function is important in preventing aspiration. The speech-language pathologist, nutritionist, and nurse have to cooperate closely to protect the patient who is prone to aspiration.

The ability to clear secretions from the airway changes as the patient progresses from airway suction while on mechanical ventilation to active expectoration of secretions after decanulation. Different requirements have to be met at each step. For example, although suctioning temporarily interferes with breathing and tires the patient, it must be done faithfully while the endotracheal tube and the tracheostomy tube are in place since allowing secretions to collect predisposes the patient to an increase in the work of breathing (24–26). This increase in the work of breathing may then limit the activity session and subsequent weaning attempts during a given day. Chest physical therapy is a mainstay for this population of patients. The staff that administers chest physical therapy varies from hospital to hospital. In some hospitals the chest physical therapy is done by respiratory therapists; in others, by nurses or physical therapists.

For the patient who is being mechanically ventilated, communication with support personnel and family depends on either mouthing words, or a word board, or gestures. All who are involved become frustrated if needs can-

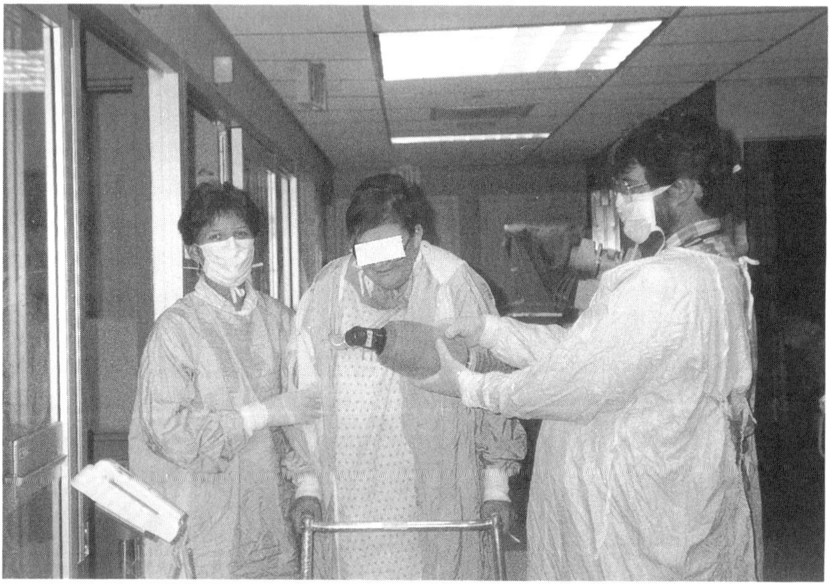

(a)

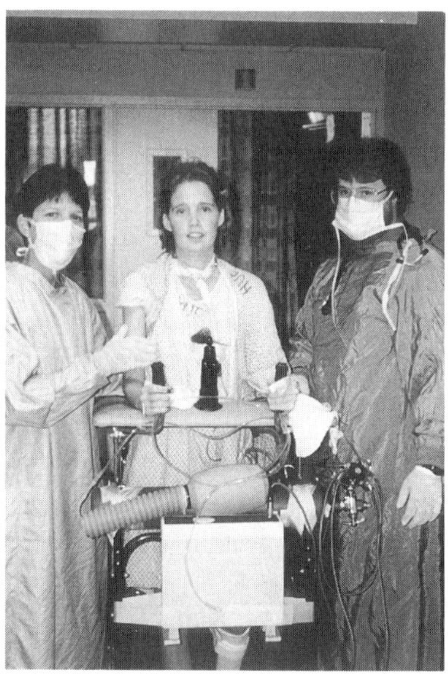

(b)

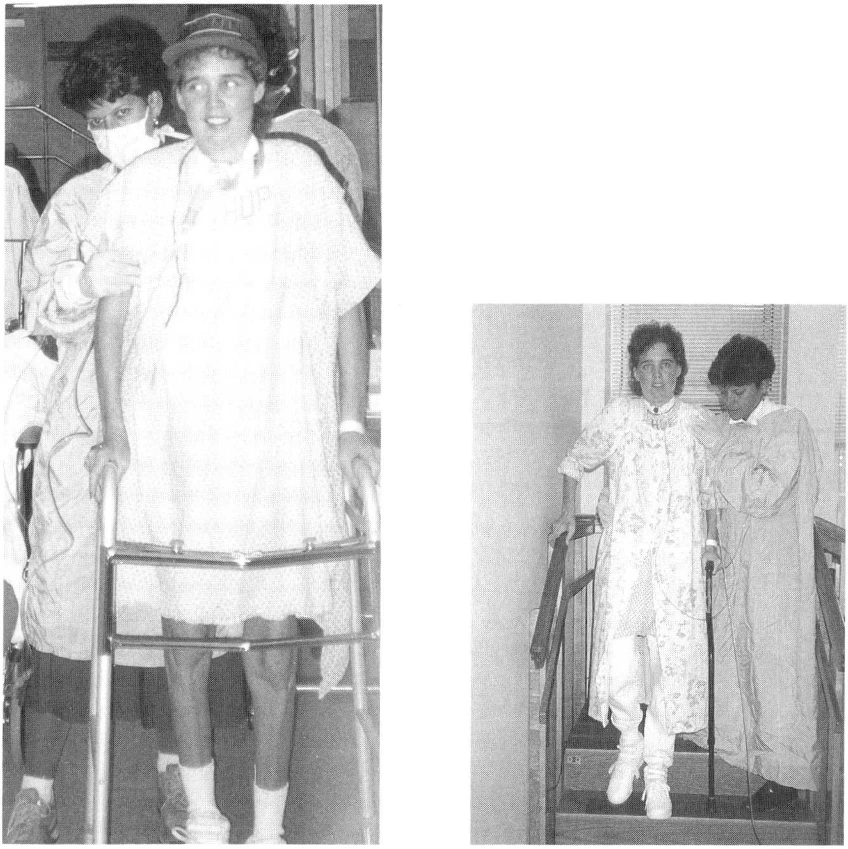

(c) (d)

Figure 1 Proposed progression of activity level for the patient in the intensive care unit. (a) Phase 1: Patient no longer on mechanical ventilator during exercise. Manual ventilation breathing 100% oxygen. Ambulation with a walker. (b) Phase 2: Independent ventilation while breathing 50% oxygen via a tracheal mask setup. Manual ventilator at hand. Ambulating with a rolling platform walker. Orthosis on left lower extremity for footdrop. (c) Phase 3: Tracheostomy still open but inspired oxygen is lower. Ambulating with a walker. Orthosis is no longer needed. (d) Phase 4: Tracheostomy buttoned. Continuing decrease in concentration of oxygen in inspired air. Oxygen delivery via nasal prongs. Ambulating with a straight cane.

not be expressed clearly. Patients are seen to wave a hand, close their eyes, shake their head in disappointment when unable to communicate their needs to staff or loved ones. Satisfying the communication needs of the patient greatly enhances the effectiveness of physical therapy as well as building a trusting relationship between the staff, patient, and family.

Malnutrition has a major impact on limiting exercise performance as well as on life expectancy in patients with end-stage chronic obstructive lung disease (27). Nutritional requirements fluctuate with the level of metabolic demands. These demands include infection, the disease process, weaning, the level of activity, the ability to absorb nutrients, and, in some instances, drug-induced diarrhea (28,29). With respect to physical therapy, the process of promoting activity may be seriously compromised by malnutrition.

Other obstacles to physical rehabilitation include sleep deprivation, anxiety, psychosis, side effects of medications, multiorgan failure, inadequate access routes for parenteral therapy, and malabsorption (23,24,26,30,31). Orthostasis often limits attempts to increase the level of activity. The orthostatic response may be minimized in a variety of ways: raising the head of the bed, manually lifting the patient out of bed to a chair, dangling the patient at the side of the bed, using tilt tables, and transferring a patient with a stand pivot to a chair. The patient must adapt to each of these sequential changes in position en route to standing and ambulation.

Musculoskeletal complications also pose challenges to the rehabilitation team in this setting. Among these complications are joint contractures and either iatrogenic or idiopathic myopathy that is induced either medically, by inactivity, or by malpositioning of the extremities (32–34). Another limiting influence on rehabilitation is a decubitus ulcer on a heel or in the sacral region. This will affect the patient's ability to ambulate or even sit up in a chair, depending on the location of the ulcer.

IX. Ventilator-Dependent Units

A. Medicare Catastrophic Act

The discharge of a patient from the intensive care or step-down unit can be slowed by complications, delay in weaning from a ventilator, loss of functional independence, and difficulties in making arrangements for discharge. These delays affect hospital costs and reimbursement. In 1988, the Medicare Catastrophic Act established five pilot ventilator-dependent units to establish criteria for reimbursement for the rehabilitation of this type of patient. The aim of this project was to evaluate the desirability of designating hospital units that deal with ventilator-dependent patients as rehabilitation units that would be exempt from limitations imposed by the reimbursement formula for diagnosis-related groups (35). These units were oriented to developing standards relating to rehabilitation rather than to acute care.

At one of these units, St. Mary's Hospital in Rochester, Minnesota, 61 patients were admitted during a period of 18 months (28). The criteria for admission included "stable medical condition, absence of the need for electrocardiographic monitoring, previous tracheostomy, and rehabilitation potential." The predominant disorder contributing to ventilator dependence was chronic obstructive pulmonary disease; this was the diagnosis in 28 of the 61 patients. Neuromuscular disorders accounted for 10 of the 61 patients. Weaning from the ventilator was successful in 53 of 58 patients. This program demonstrated that patients who had proved difficult to wean could be successfully weaned, and that savings to the institution could be substantial.

Several years before the Medicare Catastrophic Act, an inpatient unit for rehabilitation of ventilator-dependent patients was established at a university medical center in Boston (36). Sixteen patients were admitted to this unit between January 1981 and November 1982. The patients were categorized as having either chronic obstructive pulmonary disease (group 1) or restrictive lung disease (group 2). The average length of stay in acute care for the patients in group 1 was 148 days. Once on the unit the average length of stay was 133 days for group 1. In contrast to the results obtained from those at St. Mary's Hospital, none of the patients from group 1 could be completely taken off the ventilator: the time off the ventilator ranged from 2 to 14 hr and supplemental oxygen was required during the ventilator-free time.

Group 2 had an average length of stay of 43 consecutive days in the acute care hospital prior to transferring to the unit. The patients in group 2 averaged 69 days on the rehabilitation unit. Four patients in group 2 were weaned for 13 or more hours a day and one patient was liberated from the ventilator. Eleven of the 16 patients from the unit were discharged to their own homes.

Even though a limited number of patients were oxygen- and ventilator-free once inpatient rehabilitation was completed, the fact remains that ventilator-dependent patients could be discharged to home with a higher functional level than when first accepted into the rehabilitation program. Also, the level of independence improved after entry into the program. The inability to discharge some of the patients was attributed to lack of family support, on the one hand, and intractable dyspnea, on the other. Entrance criteria that identify the appropriate patient group among a disease category such as chronic obstructive lung disease, preadmission functional level, and a designated support system are critical to success of a rehabilitation program.

X. Rehabilitation in the Intensive Care Unit

Attention has been called to the fact that the earlier that pulmonary rehabilitation of the mechanically ventilated patient is begun—even in the intensive care setting—the greater its effect (25). Unfortunately, many patients have had extensive stays in the acute care setting before admission to the intensive care unit (36). During the stay in the acute care unit, consequences of limited mobility may already have set in. These effects may adversely affect the patient who survives the initial cause for admission into the intensive care unit. For example, loss of range of motion of the scapular-humoral joint may occur because of limitation in movement imposed by a central venous line or because of malpositioning that favors protraction of the scapula. Also, improper positioning in bed can result in forward flexion of the cervical spine and kyphosis of the upper thoracic spine. Because of loss of shoulder motion caused by malpositioning, the patient may subsequently have difficulty with dressing, eating, or bathing. Moreover, the patient may suffer loss of self-image and self-worth.

XI. Cost Benefits of Rehabilitation in the Intensive Care Unit

The costs for caring for the critically ill patient in the intensive care unit often exceed $1200 per day (37,38). A rehabilitation program, implemented by a multidisciplinary team, affords the prospect of shortening the hospital stay (39). As indicated above, a major effect can be the avoidance of the ill effects of prolonged immobilization. In addition, the rehabilitation team can address a variety of other preventive and therapeutic measures relating to nutrition, sleep, therapeutic levels of medication, levels of anxiety, weaning schedules, and functional demands—all of which can influence adversely the process of physical rehabilitation.

Although, in principle, the pulmonary rehabilitation team can play a major role in the cost-effective and efficient care of patients in the intensive care unit—especially those who are difficult to wean—there are a few convincing studies to support this type of intervention. The need to address this problem from a variety of perspectives has only recently begun to be appreciated (39).

References

1. Connors G, Hilling L, eds. Guidelines for Pulmonary Rehabilitation Programs. American Association of Cardiovascular and Pulmonary Rehabilitation. Champaign, IL: Human Kinetics, 1993.

2. Fishman AP. Pulmonary rehabilitation research: NIH workshop summary. Am J Respir Crit Care Med 1994; 149:825–833.
3. Bach JR, Alba AS. Noninvasive options for ventilatory support of the traumatic high level quadriplegic patient. Chest 1990; 98:613–619.
4. Foster S, Thomas HM. Pulmonary rehabilitation in lung disease other than chronic obstructive pulmonary disease. Am Rev Respir Dis 1990; 141:601–604.
5. Kaufer JM, Locker D. Rehabilitation ideology and respiratory support technology. Soc Sci Med 1990; 30(8):867–877.
6. Dail CW, Affeldt JE, Collier CR. Clinical aspects of glossopharyngeal breathing: report of use by 100 postpoliomyelitic patients. JAMA 1955; 158(6):445–449.
7. Adkins HV. Improvement of breathing ability in children with respiratory muscle paralysis. Phys Ther 1968; 48(6):577–581.
8. Dail CW. Respiratory aspects of rehabilitation in neuromuscular conditions. Arch Phys Med Rehabil 1965; 46:655–675.
9. Wenger NK. Early ambulation: the physiologic basis revisited. Adv Cardiol 1982; 31:138–141.
10. Winslow EH. Cardiovascular consequences of bed rest. Heart Lung 1985; 14(3):236–246.
11. Dean E, Ross J. Discordance between cardiovascular physiology and physical therapy. Chest 1992; 101:1694–1698.
12. Ross J, Dean E. Integrating physiological principles into the comprehensive management of cardiopulmonary dysfunction. Phys Ther 1989; 69(4):255–259.
13. Chulay M, Brown J, Summer W. Effect of postoperative immobilization after coronary artery bypass surgery. Crit Care Med 1982; 10(3):176–179.
14. Burns JR, Jones FL. Early ambulation of patients requiring ventilatory assistance. Chest 1975; 68:608.
15. Orlava OE. Therapeutic physical culture in the complex treatment of pneumonia. Phys Ther Rev 1959; 39(3):153–160.
16. Lemaire F. Respiratory muscle fatigue and acute respiratory failure, role during weaning failure. Monaldi Arch Chest Dis 1993; 48(5):494–497.
17. Spicher JE, White DP. Outcome and function following prolonged mechanical ventilation. Arch Intern Med 1987; 147:421–425.
18. Gracey DR, Naessens JM, Krishan I, Marsh HM. Hospital and post-hospital survival in patients mechanically ventilated for more than 29 days. Chest 1992; 101:211–214.
19. Warren A. Mobilization of the chest wall. Phys Ther 1968; 48(6):582–585.
20. Zadai CC. Physical therapy for the acutely ill medical patient. Phys Ther 1981; 61(12):1746–1754.
21. Kigin CM. Chest physical therapy for the postoperative or traumatic injury patient. Phys Ther 1981; 61(12):1724–1736.
22. Peirson DJ. Complications associated with mechanical ventilation. Crit Care Clin 1990; 6(3):711–724.
23. Krieger BP. Respiratory failure in the elderly. Clin Geriatr Med 1994; 10(1):103–119.
24. Witta K. New techniques for weaning difficult patients from mechanical ventilation. AACN Clin Issues 1990; 1(2):260–266.

25. Jackson NC. Pulmonary rehabilitation for mechanically ventilated patients. Crit Care Nurs Clin North Am 1991; 3(4):591–600.
26. Holtackers TR. Physical rehabilitation of the ventilator-dependent patient. In: Irwin, Tecklin, eds. Cardiopulmonary Physical Therapy, 2d ed. St Louis: CV Mosby, 1990:373–387.
27. Wouters EFM, Schols AMWJ. Metabolic support and energy supply in chronic respiratory failure. Monaldi Arch Chest Dis 1993; 48(5):530–534.
28. Gracey DR, Viggiano RW, Naessens JM, Hubmayr RD, Silverstein MD, Koenig GE. Outcomes of patients admitted to a chronic ventilator-dependent unit in an acute-care hospital. Mayo Clinic Proc 1992; 67:131–136.
29. Holtzman GM, Warner SC, Melnik G, Beer W. Nutritional support of pulmonary patients: a multidisciplinary approach. AACN Clin Issues 1990; 1(2):300–312.
30. Hammon WE. Physical therapy for the acutely ill patient in the respiratory intensive care unit. In: Irwin, Tecklin, eds. Cardiopulmonary Physical Therapy, 2d ed. St Louis: CV Mosby, 1990.
31. Knebel AR. Weaning from mechanical ventilation: current controversies. Heart Lung 1991; 20(4):321–331.
32. Bolton CF. Neuromuscular abnormalities in critically ill patients. Intens Care Med 1993; 19:309–310.
33. Isentein DA, Venner DS, Duggan J. Neuromuscular blockade in the intensive care unit. Chest 1992; 102:1258–1266.
34. Hansen-Flaschen J, Cowen J, Raps EC. Neuromuscular blockage in the intensive care unit: more than we bargained for. Am Rev Respir Dis 1993; 147:234–236.
35. O'Donohue WJ. Chronic ventilator-dependent units in hospitals: attacking the front end of a long-term problem. Mayo Clin Proc 1992; 67:198–200.
36. Make B, Gilmartin M, Brody JS, Snider GL. Rehabilitation of ventilator-dependent subjects with lung diseases: the concept and initial experience. Chest 1984; 86(3):358–365.
37. Lundberg JA, Noll ML. The long-term acute care hospital: a new option for ventilator-dependent individuals. AACN Clin Issues 1990; 1(2):280–288.
38. Rosen RL, Bone RC. Financial implications of ventilator care. Crit Care Clin 1990; 6(3):797–805.
39. Cowley RS, Swanson B, Chapman P, Kitik BA, Mackay LE. The role of rehabilitation in the intensive care unit. J Head Trauma Rehabil 1994; 9(1):32–42.

32

Pulmonary Rehabilitation Before and After Lung Transplantation

ROGER S. GOLDSTEIN

University of Toronto
Toronto, Ontario, Canada

MICHAEL J. HALL

Monash University
Alfred Hospital
Melbourne, Australia

In the 1980s, combined heart-lung transplantation was introduced for end-stage pulmonary vascular disease (1). Subsequently, single and bilateral lung transplantation have become available for a variety of respiratory conditions. Bilateral transplantation is the method of choice for conditions such as cystic fibrosis and bronchiectasis, and single lung the preferred approach for pulmonary fibrosis (2) and emphysema (3). In 1994, the St. Louis International Lung Transplant Registry reported information on 55 U.S. and 38 foreign transplant centers. Prior to September 1993, there were 1459 single lung transplants, 709 bilateral sequentials, and 157 en bloc doubles. The overall 3-year actuarial survival rate was 54%. Chronic obstructive pulmonary disease (COPD) was the most frequently listed diagnosis (27%) followed by interstitial fibrosis (16%) and cystic fibrosis (15%). For patients with COPD, the 2-year survival for those receiving a single lung ($n=704$) was 67% and for those receiving bilateral transplants ($n=190$) it was 75%. All three techniques for lung transplantation yield actuarial survivals that make them viable options for appropriately selected patients (4).

In 1993, the American Thoracic Society published guidelines in which several factors were identified as important in determining the outcome of lung transplantation (5). These included careful donor and recipient selection, attention to rejection and infection, the choice of the procedure, and the characteristics of the transplant center. Rehabilitation was not included as one of the important determinants of outcome. However, many of the criteria used to select transplant recipients were similar to those used to select patients for respiratory rehabilitation (Table 1). These included: untreatable end-stage pulmonary disease with no other significant associated medical conditions, substantial limitation of activities of daily living, and patients who are ambulatory, who have rehabilitation potential, and who have an acceptable psychosocial and nutritional profile (6). Similarly, the recommended contraindications for lung transplantation included many of the contraindications for respiratory rehabilitation, such as continued smoking, poor compliance, associated medical conditions, and a poor psychosocial situation.

Thus, in recent years, programs for respiratory rehabilitation and lung transplantation have developed in parallel although they share many of the clinical criteria for selection. It is therefore appropriate that a closer interaction between these two management approaches is fostered whereby respiratory rehabilitation would precede and follow transplantation and transplantation would be considered for patients in whom rehabilitation alone has not resulted in sufficient improvements in exercise tolerance or quality of life.

In this chapter, we explore the role of respiratory rehabilitation in preoperative and postoperative lung transplantation. In commenting on the rationale for postoperative rehabilitation, we review the limitations in exercise tolerance that persist despite successful transplantation. An understanding of these limitations will assist in planning appropriate approaches to rehabilitation that will maximize the quality of life and exercise tolerance for transplant recipients.

I. Preoperative Rehabilitation

Patients selected for respiratory rehabilitation preoperatively usually have the same characteristics as those selected for respiratory rehabilitation but who do

Table 1 General Guidelines for the Selection of Lung Transplant Recipients

Untreatable end-stage pulmonary vascular disease of any etiology
No other significant medical diseases
Substantial limitation of daily activities
Limited life expectancy
Ambulatory with rehabilitation potential
Acceptable nutritional status
Satisfactory psychosocial profile and emotional support system

Source: Ref. 5.

not undergo lung transplantation. In general, these characteristics can be divided into clinical and nonclinical components (7).

A. Clinical Components

Cessation of Smoking

Cessation of smoking is a reflection of the patient's commitment to a life-style change that needs to be continued after lung transplantation. Our experience with accepting those patients who vow to quit on the first day of the rehabilitation program is that they are highly likely to start smoking again very soon after they leave the hospital. Moreover, should supplemental oxygen be required at any stage, it is unsafe and ineffective if the subject continues to smoke. Therefore, we direct smokers to a smoking cessation program prior to accepting them for rehabilitation, admitting them to the rehabilitation program after they have discontinued smoking for at least 1 month.

Clinical Stability

Although rehabilitation is more likely to succeed in clinically stable patients, it can be introduced during the recovery phase of a treated exacerbation in a patient who is awaiting transplantation. It is, however, important that rehabilitation not be confused with convalescence or a frustrating situation can arise in which the patient, the health care team, and the family have differing expectations. Patients beginning rehabilitation after a period of hospitalization may experience gratifying increases in their exercise tolerance and quality of life.

Maximum Pharmacological Therapy

It should be emphasized that maximal therapy should precede the commencement of the rehabilitation program and should therefore be addressed at the time of the initial assessment. This includes optimizing sympathomimetics, anticholinergics, and supplemental oxygen, establishing whether airflow obstruction is clinically reversible, and minimizing the use of corticosteroids.

Associated Medical Conditions

Active associated medical conditions will influence the patient's rehabilitation potential unless treated prior to program admission. Such conditions should be minimized prior to starting rehabilitation. For example, malnutrition can be addressed at the outset of the rehabilitation program by introducing the appropriate dietary changes.

B. Nonclinical Components

Preprogram Motivation

Motivation is essential for a successful outcome. A well-motivated candidate will have recognized the existence of a substantial limitation in the quality of his/her life and the need for assistance in dealing with it. However, in some instances, attention has been diverted from this aspect of the program by the emphasis on completing the many tests associated with evaluation for transplant and on the subsequent discussions of risks and postoperative care. It may not be until the process of preoperative rehabilitation is brought to the fore that the candidate reflects on his/her quality of life and on the need to improve exercise tolerance and the sense of well-being while awaiting transplantation.

Realistic Expectations

Even well-motivated subjects should have realistic expectations both as to what is expected of them and as to what they are likely to achieve from participation in the program. If these expectations are unrealistic, an apparent lack of progress can be disruptive and detrimental to the patient, the health care team, and other patients participating in the rehabilitation program. Therefore, the patient and the health care team should agree on realistic goals at the time of commencing the rehabilitation program.

Adequate Comprehension

This is another essential component that contributes to successful rehabilitation and transplantation. Language problems can be addressed with adequate interpretation by family members or professional health care interpreters. Using this approach, receiving instruction is relatively straightforward. However, it is important to reduce the isolation that an individual will experience from being unable to communicate even basic needs during rehabilitation and, more so, during the perioperative period.

Adequate Home Situation

It should be established at the outset that there is a home for the patient to go to and that reasonable facilities exist for sleeping, cleaning, and washing. Environmental considerations such as smoke and pollution are important, as are other physical facilities, such as stairs and distance to shops. Candidates with supportive families or caregivers tend to do better than those who are socially isolated. Needless to say, the above factors are amplified when one considers that postoperatively the immunosuppressed patient will require close attention in order to recognize and manage infection and rejection.

C. Preoperative Rehabilitation Summary

The criteria used to select candidates appropriate for rehabilitation and for transplantation are so similar that, if possible, the selection should occur at the same time. Candidates ineligible for rehabilitation, for either medical or nonmedical reasons, are unlikely to be selected for transplantation.

II. Rationale for Rehabilitation

Rehabilitation is offered in an effort to maximize the benefits of lung transplantation (6). After completing a rehabilitation program, a candidate may have benefited in several different ways: (1) be so much improved that the need for transplantation could be reconsidered; (2) be better able to tolerate the waiting period for a suitable donor lung; (3) be better able to tolerate major surgery and the clinical and psychological issues that arise during the intensive perioperative period; and (4) having become familiar with an exercise routine, be more likely to continue it posttransplantation, thereby decreasing limitations in exercise tolerance that follow successful transplantation.

Unfortunately, the above rationale has not been formally tested in a prospective and randomized controlled trial. Therefore, the benefits of rehabilitation on the lung transplant recipient remain speculative. Some transplant centers insist that all patients accepted for transplantation participate in rehabilitation whereas others do not include it as part of their clinical management. Payment of the costs associated with rehabilitation vary from country to country and within a particular country, depending on the extent to which medical care has been socialized and who the third-party payer is likely to be. This clearly influences the role of rehabilitation within the overall approach to transplantation.

III. The Rehabilitation Program

The rehabilitation program itself does not differ substantially from respiratory rehabilitation offered to any patient with end-stage lung disease. Details of the team approach, breathing classes, the role of supervised exercise training and education, as well as the psychosocial supports of relaxation classes, activity tolerance, and recreation, are to be found elsewhere both in this book and in a number of authoritative reviews (8,9). However, a larger number of psychosocial stress factors may be present in patients awaiting rehabilitation prior to transplant (Table 2) (10), especially if the patients have moved from their homes to the transplant center while awaiting surgery. Such stresses may be financial, as in the personal and family expenses related to relocating, or social,

Table 2 Psychosocial Stressors in Lung Transplant Applicants

Coping with disabling or life-threatening illness
Making financial arrangements required for enrollment including:
The surgical procedure
Personal and family expenses
Postoperative medical and pharmaceutical care
Travel or moving to site of transplant program
Changes in medical management and personnel
Organizing an adequate support system
Fear of being found unsuitable for transplantation

Source: Ref. 10.

as in the changes in medical management and personnel, or in the organization of an adequate family support system. It is therefore important that the allied health personnel involved with rehabilitation, especially the social worker and psychologist, communicate freely with members of the transplant team. The duration of the initial intensive period of rehabilitation varies: some patients attend 5 days a week for 6–8 weeks of inpatient care (2) and others attend 3 times a week for 10–12 weeks on an outpatient basis. However, because the period of waiting for a suitable donor lung to materialize is unknown, there is a need for ongoing outpatient supervision (11,12). In Toronto, this takes the form of regular (at least weekly and often 2–3 times per week) outpatient attendance at the hospital until a suitable donor presents. It is expected that patients accepted for transplantation will continue to practice a daily home exercise routine; this routine includes breathing exercises, interval training, upper-extremity training, leisure walking, and either cycle or treadmill exercise, if this equipment is available.

IV. Outcome of Preoperative Rehabilitation

The influence of respiratory rehabilitation has been evaluated in a number of prospective randomized controlled trials. In patients with COPD, supervised rehabilitation, followed by compliance enhancing outpatient follow-up visits, has been shown to bring about statistically significant and clinically important improvements in quality of life and exercise tolerance compared with conventional community care (13–19). A few reports have attempted to sort out the contribution of rehabilitation, per se, from that of transplantation on the quality of life and exercise tolerance. Although problems in design or in the measures used to determine outcome limit their generalizability, the following warrant consideration.

In a report on seven subjects with end-stage fibrotic lung disease awaiting single lung transplantation, improvements in functional ability occurred as a result of a structured rehabilitation program (20). The outcome measure used was the 6-min walk test (6MW). The initial mean distance of 61 m (range 46–88) increased to 81 m (range 67–95), 3.7 months (range 1–9) later. No details were given about the circumstances of the 6MW. The differences were small and could have been attributable to test repetition. The same group has reported that only a minority of their single lung transplantation patients were able to walk less than 100 m prior to surgery, whereas most were able to walk at least 300 m after rehabilitation (6). These values suggest that the subjects in this report were probably not representative of patients with fibrotic lung disease who undergo transplantation.

In 42 patients with cystic fibrosis (mean FEV_1 26.8 ± 8% predicted) who were awaiting double lung transplantation, the mean increase in 6MW was 41 ± 91 m following rehabilitation for 1.5 hr 3 times per week. The duration of training was not stated. Nonetheless, subjects also improved their graded exercise test by 0.43 stages on a modified Bruce Protocol (21).

Sheldon (22) reported the results of respiratory rehabilitation on 28 patients who were awaiting lung transplantation. The patients undertook treadmill and upper-extremity exercises for up to 6 months while awaiting a suitable donor. The mean FEV_1 at the start of the program was 0.6 L for those with chronic obstructive pulmonary disease and 0.98 L for those with cystic fibrosis. The rehabilitation program resulted in maintenance, but no improvement, in the 6MW, treadmill load, or upper-extremity exercise.

Biggar (23) compared the functional outcome in patients with chronic obstructive pulmonary disease who underwent either single lung transplantation (SLT) or bilateral lung transplantation (BLT). Forty-four SLT recipients and 39 BLT recipients, with mean FEV_1 values of 0.5 and 0.51 L, respectively, participated in a rehabilitation program that consisted of treadmill training for 5 days a week, each session was 30 min in duration. The 6MW test was performed at 6-week intervals until the time of transplantation. Both groups improved the 6MW distance between the initial and the last tests: initial SLT = 209 m and BLT = 259 m; the last pretransplant tests, SLT = 297 m and BLT = 327 m. The method of administering the 6MW was not described nor was the duration of rehabilitation stated; no measurement was made of the quality of life.

In another report by the same group (12), 110 lung transplant recipients were divided into five groups by diagnosis and type of transplant (Table 3). Again, preoperative rehabilitation was accompanied by beneficial increments in exercise tolerance.

In a study dealing with exercise, education, and quality of life in lung transplant candidates, Manzetti (24) randomized nine subjects to receive education alone (E) (four subjects) or education plus exercise (EE) (five subjects).

Table 3 Mean 6-Min Walk Distance (m) for Patients Awaiting Transplantation Measured at the Time of Their Initial Evaluation (Eval) and Immediately Prior to Transplantation (PreTx)

Diagnosis	*n*	Eval	PreTx
COPD—single lung transplant	32	208	303*
COPD—double or bilateral lung transplant	31	266	337*
Cystic fibrosis—bilateral lung transplant	18	348	445*
Pulmonary fibrosis—single lung transplant	9	261	343
Pulmonary hypertension—single lung transplant	18	194	

*$p < 0.05$ Eval versus PreTx.
Source: Ref. 12.

The program comprised 6 weeks of lectures, 3 times a week, dealing with anatomy, physiology, home oxygen, stress reduction, bronchial hygiene, and alternative sexual techniques. In addition, subjects in the EE group also attended an exercise program twice a week that included treadmill and cycle training, interval training, and upper-extremity training with light weights. Exercise tolerance and quality of life were measured at baseline and repeated after 6 weeks of the program (Table 4).

As can be seen from Table 4, although the 6MW and the quality of well-

Table 4 Outcome Measures Before and After a Health Maintenance Program Administered 3 Times a Week for 6 Weeks to Candidates Awaiting Lung Transplantation

	Education		Education plus exercise	
Variable	Mean	SD	Mean	SD
Exercise tolerance				
Cardiopulmonary exercise (workload)				
Before	38.5	20.1	28.8	12.9
After	40.5	15.6	27.0	15.2
6-min walk distance (m)				
Before	277.5	190.6	232.2	87.4
After	350.8	132.4	299.9	161.1
Quality of life				
Quality of well-being				
Before	0.58	0.07	0.55	0.02
After	0.71	0.08	0.61	0.05

Source: Ref. 24.

being improved in both groups, there were no differences between groups as a result of adding exercise. The study design was prospective and randomized with valid outcome measures for exercise tolerance and quality of life. However, a large number of subjects were ineligible, refused to participate, or dropped out. Despite strict entry criteria and stratification based on diagnosis, the final sample size was small (nine subjects) and the variability large. The diagnoses differed between the two groups, with the E group including those with obstructive diseases, and the EE group those with restrictive diseases. Thus, it was difficult to conclude more than that rehabilitation was safe and resulted in improvements in walk distance and quality of well-being. Whether education plus exercise conferred additional benefits over education per se was not adequately tested.

In summary, reports on the effectiveness of preoperative rehabilitation have often been from trials that were uncontrolled. They have been limited by a lack of standardized measurements of exercise tolerance and quality of life and by a variable duration of rehabilitation. In a single prospective randomized controlled study, the number of subjects was small, the dropouts unequal between the two groups, and the variability of the measures large. Nevertheless, it is likely that preoperative rehabilitation will assist in maintaining function and may actually improve it. It remains to be established whether such improvements will influence the outcome of lung transplantation.

V. Early Postoperative Rehabilitation

The rehabilitation team plays an important role in the early and intermediate postoperative care. Details of the clinical goals immediately following transplantation are to be found elsewhere (11,25). In essence, good clinical care includes the early integration of chest physiotherapy, correct patient positioning, and early ambulation. Postural drainage, vibration, percussion, deep breathing, and coughing are encouraged and assisted in accordance with the usual clinical principles of postoperative thoracic care (26,27). The challenges peculiar to the posttransplant population include denervation of the lung and its influence on the cough reflex, mucous production, and clearance. Although it is possible that intensive preoperative rehabilitation could influence the course and progress of the patient within the perioperative period, there have, as yet, been no clinical trials specifically evaluating the influence of rehabilitation on outcome measures such as complication rates, length of stay, and early mobilization.

As in preoperative rehabilitation, transplant centers vary with respect to whether their patients undergo any form of structured rehabilitation program postoperatively. In some centers, no such program exists, whereas in others

(10,11), patients are encouraged to exercise for 5 days a week. They may attend a supervised exercise program and be given a written home exercise program with which to continue independently. There have been no clinical trials to determine the influence of a structured rehabilitation program on exercise tolerance or quality of life within the first 3 months of receiving a lung transplant.

VI. Exercise Tolerance Post–Lung Transplantation

After only a short postoperative period, lung transplant recipients exhibit marked improvements in measurements of pulmonary function (28–30) (Table 5). The improvements in flow rates, lung volumes, and diffusion are associated with improvements in clinical and laboratory measures of exercise tolerance. However, a number of studies have reported that notwithstanding the dramatic initial improvements in exercise tolerance, peak oxygen consumption and power output remain in the range of 40–60% of predicted maximum, with no spontaneous further improvement. This observation is consistent for all types of thoracic organ transplantation, including heart transplantation (28,30–37). The limitation in posttransplant exercise capacity appears to be independent of the age at transplantation and of the underlying condition that resulted in the need for transplantation (37,38). Therefore, when considering the rationale for rehabilitation in association with lung transplantation, it is useful to consider the mechanisms that may be responsible for this disability.

Theodore (35) compared peak exercise performance immediately prior to, and following, heart-lung transplantation in 10 subjects with pulmonary hypertension. A subset of six of these patients was available for follow-up 2 years postoperation. Prior to transplantation, all of the subjects had limitations

Table 5 Preoperative and Postoperative (6 Months) Pulmonary Function in Single Lung (SLT) and Double Lung (DLT) Transplant Recipients

	VC (L)		FEV_1 (L)		TLC (L)		DLCO (ml/min/mmHg)	
	Pre	Post	Pre	Post	Pre	Post	Pre	Post
SLT	1.7±0.5 (39)	2.7±0.7 (63)	1.5±0.4 (42)	2.1±0.5 (61)	2.7±0.5 (43)	4.1±0.7 (67)	8.1±1.5 (30)	12.9±2.8 (50)
DLT	2.0±0.6 (55)	3.1±0.5 (84)	0.5±0.2 (18)	2.6±0.5 (84)	7.2±0.5 (139)	4.9±0.4 (94)	5.1±1.3 (23)	18.3±2.3 (82)

Values in parentheses represent the percentage of predicted.
Source: Ref. 28.

in their exercise performance: peak oxygen consumption ($\dot{V}O_2$), heart rate, oxygen pulse, and ventilation were all low, as were measurements of gas exchange, consistent with the underlying pulmonary hypertension (Table 6). Not surprisingly, the pretransplant subjects were unable to exercise with sufficient intensity for their blood lactate to increase. Immediately posttransplantation, their peak $\dot{V}O_2$ almost doubled, reaching 39.3 ± 2.6% of predicted maximum. Peak heart rate increased as did the oxygen pulse. Arterial blood gases improved and the subjects could exercise with sufficient intensity to manifest an increase in blood lactate.

A number of important observations can be made from this study. First, heart-lung transplantation was associated with a significant improvement in peak exercise performance. Second, ventilatory function was not the limiting factor during activity. This finding has also been reported by Levy (37), who extended the observations to include heart-lung, double lung, and single lung transplant recipients. The single lung recipients were further divided into those who received single lungs for obstructive lung disease and those who received single lungs for restrictive lung disease. All of the groups achieved levels of ventilation that were less than 70% of the calculated maximum voluntary ventilation, indicating the presence of a ventilatory reserve at the end of exercise (Fig. 1). Third, Theodore and colleagues observed no change in peak exercise capacity between 1 and 2 years postoperation, suggesting that although patients resumed a normal life-style, the impairment in their exercise capacity persisted. The subjects in Theodore's study did not undergo respiratory rehabilitation. Of the patients in the study by Levy, only those in the double lung group participated in a supervised preoperative rehabilitation program, which was continued postoperatively, both in hospital and at home for an unspecified period. Although the double lung recipients increased their peak oxygen uptakes during

Table 6 Peak Exercise Data for Subjects with Primary Pulmonary Hypertension Pre–Heart-Lung Transplantation (HLT), Within 8 Weeks Postoperation, Within 6 Months Postoperation, and 2 Years Posttransplant

	Pretransplant	Posttransplant	Within 6 months	2 years
Peak $\dot{V}O_2$ (ml/min/kg)	9.8 ± 0.7	16.1 ± 1.3*	19.6 ± 2.2	20.2 ± 2.3
% pred. max $\dot{V}O_2$	24.2 ± 2.0	39.3 ± 2.6*	52.8 ± 4.0	55.2 ± 5.2
Peak heart rate (bpm)	116.9 ± 6.5	128.9 ± 4.8**	145.0 ± 5.6	142.0 ± 6.0
Peak O_2 pulse (ml/kg/beat)	87 ± 10	124 ± 7	139 ± 15	142 ± 14
Peak VE (L/min)	37.0 ± 4.0	41.1 ± 5.1	46.0 ± 5.2	46.7 ± 6.1
PaO_2	44.2 ± 6.8	98.9 ± 1.8*	97.2 ± 3.5	92.8 ± 6.3

*$p < 0.001$; **$p < 0.005$.
Source: Ref. 35.

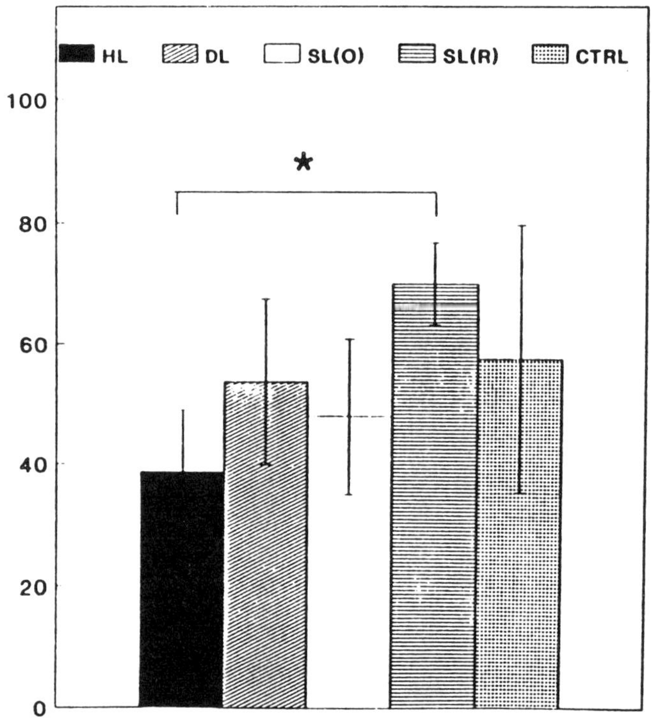

Figure 1 Values for VE/MVV (%) at peak exercise for heart-lung (HL), double lung (DL), and single lung transplant recipients with obstructive [SL(O)] and restrictive [SL(R)] lung disease compared to healthy subjects. Note the presence of adequate ventilatory reserve in all transplant groups. (From Ref. 37.)

exercise more than did the heart-lung and single lung recipients, these differences did not reach statistical significance, possibly because of the small sample sizes.

The absence of ongoing improvement has also been reported by Williams (30) in a study of six single and seven double lung transplant recipients. Assessments made 1 and 2 years after the initial exercise tests revealed no change from the low values obtained either for peak $\dot{V}O_2$ and heart rate at baseline (3 months postoperative) or for the early anaerobic threshold (Table 7). In another report from the Toronto Transplant Group, 6MW distances measured in the same group up to 2 years postoperatively showed that improvement plateaued within the first 3–6 months after transplantation; no further improvements were identified (Fig. 2). The lack of continuing improvement supports the notion that normal daily activities are insufficient to restore peak exercise capacity.

VII. Early Anaerobiosis

A recurring theme that emerges from several studies is that exercise following thoracic organ transplantation is associated with early anaerobiosis (28,36,37,39,40). Potential explanations include inadequate oxygen delivery to active muscles as a result of anemia or an inadequate cardiac output. Although the effect of anemia has not been systematically studied, the reduced oxygen-carrying capacity caused by anemia could play a role. More importantly, with respect to cardiac performance during exercise, there is a consensus that an inadequate cardiac output is not a major factor in limiting peak exercise

Table 7 Results of Maximal Exercise Tests Early (3 Months) and Late (1–2 Years) for Single (SLT) and Double (DLT) Lung Transplant Recipients

	SLT			DLT		
	Early	Late	Max. pred.	Early	Late	Max. pred.
Peak $\dot{V}O_2$ (ml/min)	1244 ±412	1180 ±500	2340	918 ±182	963 ±229	1920
Peak HR (bpm)	132.8 ± 23.6	131.5 ± 20	177	136 ± 12	129 ± 19	186
Peak VE (L/min)	54.0 ± 16.9	53.0 ± 18.4	85.8	39.0 ± 6.9	45.4 ± 6.6	93.0
AT	46.8 ± 7.4	41.0 ± 15.8		42.6 ± 3.7	43.1 ± 18.3	

AT = anaerobic threshold as a percentage of the predicted maximum $\dot{V}O_2$.
Source: Ref. 40.

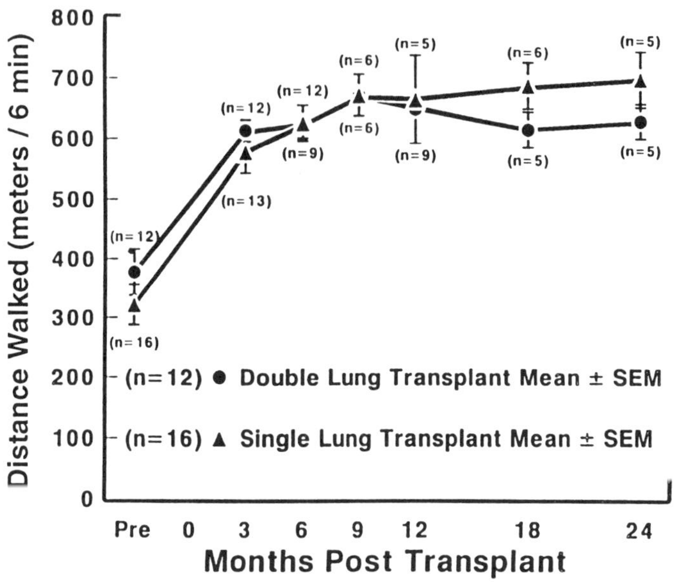

Figure 2 Six-minute walk distance post double and single lung transplantation showing a plateau in the distance walked beyond 9 months postoperation. Note both the similarity in distances walked by the single and double lung transplant groups and the lack of substantial change after 3–6 months. (From Ref. 30.)

performance in those with native or donor hearts. In fact, the evidence suggests that although the exercise response of the denervated heart is not normal, it is nevertheless adaptive: increased venous return early during exercise augments stroke volume in accord with the Starling principle, thereby compensating for the blunted increase in heart rate (41–44).

It has been speculated that muscle deconditioning may be an important factor in the exercise impairment, especially since leg fatigue is commonly stated as the reason for stopping exercise after transplantation (39,40). Indirect evidence that deconditioning is important is provided by the relationship between the length of hospital stay and the peak $\dot{V}O_2$ post–heart transplantation (45), and by the decrease in handgrip and leg extension in lung transplant recipients as compared with controls matched with respect to age and sex (46). However, no systematic evaluation has been made of the relationship between the duration of illness, inactivity, or other preoperative predictors of posttransplantation exercise capacity.

VIII. Pharmacological Effects

Cyclosporin A has recently been shown to reduce skeletal muscle mitochondrial oxidative capacity (47). This observation, plus the known influence of ongoing corticosteroids on peripheral muscle function, may have important implications in the explanation of the early anaerobic threshold observed among lung and heart transplant recipients during exercise. Although pretransplantation inactivity is almost certainly associated with deconditioning, the lack of improvement in peak exercise performance is difficult to reconcile with normal lung function and the resumption of the activities of daily living. Therefore, it is tempting to implicate one or more pharmacological explanations both for the early anaerobiosis and for what may appear to be a fixed deficit. The similarities during exercise between recipients of a variety of thoracic organ transplant techniques makes such a "posttransplant" explanation attractive.

Plasma lactate concentrations are frequently increased in individuals with heart failure during exercise. However, improvement in cardiac output and leg blood flow after administration of either hydralazine (48) or dobutamine (49) brought about no change in exercise time, peak $\dot{V}O_2$, or peak lactate, suggesting that the excessive lactate concentrations may be due to impaired oxygen utilization at the level of the muscle cell. Nuclear magnetic studies in patients with chronic respiratory or chronic cardiac disease (50–52) have disclosed depletion in ATP compatible with a decrease in oxidative metabolism. Therefore, deconditioning consequent upon long-standing respiratory dysfunction seems to be responsible for the reduction in peak $\dot{V}O_2$ and the early anaerobiosis. The postoperative contribution of cyclosporin and corticosteroids remains to be defined.

IX. Skeletal Muscle Dysfunction and Serum Potassium

Upsets in potassium balance are known to be associated with muscle fatigue (53,54), and for a given work rate, improved muscle conditioning has been associated with a lower plasma $[K^+]$. Hall et al. (55) found that both the rate of rise in plasma potassium ($\Delta[K^+]$/time) and the change in plasma potassium with respect to work performed ($\Delta[K^+]/W$) was greater during incremental exercise in heart and lung transplant recipients than in control subjects (Table 8); during the recovery period, the plasma $[K^+]$ decreased rapidly. The increased rate of rise of plasma $[K^+]$ during the active phase of muscle contraction reflected excessive K^+ release rather than impaired uptake (Fig. 3). This study provided powerful evidence for the presence of skeletal muscle deconditioning in both heart and lung transplant recipients. It was felt that peripheral muscle deconditioning was responsible for the low peak exercise capacity.

Table 8 Data Comparing the Rate of Rise of K^+ Relative to Time Exercised and Work Performed in Healthy Subjects and Heart Transplant and Lung Transplant Recipients

	Healthy subjects	Heart transplant	Lung transplant
Peak $\dot{V}O_2$ (ml/kg)	40.3 ± 4.8	16.4 ± 1.4*	15.4 ± 1.3*
% pred. $\dot{V}O_2$	101 ± 11	66 ± 6**	47 ± 4**
$[K^+]$ peak (mmol/L)	6.3 ± 0.3	6.0 ± 0.2	5.7 ± 0.1
$\Delta[K^+]$ (mmol/L)	2.5 ± 0.2	1.4 ± 0.1**	1.2 ± 0.1**
$\Delta[K^+]$/time (mmol/L/min)	18.8 ± 1.7	23.0 ± 2.2	27.0 ± 1.8*
$\Delta[K^+]$/W (mmol/L/kJ)	28.3 ± 4.9	72.7 ± 9.5**	89.4 ± 8.5**

*$p < 0.05$ versus healthy subjects; **$p < 0.001$ versus healthy subjects.
Source: Ref. 55.

In summary, even though transplantation of thoracic organs in general, and lung transplantation in particular, has been associated with dramatic improvements in pulmonary function and exercise capacity, impairment in peak oxygen uptake persists. It is likely that this impairment is closely linked to deconditioning of the peripheral muscles. If this proves to be the case, there is good reason to be optimistic that rehabilitation will be associated with improvements in exercise capacity.

X. Quality of Life Posttransplantation of Thoracic Organs

Although a major aim of any transplant program is to improve the quality of life of the recipient, few such studies pertaining to thoracic organ transplant recipients exist. Some data in the pediatric literature do suggest that developmental and cognitive function 3 months after heart or heart-lung transplantation are within the normal range (56). Also, in six adult subjects who underwent bilateral sequential lung transplantation for cystic fibrosis, improvements were reported in a number of measures of utility and quality of life (57). The changes among those receiving bilateral lung transplants were similar to those after heart transplantation. Several other studies have reported improvements after heart transplantation in a variety of outcomes, including sexual function and physical and psychiatric status (58–63).

In a cross-section survey of 200 cardiac transplant recipients 2.3 years after operation, some respondents reported scores for quality of life that were below normal and comparable to those of individuals who had experienced cardiac arrest or myocardial infarction (64). Many respondents (44%) complained of symptoms such as generalized weakness and fatigue; those who had these complaints were overrepresented in the quality-of-life scores. Despite the

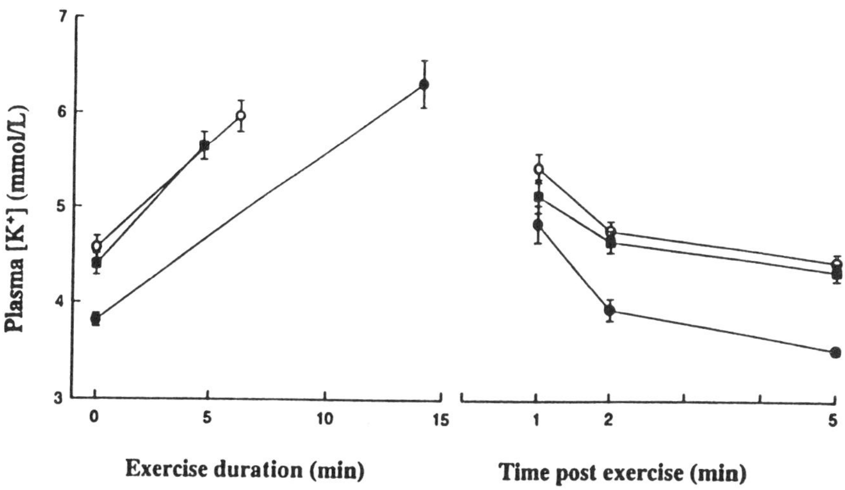

Figure 3 Plasma [K^+] at rest, peak exercise, 1 min, 2 min, and 5 min postexercise for healthy subjects (●), heart transplant (○), and lung transplant (■) subjects. Mean values for all transplant groups were higher than for the healthy group at rest ($p<0.001$). Values among both heart and lung transplant groups were also higher than for the healthy subjects at 2 min postexercise ($p<0.001$) and at 5 min postexercise ($p<0.001$). Note that while absolute differences exist during recovery, values for all groups return to baseline. (From Ref. 55.)

low response rate of those who were surveyed (48%), the study is of value because it suggests prospects for rehabilitation some time after the operative procedure, i.e., at the time of the chronic state.

An important determinant of social function appears to be the individual's perception of wellness. In one study, this perception explained why some transplant recipients did not return to work (65). In this context, carefully targeted, posttransplant psychosocial rehabilitation programs could assume great importance.

Certainly transplant survivors are challenged by the need for substantial adjustments at the time of discharge from the hospital. Such adjustments include their reintegration within their family and professional lives, coping with the threat of infection or rejection, dealing with the side effects of their medications, and the potential loss of disability-related incomes. Therefore, rehabilitation must include the psychosocial aspects of the patient's care as well as the more obvious physical needs. A life satisfaction survey, administered to all lung transplant recipients in the Toronto program (Table 9), showed that after 7 months more than 50% of surviving recipients had returned to employment. Most reported a high level of satisfaction with their physical and emotional well-being (10).

Table 9 Functional Outcome and Satisfaction of Lung Transplant Survivors[a]

Parameter	% ($n = 22$)
Vocational activity	
Full-time employee or volunteer	32
Part-time employee or volunteer	23
Full/part-time homemaker	27
None	28
Ability to work limited by physical health	
Not at all	36
Sometimes or a little	45
A lot of the time	5
Unable to work due to health	14
Satisfaction with physical health	
Excellent	27
Good	45
Satisfactory	18
Poor	9
Very poor	0
Satisfaction with emotional health	
Excellent	41
Good	45
Satisfactory	14
Poor	0
Very poor	0
Satisfaction with life	
Excellent	41
Good	32
Satisfactory	14
Poor	14
Very poor	0

[a]Excludes recipients transplanted within 6 months of survey.
Source: Ref. 10.

XI. Exercise Rehabilitation Posttransplantation of Thoracic Organs

Few reports have addressed the evaluation of rehabilitation after transplantation of a thoracic organ. However, structured programs have been evaluated for heart transplant recipients, who share many of the same issues as lung transplant recipients (reduced peak exercise $\dot{V}O_2$, early anaerobiosis, peripheral deconditioning, immunosuppression). Therefore, it is useful to consider the results of rehabilitation after heart transplantation in planning a program for the rehabilitation of individuals who have undergone lung transplantation.

A. Heart Transplantation and Exercise Training

Several studies have dealt with the effects of training on heart transplant recipients (66–72). Squires (66) described two subjects who undertook an 8-week cycle ergometer and treadmill training program comprising three 30-min sessions per week. Blood pressure and ratings of perceived exertion at submaximal workloads decreased without any change in heart rate. Subsequently, Savin (67) described five heart transplant recipients who cycled about 75% peak heart rate for 5 days per week for 16 weeks. A 44% increase in peak power output and an 18% improvement in peak $\dot{V}O_2$ was documented. Control subjects who underwent the same protocol demonstrated a decrease of 14% and an increase of 11%, respectively, in the same parameters. In addition, the submaximal heart rate decreased by 13 and 14 beats/min, respectively, for the study and control groups. Both reports suggested that substantial improvement could be achieved with exercise training. Other reports have demonstrated similar degrees of improvement in peak exercise performance (68–71).

The largest and most convincing study in this area examined the effect of a long-term walk/job training program on 36 male heart transplant recipients who were recruited 29.4 ± 24.4 weeks after transplantation (72). The exercise intensity was determined from the peak $\dot{V}O_2$ (aiming for 60–70% of peak), the anaerobic threshold, and the Borg rating of perceived exertion. The duration of the supervised training program was 16 ± 7 months. After training, the peak $\dot{V}O_2$ increased on the average by 4 ml/min/kg (19%) (Table 10) and peak power increased by 49 watts (49%). The resting heart rate decreased by 4 beats/min and the peak heart rate increased by 13 beats/min. Lean body mass increased from 46.2 kg to 58.2 kg. At equivalent submaximal workloads, there was a decrease in perceived exertion, minute ventilation, and diastolic blood pressure. Hemodynamic measurements during a steady state, before and after training, showed no differences in heart rate or stroke volume despite the increase in peak exercise performance. In a highly motivated subgroup, a 52% improvement in peak $\dot{V}O_2$ was found. Although spontaneous improvement may have played a role in the outcome of this study, this seems unlikely because of the long time that had elapsed after operation before the subjects were enrolled.

Thus, although the degree of improvement varies from study to study, exercise rehabilitation is effective in improving the submaximal and peak exercise performance among heart transplant recipients. The mechanism and site of that improvement and its influence on quality of life remain to be determined.

Table 10 Peak Exercise Pre and Post a 2-Year Training Program Among Heart Tarnsplant Recipients

	Peak HR (bpm)		Peak $\dot{V}E$ (L/min)		Peak $\dot{V}O_2$ (ml/kg/min)	
	Pre	Post	Pre	Post	Pre	Post
All ($n=36$)	103.9 ± 11.8	100.3 ± 13.4	70.5 ± 16.6	90.9 ± 23.4**	21.7 ± 4.5	25.8 ± 6.4
Mod. compliant ($n=28$)	100.3 ± 9.9	98.6 ± 14.2	70.4 ± 15.9	90.1 ± 22.6**	21.8 ± 4.4	24.5 ± 6.1**
Highly compliant ($n=8$)	116.6 ± 9.2	106.1 ± 8.7**	70.7 ± 19.9	93.8 ± 27.5**	21.3 ± 4.9	32.3 ± 5.2**

** $p < 0.001$ post versus pre.
Source: Ref. 72.

B. Lung Transplantation and Exercise Training

The similar levels of peak exercise performance demonstrated by heart and lung transplant recipients suggest that lung transplant recipients should respond to exercise rehabilitation in a similar manner. However, data confirming this hypothesis are extremely limited. The following preliminary data are available.

Stiebellehner (73) used a controlled crossover design to assess the impact of training of five lung transplant recipients, 9 ± 3 months postoperation. Subjects trained for 6 weeks at an intensity of 48 ± 8% of the difference between resting and peak heart rate. Peak $\dot{V}O_2$ increased by 18% after training while peak power increased by 35%. No other metabolic data were given, nor was any information provided about the subjects who were excluded, the characteristics of those who were included, or the type of lung transplant that was performed. The same authors reported similar findings a year later and described a fall in heart rate at equivalent submaximal workloads, suggesting that cardiac conditioning may occur (74). This finding was in keeping with that of Kavanagh (Table 11).

Although small, these studies were well designed and illustrate several important points. First, the absence of any changeover in the run-in period reinforces the idea that late spontaneous improvement in peak exercise performance, i.e., later than 3 months, does not occur. Second, the plateau in peak exercise performance appears to be reversible just as in cardiac transplant recipients. Third, although improvements were observed, the degree of change was modest, suggesting that restoration of a predicted peak exercise capacity may be an unrealistic goal. Fourth, these studies confirm that after lung transplantation, heart rate is an effective way of monitoring exercise intensity during exercise training (75).

Ambrosino (76) noted improvements in knee extensor (+18%) and flexor (+25%) torque after strength training in eight heart-lung transplant recipients who underwent training immediately after operation. The subjects were also

Table 11 Exercise Variables Before and After 6 Weeks of Aerobic Training in Seven Lung Transplant Recipients 9 ± 3 Months Posttransplant

	Baseline 1	Baseline 2	Post training
$\dot{V}O_2$max (ml/min)	1186 ± 265	1172 ± 336	1337 ± 237*†
VE (L/min)	49.1 ± 13.2	52.2 ± 13.3	40.9 ± 14.1*†
HR (bpm)	145 ± 14	143 ± 13	133 ± 16*
Lactate (mmol/L)	6.14 ± 2.35	6.48 ± 1.94	5.58 ± 2.83

*$p < 0.05$ versus baseline 1; †$p < 0.05$ versus baseline 2.
Source: Ref. 73.

able to walk further as reflected by the change in 6MW from 321 m to 436 m. Early improvements in leg strength were also reported by Fracchia among similar patients (77). However, these studies were uncontrolled and patients were assessed at a time when normal activity may have yielded similar results.

Hall (78) evaluated the response of six heart-lung transplant recipients and six heart transplant recipients to an 8-week home-based training program (Table 12). Subjects were entered more than a year after operation. Training intensity was based on perceived exertion and included step-ups in addition to cycle ergometry. Although the heart transplant patients showed improvement in peak power and peak $\dot{V}O_2$, the heart-lung group failed to do so. Significant improvement in leg strength occurred in both groups (29% and 19% in the heart and heart-lung transplant groups, respectively). Lactate concentration at peak equivalent workloads decreased in both groups. Also, the change in plasma $[K^+]$ with respect to the work performed was less after training in both groups even though the change reached statistical significance only in the heart transplant group.

Although the study was unsupervised and included relatively few subjects, objective outcome measures, such as plasma $[K^+]$ and lactate, paralleled the posttraining improvement in exercise in the heart transplant group. The improvement in leg strength in the heart transplant recipients was similar to that reported by Ambrosino (76) in lung transplant recipients. Since leg weakness is commonly reported after heart and lung transplantation, rehabilitation that is directed to improving leg strength is likely to be beneficial.

Table 12 Preliminary Data Comparing Pre- and Posttransplant Exercise for Six Heart and Six Heart-Lung Transplant Subjects Recruited More Than 1 Year Postoperation

	Heart transplant recipients		Heart-lung transplant recipients	
	Pre	Post	Pre	Post
6-min walk distance (m)	639 ± 114	632 ± 169	663 ± 112	651 ± 79
Resting HR (bpm)	102.5 ± 8.9	98.8 ± 7.1	96.7 ± 9.3	96.0 ± 11.9
Average torque (Nm)	73.3 ± 44.2	94.5 ± 43.8*	63.7 ± 30.7	75.5 ± 0.7*
Peak $\dot{V}O_2$ (ml/min/kg)	15.8 ± 4.5	18.1 ± 3.6	15.8 ± 3.4	17.0 ± 2.9
$\Delta[K^+]$ (mmol/L)	1.6 ± 0.8	1.0 ± 0.4	2.5 ± 1.9	1.9 ± 1.5
$\Delta[K^+]$/W (mmol/L/kJ)	88 ± 37	59 ± 33*	84 ± 28	71 ± 24
Lactate[a] (mmol/L)	7.4 ± 2.6	6.3 ± 1.9	6.1 ± 1.5	5.1 ± 1.4*

*$p < 0.05$ post versus pre.
[a]Lactate concentration was measured at peak equivalent workloads (isowork).
Source: Ref. 78.

In summary, despite initial improvement, the postoperative exercise capacity plateaus within the first year. Significant impairment in peak exercise performance persists despite well-functioning grafts. Although cardiac function is adequate, and even though anemia is sometimes a contributing factor, muscle deconditioning plays a significant role in limiting exercise capacity. Exercise training has been associated with improvements in both cardiac and peripheral muscle function.

XII. Conclusion

Candidates accepted for lung transplantation are often profoundly disabled and handicapped as a result both of the underlying primary physiological impairments associated with their end-stage lung disease and of the secondary physical and emotional dysfunction subsequent to deconditioning and prolonged illness. Rehabilitation is a continuum of services by a multidisciplinary team with the goal of achieving and maintaining the individual's maximum level of exercise tolerance and quality of life within the community (79). Therefore, it stands to reason that pulmonary rehabilitation may be useful to lung transplant candidates at consecutive stages in their course: preoperatively at the time of their maximum disability, perioperatively to promote early discharge from hospital, and postoperatively to address the persisting reduction in exercise capacity and the early anaerobiosis that seems to be associated with peripheral muscle deconditioning. Although preliminary results are encouraging, the effect of pulmonary rehabilitation in lung transplant recipients has not been systematically examined. Its widespread application should be preceded by appropriate clinical trials, which should include clearly defined outcome measures and economic impact.

References

1. Burke CM, Theodore J, Baldwin JC, Tazelaar HD, Morris AJ, McGregor C. Twenty-eight cases of human heart-lung transplantation. Lancet 1986; 1:517–519.
2. Toronto Lung Transplant Group. Unilateral lung transplantation for pulmonary fibrosis. N Engl J Med 1986; 314:1140–1145.
3. Trulock EP, Egan TM, Kouchoukos NT, et al. Single lung transplant for severe chronic obstructive pulmonary disease. Chest 1989; 96:738–742.
4. Pohl M, Cooper J. The international status of lung transplantation. Am J Respir Crit Care Med 1994; 149:A734 (abstract).
5. Report of the ATS workshop on lung transplantation. Am Rev Respir Dis 1993; 147:772–776.
6. Morrison DL, Maurer JR, Grossman RF. Pre-operative assessment for lung transplantation. Clin Chest Med 1990; 11:207–215.

7. Goldstein RS, Avendano MA. Candidate evaluation. In: Casaburi R, Petty TL, eds. Principles and Practice of Pulmonary Rehabilitation. Philadelphia: WB Saunders, 1993:317–321.
8. Ries AL. The team concept in pulmonary rehabilitation. In: Fishman AP, ed. Pulmonary Rehabilitation. New York: Marcel Dekker 1995.
9. Casaburi R. Principles of exercise training. Chest 1992; 101(5):263–267S.
10. Craven JL, Bright J, Lougheed Dear C. Psychiatric, psychosocial and rehabilitative aspects of lung transplantation. Pulmonary considerations in transplantation. In: Clinics in Chest Medicine. Philadelphia: WB Saunders, 1990:247–257.
11. Biggar DG, Feldman Malen J, Trulock EP, Cooper JE. Pulmonary rehabilitation before and after lung transplantation. In: Casaburi R, Petty T, eds. Principles and Practice of Pulmonary Rehabilitation. Philadelphia: WB Saunders, 1993:459–467.
12. Biggar D, Trulock E, Patterson G, et al. Medium term results of pulmonary rehabilitation prior to lung transplantation. Am Rev Respir Dis 1993; 147(4):A333 (abstract).
13. Goldstein RS, Gort EH, Stubbing D, Avendano MA, Guyatt GH. Randomised controlled trial of respiratory rehabilitation. Lancet 1994; 344:1394–1397.
14. Toshima MT, Kaplan RM, Ries AL. Experimental evaluation of rehabilitation in chronic obstructive pulmonary disease: short-term effects on exercise endurance and health status. Health Psychol 1990; 9(3):237–252.
15. Atkins CJ, Kaplan RM, Timms RM, Reinsch S, Lofback D. Behavioral exercise programs in the management of chronic obstructive pulmonary disease. J Consult Clin Psychol 1984; 52(4):591–603.
16. Mungall IPF, Hainsworth R. Assessment of respiratory function in patients with chronic obstructive airways disease. Thorax 1979; 34:254–258.
17. McGavin C, Gupta SP, Lloyd EL, McHardy GJR. Physical rehabilitation for the chronic bronchitic: results of a controlled trial of exercises in the home. Thorax 1977; 32:307–311.
18. Sinclair DJM, Ingram CG. Controlled trial of supervised exercise training in chronic bronchitis. Br Med J 1980; 23:519–521.
19. Cockcroft A, Saunders MJ, Berry G. Randomised controlled trial of rehabilitation in chronic respiratory disability. Thorax 1981; 36:200–203.
20. Dear CL, Grossman RF, Maurer JR. Preoperative evaluation of patients awaiting lung transplant. Chest 1988; 94:30S.
21. Dear CL, Thomas J, Kesten S, Maurer J. Impact of preoperative pulmonary rehabilitation on the cystic fibrosis lung transplant recipients. Am J Respir Crit Care Med 1994; 149(4):A733 (abstract).
22. Sheldon JB, Carroll BA, Ries AL, Smith CM, Kriett JM, Jamieson SW. Pulmonary rehabilitation prior to lung transplantation. Am Rev Respir Dis 1993; 147:A597 (abstract).
23. Biggar D, Trulock E, Patterson G, Cooper J. Comparison of functional results of single versus bilateral lung transplantation in COPD patients through three years. Am J Respir Crit Care Med 1994; 149(4):A740 (abstract).
24. Manzetti JD, Hoffman LA, Sereika SM, Sciurba FC, Griffith BP. Exercise, education and quality of life in lung transplant candidates. J Heart Lung Transplant 1994; 13:297–305.

25. Todd TRJ. Early postoperative management following lung transplantation. In: Clinics in Chest Medicine. Philadelphia: WB Saunders, 1990:259–267.
26. Bartlett RH, Gazzaniga AB, Geraghty T. Respiratory manoeuvres to prevent postoperative pulmonary complications. Surg Forum 1971; 22:196–201.
27. Thoren L. Post-operative pulmonary complication: observations on their prevention by means of physiotherapy. Acta Chir Scand 1954; 107:193–197.
28. Miyoshi S, Trulock EP, Schaefers H, Hsieh C, Patterson GA, Cooper JD. Cardiopulmonary exercise testing after single and double lung transplantation. Chest 1990; 97:1130–1136.
29. Burke CM, Baldwin JC, Morris AJR, et al. Twenty-eight cases of human heart-lung transplantation. Lancet 1986; 1:517–519.
30. Williams TJ, Grossman RF, Maurer JR. Long term follow-up of lung transplant recipients. In: Clinics in Chest Medicine. Philadelphia: WB Saunders, 1990:347–358.
31. Estenne M, Primo G, Yernault JC. Cardiorespiratory responses to dynamic exercise after human heart-lung transplantation. Thorax 1987; 42:629–630.
32. Pope SE, Stinson EB, Daughters GT, Schroeder JS, Ingels NB, Alderman EL. Exercise response of the denervated heart in long-term cardiac transplant recipients. Am J Cardiol 1980; 46:213–218.
33. Degre SG, Niset GL, De Smet J, et al. Cardiorespiratory response to early exercise testing after orthotopic cardiac transplantation. Am J Cardiol 1987; 60:927–928.
34. Savin WM, Haskell WL, Schroeder JS, Stinson EB. Cardiorespiratory responses of cardiac transplant patients to graded, symptom-limited exercise. Circulation 1980; 62(1):55–60.
35. Theodore J, Morris AJ, Burke CM, et al. Cardiopulmonary function at maximum tolerable work rate exercise following heart-lung transplantation. Chest 1987; 92(3):433–439.
36. Banner NR, Lloyd MH, Hamilton RD, Innes JA, Guz A, Yacoub MH. Cardiopulmonary response to dynamic exercise after heart and combined heart-lung transplantation. Br Heart J 1988; 61:215–223.
37. Levy RD, Ernst P, Levine SM, et al. Exercise performance after lung transplantation. J Heart Transplant 1993; 12:27–33.
38. Becker FS, Martinez FJ, Christensen PJ, et al. Cardiopulmonary response to exercise after double lung and single lung transplantation for different disease states. Am Rev Respir Dis 1993; 147(4):A336 (abstract).
39. Stevenson LW, Sietsema K, Tillisch JH, et al. Exercise capacity for survivors of cardiac transplantation or sustained medical therapy for stable heart failure. Circulation 1990; 81:78–85.
40. Williams TJ, Patterson GA, McClean PA, Zamel N, Maurer JR. Maximal exercise testing in single and double lung transplant recipients. Am Rev Respir Dis 1992; 145:101–105.
41. Stinson EB, Griepp RB, Schroeder JS, Dong E, Shumway NE. Hemodynamic observations one and two years after cardiac transplantation in man. Circulation 1972; 45:1183–1194.
42. Pope SE, Stinson EB, Daugters GT, Schroeder JS, Ingels NB, Alderman EL.

Exercise response of the denervated heart in long term cardiac transplant recipients. Am J Cardiol 1980; 46:213–218.
43. Younis LT, Melin JA, Schoevaerdts J, et al. Left ventricular systolic function and diastolic filling at rest and during upright exercise after orthotopic heart transplantation: comparison with young and aged normal subjects. J Heart Transplant 1992; 9:683–692.
44. Quigg RJ, Rocco MB, Gauthier DF, Creager MA, Hartley H, Colucci WS. Mechanism of the attenuated peak heart rate response to exercise after orthotopic cardiac transplantation. J Am Coll Cardiol 1989; 14(2):338–344.
45. Labovitz AJ, Drimmer AM, McBride LR, Pennington DG, Willman VL, Miller LW. Exercise capacity during the first year after cardiac transplantation. Am J Cardiol 1989; 64:642–645.
46. Quittan M, Stiebellehner L, Bochdansky T, et al. Assessment of limb muscle strength after lung transplantation amelioration by endurance training. Am J Respir Crit Care Med 1994; 149(4):A737 (abstract).
47. Mercier J, Hokanson JF, Brooks GA. Effects of cyclosporine on endurance exercise time and skeletal muscle mitochondrial respiration in rats. Am J Respir Crit Care Med 1994; 149(4, part 2):A742 (abstract).
48. Wilson JR, Martin JL, Ferraro N, Weber KT. Effect of hydralazine on perfusion and metabolism in the leg during upright bicycle exercise in patients with heart failure. Circulation 1983; 68(2):425–432.
49. Wilson JR, Martin JL, Ferraro N. Impaired skeletal muscle nutritive flow during exercise in patients with congestive heart failure: role of cardiac pump dysfunction as determined by the effect of dobutamine. Am J Cardiol 1984; 53:1308–1315.
50. Shuey CB, Pierce AK, Johnson RL Jr. An evaluation of exercise tests in chronic obstructive lung disease. J Appl Physiol 1969; 27:256–261.
51. Kutsuzawa T, Shioya S, Kurita D, Haida M, Ohta Y, Yamabayishi H. ^{31}P-NMR study of skeletal muscle metabolism in patients with chronic respiratory impairment. Am Rev Respir Dis 1992; 146:1019–1024.
52. Mancini DM, Ferraro N, Tuchler M, Chance B, Wilson JR. Detection of abnormal calf muscle metabolism in patients with heart failure using phosphorous-31 nuclear magnetic resonance. Am J Cardiol 1988; 62:1234–1240.
53. Sjøgaard G. Role of exercise-induced potassium fluxes underlying muscle fatigue: a brief review. Can J Physiol Pharmacol 1991; 69:238–245.
54. McKenna MJ. The roles of ionic processes in muscular fatigue during intense exercise. Sports Med 1992; 13(2):134–145.
55. Hall MJ, Snell GI, Side EA, Esmore DS, Walters EH, Williams TJ. Exercise, potassium and muscle deconditioning post thoracic organ transplantation. J Appl Physiol 1994b 77(6):2784–2790 (abstract).
56. Wray J, Radley-Smith R, Yacoub M. Effect of cardiac or heart-lung transplantation on the quality of life of the paediatric patient. Qual Life Res 1992; 1:41–46.
57. Busschbach JJ, Horikx PE, van den Bosch JM, Brutel de la Riviere A, deCharro FT. Measuring the quality of life before and after bilateral lung transplantation in patients with cystic fibrosis. Chest 1994; 105:911–917.

58. Bunzel B, Grundbock A, Laczkovics A, Holzinger C, Teufelsbauer H. Quality of life after orthotopic heart transplantation. J Heart Lung Transplant 1991; 10:455–459.
59. Mai FM, McKenzie FN, Kostuk WJ. Psychosocial adjustment and quality of life following heart transplantation. Can J Psychiatry—Rev Can Psychiatrie 1990; 35:223–227.
60. Jones BM, Taylor F, Downs K, Spratt P. Longitudinal study of quality of life and psychological adjustment after cardiac transplantation. Med J Aust 1992; 157:24–26.
61. Rector TS, Ormaza SM, Kubo SH. Health status of heart transplant recipients versus patients awaiting heart transplantation: a preliminary evaluation of the SF-36 questionnaire. J Heart Lung Transplant 1993; 12:983–986.
62. Niset G, Coustry-Degre C, Degre S. Psychosocial and physical rehabilitation after heart transplantation. Cardiology 1988; 75:311–317.
63. Jones BM, Chang VP, Esmore D, et al. Psychological adjustment after cardiac transplantation. Med J Aust 1988; 149:118–122.
64. Rosenblum DS, Rosen ML, Pine ZM, Rosen SH, Borg-Stein J. Health status and quality of life following cardiac transplantation [published erratum appears in Arch Phys Med Rehabil 1993; 74(7):701]. Arch Phys Med Rehabil 1993; 74:490–493.
65. Paris W, Woodbury A, Thompson S, et al. Social rehabilitation and return to work after cardiac transplantation—a multicenter survey. Transplantation 1992; 53:433–438.
66. Squires RW, Arthur PR, Gau GT, Muri A, Lambert WB. Exercise after cardiac transplantation: a report of two cases. J Cardiac Rehabil 1983; 3:570–574.
67. Savin WM, Gordon E, Green S, et al. Comparison of exercise training effects in denervated and innervated humans. J Am Coll Cardiol 1983; 1(2):722.
68. Degre S. Rehabilitation and psycho-social factors after heart transplantation. Presented at the XIth Congress of the European Society of Cardiology, Nice, France, September 10–14, 1989.
69. Keteyian SJ, Ehrman JK, Fedel FJ, Rhoads KL. Rehabilitation following heart transplantation. Med Sci Sports Exerc 1989; 21:S55.
70. Keteyian S, Shephard R, Ehrman J, et al. Cardiovascular responses of heart transplant patients to exercise training. J Appl Physiol 1991; 70(6):2627–2631.
71. Shephard RJ. Responses of the cardiac transplant patient to exercise and training. Exerc Sports Sci Rev 1992; 20:297–320.
72. Kavanagh T, Yacoub MH, Mertens DJ, Kennedy J, Campbell RB, Sawyer P. Cardiorespiratory responses to exercise training after orthotopic cardiac transplantation. Circulation 1988; 77(1):162–171.
73. Stiebellehner L, Quittan M, End A, et al. Effect of aerobic endurance training on reduced exercise capacity in patients after lung transplantation. Am Rev Respir Dis 1993; 147(4):A333 (abstract).
74. Stiebellehner L, Quittan M, End A, et al. Lung transplant recipients benefit from aerobic endurance training program. Am J Respir Crit Care Med 1994; 149(4):A742 (abstract).
75. Ketteyian S, Ehrman J, Fedel F, Roades K. Heart rate perceived exertion relation-

ship during exercise in orthotopic heart transplant patients. J Cardiac Rehabil 1990; 10:287–293.
76. Ambrosino N, Callegari G, Baiocchi S, et al. Postoperative rehabilitation of the first patients undergoing heart-lung transplantation in Italy. Am Rev Respir Dis 1993; 147(4):A333 (abstract).
77. Fracchia C, Baiocchi S, Callegari G, et al. Heart-lung transplantation in Italy: time-course of exercise, skeletal and respiratory muscle function. Am J Respir Crit Care Med 1994; 149:A742 (abstract).
78. Hall MJ, Side EA, Snell GI, Walters EH, Esmore DS, Williams TJ. Exercise training post heart and heart-lung transplantation. Am J Respir Crit Care Med 1994a; 149:A741 (abstract).
79. Fishman AP. NIH Workshop Summary. Pulmonary rehabilitation research. Am J Respir Crit Care Med 1994; 149:825–833.

AUTHOR INDEX

Italic numbers give the page on which the complete reference is listed.

A

D

E

F

I

L

M

O

P

S

T

X

Y

SUBJECT INDEX

Q

R

S

T

V

W